Physicochemical Principles of Pharmacy

FOURTH EDITION

Alexander T Florence
CBE, DSc, FRSC, FRSE, FRPharmS
School of Pharmacy, University of London, UK

David Attwood
PhD, DSc, CChem FRSC
School of Pharmacy and Pharmaceutical Sciences
University of Manchester, UK

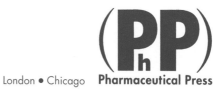

London • Chicago

Published by the Pharmaceutical Press
Publications division of the Royal Pharmaceutical Society of Great Britain

1 Lambeth High Street, London SE1 7JN, UK
100 South Atkinson Road, Suite 206, Grayslake, IL 60030–7820, USA

© Pharmaceutical Press 2006

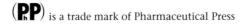 is a trade mark of Pharmaceutical Press

First, second and third editions published by Palgrave
(formerly Macmillan Press Ltd) 1981, 1988, 1998
Third edition reprinted 2004, 2005
Fourth edition 2006

Typeset by MCS Publishing Services Ltd, Salisbury, Wiltshire
Printed in Great Britain by Butler & Tanner, Frome, Somerset

ISBN 0 85369 608 X

A catalogue record for this book is available from the British Library

Cover image: Polarised light micrograph of liquid crystals.
Magnification ×100 at 35 mm size. Reproduced with permission
from James Bell/Science Photo Library.

Contents

Preface

Physicochemical Principles of Pharmacy emerged first in 1981, partly as a result of the authors' frustration when teaching physical pharmacy to undergraduate pharmacy students that there was no European book which covered the subject using pharmaceutical examples to illustrate the topics. Having been brought up ourselves on a diet of physical chemistry of little implicit pharmaceutical relevance, we decided that a book should be compiled which illustrated pharmaceutical not chemical themes. We argued that if a particular concept had never been used in a published pharmacy or pharmaceutical science paper, then it perhaps could be ignored. For too long pharmacy students have been subjected to shards of material more suited for honours students in pure disciplines. We have felt that the book served as a component of the science of pharmacy, as opposed to science for pharmacy. The first edition was well received and a second and third followed. It was encouraging that the text was used widely throughout the world in spite of it being difficult to purchase in the Americas and elsewhere. Charles Fry in a previous existence encouraged us to publish the book. His career took him away from Macmillan Press, who published the first three editions, but in his senior capacity at the Pharmaceutical Press he negotiated the rights of the book and reapplied the ever so gentle pressure for us to complete the fourth edition.

We thank Charles Fry and Paul Weller for their patience and faith in the text.

The present edition has of course been updated. Some students have found 'Florence and Attwood' difficult and prefer simpler texts, but we have not pandered and have not reduced the rigour of the material, in the firm belief of the vital importance of the physicochemical basis of pharmacy to the future strength of pharmacy. We have tried wherever possible to make links with real situations that occur with medicines or that might be important in the future. Some of the examples we have used are those in the original editions, because they have now become classics. New material has been added, but we have always reminded ourselves that this is not a monograph on the latest advances but a textbook for undergraduates and postgraduates.

We hope that the book will continue to be used in undergraduate and postgraduate pharmacy courses and by students of pharmaceutical science and the increasing number of students of cognate disciplines interested in pharmaceutical formulation and medicines.

Alexander T Florence
London
David Attwood
Manchester
September 2005

Acknowledgements

THE NEW EDITION has taken many hours of patient work by Bridget Perez at the School of Pharmacy in London interpreting scribbled insertions and deletions and carrying out detective work on myriad queries. Useful comments have been received over the years from users of previous editions.

We thank Charles Fry and Paul Weller for gentle encouragement and understanding when deadlines were missed and all those at Pharmaceutical Press who have nursed the book through various stages.

About the authors

ALEXANDER FLORENCE is Dean of The School of Pharmacy at the University of London; he was previously James P. Todd Professor of Pharmaceutics at the University of Strathclyde. His research and teaching interests are drug delivery and targeting, dendrimers, nanoparticles, non-aqueous emulsions, novel solvents for use in pharmacy and general physical pharmaceutics. He co-authored the book *Surfactant Systems: their Chemistry, Pharmacy and Biology* with David Attwood.

DAVID ATTWOOD is Professor of Pharmacy at the University of Manchester; he previously lectured at the University of Strathclyde. His research interests are in the physicochemical properties of drugs and surfactants, and in polymeric drug delivery systems. He has many years' experience in the teaching of physical pharmacy.

Introduction

Pharmacy has one unique scientific discipline – pharmaceutics – which is the study of drug formulations and their design, manufacture and delivery to the body. In brief, pharmaceutics is about the conversion of drug substances into medicines suitable for administration by or to patients. There are other vital component disciplines in pharmacy. The way drugs act in and on the body is the domain of pharmacology; the science of drug design and analysis is that of medicinal and pharmaceutical chemistry. There is no clear dividing line between these subject areas. One cannot design formulations without a comprehensive knowledge of the chemistry of the drug substance, nor study how medicines behave in the laboratory or in patients without good analytical methodology. An understanding of the pharmacology of a drug is crucial not only to the proper design of an optimal delivery system, but also to the practice of pharmacy. There is certainly no dividing line in the sciences underlying these subjects, and the physical chemistry that operates in the formulation laboratory is the same that holds within the human body. The forces acting between suspension particles and the walls of a container are the same as those acting on bacteria adsorbing onto a catheter or intestinal wall. The boundary conditions might differ, but the principles are the same. An understanding of the rules that govern what keeps drugs in solution in an infusion fluid allows us to predict the extent to which a drug might precipitate in the renal tubules or in the blood after injection. Studying the solid state properties of drugs should not only provide vital information for formulators but might also help us to understand the formation of crystals in joints or in the kidneys, and how to dissolve them or prevent their formation. You will find many such examples in this book.

Physical chemistry and pharmacy

Undergraduates beginning their study of pharmacy have often been surprised at the amount of physical chemistry they are expected to absorb, when they had expected a more biological flavour to their diet. But the biological processes in the body do not operate and exist in some special nonphysical world, although it is true that they are usually more complex than the processes we control in the test tube. So in this book we not only try to give the physicochemical basis for understanding pharmaceutical formulation and drug delivery but we also stray, as we must, into areas which in the past others would have called pharmaceutical chemistry and pharmacology, biochemistry even. It is important that the underpinning sciences are used intelligently by pharmacy graduates, and not separated into compartments.

Although in the book we have minimised the derivation of equations, the value of appreciating the way in which an equation is derived is that one understands its limitations. Sometimes it is useful to be able to derive an equation from first principles. It would be sad if the modern pharmacist were an empiricist at a time when the science of drug development and drug therapy has become much more quantitative and predictable. It is, of course, not always possible to apply precisely the equations in this book in the complex world of multicomponent medicines, especially after their administration, but rigorous physical chemistry is the starting point for quantitative understanding. Equations often apply only in extremely dilute solutions, so the caveats in the derivations of equations must be noted. Nevertheless, the knowledge of the way in which the solubility of a drug increases or decreases with change in the acidity of the stomach or the intestine is a useful beginning in the understanding of the complex process of drug absorption.

This book is not a complete survey of all the physical chemistry underlying pharmacy, but we have selected the most important in pharmaceutics and biopharmaceutics, without dealing with pharmacokinetics or with many aspects of pharmaceutical production, which are covered in specialised textbooks.

Adjuvants or excipients

In any medicine, the drug molecule is central, whether we are dealing with its formulation, its delivery, its analysis or its activity. The formulation itself might simply be a means of delivering the dose conveniently to the patient, or it might have an influence on the site of delivery or the time course of action. Rational formulation requires a firm understanding of the physical mode of action of excipients in formulations. It is therefore vital that we understand the physical chemistry of materials used in formulations to control the rate of release or to solubilise insoluble molecules, to stabilise or to suspend or to form microspheres and nanoparticles. These so-called adjuvants or excipients are generally regarded as inert, but few substances are totally inert and some, such as a number of surfactants, may be biologically active and indeed harmful if used inappropriately. Surfactant toxicity has its roots in surface activity and hence membrane activity.

Arrangement of the book

How is the book arranged? In the first few chapters we examine the properties of drugs and excipients in the solid state and in solution. Gases also are treated because of their importance in the design and use of therapeutic pressurised aerosols, which until recently have been derived from chlorinated fluorocarbons (CFCs), but now are based on volatile fluorinated hydrocarbons (HFAs).

Special classes of materials are also considered in separate chapters. Colloidal systems (which are those comprising particulates generally below 1 μm in diameter), including many suspensions and emulsions, are experiencing a renaissance in pharmacy because of the use of microparticles and nanoparticles in drug targeting and controlled drug delivery. Polymers and macromolecules, used widely in pharmaceutical formulations as excipients in many forms, as hydrogels, lipogels, viscous solutions and solid matrices or membranes, are treated in one chapter. Proteins, peptides and oligonucleotides have a chapter devoted to the pharmaceutical challenges they pose because of their size, lability and physical properties.

Surface activity is a phenomenon that has widespread consequences. Surface-active substances are those which adsorb at surfaces and lower surface tension; these so-called surfactant materials have a wide applicability in pharmacy. In micellar form they can solubilise water-insoluble drugs and many at low concentrations can increase membrane permeability and aid the transport of drugs across biological barriers. Many drugs have surface-active properties and this might have consequences for their activity and behaviour. The topic is summarised in a chapter on surface activity and surfactants.

Crucial to the whole subject is the process of drug absorption, and how the physical properties of drugs and their formulation can influence the rate and extent (and sometimes site) of absorption. The oral route and the many alternative routes to achieving systemic levels of drugs are reviewed in a chapter which deals with the basics of the absorption process common to all routes of delivery, and then with the individual routes of administration and the way in which the physiology of the route influences the design of formulations and the behaviour of drugs.

Drugs are frequently given together and some interact with clinically important consequences. Often these interactions are pharmacological, but some have a basis in physical chemistry. Incompatibilities might arise from electrostatic interactions between oppositely charged drugs, or from complexation between drugs and ions or drugs and polymers; these and a variety of other interactions are discussed in the book.

It is not always possible to predict the behaviour of drugs and formulations in the complicated environments in which they find themselves *in vivo*, but this should not deter us from at least attempting to rationalise events once they have become known; in this way our predictive powers will be honed and will allow us to prevent adverse events in the future. Some unwanted effects are due to the degradation of drugs and drug formulations; the examination of stability is an important part of assessing the suitability of formulations. This requires a good understanding of the chemistry of the drug substance and reaction kinetics. This too is the subject of a chapter.

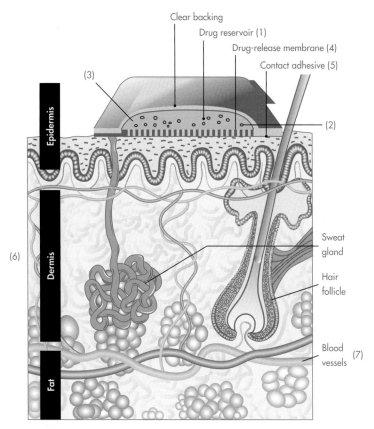

Figure I.1   A drawing of a typical transdermal patch system to deliver drug into the systemic circulation by way of the skin. Drawn here is the system with (1) a reservoir containing the drug adsorbed to (2) lactose particles in (3) an oil; (4) the rate-controlling membrane, a copolymer whose thickness and composition are altered to achieve the desired rate of transport of the drug; and (5) the adhesive layer, also a polymer, although liquid, which attaches the patch to the skin. The basic structure of the skin (6) illustrates the routes of penetration of the drug through this barrier layer into the systemic circulation via the capillary blood supply (7).

Objective of this book

Almost any of the topics discussed could be the subject of a complete textbook in its own right. The objective of this book is to present sufficient of the physical chemistry in context to illustrate the many and varied areas of pharmacy which the subject can illuminate. If we wish to understand what makes modern delivery systems work at more than a superficial level, we would advocate close reading of all the pharmaceutical sciences, of which the topic of physical chemistry forms one important part. Examination of just one such delivery system (Fig. I.1), a transdermal patch, can bring into focus the diversity of physical phenomena that are involved in the design, use and action of delivery systems. One could list these as adsorption, the stability of suspensions, molecular transport through polymeric membranes, adhesion, the interaction of drugs with polymers, the physicochemical properties of the skin and the diffusional characteristics of drugs in the subsections of the skin, including crossing the capillary membrane into the blood. Perhaps enough, we hope, to convince you that reading the rest of the book is necessary.

'Reading' structures and formulae

Throughout this book you will come across two types of formulae: chemical (structural) formulae and physicochemical equations. 'Reading' and understanding formulae – of both kinds – is like learning a language. We often equate reading chemical formulae to reading Chinese characters. To a person without any knowledge of the components of Chinese pictograms, the beautiful shapes mean nothing. A physical equation, similarly, is possibly more akin to the first sight of Arabic: a jumble of letters and numbers to the unversed. Before we delve into the book proper, we wish to rehearse how to see the important features of chemical structures and equations.

Chemical structures

It is not necessary always to understand how a drug was synthesised, but it is important to know about the chemistry of a drug as this determines so many features important in its formulation: solubility in water, solubility in lipid phases, stability, interaction with excipients and of course absorption, not to mention ultimate metabolism. Often one can take a drug molecule and determine which is the main scaffold on which the whole molecule is built; there are of course classes of drugs with the same central 'core' to which are added substituents. It is important that we have a feel for the properties of the 'core' and the substituent groups, that is whether they are polar or nonpolar, water soluble or hydrophobic, (these terms are explained later). A hydrophobic aromatic ring can have substituents which make the molecule water soluble. Much of this is discussed in the text itself. This section simply asks that you look at the drug molecule (or an excipient or an additive molecule) in a certain way. Two drugs – meperidine (pethidine) (**I**) and procainamide – are shown below. Meperidine possesses an aromatic hydrocarbon ring and a piperidine ring and it is a carboxylic acid ester. The nitrogen is a tertiary amine and will be protonated at low pH; the ester is neutral. So one can predict something about the way the molecule will behave in solution and its relative hydrophobicity once the influence of substituent groups are realized. Also, a drug's name will often reveal something of its structure, hence the piperidine clue in meperidine. So too with procainamide (**II**), which is an amide with a primary amine group and a tertiary alkylamine as well. This drug will have two pK_a

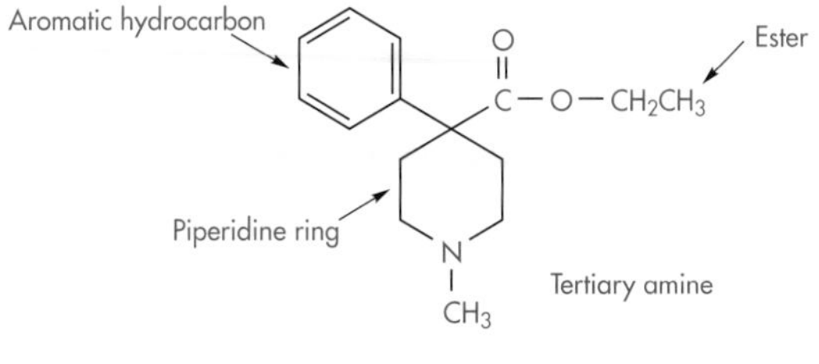

Structure **I**   Meperidine

NH$_2$ Aryl primary amine

Amide O   N—CH$_2$CH$_2$—N   Tertiary alkyl amine
          H
          C$_2$H$_5$
          C$_2$H$_5$

Structure II Procainamide

values (or pK_b values) and this will have consequences for its solubility and absorption.

Equations

One equation, which you will find on page 22, is the Noyes–Whitney equation, which relates the surface area of a drug powder to its rate of solution. Some equations are phenomenological (that is they are derived as a result of experiment and observation) and do not necessarily have a deep theoretical base, so there is no need to be frightened of them. These are often intuitive equations, quite logical, as this one is:

$$\frac{dw}{dt} = \frac{DA}{\delta}(c_s - c)$$

where dw is the increase of the mass of material going into solution with increase of time dt; D is the diffusion coefficient of the molecules escaping from the crystal surface; A is

the surface area of the powder or of the crystal (if it is a single crystal); δ is the diffusion layer thickness; c_s is the saturation solubility of the drug; and c is the concentration of drug at any time point, t.

It is quite logical that the rate of solution should increase as the available surface area for dissolution increases, so you would expect dw/dt to be directly proportional to A. D is a property of the drug molecule diffusing in concentrated drug solution. As the diffusion coefficient increases, one would expect the rate to increase. Diffusion takes place through a concentrated layer – the diffusion layer – and the thicker this is (i.e. the larger δ is), the further the drug has to diffuse to reach the bulk of the solution, hence dw/dt is proportional to $1/\delta$. The more soluble a compound is (i.e. the higher c_s is), the higher the rate of solution; it is clear that if $c_s = c$, then the dissolution stops.

So, by thinking of a process logically, one can almost formulate the equation. Noyes and Whitney did this for us, and precisely, although each equation operates only under certain boundary conditions. Nevertheless, from the Noyes–Whitney equation one can predict accurately what the effect on dissolution will be if the solubility of the drug in the medium is increased, for example, by a change in pH. There are other equations for calculating the effect of pH on the equilibrium solubility, so this helps us get a quantitative view of the world.

1

Solids

The physical properties of the solid state seen in crystals and powders of both drugs and pharmaceutical excipients are of interest because they can affect both the production of dosage forms and the performance of the finished product. Powders, as Pilpel[1] reminded us, 'can float like a gas or flow like a liquid' but when compressed can support a weight. Fine powders dispersed as suspensions in liquids are used in injections and aerosol formulations. Both liquid and dry powder aerosols are available and are discussed in Chapter 9; some properties of compacted solids are dealt with in Chapter 6. In this chapter we deal with the form and particle size of crystalline and amorphous drugs and the effect these characteristics have on drug behaviour, especially on drug dissolution and bioavailability.

The nature of the crystalline form of a drug substance may affect its stability in the solid state, its solution properties and its absorption. It is with this last topic that we start, to consider later other properties of the solid state important in production and formulation. Recently, nanoparticles have been produced to improve the absorption of poorly soluble drugs.

1.1 Crystal structure

Crystals contain highly ordered arrays of molecules and atoms held together by non-covalent interactions. We can consider as a simple example the unit cell of an inorganic salt, sodium chloride. Figure 1.1 shows the ordered arrangement of Cl^- ions and Na^+ ions

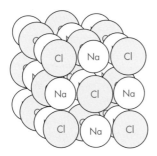

Figure 1.1 Space lattice of sodium chloride crystal. Each sodium ion is octahedrally surrounded by six chloride ions and each chloride ion is octahedrally surrounded by six sodium ions.

which make up the sodium chloride crystal structure. We can draw a square on one side connecting the sodium ions. Similar squares could be drawn on all the sides to form a cubic repeating unit, which we call the *unit cell*. Within a specific crystal, each unit cell is the same size and contains the same number of molecules or ions arranged in the same way. It is usually most convenient to think of the atoms or molecules as points and the crystal as a three-dimensional array of these points, or a *crystal lattice*.

For all possible crystals there are seven basic or primitive unit cells, which are shown in Fig. 1.2. We will represent the lengths of the sides as *a*, *b* and *c* and the angles as

α (between sides *b* and *c*)
β (between sides *a* and *c*)
γ (between sides *a* and *b*)

Figure 1.2 shows the characteristic side lengths and angles for these 'primitive' unit cells.

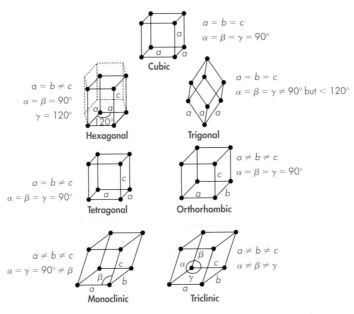

Figure 1.2 The seven possible primitive unit cells with atoms or molecules only at each corner of the unit cell. Drug molecules will typically form triclinic, monoclinic and orthorhombic unit cells.

The structures in Fig. 1.2 have atoms or molecules only at each corner of the unit cell. It is possible to find unit cells with atoms or molecules also at the centre of the top or bottom faces (*end-centred*), at the centre of every face (*face-centred*) or with a single atom in the centre of the cell (*body-centred*), as in Fig. 1.3.

Note that these variations do not occur with every type of unit cell: we find

> End-centred monoclinic and
>   orthorhombic
> Face-centred cubic and orthorhombic
> Body-centred, cubic tetragonal and
>   orthorhombic

Altogether there are 14 possible types of unit cell and we call these the *Bravais lattices*. For drugs there are three common types of unit cell: triclinic, monoclinic and orthorhombic.

Miller indices

We can identify the various planes of a crystal using the system of *Miller indices*. To understand how this system is used, let us consider the plane drawn through the cubic crystal shown in Fig. 1.4(a). The plane cuts the *a* axis at one unit length and also the *c* axis at one unit length. It does not, however, cut the *b* axis, and hence the intercept to this axis is infinity. One way we could label planes is to denote each set by the distances along the axes to the point where the plane crosses the axis. So, for example, the planes marked in Fig. 1.4(a) would have intercept lengths of $a = 1$, $b = \infty$, $c = 1$. This system of labelling the faces is inconvenient because of the appearance of ∞. A way around this problem is to take the reciprocals of the numbers (since the reciprocal of $\infty = 0$). The plane shown then becomes $1/1$, $1/\infty$, $1/1$ for the *a*, *b* and *c* axes, i.e. 1, 0, 1. The Miller indices for this plane are then written as (101).

A second example is illustrated in Fig. 1.4(b). This plane does not cut the *a* axis; it cuts the *b* axis at a unit cell length of $\frac{1}{2}$, and does not cut the *c* axis. The intercept lengths are therefore $a = \infty$, $b = \frac{1}{2}$, $c = \infty$ which on taking reciprocals become 0, 2, 0. A second rule of Miller indices is now applied, that is to reduce the numbers to the lowest terms, i.e. in this case by dividing them all by 2. The Miller indices for this plane are therefore (010).

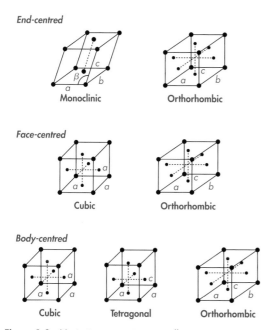

Figure 1.3   Variations on primitive cells

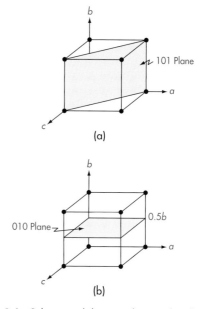

Figure 1.4   Cubic crystal showing planes with Miller indices of (a) (101) and (b) (010).

Other rules for applying Miller indices are shown by the following examples, which for ease of illustration are shown using a two-dimensional array (the *c* axis can be imagined to be at right angles to the page). None of the sets of planes we will consider crosses the *c* axis, i.e. we consider them to intersect it at ∞. The plane x in Fig. 1.5 has *a*, *b* and *c* intercepts of 3, 2, and ∞, giving reciprocals of $\frac{1}{3}$, $\frac{1}{2}$ and 0. The procedure is now to clear the fractions, in this case by multiplying each term by 6, giving 2, 3, and 0. It is not possible to reduce these further, and the Miller indices are therefore (230). The plane y in Fig. 1.5 shows an example of a negative intercept where the *a* axis is crossed. The reciprocals of the *a*, *b* and *c* intercepts are −1, 1, and 0. The procedure that is now used is to write the negative number using a bar above it, giving Miller indices for this plane of ($\bar{1}$10).

Summarising the general rules for expressing planes using the system of Miller indices:

- Determine the intercepts of the plane on the *a*, *b*, and *c* axes in terms of unit cell lengths.
- Take the reciprocals of the intercepts.
- Clear the fractions by multiplying by the lowest common denominator.
- Reduce the numbers to the lowest terms.
- Indicate negative numbers with a bar above the number.

We should notice that the smaller the number in the Miller index for a particular axis, the more parallel is the plane to that axis, a zero value indicating a plane exactly parallel to that axis. The larger a Miller index, the more nearly perpendicular a plane is to that axis.

1.2   Crystal form

The solid state is important for a variety of reasons, summarized in Fig. 1.6: morphology, particle size, polymorphism, solvation or hydration can affect filtration, flow, tableting, dissolution and bioavailability. These are described below.

The crystals of a given substance may vary in size, the relative development of the given faces and the number and kind of the faces (or forms) present; that is, they may have different crystal *habits*. The habit describes the overall shape of the crystal in rather general terms and includes, for example, acicular (needle-like), prismatic, pyramidal, tabular, equant, columnar and lamellar types. Figure 1.7 shows the crystal habits of a hexagonal crystal.

Although there may not be significant differences in the bioavailability of drugs with different crystal habits, the crystal habit is of importance from a technological point of view. The ability to inject a suspension

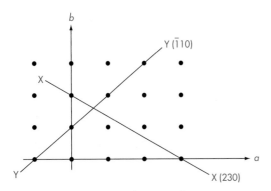

Figure 1.5   Planes in a two-dimensional array.

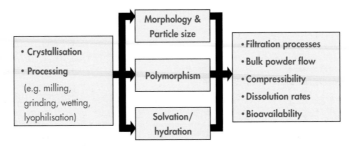

Figure 1.6   The solid state in pharmaceutical science: potential causes and effects of structural change (after A.J. Florence).

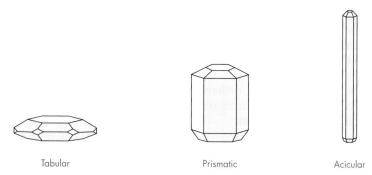

Tabular   Prismatic   Acicular

Figure 1.7 Crystal habits of a hexagonal crystal.

containing a drug in crystal form will be influenced by the habit: plate-like crystals are easier to inject through a fine needle than are needle-like crystals. The crystal habit can also influence the ease of compression of a tablet and the flow properties of the drug in the solid state. The plate-like crystals of tolbutamide, for example, cause powder bridging in the hopper of the tablet machine and also capping problems during tableting. Neither of these problems occurs with tolbutamide in other crystal habits. The habits acquired depend on the conditions of crystallisation, such as solvent used, the temperature, and the concentration and presence of impurities. Ibuprofen is usually crystallised from hexane as elongated needle-like crystals, which have been found to have poor flow properties; crystallisation from methanol produces equidimensional crystals with better flow properties and compaction characteristics, making them more suitable for tableting. The crystal morphology of the excipients (such as powdered cellulose) included in tablet formulations can also have a significant influence on the strength and disintegration time of tablets.

1.2.1 Crystallisation and factors affecting crystal form[2]

Crystallisation from solution can be considered to be the result of three successive processes:

- Supersaturation of the solution
- Formation of crystal nuclei
- Crystal growth round the nuclei

Supersaturation can be achieved by cooling, by evaporation, by the addition of a precipitant or by a chemical reaction that changes the nature of the solute. Supersaturation itself is insufficient to cause crystals to form; the crystal embryos must form by collision of molecules of solute in the solution, or sometimes by the addition of seed crystals, or dust particles, or even particles from container walls. Deliberate seeding is often carried out in industrial processes; seed crystals do not necessarily have to be of the substance concerned but may be isomorphous substances (i.e. of the same morphology). As soon as stable nuclei are formed, they begin to grow into visible crystals.

Crystal growth can be considered to be a reverse dissolution process and the diffusion theories of Noyes and Whitney, and of Nernst, consider that matter is deposited continuously on a crystal face at a rate proportional to the difference of concentration between the surface and the bulk solution. So an equation for crystallisation can be proposed in the form

$$\frac{dm}{dt} = A k_m (c_{ss} - c_s) \qquad (1.1)$$

where m is the mass of solid deposited in time t, A is the surface area of the crystal, c_s is the solute concentration at saturation and c_{ss} is the solute concentration at supersaturation. As $k_m = D/\delta$ (D being the diffusion coefficient of the solute and δ the diffusion layer thickness; see Fig. 1.15), the degree of agitation of the system, which affects δ, also influences crystal growth. Crystals generally dissolve

are almost planar and perpendicular to the E ring and to the 7α-acetothio side-chain. The packing of the molecules in the two polymorphs is compared in Fig. 1.9. Both unit cells are orthorhombic but they differ in their dimensions. The *a*, *b* and *c* axes of Form 1 were found to be 0.998, 3.557 and 0.623 nm respectively, compared with equivalent lengths for Form 2 of 1.058, 1.900 and 1.101 nm. There are also differences in the crystal habits: Form 1 crystals are needle-like, while those of Form 2 are prisms (see Fig. 1.10). The melting points are slightly different: Form 1 melts at 205°C whereas Form 2 has a melting point of 210°C.

Our second example of a drug exhibiting polymorphism is paracetamol (**II**). This drug is known to exist in two polymorphic forms, monoclinic (Form 1) and orthorhombic (Form 2), of which Form 1 is the more thermo-

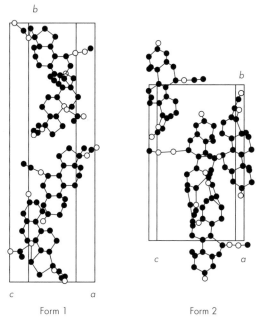

Form 1   Form 2

Figure 1.9 Unit cells of spironolactone.
Reproduced from reference 5 with permission.

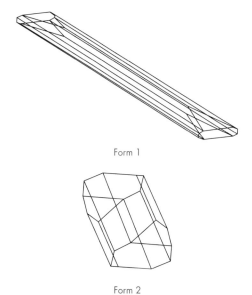

Form 1

Form 2

Figure 1.10 Crystal forms of spironolactone.
Reproduced from reference 5 with permission.

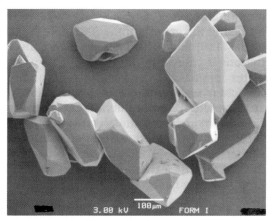

(a)

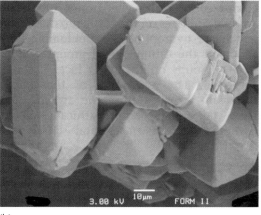

(b)

Figure 1.11 Scanning electron micrographs showing the crystal habit of (a) Form 1 and (b) Form 2 of paracetamol grown from supersaturated IMS.
Reproduced from reference 6 with permission.

Structure II Paracetamol

dynamically stable at room temperature and is the commercially used form.[6] However, this form is not suitable for direct compression into tablets and has to be mixed with binding agents before tableting, a procedure that is both costly and time-consuming. In contrast, Form 2 can readily undergo plastic deformation upon compaction and it has been suggested that this form may have distinct processing advantages over the monoclinic form. Monoclinic paracetamol is readily produced by crystallisation from aqueous solution and many other solvents; production of the orthorhombic form has proved more difficult but may be achieved, at least on a laboratory scale, by nucleating a supersaturated solution of paracetamol with seeds of Form 2 (from melt-crystallised paracetamol). Figure 1.11 shows scanning electron micrographs of the two polymorphic forms

when crystallised from industrial methylated spirits (IMS). Form 1 is described as having a prismatic to plate-like habit that is elongated in the direction of the c-axis, while Form 2 crystallises as prisms that are elongated along the c-axis.

Polymorphism is common with pharmaceutical compounds. Although we do not yet understand the process sufficiently well to predict which drugs are likely to exhibit this phenomenon, it is clear that certain classes of drug are particularly susceptible. Eight crystal modifications of phenobarbital have been isolated but 11 have been identified with melting points ranging from 112 to 176°C. Of the barbiturates used medicinally, about 70% exhibit polymorphism. The steroids frequently possess polymorphic modifications, testosterone having four: these are cases of true polymorphism and not pseudopolymorphism in which solvent is the cause (see section 1.4). Of the commercial sulfonamides, about 65% are found to exist in several polymorphic forms. Examples of the differing solubilities and melting points of polymorphic sulfonamides and steroids are given in Table 1.1.

Predictability of the phenomenon is difficult

Table 1.1   Melting points of some polymorphic forms of steroids, sulfonamides and riboflavin[a]

Compound	Form and or melting point (°C)			
Polymorphic steroids	(I)	(II)	(III)	(IV)
Corticosterone	180–186	175–179	163–168	155–160
β-Estradiol	178	169		
Estradiol	225	223		
Testosterone	155	148	144	143
Methylprednisolone	I (205, aqueous solubility 0.075 mg cm^{-3})			
	II (230, aqueous solubility 0.16 mg cm^{-3})			
Polymorphic sulfonamides				
Sulfafurazole	190–195	131–133		
Acetazolamide	258–260	248–250		
Tolbutamide	127	117	106	
Others				
Riboflavin				
	I (291, aqueous solubility 60 mg cm^{-3})			
	II (278, aqueous solubility 80 mg cm^{-3})			
	III (183, aqueous solubility 1200 mg cm^{-3})			

[a] Reproduced from M. Kuhnert-Brandstatter, *Thermomicroscopy in the Analysis of Pharmaceuticals*, Pergamon Press, New York, 1971.

except by reference to past experience. Its pharmaceutical importance depends very much on the stability and solubility of the forms concerned. It is difficult, therefore, to generalise, except to say that where polymorphs of insoluble compounds occur there are likely to be biopharmaceutical implications. Table 1.2 is a partial listing of the drugs for which polymorphic and pseudopolymorphic states have been identified or for which an amorphous state has been reported.

1.3.1 Pharmaceutical implications of polymorphism

We have already considered the problems in tableting and injection which may result from

Table 1.2 Polymorphic and pseudopolymorphic drugs[a].

Compound	Number of forms		
	Polymorphs	Amorphous	Pseudopolymorphs
Amipicillin	1	–	1
Beclometasone dipropionate	–	–	2
Betamethasone	1	1	–
Betamethasone 21-acetate	1	1	–
Betamethasone 17-valerate	1	1	–
Caffeine	1	–	1
Cefaloridine	4	–	2
Chloramphenicol palmitate	3	1	–
Chlordiazepoxide HCl	2	–	1
Chlorthalidone	2	–	–
Dehydropregnenolone	1	–	7
Dexamethasone acetate	3	–	1
Dexamethasone pivalate	4	–	7
Digoxin	–	1	–
Erythromycin	2	–	–
Fludrocortisone acetate	3	1	–
Fluprednisolone	3	–	2
Glutethimide	1	–	1
Hydrocortisone TBA[b]	1	–	3
Indometacin	3		
Mefenamic acid	2	–	–
Meprobamate	2	–	–
Methyl p-hydroxybenzoate	6	–	–
Methylprednisolone	2	–	–
Novobiocin	1	1	–
Prednisolone	2	–	–
Prednisolone TBA[b]	2	–	2
Prednisolone TMA[c]	3	–	–
Prednisolone acetate	2	–	–
Prednisone	1	–	1
Progesterone	2	–	–
Sorbitol	3	–	–
Testosterone	4	–	–
Theophylline	1	–	1
Triamcinolone	2	–	–

[a] Modified from R. Bouché and M. Draguet-Brughmans, *J. Pharm. Belg.*, 32, 347 (1977) with additions.

[b] Tertiary butyl acetate (tebutate).

[c] Trimethyl acetate.

differences in crystal habit (see section 1.2). Since polymorphs frequently have different habits, they too will be subject to these same problems. However, polymorphs also have different crystal lattices and consequently their energy contents may be sufficiently different to influence their stability and biopharmaceutical behaviour.

As the different polymorphs arise through different arrangement of the molecules or ions in the lattice, they will have different inter-action energies in the solid state. Under a given set of conditions the polymorphic form with the lowest free energy will be the most stable, and other polymorphs will tend to transform into it. We can determine which of two polymorphs is the more stable by a simple experiment in which the polymorphs are placed in a drop of saturated solution under the microscope. The crystals of the less stable form will dissolve and those of the more stable form will grow until only this form remains. Figure 1.12 shows this process occurring with the two polymorphs of paracetamol discussed earlier. Figure 1.12(a) shows the presence of both forms of paracetamol at room temper-ature in saturated benzyl alcohol. Over a time interval of 30 min the less stable of the two forms, the orthorhombic Form 2, has com-pletely converted to the more stable mono-clinic Form 1 (Fig. 1.12b). For drugs with more than two polymorphs we need to carry out this experiment on successive pairs of the polymorphs of the drug until we eventually arrive at their rank order of stability.

Transformations

The transformation between polymorphic forms can lead to formulation problems. Phase transformations can cause changes in crystal size in suspensions and their eventual caking. Crystal growth in creams as a result of phase transformation can cause the cream to become gritty. Similarly, changes in polymorphic forms of vehicles, such as theobroma oil used to make suppositories, could cause products with different and unacceptable melting characteristics.

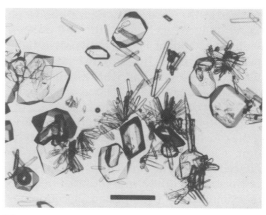
(a)

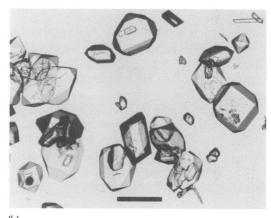
(b)

Figure 1.12 Photomicrographs showing the solution phase polymorphic conversion of orthorhombic paracetamol (needles) to monoclinic paracetamol (prisms and plates). Micrograph (a) was taken at $t = 0$ and (b) was taken at $t = 30$ min. Scale bars = 250 μm.
Reproduced from reference 6 with permission.

Analytical issues

For analytical work it is sometimes necessary to establish conditions whereby different forms of a substance, where they exist, might be converted to a single form to eliminate differences in the solid-state infrared spectra which result from the different internal struc-tures of the crystal forms. As different crystal forms arise through different arrangements of the molecules or ions in a three-dimensional array, this implies different interaction energies in the solid state. Hence one would expect different melting points and different solubilities (and of course different infrared spectra). Changes in infrared spectra of steroids due to grinding with KBr have been reported; changes in the spectra of some substances have been ascribed to conversion of a crystalline form into an amorphous form (as in the case of digoxin), or into a second crystal form. Changes in crystal form can also be induced by solvent extraction methods used for isolation of drugs from formulations prior to examination by infrared spectroscopy. Difficulties in identification arise when samples that are thought to be the same substance give different spectra in the solid state; this can happen, for example, with cortisone acetate, which exists in at least seven forms, or dexamethasone acetate, which exists in four. Therefore, where there is a likelihood of polymorphism it is best where possible to record solution spectra if chemical identification only is required. The normal way to overcome the effects of polymorphism is to convert both samples into the same form by recrystallisation from the same solvent, although obviously this technique should not be used to hide the presence of polymorphs.

Consequences

The most important consequence of polymorphism is the possible difference in the bioavailability of different polymorphic forms of a drug; particularly when the drug is poorly soluble. The rate of absorption of such a drug is often dependent upon its rate of dissolution. The most stable polymorph usually has the lowest solubility and often the slowest dissolution rate. Fortunately, the difference in the bioavailability of different polymorphic forms of a drug is usually insignificant. It has been proposed that when the free energy differences between the polymorphs are small there may be no significant differences in their biopharmaceutical behaviour as measured by the blood levels they achieve. Only when the differences are large may they affect the extent of absorption. For example, $\Delta G_{B \to A}$ for the transition of chloramphenicol palmitate

Form B to Form A is -3.24 kJ mol^{-1}; ΔH is -27.32 kJ mol^{-1}. For mefenamic acid $\Delta G_{II \to I}$ is -1.05 kJ mol^{-1} and ΔH is -4.18 kJ mol^{-1}. Whereas differences in biological activity are shown by the palmitate polymorphs, no such differences are observed with the mefenamic acid polymorphs. When little energy is required to convert one polymorph into another, it is likely that the forms will interconvert *in vivo* and that the administration of one in place of the other form will be clinically unimportant.

Particle size reduction may lead to fundamental changes in the properties of the solid. Grinding of crystalline substances such as digoxin can lead to the formation of amorphous material that has an intrinsically higher rate of solution and therefore apparently greater activity. Such is the importance of the polymorphic form of poorly soluble drugs that it has to be controlled. For instance, there is a limit on the inactive polymorph of chloramphenicol palmitate. Of the three polymorphic forms of chloramphenicol palmitate Form A has a low biological activity because it is so slowly hydrolysed *in vivo* to free chloramphenicol.[7] We can see from Fig. 1.13 that the maximum blood levels attained with 100% Form B polymorph are about seven times greater than with 100% Form A polymorph, and that with mixtures of A and B the blood levels vary in proportion to the percentage of B in the suspension.[8]

During formulation development it is vital that sufficient care is taken to determine polymorphic tendencies of poorly soluble drugs. This is so that formulations can be designed to release drug at the correct rate and so that intelligent guesses can be made before clinical trial about possible influences of food and concomitant therapy on drug absorption. As will be seen later, particle characteristics (of nitrofurantoin, for example) can affect drug interaction as well as drug absorption. Above all, it is important that during toxicity studies care is given to the characterisation of the physical state of the drug, and that during development the optimal dosage form is attained. It is insufficient that drug is 'available' from the dosage form; on both economic

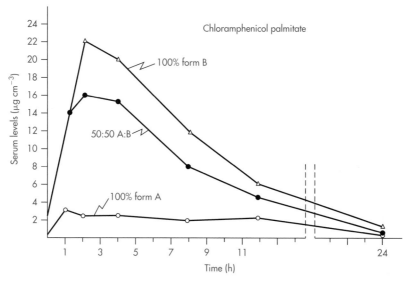

Figure 1.13 Comparison of serum levels (μg cm^{-3}) obtained with suspensions of chloramphenicol palmitate after oral administration of a dose equivalent to 1.5 g of chloramphenicol.
Redrawn from reference 8.

and biological grounds, the maximum response must be achieved with the minimum amount of drug substance.

1.4   Crystal hydrates

When some compounds crystallise they may entrap solvent in the crystal. Crystals that contain solvent of crystallisation are called crystal *solvates*, or crystal *hydrates* when water is the solvent of crystallisation. Crystals that contain no water of crystallisation are termed *anhydrates*.

Crystal solvates exhibit a wide range of behaviour depending on the interaction between the solvent and the crystal structure. With some solvates the solvent plays a key role in holding the crystal together; for example, it may be part of a hydrogen-bonded network within the crystal structure. These solvates are very stable and are difficult to desolvate. When these crystals lose their solvent they collapse and recrystallise in a new crystal form. We can think of these as *polymorphic solvates*. In other solvates, the solvent is not part of the crystal bonding and merely occupies voids in the crystal. These solvates lose their solvent more readily and desolvation does not destroy the crystal lattice. This type of solvate has been called a *pseudopolymorphic solvate*.

By way of illustration of this phenomenon, we return to the case of spironolactone which we considered earlier. As well as the two polymorphs, this compound also possesses four solvates, depending on whether it is crystallised from acetonitrile, ethanol, ethyl acetate or methanol. Each of these solvates is transformed to the polymorphic Form 2 on heating, indicating that the solvent is involved in the bonding of the crystal lattice.

The stoichiometry of some of the solvates is unusual. Fludrocortisone pentanol solvate, for example, contains 1.1 molecules of pentanol for each steroid molecule, and its ethyl acetate solvate contains 0.5 molecules of ethyl acetate per steroid molecule. A succinylsulfathiazole solvate appears to have 0.9 moles of pentanol per mole of drug. Beclometasone dipropionate forms solvates with chlorofluorocarbon propellants.

Infrared measurements show that cefaloridine exists in α, β, δ, ε, ζ and μ forms (that is, six forms after recrystallisation from different solvents).[9]   Proton   magnetic   resonance spectroscopy showed that although the μ form contained about 1 mole of methanol and the ε form about 1 mole of dimethyl sulfoxide, ethylene glycol or diethylene glycol (depending on the solvent), the α, β, anhydrous δ and ε forms contained less than 0.1 mole, that is nonstoichiometric amounts of solvent. The α form is characterised by containing about 0.05 mole of N,N-dimethylacetamide. This small amount of 'impurity', which cannot be removed by prolonged treatment under vacuum at 10^{-5}–10^{-6} torr, is apparently able to 'lock' the cefaloridine molecule in a particular crystal lattice.

1.4.1 Pharmaceutical consequences of solvate formation

Modification of the solvent of crystallisation may result in different solvated forms. This is of particular relevance because the hydrated and anhydrous forms of a drug can have melting points and solubilities sufficiently different to affect their pharmaceutical behaviour. For example, glutethimide exists in both an anhydrous form (m.p. 83°C, solubility 0.042% at 25°C) and a hydrated form (m.p. 68°C, solubility 0.026% at 25°C). Other anhydrous forms show similar higher solubilities than the hydrated materials and, as expected, the anhydrous forms of caffeine, theophylline, glutethimide and cholesterol show correspondingly higher dissolution rates than their hydrates.

One can assume that as the hydrate has already interacted intimately with water (the solvent), then the energy released for crystal break-up, on interaction of the hydrate with solvent, is less than for the anhydrous material. The nonaqueous solvates, on the other hand, tend to be more soluble in water than the nonsolvates. The n-amyl alcohol solvate of fludrocortisone acetate is at least five times as soluble as the parent compound, while the ethyl acetate solvate is twice as soluble.

The equilibrium solubility of the nonsolvated form of a crystalline organic compound which does not dissociate in the solvent (for example, water) can be represented as

$$A_{(c)} \xrightleftharpoons{K_s} A_{(aq)}$$

where K_s is the equilibrium constant. This equilibrium will of course be influenced by the crystal form, as we have seen, as well as by temperature and pressure. For a hydrate $A \cdot xH_2O$, we can write

$$A \cdot xH_2O_{(c)} \xrightleftharpoons{K_{sh}} A_{(aq)} + xH_2O$$

K_{sh} is then the solubility of the hydrate. The process of hydration of an anhydrous crystal in water is represented by an equation of the type

$$\underset{\text{(anhydrate)}}{A_{(c)} + xH_2O_{\text{liquid}}} \underset{K_{sh}}{\overset{K_s}{\rightleftharpoons}} \underset{\text{(hydrate)}}{A \cdot xH_2O_{(c)}}$$

and the free energy of the process is written

$$\Delta G_{\text{trans}} = RT \ln \frac{K_{sh}}{K_s} \tag{1.3}$$

ΔG_{trans} can be obtained from the solubility data of the two forms at a particular temperature, as for theophylline and glutethimide in Table 1.3.

The dissolution rates of solvates can vary considerably. Table 1.4 shows the range of intrinsic dissolution rates reported for solvates of oxyphenbutazone into a dissolution medium containing a surface active agent (to avoid wetting problems). The superior

Table 1.3 Solubility of theophylline and glutethimide forms at various temperatures[a]

	Temperature (°C)	Solubility	
		Hydrate (mg cm^{-3})	Anhydrate (mg cm^{-3})
Theophylline	25	6.25	12.5
	35	10.4	18.5
	45	17.6	27.0
	55	30	38
Glutethimide		(%w/v)	(%w/v)
	25	0.0263	0.042
	32	0.0421	0.0604
	40	0.07	0.094

[a] Reproduced from S. P. Eriksen, *Am. J. Pharm. Educ.*, **28**, 47 (1964).

Table 1.4   Intrinsic dissolution rates of the crystal forms of oxyphenbutazone[a]

Sample	Intrinsic dissolution rate[b] (μg min^{-1} cm^{-2})
Solvate C	21.05 ± 0.02
Solvate B	18.54 ± 0.47
Anhydrate	14.91 ± 0.47
Hemihydrate	17.01 ± 0.78
Monohydrate	9.13 ± 0.23

[a] Reproduced from A. P. Lotter and J. G. van der Walt, J. Pharm. Sci., 77, 1047 (1988).
[b] Mean ± range of uncertainty of two determinations.

Table 1.5   Absorption rate of hydrocortisone tertiary butyl acetate and prednisolone tertiary butyl acetate (mg h^{-1} cm^{-2})[a]

Compound	Absorption rate (mg h^{-1} cm^{-2})
Prednisolone tertiary butyl acetate	
Anhydrous	1.84 ± 10^{-3}
Monoethanol solvate	8.7 ± 10^{-3}
Hemiacetone solvate	2.2 ± 10^{-1}
Hydrocortisone tertiary butyl acetate	
Anhydrous	4.74 ± 10^{-3}
Monoethanol solvate	1.83 ± 10^{-3}
Hemichloroform solvate	7.40 ± 10^{-1}

[a] Modified from B. E. Ballard and J. Biles, Steroids, 4, 273 (1964).

dissolution rates of the benzene and cyclo-hexane solvates (B and C respectively) are apparent but, of course, the possible use of the solvates is prohibited because of their likely toxicity.

Differences in solubility and dissolution rate between solvates can lead to measurable differences in their bioavailabilities. You can see in Table 1.5 the differences in *in vivo*

absorption rates of solvates of prednisolone tertiary butyl acetate and hydrocortisone tertiary butyl acetate after implantation of pellets of these compounds. Note, for example, that the monoethanol solvate of prednisolone has an absorption rate *in vivo* which is nearly five times greater than that of the anhydrous

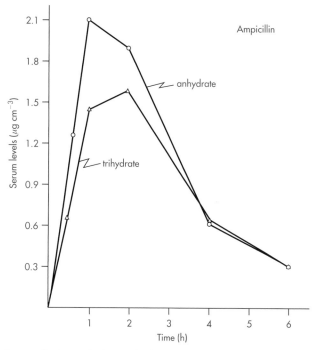

Figure 1.14   Serum levels (μg cm^{-3}) obtained after oral administration of a suspension containing 250 mg ampicillin as the anhydrate and as the trihydrate.
Reproduced from J. W. Poole et al., Curr. Ther. Res., 10, 292 (1968).

tertiary butyl acetate. Differences in the absorption of ampicillin and its trihydrate can be observed (Fig. 1.14), but the extent of the difference is of doubtful clinical significance. The more soluble anhydrous form appears at a faster rate in the serum and produces higher peak serum levels.

1.5 Dissolution of solid drugs

Whether the solution process takes place in the laboratory or *in vivo*, there is one law which defines the rate of solution of solids when the process is diffusion-controlled and involves no chemical reaction. This is the Noyes–Whitney equation, which may be written

$$\frac{dw}{dt} = k(c_s - c) \qquad (1.4)$$

where $k = DA/\delta$. The equation is the analogue of equation (1.1) discussed previously. Figure 1.15 shows the model on which this equation is based. The terms of the equation are: dw/dt, the rate of increase of the amount of material in solution dissolving from a solid; k, the rate constant of dissolution (time^{-1}); c_s, the saturation solubility of the drug in solution in the diffusion layer; and c the concentration of the drug in the bulk solution. A is the area of the solvate particles exposed to the solvent, δ is the thickness of the diffusion

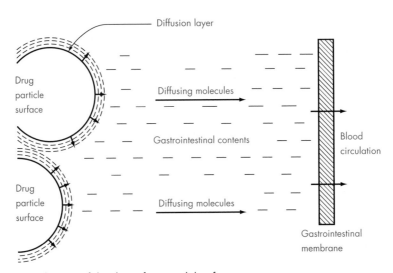

Figure 1.15 Schematic diagram of dissolution from a solid surface.

Table 1.6 How the parameters of the dissolution equation can be changed to increase (+) or decrease (–) the rate of solution

Equation parameter	Comments	Effect on rate of solution
D (diffusion coefficient of drug)	May be decreased in presence of substances which increase viscosity of the medium	(–)
A (area exposed to solvent)	Increased by micronisation and in 'amorphous' drugs	(+)
δ (thickness of diffusion layer)	Decreased by increased agitation in gut or flask	(+)
c_s (solubility in diffusion layer)	That of weak electrolytes altered by change in pH, by use of appropriate drug salt or buffer ingredient	(–)(+)
c (concentration in bulk)	Decreased by intake of fluid in stomach, by removal of drug by partition or absorption	(+)

layer, and D is the diffusion coefficient of the dissolved solute. The relevance of polymorphism and solid-state properties to this equation lies in the fact that A is determined by particle size. Particle size reduction, if it leads to a change in polymorph, results in a change in c_s, and if dissolution is the rate-limiting step in absorption then bioavailability is affected. In more general terms, one can use the equation to predict the effect of solvent change or other parameters on the dissolution rate of solid drugs. These factors are listed in Table 1.6.

1.6   Biopharmaceutical importance of particle size

It has generally been believed that only substances in the molecularly dispersed form (that is, in solution) are transported across the intestinal wall and absorbed into the systemic circulation. This is the premise on which much thinking on bioavailability from pharmaceutical dosage forms is based. While this is generally true, it has, however, been shown that very small particles in the nanometre size range can also be transported through enterocytes by way of pinocytosis, and that solid particles of starch, for example, in the micrometre size range enter by a mechanism involving passage of particles between the enterocytes.[10] Submicrometre particulate uptake by the M-cells of the gut-associated lymphoid tissue (GALT) is a phenomenon of increasing importance.[11] Because of the much greater absorptive area available to molecules, however, the opportunity for molecules to penetrate the cell membrane is obviously higher than that for particles.

The rate of absorption of many slightly soluble drugs from the gastrointestinal tract and other sites is limited by the rate of dissolution of the drug. The particle size of a drug is therefore of importance if the substance in question has a low solubility.

The Noyes–Whitney equation demonstrates that solubility is one of the main factors determining rate of solution. When the rate of solution is less than the rate of absorption, the solution process becomes rate limiting. Generally speaking, it should become so only when the drug is of low solubility at the pH of the stomach and intestinal contents. The rate of absorption, the speed of onset of effect and

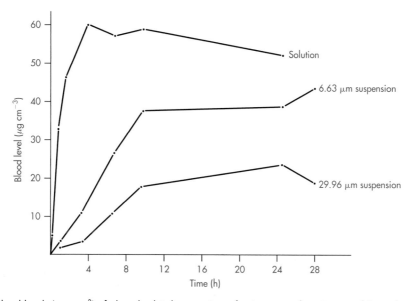

Figure 1.16   Blood levels (μg cm^{-3}) of phenobarbital versus time after intramuscular injection of three dosage forms.
Redrawn from L. G. Miller and J. H. Fincher, *J. Pharm. Sci.*, 60, 1733 (1971).

the duration of therapeutic response can all be determined by particle size for most routes of administration. Figure 1.16 shows the effect of particle size of phenobarbital suspensions on the drug's bioavailability after intramuscular injection, compared with a solution of the drug, which probably precipitates in fine crystal form at the site of injection. The rate of solution of the drug crystals controls the extent of absorption from the intramuscular site.

The vital influence (for mainly aerodynamic reasons) of particle size in the activity of inhaled drug particles is discussed in Chapter 9, section 9.9.

The range of substances over which there is pharmacopoeial control of particle size is shown in Table 1.7; sometimes the aim is to achieve uniformity in a product rather than any direct benefit. The control exercised over the particle size of cortisone acetate and griseofulvin is due to their very low solubility; the experience is that if the solubility of a drug substance is about 0.3% or less then the dissolution rate *in vivo* may be the rate-controlling step in absorption.

The effect of particle size reduction on dissolution rate is one of exposure of increasing amounts of surface of the drug to the solvent. It is only when comminution reduces particle size below 0.1 μm that there is an effect on the intrinsic solubility of the substance (see Chapter 5), and thus on its intrinsic dissolution rate. Very small particles have a very high surface/bulk ratio. If the surface layer has a higher energy than the bulk, as is the case with these small particles, they will interact more readily with solvent to produce higher degrees of solubility.

It was with the action of phenothiazine that the importance of particle size was first recognised, in 1939, in relation to its toxicity to codling moth larvae, and in 1940 in relation to its anthelmintic effect, in both of which it was shown that reduction in particle size increased activity. The improvement in biological response to griseofulvin on micronisation is well known; similar blood levels of the drug were obtained with half the dose of micronised drug compared to those of non-micronised griseofulvin.[12] The influence of particle size on the bioavailability of digoxin[13] and dicoumarol (bishydroxycoumarin)[14] has also been investigated. In both cases, plasma levels of drug are of high significance in clinical and toxic responses.

In the case of digoxin there is evidence that milling to reduce particle size can produce an amorphous modification of the drug with enhanced solubility and hence increased bioavailability. The possibility of changing the crystal structure during processing is therefore important: comminution, recrystallisation and drying can all affect crystal properties.

During the pharmacological and toxicological testing of drugs before formal formulation exercises have been carried out, insoluble drugs are frequently administered in suspension form, often routinely in a vehicle containing gum arabic or methylcellulose. Without adequate control of particle size or adequate monitoring, the results of these tests must sometimes be in doubt, as both pharmacological activities and toxicity generally result from absorption of the drug. In a few cases particle size influences side-effects such as gastric bleeding or nausea. Gastric bleeding may in part be the direct result of contact of acidic particles of aspirin or nonsteroidal anti-inflammatory agents with the mucosal wall. The influence of drug form on the LD_{50} of pentobarbital in mice is shown in Table 1.8. A twofold range of LD_{50} values is obtained by the use of different, simple formulations of the barbiturate. Even in solution form, sodium carboxymethylcellulose affects the LD_{50} by mechanisms which are not confirmed. Adsorption of the polymer at the intestinal surface may retard absorption, or some of the drug may be adsorbed onto the polymer.

The deliberate manipulation of particle size leads to a measure of control of activity and side-effects. Rapid solution of nitrofurantoin from tablets of fine particulate material led to a high incidence of nausea in patients, as local high concentrations of the drug produce a centrally mediated nausea. Development of macrocrystalline nitrofurantoin (as in Macrodantin) has led to the introduction of a form of therapy in which the incidence of nausea is reduced. Capsules are used to avoid compression of the

Table 1.7 Particle size control of drugs and adjuvants in compendia[a]

Substance or preparation	Pharmacopoeia	Remarks
Aspirin	BP	In fine powder[b] form for preparation of Soluble Aspirin Tablets and Soluble Aspirin, Phenacetin and Codeine Tablets
Bephenium Hydroxynaphthoate	BP	Surface area of not less than 7000 $cm^2 g^{-1}$ determined by air permeability method
Betamethasone	EP & PC	Ultrafine powder to be used for preparation of solid dosage forms to achieve a satisfactory rate of solution
Cellulose Microcrystalline	PC	Colloidal water-miscible type differentiated from nondispersible form by size
Cortisone Acetate	PC	Fine powder to be used for preparation of solid dosage forms
Dithranol Ointment	BP	Prepared from dithranol in fine powder form
Ergotamine Aerosol Inhalation	BPC	Most of the individual particles have a diameter not greater than 5 μm; no individual particle has a length greater than 20 μm
Fusidic Acid Mixture	BPC	95% of particles have a maximum diameter of not more than 5 μm
Griseofulvin Tablets	PC & EP	Particle size determined from disintegrated tablet generally up to 5 μm in maximum dimension although larger particles may occasionally be greater than 30 μm
Hydrocortisone preparations	BP & PC	All subject to limit on particle size of Hydrocortisone or Hydrocortisone Acetate. See Hydrocortisone Acetate Ointment BP, Hydrocortisone Cream BPC, Hydrocortisone and Neomycin Cream BPC, Hydrocortisone and Neomycin Ear Drops and Eye Drops BPC, Hydrocortisone Eye Ointment BPC, Hydrocortisone Lotion BPC and Hydrocortisone Suppositories BPC
Insulin preparations	BP	See Insulin Zinc Suspension (Crystalline) BP, Insulin Zinc Suspension (Amorphous) BP, Biphasic Insulin Injection BP
Isoprenaline Inhalation Aerosol	BPC	As for Ergotamine Aerosol Inhalation BPC
Nystatin Ointment	BPC	No particle of nystatin has a maximum diameter greater than 75 μm
Orciprenaline Aerosol Inhalation	BPC	As for Ergotamine Aerosol Inhalation BPC
Phenolphthalein		Microcrystalline phenolphthalein[c] to be used in Liquid Paraffin Emulsion with Phenolphthalein BPC to prevent sedimentation of the phenolphthalein
Salbutamol Aerosol Inhalation	BPC	As for Ergotamine Aerosol Inhalation BPC

[a] Modified from E. G. Salole, in *Practical Pharmaceutical Chemistry* (ed. A. H. Beckett and J. B. Stenlake), vol. 2, Athlone Press, London, 1987.
[b] The following terms, *inter alia*, are used in the description of powders in the British Pharmacopoeia and the Pharmaceutical Codex 1994:
Coarse powder: a powder all the particles of which pass through a sieve with a nominal mesh aperture of 1700 μm and not more than 40% by weight pass through a sieve with a nominal aperture of 355 μm.
Moderately coarse powder: a powder all the particles of which pass through a sieve with a nominal mesh aperture of 710 μm and not more than 40% by weight pass through a sieve with a nominal aperture of 250 μm.
Moderately fine powder: a powder all the particles of which pass through a sieve with a nominal mesh aperture of 355 μm and not more than 40% by weight pass through a sieve with a nominal aperture of 180 μm.
Fine powder: a powder all the particles of which pass through a sieve with a nominal mesh aperture of 180 μm and not more than 40% by weight pass through a sieve with a nominal aperture of 125 μm.
Very fine powder: a powder all the particles of which pass through a sieve with a nominal mesh aperture of 125 μm and not more than 40% by weight pass through a sieve with a nominal aperture of 45 μm.
Microfine powder: a powder of which not less than 90% by weight of the particles pass through a sieve with a nominal mesh diameter of 45 μm.
Superfine powder: a powder of which not less than 90% by number of the particles are less than 10 μm in size.
Ultrafine powder: a powder of which the maximum diameter of 90% of the particles is not greater than 5 μm and of which the diameter of none is greater than 50 μm.
[c] BPC 1973, p. 679.
BP, British Pharmacopoeia; EP, European Pharmacopoeia; PC, Pharmaceutical Codex, 12th edn, 1994; BPC, British Pharmacopoeial Codex.

Table 1.8 Influence of formulation on the potency ratios of pentobarbital in the form of the sodium salt and the free acid[a]

Pentobarbital form	Dosage form	Vehicle	Particle size (μm)	LD_{50}	Potency ratio[b]
Sodium salt	Solution	Water	–	132	1
Sodium salt	Solution	1%NaCMC[c]	–	170	0.78
Free acid	Suspension	1%NaCMC[c]	<44	189	0.70
Free acid	Suspension	1%NaCMC[c]	297–420	288	0.46

[a] Reproduced from W. A. Ritschel *et al.*, *Arzneim. Forsch.*, 25, 853 (1975).

[b] Relative to aqueous solution of the sodium salt.

[c] Aqueous solution of sodium carboxymethylcellulose.

large crystals during manufacture. Although the urinary levels of the antibacterial are also lowered by the use of a more slowly dissolving form of the drug, levels are still adequate to produce efficient antibacterial effects.[15]

1.7 Wetting of powders

Penetration of water into tablets or into granules precedes dissolution. The wettability of the powders, as measured by the contact angle (θ) of the substance with water (Fig. 1.17), therefore determines the contact of solvent with the particulate mass. The measurement of the contact angle gives an indication of the nature of the surface. The behaviour of crystalline materials can be related to the chemical structure of the materials concerned, as is shown by the results in Table 1.9 on a series of substituted barbiturates. The more hydrophobic the individual barbiturate molecules, the more hydrophobic the crystal which

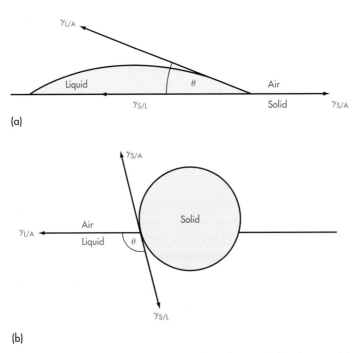

Figure 1.17 Equilibrium between forces acting on (a) a drop of liquid on a solid surface, and (b) a partially immersed solid.

Table 1.9 Relationship between chemical structure of barbiturates and contact angle (θ) with water[a]

R^1	R^2	θ (deg)
Et	Et	70
Et	Bu	78
Et	$CH_2CH_2CH_2(CH)_2$	102
$-CH-CH_3$ $\quad\vert$ $\quad CH_3$	$CH_2-CH=CH_2$	75
$-CH_2CH\ CH_3$ $\qquad\vert$ $\qquad CH_3$	$CH_2-CH=CH_2$	87

[a] Reproduced from C. F. Lerk et al., J. Pharm. Sci., 66, 1480 (1977).

forms, although this would not be necessarily a universal finding but one dependent on the orientation of the drug molecules in the crystal and the composition of the faces, as we have already seen with adipic acid. Thus, hydrophobic drugs have dual problems: they are not readily wetted, and even when wetted they have low solubility. On the other hand, because they are lipophilic, absorption across lipid membranes is facilitated.

1.7.1 Contact angle and wettability of solid surfaces

A representation of the several forces acting on a drop of liquid placed on a flat, solid surface is shown in Fig. 1.17(a). The surface tension of the solid, $\gamma_{S/A}$, will favour spreading of the liquid, but this is opposed by the solid–liquid interfacial tension, $\gamma_{S/L}$, and the horizontal component of the surface tension of the liquid $\gamma_{L/A}$ in the plane of the solid surface, that is $\gamma_{L/A} \cos\theta$. Equating these forces gives

$$\gamma_{S/A} = \gamma_{S/L} + \gamma_{L/A} \cos\theta \qquad (1.5)$$

Equation (1.5) is generally referred to as *Young's equation*. The angle θ is termed the *contact angle*. The condition for complete wetting of a solid surface is that the contact angle should be zero. This condition is fulfilled when the forces

of attraction between the liquid and solid are equal to or greater than those between liquid and liquid.

The type of wetting in which a liquid spreads over the surface of the solid is referred to as *spreading wetting*. The tendency for spreading may be quantified in terms of the spreading coefficient S, where

$$S = \gamma_{L/A}(\cos\theta - 1) \qquad (1.6)$$

If the contact angle is larger than 0°, the term $(\cos\theta - 1)$ will be negative, as will the value of S. The condition for complete, spontaneous wetting is thus a zero value for the contact angle.

1.7.2 Wettability of powders

When a solid is immersed in a liquid, the initial wetting process is referred to as *immersional wetting*. The effectiveness of immersional wetting may be related to the contact angle that the solid makes with the liquid–air interface (see Fig. 1.17b). The condition for complete immersion of the solid in the liquid is that there should be a decrease in surface free energy as a result of the immersion process. Once the solid is submerged in the liquid, the process of *spreading wetting* (see previous section) becomes important.

Table 1.10 gives the contact angles of a series of pharmaceutical powders. These values were determined using compacts of the powder (produced by compressing the powder in a large-diameter tablet die) and a saturated aqueous solution of each compound as the test liquid. Many of the powders are slightly hydrophobic (for example, indometacin and stearic acid), or even strongly hydrophobic (for example, magnesium stearate, phenylbutazone and chloramphenicol palmitate). Formulation of these drugs as suspensions (for example, Chloramphenicol Palmitate Oral Suspension USP) presents wetting problems. Table 1.10 shows that θ can be affected by the crystallographic structure, as for chloramphenicol palmitate. Surface modification or changes in crystal structure are clearly not routine methods of lowering the contact angle

Table 1.10 Contact angles of some pharmaceutical powders[a]

Material	Contact angle θ (deg)	Material	Contact angle θ (deg)
Acetylsalicylic acid (aspirin)	74	Lactose	30
Aluminium stearate	120	Magnesium stearate	121
Aminophylline	47	Nitrofurantoin	69
Ampicillin (anhydrous)	35	Phenylbutazone	109
Ampicillin (trihydrate)	21	Prednisolone	43
Caffeine	43	Prednisone	63
Calcium carbonate	58	Salicyclic acid	103
Calcium stearate	115	Stearic acid	98
Chloramphenicol	59	Succinylsulfathiazole	64
Chloramphenicol palmitate (α form)	122	Sulfadiazine	71
Chloramphenicol palmitate (β form)	108	Sulfamethazine	48
Diazepam	83	Sulfathiazole	53
Digoxin	49	Theophylline	48
Indometacin	90	Tolbutamide	72
Isoniazid	49		

[a] Selected values from C. F. Lerk *et al.*, *J. Pharm. Sci.*, 65, 843 (1976); *J. Pharm. Sci.*, 66, 1481 (1977).

and the normal method of improving wettability is by the inclusion of surfactants in the formulation. The surfactants not only reduce $\gamma_{L/A}$ but also adsorb onto the surface of the powder, thus reducing $\gamma_{S/A}$. Both of these effects reduce the contact angle and improve the dispersibility of the powder.

1.8 Solid dispersions

Over the past few years interest has been shown in *solid solutions* of drugs in attempts to change the biopharmaceutical properties of drugs which are poorly soluble or difficult to wet. The object is usually to provide a system in which the crystallinity of the drug is so altered as to change its solubility and solution rate, and to surround the drug intimately with water-soluble material. A solid solution comprises solute and solvent – a solid solute molecularly dispersed in a solid solvent. These systems are sometimes termed *mixed crystals* because the two components crystallise together in a homogeneous one-phase system. For understanding of the systems and their potential use, an arbitrary system might be considered.

In Fig. 1.18, the melting temperature of mixtures of A and B is plotted against mixture composition. On addition of B to A or of A to B, melting points are reduced. At a particular composition the *eutectic point* is reached, the eutectic mixture (the composition at that point) having the lowest melting point of any mixture of A and B. Below the eutectic temperature, no liquid phase exists. The phenomenon is important because of the change in the crystallinity at this point. If we cool a solution of A and B which is richer in A than the eutectic mixture (see M in Fig. 1.18), crystals of pure A will appear. As the solution is cooled further, more and more A crystallises out and the solution becomes richer in B. When the eutectic temperature is reached, however, the remaining solution crystallises out, forming a microcrystalline mixture of pure A and pure B, differing markedly at least in superficial characteristics from either of the pure solids. This has obvious pharmaceutical possibilities. This method of obtaining microcrystalline dispersions for administration of drugs involves the formation of a eutectic mixture composed of drug and a substance readily soluble in water. The soluble 'carrier' dissolves, leaving the drug in a fine state of solution *in vivo*, usually in a state which predisposes to rapid solution.

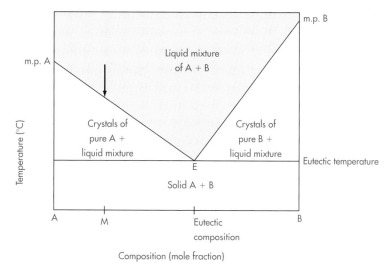

Figure 1.18 Phase diagram (temperature versus composition) showing boundaries between liquid and solid phases, and the eutectic point, E.

This technique has been applied to several poorly soluble drugs such as griseofulvin. A griseofulvin–succinic acid (soluble carrier) system has a eutectic point at 0.29 mole fraction of drug (55% w/w griseofulvin) (Fig. 1.19a). The eutectic mixture consists here of two physically separate phases; one is almost pure griseofulvin, while the other is a saturated solid solution of griseofulvin in succinic acid. The solid solution contains about 25% griseofulvin; the eutectic mixture, which has a fixed ratio of drug to carrier, thus comprises 60% solid solution and 40% almost pure griseofulvin. As can be seen from Fig. 1.19(b), which shows the solution profiles of the different forms, the solid solution dissolves 6–7 times faster than pure griseofulvin.

The simplest eutectic mixtures are usually prepared by the rapid solidification of the fused liquid mixture of the components which show complete miscibility in the liquid state and negligible solid–solid solubility. In addition to the reduction in crystalline size, the following factors may contribute to faster dissolution rate of drugs in eutectic mixtures:

- An increase in drug solubility because of the extremely small particle size of the solid
- A possible solubilisation effect by the carrier, which may operate in the diffusion layer immediately surrounding the drug particle

- Absence of aggregation and agglomeration of the particles
- Improved wettability in the intimate drug–carrier mixture
- Crystallisation in metastable forms

Where more complex solubility patterns emerge, as with the griseofulvin and succinic acid phase, the phase diagram becomes correspondingly more complex. Figure 1.20 shows one example of a system in which each component dissolves in the other above and below the eutectic temperature.

Other systems that form eutectic mixtures are chloramphenicol–urea, sulfathiazole–urea, and niacinamide–ascorbic acid. The solid solution of chloramphenicol in urea was found to dissolve twice as rapidly as a physical mixture of the same composition and about four times as rapidly as the pure drug. *In vivo*, however, the system failed to display improved bioavailability. On the other hand, the eutectic mixture of sulfathiazole–urea did give higher blood levels than pure sulfonamide.

A formulation containing a eutectic

A topical preparation for intradermal anaesthesia to reduce the pain of venepuncture is available. The cream, Emla (Eutectic Mixture

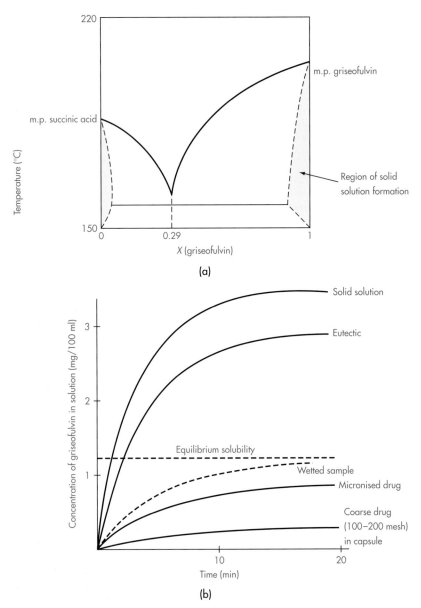

Figure 1.19 (a) Griseofulvin–succinic acid phase diagram. (b) Rate of solution of griseofulvin solid solutions, eutectic and crystalline material.

of Local Anaesthetics) (AstraZeneca), contains a eutectic of procaine and lidocaine.[16]. The eutectic mixture (50 : 50 mixture) is an oil, which is then formulated as an oil-in-water emulsion. This allows much higher concentrations than would have been possible by using the individual drugs dissolved in an oil.

1.8.1 Eutectics and drug identification

As the eutectic temperature of a substance in mixtures with other compounds is, as a rule, different even when the other substances have the same melting point, this parameter can be used for identification purposes. Benzanilide

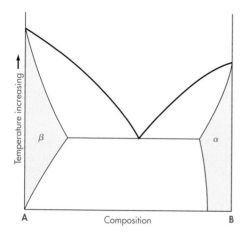

Figure 1.20 Melting point–composition plot for a system in which α and β are regions of solid solution formation. Each component dissolves the other component to some extent above the eutectic temperature. As the temperature is lowered, the solid solution regions become narrower.

(m.p. 163°C), phenacetin (m.p. 134.5°C) and salophen (m.p. 191°C) are often used as test substances. The eutectic temperatures of mixtures of benzanilide with various drugs are shown in Table 1.11. Substances of identical melting points can be distinguished by measurement of the eutectic temperature with another suitable compound.

Ternary eutectics are also possible. The binary eutectic points of three mixtures are as follows: for aminophenazone–phenacetin 82°C; for aminophenazone–caffeine 103.5°C; and for phenacetin–caffeine 125°C. The ternary eutectic temperature of aminophenazone–phenacetin–caffeine is 81°C. In this mixture the presence of aminophenazone and phenacetin can be detected by the mixed melting point

Table 1.11 Eutectic temperatures of drugs with benzanilide[a]

Compound	Melting point (°C)	Eutectic temperature (°C)
Allobarbital	173	144
Ergotamine	172–174	135
Imipramine HCl	172–174	109

[a] From M. Kuhnert-Brandstatter, *Thermomicroscopy in the Analysis of Pharmaceuticals*, Pergamon, New York, 1971.

test, but the caffeine causes little depression of the eutectic given by the other two components.

The possibility of determining eutectic temperatures of multicomponent mixtures has practical value in another respect. During tableting, for example, heat is generated in the punch and die and in the powder compact; measurement of the eutectic temperature can give information on whether this rise in temperature is likely to cause problems of melting and fusion.

Summary

- The crystal lattices of drugs are constructed from repeating units called unit cells. All unit cells in a specific crystal are the same size and contain the same number of molecules or ions arranged in the same way. For all crystals there are seven primitive unit cells: cubic, orthorhombic, monoclinic, hexagonal, tetragonal, triclinic and trigonal. Certain of these may also be end-centred, body-centred or face-centred, making a total of 14 possible unit cells or Bravais lattices. The various planes of the crystal lattice can be identified using the system of Miller indices.
- The external shape of the crystal can be described in terms of its habit, which is affected by the rate of crystallisation and by the presence of impurities, particularly surfactants. The habit of a crystal is of pharmaceutical importance, since it affects the compression characteristics and flow properties of the drug during tableting and also the ease with which the suspensions of insoluble drugs will pass through syringe needles.
- Many drugs exist in several polymorphic forms. The various polymorphs of a drug differ in the packing of the molecules in the crystal lattice or in the conformation of the molecules at the lattice sites. The different polymorphs have different physical and chemical properties and usually exist in different habits. The transformation between

polymorphic forms can cause formulation problems. Phase transformations can cause changes in crystal size, which in suspensions can eventually cause caking, and in creams can cause detrimental changes in the feel of the cream. Changes in polymorphic form of vehicles, such as theobroma oil used to make suppositories, can result in unacceptable melting characteristics. Problems may also result from phase transformation when attempting to identify drugs using infrared spectroscopy. The most significant consequence of polymorphism is the possible difference in the bioavailability of the different polymorphic forms of a drug, as for example, in the case of polymorphs of chloramphenicol palmitate.

• When some drugs crystallise they may entrap solvent in their crystals and so form different crystal solvates. In some solvates the solvent plays an important role in holding the crystal together. These solvates, called polymorphic solvates, are very stable, and when they lose their solvent they recrystallise in a different crystal form. In other solvates, referred to as pseudopolymorphic solvates, the solvent is not part of the crystal bonding and merely occupies voids in the crystal. These solvates can lose their solvent more readily and desolvation does not alter the crystal lattice. Solvated and anhydrous forms of a drug differ in

their aqueous solubilities. Anhydrous forms are generally more soluble than hydrates of the same drug, but less soluble than non-aqueous solvates of the drug. The dissolution rates of the various solvates of a drug may differ significantly, and with poorly soluble drugs this may result in differences in their absorption rates.

• The rate of dissolution of a solid can be increased by reduction in the particle size, providing that this does not induce changes in polymorphic form which could alter the drug's solubility. The reduction of particle size of some drugs to below 0.1 μm can cause an increase in the intrinsic solubility. This is the basis of a method for increasing the rate of dissolution and solubility of poorly soluble drugs such as griseofulvin, by forming a eutectic mixture or solid dispersion with a highly soluble carrier compound.

• The contact angle is an indicator of the ability of a liquid to wet a solid surface; for complete, spontaneous wetting the contact angle should be zero. There are two types of wetting – spreading wetting, in which a liquid spreads over the surface of a solid, and immersional wetting, which is the initial wetting process that occurs when a solid is immersed in a liquid. Several pharmaceutical powders have been identified which, because of their high contact angle, present wetting problems.

References

1. N. Pilpel. Powders – gaseous, liquid and solid. *Endeavour (NS)*, 6, 183–8 (1982)

2. J. W. Mullin. *Crystallization*, 4th edn, Butterworth-Heinemann, London, 2001

3. A. S. Michaels and A. R. Colville. The effect of surface-active agents on the crystal growth rate and habit. *J. Phys. Chem.*, 64, 13–19 (1960)

4. S. R. Vippagunta, H. G. Britain and D. J. W. Grant. Crystalline solids. *Adv. Drug Deliv. Rev.*, 48, 3–26 (2001)

5. V. Agafonov, B. Legendre, N. Rodier, *et al.* Polymorphism of spironolactone. *J. Pharm. Sci.*, 80, 181–5 (1991)

6. G. Nichols and C. S. Frampton. Physicochemical characterization of the orthorhombic polymorph of paracetamol crystallized from solution. *J. Pharm. Sci.*, 87, 684–93 (1998)

7. A. Koda, S. Ito, S. Itai and K. Yamamoto. Characterization of chloramphenicol palmitate form C and absorption assessments of chloramphenicol palmitate polymorphs. *J. Pharm. Sci. Technol. Jpn.*, 60, 43–52 (2000)

8. A. J. Aiguiar and J. E. Zelmer. Dissolution behaviour of polymorphs of chloramphenicol palmitate and mefanamic acid. *J. Pharm. Sci.*, 58, 983–7 (1969)

9. J. H. Chapman, J. E. Page, A. C. Parker, *et al.* Polymorphism of cephaloridine. *J. Pharm. Pharmacol.*, 20, 418–29 (1968)

10. G. Volkheimer. Persorption of particles: physiology and pharmacology. *Adv. Pharmacol. Chemother.*, 14, 163–87 (1977)

11. A. T. Florence. The oral absorption of micro- and nanoparticulates: neither exceptional nor unusual. *Pharm. Res.*, 14, 259–66 (1997)

12. R. M. Atkinson, C. Bedford, K. J. Child and E. G. Tomich. Effect of particle size on blood griseofulvin-levels in man. *Nature*, 193, 588–9 (1962)

13. T. R. D. Shaw, J. E. Carless, M. R. Howard and K. Raymond. Particle size and absorption of digoxin. *Lancet*, 2, 209–10 (1973)

14. J. F. Nash, L. D. Bechtel, L. R. Lowary, *et al.* Relation between the particle size of dicumarol and its bioavailability in dogs. I. Capsules. *Drug Dev. Commun.*, 1, 443–57 (1975)

15. J. H. Fincher. Particle size of drugs and its relationship to absorption and activity. *J. Pharm Sci.*, 57, 1825–35 (1968)

16. B. F. J. Broberg and H. C. A. Evers. Local anaesthetic emulsion cream. Eur. Pat. 0 002 425 (1981)

2

Gases and volatile agents

Gases and volatile substances are encountered in pharmacy mainly as anaesthetic gases, volatile drugs and aerosol propellants. This chapter deals with the properties of gases and vapours, including the way in which the vapour pressure above solutions varies with the composition of the solution and the temperature. The factors governing the solubility of gases in liquids are reviewed and related to the solubility of anaesthetic gases in the complex solvent systems comprising blood and tissues. Formulation issues arise from the replacement of chlorofluorocarbons (CFCs) by hydrofluorocarbons – not only because of differences in vapour pressure but also because of the changes in solvency of the propellants.

properties of CFCs, led to a substantial review of the formulation of these devices as a consequence of major differences in physical and chemical properties of these propellants.[1] The properties of the two most widely used HFAs (HFA 227 and HFA 134a) are summarised in Table 2.2. The vapour pressure of metered-dose inhalers determines the aerosol droplet size and consequently has an important influence on the efficiency of deposition in the lungs (see Chapter 9, section 9.9). Its application to the type of aerosol system in which there is an equilibrium between the liquefied propellant and its vapour is illustrated in Example 2.2. It is instructive to consider how the composition of the vapour can be calculated since similar principles can be applied to other vaporising devices such as those used to deliver anaesthetic gases.

•••••••••••••••••••••••••••••••••••••••

EXAMPLE 2.2 Calculation of the vapour pressure of a mixture of hydrofluoroalkanes

Calculate the vapour pressure (in Pa) at 20°C above an aerosol mixture consisting of 30% w/w of HFA 134a (tetrafluoroethane, molecular weight 102) with a vapour pressure of 68.4 psig and 70% w/w of HFA 227 (heptafluoropropane, molecular weight 170) with a vapour pressure of 56.0 psig. Assume ideal behaviour.

Answer
For the two propellants HFA 134a and HFA 227 with respective vapour pressures $p_{134}^{\ominus}$ and $p_{227}^{\ominus}$ we have

$$p_{134} = p_{134}^{\ominus} x_{134}$$
$$p_{227} = p_{227}^{\ominus} x_{227}$$

where p_{134} and p_{227} are the partial pressures of components HFA 134a and HFA 227 respectively, and x_{134} and x_{227} are the mole fractions of these components in the liquid phase.

No. of moles of HFA 134a in 100 g mixture = 30/102 = 0.2941 moles

No. of moles of HFA 227 in 100 g mixture = 70/170 = 0.4118 moles

$x_{134} = 0.2941/0.7059 = 0.4166$

$x_{227} = 0.4118/0.7059 = 0.5834$

From Dalton's law of partial pressures, the total vapour pressure P is the sum of the partial pressures of the component gases, assuming ideal behaviour. Thus,

$$P = p_{134}^{\ominus} x_{134} + p_{227}^{\ominus} x_{227}$$

and hence

$$P = (68.4 \times 0.4166) + (56.0 \times 0.5834)$$
$$= 61.17 \text{ psig}$$

Converting pressures into Pa using

psia = psig + 14.7   and   1 psia = 6894.76 Pa
$P = 5.23 \times 10^5$ Pa
•••••••••••••••••••••••••••••••••••••••

An interesting application of aerosol propellants which exploits the constant vapour pressure above a liquid propellant is in the design of totally implantable infusion pumps. Such devices are implanted under the skin in the lower abdomen and are designed to deliver infusate containing the appropriate drug at a constant rate (usually 1 cm³ per day) into an artery or vein. The Infusaid implantable pump was originally devised for the long-term administration of heparin but has since found application for a wide variety of drugs.[2] The

Table 2.2 Physicochemical properties of hydrofluoroalkanes[a]

Propellant	Molecular formula	Molecular weight	Boiling point (°C) at 1.013 bar (1 atm)	Gauge vapour pressure (psig) at 20°C
HFA 134a	$C_2H_2F_4$	102.0	−26.5	68.4
HFA 227	C_3HF_7	170.0	−17.3	56.0

[a] Data from reference 1.

device consists of a relatively small (9 × 2.5 cm) titanium disc which is divided into two chambers by cylindrical titanium bellows that form a flexible but impermeable barrier between the compartments (Fig. 2.2). The outer compartment contains Freon (chlorofluorocarbon propellant); the inner compartment contains the infusate and connects via a catheter to a vein or artery through a series of filters and flow-regulating resistant elements. The vapour pressure above the liquid propellant remains constant because of the relatively constant temperature of the body, and hence a constant pressure is exerted on the bellows, ensuring a constant rate of delivery of infusate into the bloodstream. The propellant is replenished as required by a simple percutaneous injection through the skin.

Binary mixtures of hydrofluoroalkanes show behaviour which approaches ideality.[3] Figure 2.3(a) shows the vapour pressure–composition plots for a mixture of the propellants HFA 134a (tetrafluoroethane) and HFA 227 (heptafluoropropane); the linearity of the plots indicates that Raoult's law is obeyed over the temperature range examined. It is frequently necessary to include a cosolvent such as alcohol in the aerosol formulation to

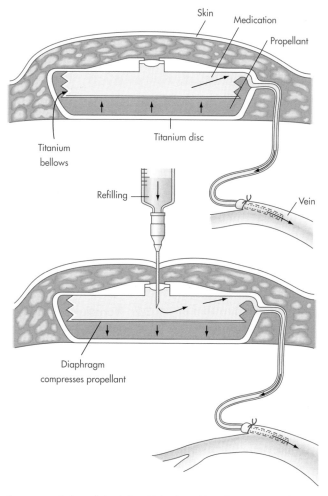

Figure 2.2 Diagrammatic representation of the Infusaid implantable infusion pump during operation (top) and during refilling (bottom).

Reproduced from P. J. Blackshear and T. H. Rhode, in *Controlled Drug Delivery*, vol. 2. *Clinical Applications* (ed. S. D. Burk), Boca Raton, FL, CRC Press, p. 11.

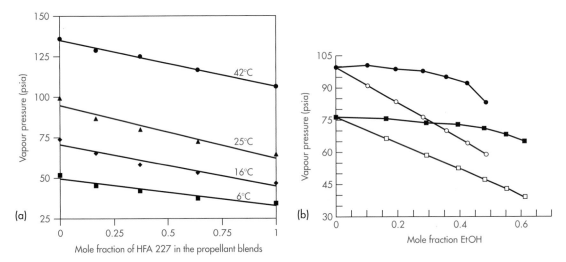

Figure 2.3 (a) Plots of vapour pressure versus mole fraction of HFA 227 for propellant systems composed of HFA 134a and HFA 227 at 6, 16, 25 and 42°C showing ideality of mixing (Raoult's law obeyed). (Reproduced from reference 3 with permission.) (b) Plots of vapour pressure of HFA 134a (circles) and HFA 227 (squares) versus mole fraction of ethanol at 21.5°C. Solid symbols represent experimental data; open symbols represent theoretical values calculated assuming ideal (Raoult's law) behaviour. (Reproduced from reference 4 with permission.)

enhance the solvent power of the propellant blend.[4] Figure 2.3(b) shows large positive deviations from Raoult's law due to interactions between the components of the formulation. In practical terms such behaviour is beneficial as it enables substantial addition of ethanol without reduction in vapour pressure and aerosol performance.

Vapour pressure–concentration curves for mixtures of two anaesthetic agents often show positive deviations from ideality. For example in enflurane–halothane mixtures (Fig. 2.4). there is a very much larger positive deviation from ideality of enflurane compared to that of halothane. Such positive deviations usually arise when the attraction between molecules of one component is greater than that between the molecules of the two components. This form of interaction is referred to as *association*. Such curves are of value in assessing errors which may arise through the incorrect usage of agent-specific anaesthetic vaporisers. As the name suggests, these vaporisers are specifically calibrated for a particular anaesthetic gas. If a vaporiser partly filled with the correct gas is mistakenly replenished with another, then it is clear from Fig. 2.4 that, because of the facilitation of vaporisation in the gas mixtures, more

of each agent will be delivered than would be the case if ideal mixtures were formed. The clinical consequences of this error will of course depend upon the potency of each agent as well as the delivered vapour concentration.

Negative deviations from Raoult's law may arise when the specific attractions between the component molecules exceed the normal attractions which exist between the molecules of each pure component. A typical example is a solution of the ethanol and water.

2.3.2 Variation of vapour pressure with temperature: Clausius–Clapeyron equation

The increased motion of the molecules of the liquid following an increase of temperature leads to a greater tendency for escape of molecules into the vapour phase with a consequent increase of vapour pressure. The variation of vapour pressure with temperature may be expressed in terms of the molar enthalpy of vaporisation of the liquid, ΔH_{vap}, using the Clapeyron equation

$$\frac{dP}{dT} = \frac{\Delta H_{vap}}{T\,\Delta V} \tag{2.4}$$

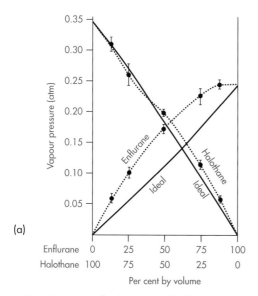
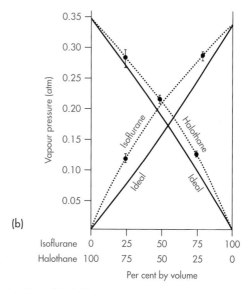

(a)

| Enflurane | 0 | 25 | 50 | 75 | 100 |
| Halothane | 100 | 75 | 50 | 25 | 0 |

Per cent by volume

(b)

| Isoflurane | 0 | 25 | 50 | 75 | 100 |
| Halothane | 100 | 75 | 50 | 25 | 0 |

Per cent by volume

Figure 2.4 Experimentally determined (broken lines) and calculated ideal (solid lines) vapour pressures of (a) halothane and enflurane and (b) halothane and isoflurane when combined at 760 torr and 22°C.
From D. L. Bruce and H. W. Linde, *Anesthesiology*, 60, 342 (1984).

In this equation ΔV is the difference in molar volumes of the two phases. Since the molar volume of the vapour, V_v, is very much larger than that of the liquid, ΔV may be approximately equated with V_v. If it is also assumed that the vapour obeys the ideal gas equation, so that V_v may be replaced by RT/P, equation (2.4) reduces to

$$\frac{\mathrm{d}P}{\mathrm{d}T} = \frac{P\,\Delta H_{vap}}{RT^2}$$

or

$$\frac{\mathrm{d}\ln P}{\mathrm{d}T} = \frac{\Delta H_{vap}}{RT^2} \qquad (2.5)$$

Equation (2.5) is the Clausius–Clapeyron equation. General integration, assuming ΔH_{vap} to be constant, gives

$$\log P = \frac{-\Delta H_{vap}}{2.303RT} + \text{constant} \qquad (2.6)$$

A plot of log vapour pressure versus reciprocal temperature should be linear with a slope of $-\Delta H_{vap}/2.303R$, from which values of enthalpy of vaporisation may be determined.

The Clausius–Clapeyron equation is useful in the calculation of the enthalpy of vaporisation,

and also in the study of phase transitions, for example, the melting of a solid or vaporisation of a liquid. An example of the application of the Clausius–Clapeyron equation to solid–vapour phase transition is seen from a consideration of the sublimation of ibuprofen.[5] Glass vials containing solid ibuprofen develop a haze on their inner walls when stored at 40°C, which is a consequence of sublimation. Ibuprofen vapour pressure– temperature data obey equation (2.6) over the temperature range 23–64°C as seen from Fig. 2.5, with a molar enthalpy of vaporisation of 121 kJ mol^{-1}. Although the vapour pressure exerted at 25°C is negligible (9×10^{-6} torr), the value increases by several orders of magnitude as the temperature is increased and at higher temperatures the rate of loss of ibuprofen becomes significant. For example, the measured weight loss at 55°C is 4.15 mg day^{-1}. Weight losses of this magnitude are significant during drying and coating processes and during accelerated stability testing procedures.

A further example of the applicability of the Clausius–Clapeyron equation is in the assessment of risk associated with the handling of hazardous drugs, particularly by personnel who are potentially exposed to cytostatic

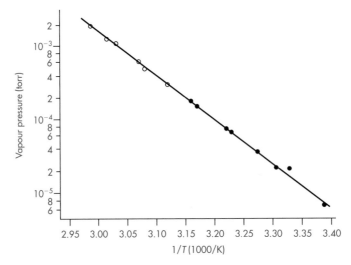

Figure 2.5 Ibuprofen vapour pressure data plotted according to the Clausius–Clapeyron equation (equation 2.6).
Reproduced from reference 5 with permission.

agents routinely used for cancer chemotherapy. Most of the contamination detected with cytostatics occurs because of spillage, inhalation of aerosolised liquid (which can occur for example when a needle is withdrawn from a drug vial) or direct contact with contaminated material such as gloves. There is, however, also evidence that cytotoxic agents evaporate and form a vapour during normal handling, which presents a risk to personnel from inhalation of this vapour.[6] Two factors – the vapour pressure of the drug and the particle size – are influential in determining the rate of evaporation of the drug in powdered form. Table 2.3 shows the significantly higher evaporation times calculated for several widely used antineoplastic agents when the

mean particle size is 1 μm compared to those of 100 μm particles and emphasises the greatly increased risks involved when handling fine powder.

The influence of temperature on the vapour pressure of these drugs is plotted according to equation (2.6) in Fig. 2.6. The vapour above the drugs behaves as an ideal gas because of the low quantity of drug transferred to the gaseous phase and the Clausius–Clapeyron equation is obeyed in all cases. The vapour pressure of carmustine is about 10–100 times greater than that of the other antineoplastic agents and approaches that of mercury (1.0 Pa at 40°C) at elevated temperature, with implications for occupational safety when handling this drug.

Table 2.3 Vapour pressure and evaporation time for drug particles of diameter, d[a]

Compound	Measured vapour pressure (Pa)		Calculated evaporation time (s)	
	20°C	40°C	$d = 1$ μm	$d = 100$ μm
Carmustine	0.019	0.530	12	1.2×10^5
Cisplatin	0.0018	0.0031	110	11.0×10^5
Cyclophosphamide	0.0033	0.0090	44	4.4×10^5
Etoposide	0.0026	0.0038	51	5.1×10^5
Fluorouracil	0.0014	0.0039	210	21.0×10^5

[a] Reproduced from reference 6.

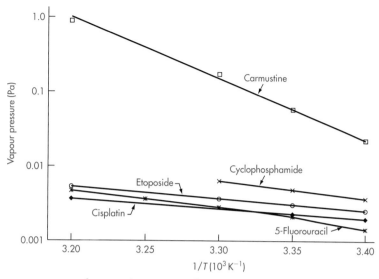

Figure 2.6 The vapour pressures of antineoplastic agents plotted according to the Clausius–Clapeyron equation. Redrawn from reference 6.

EXAMPLE 2.3 Calculation of the molar enthalpy of vaporisation

The slope of a plot of $\log P$ against $1/T$ for metamfetamine is -2.727×10^3 K. Calculate the molar enthalpy of vaporisation of this compound over the given temperature range.

Answer

From the form of the Clausius–Clapeyron equation given by equation (2.6), the slope of a plot of $\log P$ against $1/T$ is

$$\text{Slope} = \frac{-\Delta H_{\text{vap}}}{2.303RT} = -2.727 \times 10^3 \text{ K}$$

$$\therefore \quad \Delta H_{\text{vap}} = -2.727 \times 10^3 \times 2.303 \times 8.314$$

$$= -52.2 \times 10^3 \text{ J mol}^{-1}$$

The molar enthalpy of vaporisation of metamfetamine is 52.2 kJ mol^{-1}.

Gaseous anaesthesia in mice is an equilibrium process between the anaesthetic gas and the phase in which the gas exerts its effect (the *biophase*). As such, it should be amenable to treatment by the Clausius–Clapeyron equation. Modification of this equation is required when the distribution of a series of gases is to

be compared. So that the same equation of state will apply to each gas, it is necessary to use 'reduced' thermodynamic variables. The reduced physiological temperature T_r may be obtained by dividing the physiological temperature for mice (310 K) by the critical temperature of each gas, or, as an approximation, by the boiling point of the gas. Equation (2.6) now becomes

$$\log P = \frac{-\Delta H_{\text{vap}}}{2.303RT_r} + \text{constant} \qquad (2.7)$$

Figure 2.7 shows the logarithm of the partial pressure of each anaesthetic gas required to produce a given level of anaesthesia plotted against the reciprocal of its reduced physiological temperature. Apart from the fluorinated compounds (which possess unique solubility properties), a close adherence to equation (2.7) is noted.

2.3.3 Vapour pressure lowering

The change of vapour pressure following the addition of a nonvolatile solute to a solvent may be determined by application of Raoult's law. Since the solute is nonvolatile, the total vapour pressure, P, above the dilute solution is

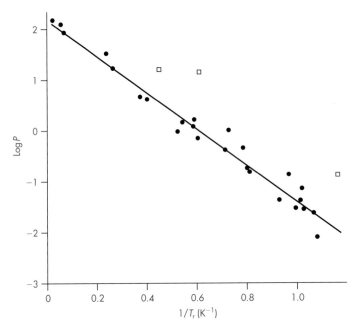

Figure 2.7 Graph of anaesthetic pressure P against the reciprocal of the reduced physiological temperature, T_r. Compounds not following the relationship (fluoromethane, perfluoromethane and perfluoroethane) are identified by the symbol □.

Reproduced from A. Cammarata, *J. Pharm. Sci.*, 64, 2025 (1975) with permission.

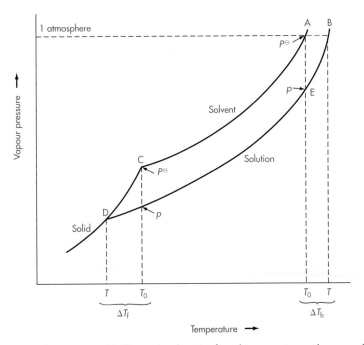

Figure 2.8 Freezing point depression and boiling point elevation for a binary system with a nonvolatile solute.

due entirely to the solvent and may be equated with p_1, the vapour pressure of the solvent. From Raoult's law we have

$$P = p_1 = p_1^{\ominus} x_i = p_1^{\ominus}(1 - x_2) \qquad (2.8)$$

where x_2 is the mole fraction of the added solute. Rearranging gives

$$\frac{p_1^{\ominus} - p_1}{p_1^{\ominus}} = x_2 \qquad (2.9)$$

That is, the relative lowering of the vapour pressure is equal to the mole fraction of the solute.

A direct consequence of the reduction of vapour pressure by the added solute is that the temperature at which the vapour pressure of the solution attains atmospheric pressure (that is, the boiling point) must be higher than that of the pure solvent.

In Fig. 2.8, points A and B represent the boiling points of pure solvent and solution respectively. The boiling point is thus raised by an amount $T - T_0 = \Delta T_b$. A–E represents the lowering of vapour pressure, $p^{\ominus} - p$, by the solution.

An expression for the boiling point elevation may readily be derived using the Clausius–Clapeyron equation (see Box 2.1). This expression allows the calculation of the increase of boiling point, ΔT_b, from the molality, m, of the solution using

$$\Delta T_b = K_b m$$

where K_b is the molal elevation constant, which has the value $0.511 \text{ K mol}^{-1} \text{ kg}$ for water.

Another consequence of lowering of vapour pressure is that the freezing point of the solution is lower than that of the pure solvent. The freezing point of a solution is the temperature at which the solution exists in equilibrium with solid solvent. In such an equilibrium, the solvent must have the same vapour pressure in both solid and liquid states. Consequently, the freezing point is the temperature at which the vapour pressure curves of the solvent and solution intersect the sublimation curve of the solid solvent; that is, points C and D, respectively, in Fig. 2.8. The freezing point depression is $T - T_0 = \Delta T_f$. An expression for freezing

---

Box 2.1   Boiling point elevation

The vapour pressure of the solution is p at temperature T_0 and $p^{\ominus}$ (equal to that of pure solvent) at temperature T. According to the Clausius–Clapeyron equation we may write

$$\ln \frac{p}{p^{\ominus}} = \frac{\Delta H_{vap}}{R}\left[\frac{T - T_0}{T T_0}\right] \qquad (2.10)$$

Assuming that the magnitude of the elevation is small, T may be replaced by T_0 in the denominator and hence

$$\ln \frac{p}{p^{\ominus}} = \frac{\Delta H_{vap} \Delta T_b}{R T_0^2} \qquad (2.11)$$

According to Raoult's law, the relative lowering of the vapour pressure is equal to the mole fraction of solute; that is $(p^{\ominus} - p)/p^{\ominus} = x_2$, or $p/p^{\ominus} = 1 - x_2$. Thus,

$$\ln(p/p^{\ominus}) = \ln(1 - x_2)$$

For small values of x_2 (that is, dilute solutions), $\ln(1 - x_2) \approx -x_2$, and equation (2.11) becomes

$$\Delta T_b = \frac{x_2 T_0^2 R}{\Delta H_{vap}} \qquad (2.12)$$

Mole fraction may be replaced by molality, m, using the relationship

$$x_2 = m M_1 / 1000$$

Therefore,

$$\Delta T_b = \frac{R T_0^2 M_1 m}{1000 \, \Delta H_{vap}} = K_b m \qquad (2.13)$$

where K_b is the molal elevation constant, which has the value $0.511 \text{ K mol}^{-1} \text{ kg}$ for water, and M_1 is the molecular weight of the solvent.

---

point lowering can be derived in a similar manner to that for boiling point elevation, giving

$$\Delta T_f = \frac{R T_0^2 M_1 m}{1000 \, \Delta H_{fus}} \qquad (2.14)$$

where ΔH_{fus} is the molal heat of fusion. Therefore,

$$\Delta T_f = K_f m \qquad (2.15)$$

where K_f is the molal freezing point constant, which is $1.86 \text{ K mol}^{-1} \text{ kg}$ for water.

2.4   Solubility of gases in liquids

The amount of gas which can be dissolved by a particular liquid depends on the temperature, the pressure and the nature of both the gas and the liquid solvent. The solubility may be expressed by *Bunsen's absorption coefficient, a*, which is the volume of gas reduced to 273 K and a pressure of 1 bar which dissolves in a unit volume of the liquid at the given temperature when the partial pressure of the gas is 1 bar.

∙∙∙∙∙∙∙∙∙∙∙∙∙∙∙∙∙∙∙∙∙∙∙∙∙∙∙∙∙∙∙∙∙∙∙∙∙∙

EXAMPLE 2.4 Calculation of the Bunsen absorption coefficient

If the solubility of N_2 in water at 25°C and a nitrogen pressure of 450 torr is 0.378 mol m^{-3}, calculate the Bunsen coefficient.

Answer
The volume, V, of dissolved nitrogen at 0°C and a pressure of 760 torr (1.013×10^5 N m^{-2}), assuming ideality, is given by equation (2.1) as

$$V = \frac{0.378 \times 8.314 \times 273.16}{1.013 \times 10^5}$$

$$= 8.474 \times 10^{-3}\, \text{m}^3$$

The volume of N_2 that would dissolve at a nitrogen pressure of 760 torr is

$$V = 8.474 \times 10^{-3} \times (760/450)$$

$$= 0.0143\, \text{m}^3$$

That is, the Bunsen absorption coefficient for N_2 at 25°C is 0.0143.

∙∙∙∙∙∙∙∙∙∙∙∙∙∙∙∙∙∙∙∙∙∙∙∙∙∙∙∙∙∙∙∙∙∙∙∙∙∙

In anaesthetic practice, an alternative solubility coefficient, the *Ostwald solubility coefficient*, is preferred. This coefficient is defined as the volume of gas which dissolves in a unit volume of the liquid at the given temperature. The volume of gas is not corrected to standard temperature and pressure but instead is measured at the temperature and pressure concerned. The important difference between these two coefficients is that the Ostwald coefficient is independent of pressure, as we can see from the following example.

Consider a closed vessel containing 1 dm^3 (1 litre) of water above which is nitrogen at a pressure of 1 bar at room temperature. The volume of nitrogen dissolved at equilibrium is 0.016 dm^3. If the pressure is increased to 2 bar at the same temperature, then the amount of nitrogen which dissolves is doubled, according to Henry's law (see section 2.4.2). The resultant volume of nitrogen dissolved is 0.032 dm^3 when measured at 1 bar but 0.016 dm^3 when measured at the ambient pressure of 2 bar (according to the ideal gas law). Consequently, the volume of nitrogen dissolved measured at ambient pressure, and hence the Ostwald coefficient, remains unchanged even though the partial pressure of the nitrogen and also the number of dissolved molecules are doubled.

2.4.1   Effect of temperature on solubility

When gases dissolve in water without chemical reaction there is generally an evolution of heat. Hence by Le Chatelier's principle an increase in temperature usually leads to a decreased solubility. The effect of temperature on the absorption coefficient may be determined from an equation analogous to the van't Hoff equation:

$$\log \frac{a_2}{a_1} = \frac{\Delta H}{2.303R} \left[\frac{T_2 - T_1}{T_1 T_2} \right] \qquad (2.16)$$

where a_1 and a_2 are the absorption coefficients at temperature T_1 and T_2, respectively, and ΔH is the change in enthalpy accompanying the solution of 1 mole of gas.

A practical illustration of the decreased solubility of gases with increase of temperature is the appearance of gas bubbles on the sides of a vessel containing water when the vessel is heated; the water is saturated with air at lower temperatures and the amount of air that it can contain decreases with increase of temperature, resulting in bubble formation.

2.4.2   Effect of pressure on solubility

The influence of pressure on solubility is expressed by Henry's law, which states that the mass of gas dissolved by a given volume of solvent at a constant temperature is proportional to the pressure of the gas in equilibrium with the solution. If w is the mass of gas dissolved by unit volume of solvent at an equilibrium pressure, p, then from Henry's law,

$$w = kp \qquad (2.17)$$

where k is a proportionality constant. Most gases obey Henry's law under normal conditions of temperature and at reasonable pressures, providing the solubility is not too high. If a mixture of gases is equilibrated with a liquid, the solubility of each component gas is proportional to its own partial pressure; that is, Henry's law may be applied independently to each gas.

In practice, Henry's law explains the often violent release of gas that occurs as a consequence of the decrease of solubility of a gas when the pressure above the gas is released suddenly, for example when the cap of a bottle of sparkling water is unscrewed quickly.

The application of Henry's law in the calculation of the effect of pressure on the solubility of gases in liquids is illustrated in Example 2.5.

· ·

EXAMPLE 2.5   Henry's law calculation

The solubility of oxygen in water at a partial pressure of 25 torr is 8.31 mg dm^{-3} at 25°C. Calculate the solubility if the partial pressure is increased to 100 torr at the same temperature.

Answer
Applying equation (2.17) at the two partial pressures, noting that k is the same at both:

$$w_1/p_1 = w_2/p_2$$

where

$p_1 = 25$ torr   and $w_1 = 8.31$ mg dm^{-3}
$p_2 = 100$ torr   and $w_2 = ?$

gives

$$w_2 = 100 \times 8.31/25 = 33.2 \text{ mg dm}^{-3}$$

The solubility of oxygen at a partial pressure of 100 torr is 33.2 mg dm^{-3}.

· ·

Rather than considering equation (2.17) as a means of expressing the solubility of a gas in terms of vapour pressure, we could also view it as a way of expressing the vapour pressure developed by a given concentration of dissolved gas, as explained in Box 2.2.

Box 2.2   Relationship between Henry's law and Raoult's law

By expressing the solubility of a gas in terms of vapour pressure, we invoke an analogy with Raoult's law which gives the vapour pressure p_1 of the solvent in equilibrium with a solution in which the solvent mole fraction is x_1, as

$$p_1 = x_1 p_1^{\ominus} \qquad (2.18)$$

where $p_1^{\ominus}$ is the vapour pressure of pure solvent. Assuming the solute rather than the solvent to be the volatile component, we may write

$$p_2 = x_2 p_2^{\ominus} \qquad (2.19)$$

For a dilute solution of a gas we may express the concentration of gas in terms of the mole fraction and thus Henry's law may be written

$$x_2 = k' p_2$$

or $\qquad (2.20)$

$$p_2 = \frac{x_2}{k'}$$

Comparing equations (2.19) and (2.20), it is clear that the Henry's law and Raoult's law expressions would become identical if k' could be equated with $1/p_2^{\ominus}$. Such an equating of terms is valid in the case of ideal solutions only, and in most solutions of gases in liquids, although k' is constant, it is not equal to $1/p_2^{\ominus}$.

Figure 2.9 shows the plot of the partial pressure of chloroform in an oleyl alcohol–chloroform mixture as a function of the percentage of chloroform in the gas phase. Significant departures from Raoult's law are apparent when the amount of dissolved chloroform exceeds about 20%.

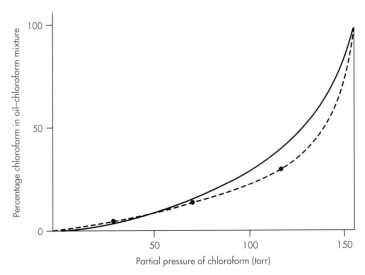

Figure 2.9 Plot of the partial pressure of chloroform in the gas phase over an oleyl alcohol–chloroform mixture at 20°C as a function of the percentage of chloroform in the mixture; solid circles represent experimental results; full curve is the Raoult's law plot.
Reproduced from J. F. Nunn, *Br. J. Anaesth.*, 32, 346 (1960) with permission.

2.4.3 The solubility of volatile anaesthetics in oil

The oil solubility of an anaesthetic is of interest, not only because it governs the passage of the anaesthetic into and out of the fat depots of the body, but also because there is a well-established correlation between anaesthetic potency and oil solubility. Figure 2.10 shows a linear inverse relationship between log narcotic concentration and log solubility in oleyl alcohol for a series of common anaesthetic gases. The ordinate of the graph represents the minimum alveolar concentration (MAC), which is that concentration of anaesthetic at which 50% of the patients cease to move in response to a stimulus. The abscissa shows the solubility expressed in terms of the oil/gas partition coefficient. Partition coefficients are widely used to express solubility and are the ratios of the concentration of the gas in the two phases in equilibrium at a given temperature. When, as in this case, one of the phases is the gas itself, the partition coefficient expressed as the liquid/gas (note the order of the phases) concentration ratio is equal to the

Ostwald solubility coefficient. The graph shows that an anaesthetic gas with a high oil solubility is effective at a low alveolar concentration and has a high potency. This relationship is the basis of the Meyer–Overton hypothesis of anaesthesia.

The correlation between anaesthetic potency and lipid solubility shown in Fig. 2.10 is valid for most inhaled anaesthetics and the product MAC × oil/gas partition coefficient (which should of course be a constant) varies by only a factor of 2 or 3 for potencies ranging over 100 000-fold. This constancy implies that inhaled anaesthetics act in the same manner at a specific hydrophobic site (the so-called unitary theory of anaesthesia). This has been challenged by more recent work that has identified compounds, including alkanes[7] and polyhalogenated and perfluorinated compounds,[8] which do not obey the Meyer–Overton hypothesis. It has been suggested that a contributory cause of deviation from this hypothesis may be the choice of lipid to represent the anaesthetic site of action of these compounds, implying that there may be multiple sites of action for inhaled anaesthetics.

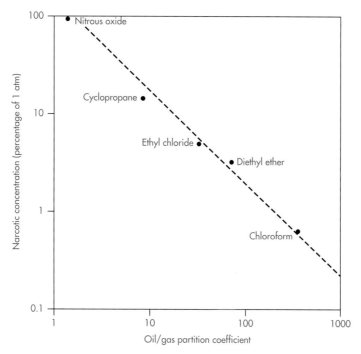

Figure 2.10 Narcotic concentrations of various anaesthetic agents plotted against solubility in oleyl alcohol (expressed as oil/gas partition coefficient).
Reproduced from J. F. Nunn, *Br. J. Anaesth.*, 32, 346 (1960) with permission.

2.5 The solubility of gases in blood and tissues

The application of physicochemical principles in the consideration of the solubility of gases in blood and tissues is complicated by the complex nature of these solvent systems.

2.5.1 The solubility of oxygen in the blood

The major respiratory function of the lungs is to add oxygen to the blood and to remove carbon dioxide from it. Thus the measurement of the concentration of these gases in the arterial blood leaving the lungs, combined with a knowledge of the partial pressure of oxygen in the inspired air (approximately 147 torr at 37°C), allows an assessment of the gas exchanging function of the lungs.

The solubility of oxygen in the blood is dependent upon the concentration of haemo-globin, each gram of which can combine with 1.34 cm^3 of oxygen at 37°C, and upon the presence of other ligands which combine with haemoglobin and affect oxygen binding. The oxygen saturation, S_{O_2}, of a particular blood sample, which determines the colour of the blood, is defined by the ratio of the oxygen concentration in the blood sample to the oxygen concentration when that blood is fully saturated (i.e. the oxygen capacity of the blood). Defined in this manner, it is clear that S_{O_2} for an anaemic patient, where there is a low haemoglobin content, may be the same as that for a patient with polycythaemia, but the oxygen concentration of the blood would be much less in the anaemic patient.

The partial pressure, P_{O_2}, of the oxygen in the blood (oxygen tension) is related to S_{O_2} by the oxygen dissociation curve (Fig. 2.11). The shape and position of this sigmoidal curve depend on the temperature, the hydrogen ion concentration and the concentration within the red cells of other ligands of haemoglobin

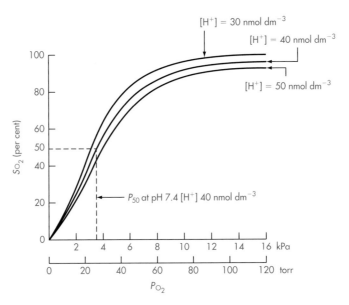

Figure 2.11 The oxygen dissociation curve relating blood oxygen saturation, S_{O_2}, to oxygen tension, P_{O_2}, at three different hydrogen ion concentrations [H+].
Reproduced from D. C. Flenley, *Br. J. Clin. Pharm.*, 9, 129 (1980).

which may also bind to this molecule in addition to oxygen. The position of the curve is defined by the P_{O_2} at 50% saturation, which is denoted as P_{50}. An alternative method of plotting the data uses the logarithmic equation

$$\log\left[\frac{S_{O_2}}{1 - S_{O_2}}\right] = n \log P_{O_2} \qquad (2.21)$$

Plots of $\log[S_{O_2}/(1 - S_{O_2})]$ against $\log P_{O_2}$ are linear over most of the range with a gradient n.

As seen from Fig. 2.11, the P_{50} value is affected by pH change. Oxygenation of the haemoglobin molecule releases hydrogen ions, i.e. oxygenated haemoglobin behaves as a stronger acid (proton donor) than reduced haemoglobin. The ratio of ΔP_{50} to ΔpH (where Δ refers to the change in the property) is referred to as the *Bohr effect* and normally has a value of 0.5. It is usual to correct the P_{50} value to a plasma pH of 7.4 (although the pH in the red blood cell is about 7.18).

Normal haemoglobin has a P_{50} of 3.4 kPa and n of 2.6–3.0 at pH 7.4. Values of both P_{50} and n are affected by genetic abnormalities in haemoglobin synthesis that alter the amino acid sequence. Over 190 such variants are known, with a wide range of P_{50} and n values.

Other ligands of the haemoglobin molecule apart from oxygen which can affect these values include 2,3-diphosphoglycerate, a by-product within the Embden–Meyerhof glycolytic pathway in the red cell. This is normally present in equimolar concentrations to haemoglobin. Transfused blood stored in acid-citrate dextrose, however, contains very little of this compound, and a lowering of P_{50} is noted over several hours in patients receiving massive blood transfusions. P_{50} is also affected by the presence of carbon monoxide, which may result from heavy smoking or endogenous haemolysis.

2.5.2 The solubility of anaesthetic gases in blood and tissues

Blood solubility and anaesthetic action

Anaesthetic gases such as ether which have a high blood solubility (Ostwald solubility coefficient in blood is 12) are transported away from the lungs more rapidly than those such as halothane (Ostwald coefficient = 2.3) and nitrous oxide (Ostwald coefficient = 0.47). As a consequence, the concentration of ether in alveolar air builds up more slowly than that of the more poorly soluble anaesthetic gases and is only slightly above the level in the tissues. Figure 2.12 shows the way in which the alveolar concentrations of anaesthetic gases with a range of blood solubilities (expressed as a percentage of their final values) change with time after administration. We can see that soluble anaesthetics such as ether are very slow to approach their equilibrium value compared with those of lower solubility; nitrous oxide, for example, reaches an equilibrium value in 10–15 minutes. Because the concentrations of anaesthetics in the blood and brain are close to the alveolar concentrations, there is a rapid onset of anaesthesia in the case of nitrous oxide and a relatively slow induction of anaesthesia with ether.

Increases in blood solubility without corresponding increases in tissue solubility slow the rate at which halothane increases in the alveoli. Because of the increased content of this anaesthetic in the blood flowing through the tissues, however, the halothane partial pressure in the tissues approaches equilibrium more rapidly than in the alveoli. The net consequence is that the time for induction with halothane is not greatly affected by changes in blood solubility, although the

depth of anaesthesia achieved after 10–30 minutes may be considerably affected.

Influence of blood and tissue composition on solubility

The solubility of an anaesthetic gas in the *blood* is mainly a consequence of its higher solubility in the lipids and proteins than in aqueous solution. Consequently, changes in the amounts of these components in the blood can alter the anaesthetic solubility in this solvent. The influence of the composition of the blood on the solubility of anaesthetic gases has been studied by several workers;[9] we will consider a few examples here. In many cases anaemia leads to a decrease in blood solubility through a reduction in haemoglobin and in the protein and lipids which form the red cells. Changes in the concentration and type of plasma proteins have been reported to affect the solubility of halothane.[10] Some workers have correlated the solubility of halothane with the concentration of plasma triglycerides in the blood of dogs and humans[11, 12] and also of horses.[13] Changes in serum constituents with age lead to concomitant changes in the blood/gas partition coefficient, $\lambda_{\text{blood/gas}}$. A patient who has recently eaten will have a higher blood lipid content than a fasting patient, and this results

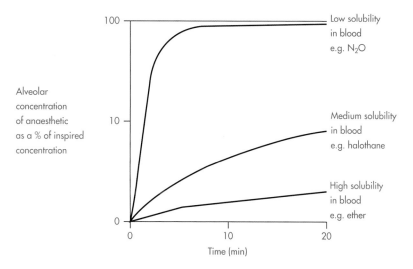

Figure 2.12   Graph of alveolar concentration of anaesthetic gases against time during anaesthetic uptake.

in a greater concentration of anaesthetic in the blood (Fig. 2.13).

The high lipid solubility of anaesthetics is an important factor in determining their solubility in *tissue fluids*. The solubility of xenon and krypton in human liver tissue has been found to be proportional to its triglyceride content.[14] Halothane solubility has been correlated with the fat content of the muscles of horses.[13] This relationship between solubility and fat content implies a greater muscle solubility in adults than in children because of a greater infiltration of fat in adult muscles. The consequence of increased tissue solubility on the depth and rate of onset of anaesthesia is different from that caused by increased blood solubility. Although a similar slowing of the rate of rise of anaesthetic in the alveoli is observed, the increased capacity of the tissues for the anaesthetic leads to an increase in the time required for the partial pressure in the tissues to approach that in the alveoli. The resultant effect of increased tissue solubility is a delayed onset of anaesthesia and also a decreased eventual depth of anaesthesia produced by a given inspired concentration.

Influence of pressure

It is perhaps not surprising, bearing in mind the complexity of blood and tissue fluids, that Henry's law is frequently disobeyed. For example, departures of the solubility versus pressure relationships from Henry's law have been reported for cyclopropane in blood,[15] which have been attributed to the binding of the cyclopropane by the haemoglobin molecule. An increase in pressure at low partial pressures of cyclopropane simply results in an increase in the proportion of cyclopropane-binding sites on the haemoglobin molecule that are occupied. At higher pressures, however, nearly all the sites become occupied and further pressure increases cannot further increase the extent of cyclopropane binding, and a deviation from Henry's law becomes apparent. Similar deviations from Henry's law have been reported for xenon in the presence of myoglobin.[16] In contrast, a study of the solubility of isoflurane and halothane in rabbit blood and human or rabbit brain has shown Henry's law to be obeyed over a wide range of partial pressures.[17] The authors have concluded that there was no evidence of saturable binding sites for these anaesthetic gases.

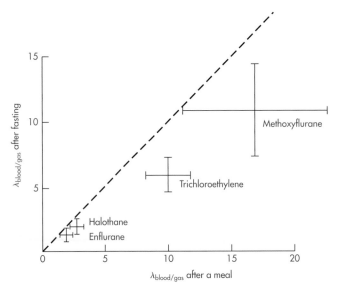

Figure 2.13   Postprandial and fasting effects on blood/gas partition coefficients (λ): the broken line represents the situation in which the values of the two blood/gas partition coefficients are identical.
The data are taken from V. Fiserova, J. Vlach and J. C. Cassady, *Br. J. Ind. Med.*, 37, 42 (1980).

Table 2.4 Variation of partition coefficients with temperature[a]

Agent	$\lambda_{water/gas}$ at 20°C	Aqueous temperature coefficient (% per °C)	$\lambda_{oil/gas}$ at 20°C	Oil temperature coefficient (% per °C)
Methoxyflurane	9.3	−4.18	2108	−4.58
Trichloroethylene	3.4	−3.94	1570	−4.53
Chloroform	7.7	−3.76	881	−4.54
Halothane	1.6	−4.01	469	−4.36
Enflurane	1.4	−3.22	180	−3.51
Diethyl ether	30.5	−4.89	117	−3.39
Cyclopropane	0.3	−2.11	16.7	−2.18
Nitrous oxide	0.7	−2.33	1.7	−1.13

[a] Reproduced from M. J. Halsey, in *General Anaesthesia*, 5th edn (ed. J. F. Nunn, J. E. Utting and B. R. Brown), Butterworths, London, 1989, Ch. 2.

Influence of body temperature

Temperature also influences anaesthetic solubility; temperature increase leads to a decrease in solubility as expected from section 2.4.1. Table 2.4 shows the temperature coefficients of the both water/gas, $\lambda_{water/gas}$, and oil/gas, $\lambda_{oil/gas}$, partition coefficients for a range of anaesthetic gases.

These data are relevant clinically because of possible wide variation of body temperature in the surgical patient. Body temperature may be lowered as a result of preoperative sedation, by cutaneous vasodilation, by the infusion of cold fluids and by reduced metabolism under operating conditions. The increase in oil/gas partition coefficient with decreasing temperature means that the effective concentration at the hydrophobic site of action is increasing and hence the apparent potency of the anaesthetic increases.

Summary

- Raoult's law can be used to calculate the partial pressure of a component in the vapour phase above a liquid under conditions of equilibrium if the composition of the liquid is known and if the system is assumed to be ideal. Mixtures of the hydrofluoroalkane propellants HFA 134a and HFA 227 obey Raoult's law over a wide concentration range, but positive deviations from this law occur when the cosolvent alcohol is included in the formulation.
- The variation of vapour pressure with temperature is described by the Clausius–Clapeyron equation; an equation, which provides a useful method for the experimental determination of the enthalpy changes accompanying phase transitions.
- The relative lowering of the vapour pressure following the addition of a solute to a solvent is equal to the mole fraction of the solute. A consequence of this change of vapour pressure is that the boiling point of the solution is increased and its freezing point decreased.
- The solubility of a gas in a liquid may be expressed by the Ostwald solubility coefficient, which is the volume of gas dissolved in unit volume of liquid at a given temperature, or as the Bunsen's absorption coefficient, in which the temperature and pressure are reduced to standard conditions.
- The solubility of a gas in a liquid decreases with increase of temperature at constant pressure and is directly proportional to pressure at a constant temperature (Henry's law).
- Application of temperature and pressure relationships in the prediction of the solubility of anaesthetic gases *in vivo* is complicated by the interaction of these gases with the lipids and proteins in the blood and in tissue fluids.

References

1. K. J. McDonald and G. P. Martin. Transition to CFC-free metered dose inhalers – into the new millennium. *Int. J. Pharm.*, 201, 89–107 (2000)

2. C. M. Balch, M. U. Urist and M. L. McGregor. Continuous regional chemotherapy for metastatic colorectal cancer using a totally implantable infusion pump. A feasibility study in 50 patients. *Am. J. Surg.*, 145, 285–90 (1983)

3. R. O. Williams and J. Lie. Influence of formulation additives on the vapor pressure of hydrofluoroalkane propellants. *Int. J. Pharm.*, 166, 99–103 (1998)

4. C. Vervaet and P. Byron. Drug–surfactant–propellant interactions in HFA-formulations. *Int. J. Pharm.*, 186, 13–30 (1999)

5. K. D. Ertel, R. A. Heasley, C. Koegel, *et al.* Determination of ibuprofen vapor pressure at temperatures of pharmaceutical interest. *J. Pharm. Sci.*, 79, 552 (1990)

6. T. K. Kiffmeyer, C. Kube, S. Opiolka, K. G., *et al. Pharm. J.*, 268, 331 (2002)

7. J. Liu, M. J. Laster, S. Taheri, E. I. *et al.* Effect of *n*-alkane kinetics in rats on potency estimations and the Meyer–Overton hypothesis. *Anesth. Analg.*, 79, 1049–55 (1994)

8. D. D. Koblin, B. S. Chortkoff, M. J. Laster, *et al.* Polyhalogenated and perfluorinated compounds that disobey the Meyer–Overton hypothesis. *Anesth. Analg.*, 79, 1043–8 (1994)

9. E. I. Eger. *Anaesthetic Uptake and Action*, Williams and Wilkins, Baltimore, 1974, chapter 9

10. L. H. Laasberg and J. Hedley-Whyte. Halothane solubility in blood and solutions of plasma proteins: effects of temperature, protein composition, and hemoglobin concentration. *Anesthesiology*, 32, 351–6 (1970)

11. P. D. Wagner, P. F. Naumann and R. B. Laravuso. Simultaneous measurement of eight foreign gases in blood by gas chromatography. *J. Appl. Physiol.*, 36, 600–5 (1974)

12. R. A. Saraiva, B. A. Willis, A. Steward, *et al.* Halothane solubility in human blood. *Br. J. Anaesth.*, 49, 115–9 (1977)

13. B. M. Q. Weaver and A. I. Webb. Tissue composition and halothane solubility in the horse. *Br. J. Anaesth.*, 53, 487–93 (1981)

14. K. Kitani and K. Winkler. *In vitro* determination of solubility of 133xenon and 85krypton in human liver tissue with varying triglyceride content. *Scand. J. Clin. Lab. Invest.*, 29, 173–6 (1972)

15. H. J. Lowe and K. Hagler. In *Gas Chromatography in Biology and Medicine* (ed. R. Porter), Churchill, London, 1969, pp. 86–112

16. B. P. Schoenborn. Binding of cyclopropane to sperm whale myoglobin. *Nature*, 214, 1120–2 (1967)

17. C. M. Coburn and E. I. Eger. The partial pressure of isoflurane or halothane does not affect their solubility in rabbit blood or brain or human brain: inhaled anesthetics obey Henry's law. *Anesth. Analg.*, 65, 960–2 (1986)

3

Physicochemical properties of drugs in solution

In this chapter we examine some of the important physicochemical properties of drugs in aqueous solution which are of relevance to such liquid dosage forms as injections, solutions, and eye drops. Some basic thermodynamic concepts will be introduced, particularly that of thermodynamic activity, an important parameter in determining drug potency. It is important that parenteral solutions are formulated with osmotic pressure similar to that of blood serum; in this chapter we will see how to adjust the tonicity of the formulation to achieve this aim. Most drugs are at least partially ionised at physiological pH and many studies have suggested that the charged group is essential for biological activity. We look at the influence of pH on the ionisation of several types of drug in solution and consider equations that allow the calculation of the pH of solutions of these drugs.

First, however, we recount the various ways to express the strength of a solution, since it is of fundamental importance that we are able to interpret the various units used to denote solution concentration and to understand their interrelationships, not least in practice situations.

3.1 Concentration units

A wide range of units is commonly used to express solution concentration, and confusion often arises in the interconversion of one set of units to another. Wherever possible throughout this book we have used the SI system of units. Although this is the currently recommended system of units in Great Britain, other more traditional systems are still widely used and these will be also described in this section.

3.1.1 Weight concentration

Concentration is often expressed as a weight of solute in a unit volume of solution; for example, $g\ dm^{-3}$, or % w/v, which is the number of grams of solute in $100\ cm^3$ of solution. This is not an exact method when working at a range of temperatures, since the volume of the solution is temperature-dependent and hence the weight concentration also changes with temperature.

Whenever a hydrated compound is used, it is important to use the correct state of hydration in the calculation of weight concentration. Thus 10% w/v $CaCl_2$ (anhydrous) is approximately equivalent to 20% w/v $CaCl_2 \cdot 6H_2O$ and consequently the use of the vague statement '10% calcium chloride' could result in gross error. The SI unit of weight concentration is $kg\ m^{-3}$ which is numerically equal to $g\ dm^{-3}$.

3.1.2 Molarity and molality

These two similar-sounding terms must not be confused. The *molarity* of a solution is the number of moles (gram molecular weights) of solute in 1 litre ($1\ dm^3$) of *solution*. The *molality* is the number of moles of solute in 1 kg of *solvent*. Molality has the unit, $mol\ kg^{-1}$, which

is an accepted SI unit. Molarity may be converted to SI units using the relationship $1\ mol\ litre^{-1} = 1\ mol\ dm^{-3} = 10^3\ mol\ m^{-3}$. Interconversion between molarity and molality requires a knowledge of the density of the solution.

Of the two units, molality is preferable for a precise expression of concentration because it does not depend on the solution temperature as does molarity; also, the molality of a component in a solution remains unaltered by the addition of a second solute, whereas the molarity of this component decreases because the total volume of solution increases following the addition of the second solute.

3.1.3 Milliequivalents

The unit milliequivalent (mEq) is commonly used clinically in expressing the concentration of an ion in solution. The term 'equivalent', or gram equivalent weight, is analogous to the mole or gram molecular weight. When monovalent ions are considered, these two terms are identical. A 1 molar solution of sodium bicarbonate, $NaHCO_3$, contains 1 mol or 1 Eq of Na^+ and 1 mol or 1 Eq of HCO_3^- per litre (dm^{-3}) of solution. With multivalent ions, attention must be paid to the valency of each ion; for example, 10% w/v $CaCl_2 \cdot 2H_2O$ contains 6.8 mmol or 13.6 mEq of Ca^{2+} in $10\ cm^3$.

The Pharmaceutical Codex[1] gives a table of milliequivalents for various ions and also a simple formula for the calculation of milliequivalents per litre (see Box 3.1).

In analytical chemistry a solution which contains $1\ Eq\ dm^{-3}$ is referred to as a *normal* solution. Unfortunately the term 'normal' is also used to mean physiologically normal with reference to saline solution. In this usage, a physiologically normal saline solution contains 0.9 g NaCl in $100\ cm^3$ aqueous solution and *not* 1 equivalent (58.44 g) per litre.

Box 3.1   Calculation of milliequivalents

The number of milliequivalents in 1 g of substance is given by

$$mEq = \frac{valency \times 1000 \times no.\ of\ specified\ units\ in\ 1\ atom/molecule/ion}{atomic,\ molecular\ or\ ionic\ weight}$$

For example, $CaCl_2 \cdot 2H_2O$ (mol. wt. = 147.0)

$$mEq\ Ca^{2+}\ in\ 1\ g\ CaCl_2 \cdot 2H_2O = \frac{2 \times 1000 \times 1}{147.0}$$
$$= 13.6\ mEq$$

and

$$mEq\ Cl^-\ in\ 1\ g\ CaCl_2 \cdot 2H_2O = \frac{1 \times 1000 \times 2}{147.0}$$
$$= 13.6\ mEq$$

that is, each gram of $CaCl_2 \cdot 2H_2O$ represents 13.6 mEq of calcium and 13.6 mEq of chloride

---

3.1.4   Mole fraction

The mole fraction of a component of a solution is the number of moles of that component divided by the total number of moles present in solution. In a two-component (binary) solution, the mole fraction of solvent, x_1, is given by $x_1 = n_1/(n_1 + n_2)$, where n_1 and n_2 are respectively the numbers of moles of solvent and of solute present in solution. Similarly, the mole fraction of solute, x_2, is given by $x_2 = n_2/(n_1 + n_2)$. The sum of the mole fractions of all components is, of course, unity, i.e. for a binary solution, $x_1 + x_2 = 1$.

• •

EXAMPLE 3.1   Units of concentration

Isotonic saline contains 0.9% w/v of sodium chloride (mol. wt. = 58.5). Express the concentration of this solution as: (a) molarity; (b) molality; (c) mole fraction and (d) milliequivalents of Na^+ per litre. Assume that the density of isotonic saline is 1 g cm^{-3}.

Answer
(a) 0.9% w/v solution of sodium chloride contains 9 g dm^{-3} = 0.154 mol dm^{-3}.

(b) 9 g of sodium chloride are dissolved in 991 g of water (assuming density = 1 g dm^{-3}).

Therefore 1000 g of water contains 9.08 g of sodium chloride = 0.155 moles, i.e. molality = 0.155 mol kg^{-1}.

(c) Mole fraction of sodium chloride, x_1, is given by

$$x_1 = \frac{n_1}{n_1 + n_2} = \frac{0.154}{0.154 + 55.06} = 2.79 \times 10^{-3}$$

(Note 991 g of water contains 991/18 moles, i.e. $n_2 = 55.06$.)

(d) Since Na^+ is monovalent, the number of milliequivalents of Na^+ = number of millimoles.

Therefore the solution contains 154 mEq dm^{-3} of Na^+.

• •

3.2   Thermodynamics – a brief introduction

The importance of thermodynamics in the pharmaceutical sciences is apparent when it is realised that such processes as the partitioning of solutes between immiscible solvents, the solubility of drugs, micellisation and drug–receptor interaction can all be treated in thermodynamic terms. This brief section merely introduces some of the concepts of thermodynamics which are referred to throughout the book. Readers requiring a greater depth of treatment should consult standard texts on this subject.[2, 3]

3.2.1   Energy

Energy is a fundamental property of a system. Some idea of its importance may be gained by considering its role in chemical reactions, where it determines what reactions may occur, how fast the reaction may proceed and in which direction the reaction will occur. Energy takes several forms: kinetic energy is that which a body possesses as a result of its motion; potential energy is the energy which a body has due to its position, whether gravitational potential energy or coulombic potential energy which is associated with charged particles at a given distance apart. All forms of energy are related, but in converting between the various types it is not possible to create or destroy energy. This forms the basis of the *law of conservation of energy*.

The *internal energy U* of a system is the sum of all the kinetic and potential energy contributions to the energy of all the atoms, ions and molecules in that system. In thermodynamics we are concerned with *change* in internal energy, ΔU, rather than the internal energy itself. (Notice the use of Δ to denote a finite change). We may change the internal energy of a closed system (one that cannot exchange matter with its surroundings) in only two ways: by transferring energy as *work* (*w*) or as *heat* (*q*). An expression for the change in internal energy is

$$\Delta U = w + q \qquad (3.1)$$

If the system releases its energy *to* the surroundings ΔU is negative, i.e. the total internal energy has been reduced. Where heat is absorbed (as in an endothermic process) the internal energy will increase and consequently *q* is positive. Conversely, in a process which releases heat (an exothermic process) the internal energy is decreased and *q* is negative. Similarly, when energy is supplied *to* the system as work, *w* is positive; and when the system loses energy by doing work, *w* is negative.

It is frequently necessary to consider infinitesimally small changes in a property; we denote these by the use of d rather than Δ. Thus for an infinitesimal change in internal energy we write equation (3.1) as

$$dU = dw + dq \qquad (3.2)$$

We can see from this equation that it does not really matter whether energy is supplied as heat or work or as a mixture of the two: the change in internal energy is the same. Equation (3.2) thus expresses the principle of the law of conservation of energy but is much wider in its application since it involves

changes in heat energy, which were not encompassed in the conservation law.

It follows from equation (3.2) that a system which is completely isolated from its surroundings, such that it cannot exchange heat or interact mechanically to do work, cannot experience any change in its internal energy. In other words *the internal energy of an isolated system is constant* – this is the *first law of thermodynamics*.

3.2.2 Enthalpy

Where a change occurs in a system at *constant pressure* as, for example, in a chemical reaction in an open vessel, then the increase in internal energy is not equal to the energy supplied as heat because some energy will have been lost by the work done (against the atmosphere) during the expansion of the system. It is convenient, therefore, to consider the heat change in isolation from the accompanying changes in work. For this reason we consider a property that is equal to the heat supplied at constant pressure: this property is called the *enthalpy* (*H*). We can define enthalpy by

$$\Delta H = q \text{ at constant pressure} \qquad (3.3)$$

ΔH is positive when heat is supplied to a system which is free to change its volume and negative when the system releases heat (as in an exothermic reaction). Enthalpy is related to the internal energy of a system by the relationship

$$H = U + pV \qquad (3.4)$$

where *p* and *V* are respectively the pressure and volume of the system.

Enthalpy changes accompany such processes as the dissolution of a solute, the formation of micelles, chemical reaction, adsorption onto solids, vaporisation of a solvent, hydration of a solute, neutralisation of acids and bases, and the melting or freezing of solutes.

3.2.3 Entropy

The first law, as we have seen, deals with the conservation of energy as the system changes from one state to another, but it does not specify which particular changes will occur spontaneously. The reason why some changes have a natural tendency to occur is not that the system is moving to a lower-energy state but that there are changes in the randomness of the system. This can be seen by considering a specific example: the diffusion of one gas into another occurs without any external intervention – i.e. it is spontaneous – and yet there are no differences in either the potential or kinetic energies of the system in its equilibrium state and in its initial state where the two gases are segregated. The driving force for such spontaneous processes is the tendency for an increase in the chaos of the system – the mixed system is more disordered than the original.

A convenient measure of the randomness or disorder of a system is the *entropy* (S). When a system becomes more chaotic, its entropy increases in line with the degree of increase in disorder caused. This concept is encapsulated in the *second law of thermodynamics* which states that *the entropy of an isolated system increases in a spontaneous change.*

The second law, then, involves entropy change, ΔS, and this is defined as the heat absorbed in a *reversible* process, q_{rev}, divided by the temperature (in kelvins) at which the change occurred.

For a finite change

$$\Delta S = \frac{q_{rev}}{T} \tag{3.5}$$

and for an infinitesimal change

$$dS = \frac{dq_{rev}}{T} \tag{3.6}$$

By a 'reversible process' we mean one in which the changes are carried out infinitesimally slowly, so that the system is always in equilibrium with its surroundings. In this case we infer that the temperature of the surroundings is infinitesimally higher than that of the system, so that the heat changes are occurring at an infinitely slow rate, so that the heat transfer is smooth and uniform.

We can see the link between entropy and disorder by considering some specific examples.

For instance, the entropy of a perfect gas changes with its volume V according to the relationship

$$\Delta S = nR \ln \frac{V_f}{V_i} \tag{3.7}$$

where the subscripts f and i denote the final and initial states. Note that if $V_f > V_i$ (i.e. if the gas expands into a larger volume) the logarithmic (ln) term will be positive and the equation predicts an increase of entropy. This is expected since expansion of a gas is a spontaneous process and will be accompanied by an increase in the disorder because the molecules are now moving in a greater volume.

Similarly, increasing the temperature of a system should increase the entropy because at higher temperature the molecular motion is more vigorous and hence the system more chaotic. The equation which relates entropy change to temperature change is

$$\Delta S = C_V \ln \frac{T_f}{T_i} \tag{3.8}$$

where C_V is the molar heat capacity at constant volume. Inspection of equation (3.8) shows that ΔS will be positive when $T_f > T_i$, as predicted.

The entropy of a substance will also change when it undergoes a phase transition, since this too leads to a change in the order. For example, when a crystalline solid melts, it changes from an ordered lattice to a more chaotic liquid (see Fig. 3.1) and consequently an increase in entropy is expected. The entropy change accompanying the melting of a solid is given by

$$\Delta S = \frac{\Delta H_{fus}}{T} \tag{3.9}$$

where ΔH_{fus} is the enthalpy of fusion (melting) and T is the melting temperature. Similarly, we may determine the entropy change when a liquid vaporises from

$$\Delta S = \frac{\Delta H_{vap}}{T} \tag{3.10}$$

where ΔH_{vap} is the enthalpy of vaporisation and T now refers to the boiling point. Entropy

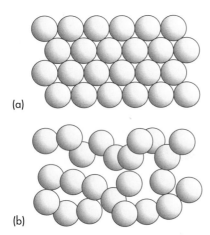

(a)

(b)

Figure 3.1 Melting of a solid involves a change from an ordered arrangement of molecules, represented by (a), to a more chaotic liquid, represented by (b). As a result, the melting process is accompanied by an increase in entropy.

changes accompanying other phase changes, such as change of the polymorphic form of crystals (see section 1.2), may be calculated in a similar manner.

At absolute zero all the thermal motions of the atoms of the lattice of a crystal will have ceased and the solid will have no disorder and hence a zero entropy. This conclusion forms the basis of the *third law of thermodynamics*, which states that *the entropy of a perfectly crystalline material is zero when $T = 0$.*

3.2.4 Free energy

The free energy is derived from the entropy and is, in many ways, a more useful function to use. The free energy which is referred to when we are discussing processes at constant pressure is the *Gibbs free energy (G)*. This is defined by

$$G = H - TS \qquad (3.11)$$

The change in the free energy at constant temperature arises from changes in enthalpy and entropy and is

$$\Delta G = \Delta H - T \Delta S \qquad (3.12)$$

Thus, at constant temperature and pressure,

$$\Delta G = -T \Delta S \qquad (3.13)$$

from which we can see that the change in free energy is another way of expressing the change in overall entropy of a process occurring at constant temperature and pressure.

In view of this relationship we can now consider changes in free energy which occur during a spontaneous process. From equation (3.13) we can see that ΔG will decrease during a spontaneous process at constant temperature and pressure. This decrease will occur until the system reaches an equilibrium state when ΔG becomes zero. This process can be thought of as a gradual using up of the system's ability to perform work as equilibrium is approached. Free energy can therefore be looked at in another way in that it represents the maximum amount of work, w_{max} (other than the work of expansion), which can be extracted from a system undergoing a change at constant temperature and pressure; i.e.

$$\Delta G = w_{max} \qquad (3.14)$$

at constant temperature and pressure

This nonexpansion work can be extracted from the system as electrical work, as in the case of a chemical reaction taking place in an electrochemical cell, or the energy can be stored in biological molecules such as adenosine triphosphate (ATP).

When the system has attained an equilibrium state it no longer has the ability to reverse itself. Consequently *all spontaneous processes are irreversible.* The fact that all spontaneous processes taking place at constant temperature and pressure are accompanied by a negative free energy change provides a useful criterion of the spontaneity of any given process.

By applying these concepts to chemical equilibria we can derive (see Box 3.2) the following simple relationship between free energy change and the equilibrium constant of a reversible reaction, K:

$$\Delta G^{\ominus} = -RT \ln K$$

where the standard free energy $G^{\ominus}$ is the free energy of 1 mole of gas at a pressure of 1 bar.

A similar expression may be derived for reactions in solutions using the *activities* (see

---

Box 3.2   Relationship between free energy change and the equilibrium constant

---

Consider the following reversible reaction taking place in the gaseous phase

$$aA + bB \rightleftharpoons cC + dD$$

According to the law of mass action, the equilibrium constant, K, can be expressed as

$$K = \frac{(p'_C)^c (p'_D)^d}{(p'_A)^a (p'_B)^b} \tag{3.15}$$

where p' terms represent the partial pressures of the components of the reaction at equilibrium.

The relationship between the free energy of a perfect gas and its partial pressure is given by

$$\Delta G = G - G^\ominus = RT \ln p \tag{3.16}$$

where $G^\ominus$ is the free energy of 1 mole of gas at a pressure of 1 bar.

Applying equation (3.16) to each component of the reaction gives

$$aG_A = a(G_A^\ominus + RT \ln p_A)$$
$$bG_B = b(G_B^\ominus + RT \ln p_B)$$
$$\vdots$$

etc.

As

$$\Delta G = \Sigma G_{prod} - \Sigma G_{react}$$

so

$$\Delta G = \Delta G^\ominus + RT \ln \frac{(p_C)^c (p_D)^d}{(p_A)^a (p_B)^b} \tag{3.17}$$

$\Delta G^\ominus$ is the standard free energy change of the reaction, given by

$$\Delta G^\ominus = cG_C^\ominus + dG_D^\ominus - aG_A^\ominus - bG_B^\ominus$$

As we have noted previously, the free energy change for systems at equilibrium is zero, and hence equation (3.17) becomes

$$\Delta G^\ominus = -RT \ln \frac{(p'_C)^c (p'_D)^d}{(p'_A)^a (p'_B)^b} \tag{3.18}$$

Substituting from equation (3.15) gives

$$\Delta G^\ominus = -RT \ln K \tag{3.19}$$

Substituting equation (3.19) into equation (3.17) gives

$$\Delta G = -RT \ln K + RT \ln \frac{(p_C)^c (p_D)^d}{(p_A)^a (p_B)^b} \tag{3.20}$$

Equation (3.20) gives the change in free energy when a moles of A at a partial pressure p_A and b moles of B at a partial pressure p_B react together to yield c moles of C at a partial pressure p_C and d moles of D at a partial pressure p_D. For such a reaction to occur spontaneously, the free energy change must be negative, and hence equation (3.20) provides a means of predicting the ease of reaction for selected partial pressures (or concentrations) of the reactants.

---

section 3.3.1) of the components rather than the partial pressures. $\Delta G^\ominus$ values can readily be calculated from the tabulated data and hence equation (3.19) is important because it provides a method of calculating the equilibrium constants without resort to experimentation.

A useful expression for the temperature dependence of the equilibrium constant is the *van't Hoff equation* (equation 3.23), which may be derived as outlined in Box 3.3. A more general form of this equation is

$$\log K = \frac{-\Delta H^\ominus}{2.303RT} + \text{constant} \tag{3.24}$$

Plots of $\log K$ against $1/T$ should be linear with a slope of $-\Delta H^\ominus/2.303R$, from which $\Delta H^\ominus$ may be calculated.

Equations (3.19) and (3.24) are fundamental equations which find many applications in the broad area of the pharmaceutical sciences: for example, in the determination of equilibrium constants in chemical reactions and for micelle formation; in the treatment of stability data for some solid dosage forms (see section 4.4.3); and for investigations of drug–receptor binding.

From equation (3.19),

$$\frac{-\Delta G^{\ominus}}{RT} = \ln K$$

Since

$$\Delta G^{\ominus} = \Delta H^{\ominus} - T\Delta S^{\ominus}$$

then at a temperature T_1

$$\ln K_1 = \frac{-\Delta G^{\ominus}}{RT_1} = \frac{-\Delta H^{\ominus}}{RT_1} + \frac{\Delta S^{\ominus}}{R} \qquad (3.21)$$

and at temperature T_2

$$\ln K_2 = \frac{-\Delta G^{\ominus}}{RT_2} = \frac{-\Delta H^{\ominus}}{RT_2} + \frac{\Delta S^{\ominus}}{R} \qquad (3.22)$$

If we assume that the standard enthalpy change $\Delta H^{\ominus}$ and the standard entropy change $\Delta S^{\ominus}$ are independent of temperature, then subtracting equation (3.21) from equation (3.22) gives

$$\ln K_2 - \ln K_1 = -\frac{\Delta H^{\ominus}}{R}\left(\frac{1}{T_2} - \frac{1}{T_1}\right)$$

or

$$\log \frac{K_2}{K_1} = \frac{\Delta H^{\ominus}}{2.303R}\frac{(T_2 - T_1)}{T_1\,T_2} \qquad (3.23)$$

Equation (3.23), which is often referred to as the *van't Hoff equation*, is useful for the prediction of the equilibrium constant K_2 at a temperature T_2 from its value K_1 at another temperature T_1.

3.3 Activity and chemical potential

3.3.1 Activity and standard states

The term *activity* is used in the description of the departure of the behaviour of a solution from ideality. In any real solution, interactions occur between the components which reduce the *effective concentration* of the solution. The activity is a way of describing this effective concentration. In an ideal solution or in a real solution at infinite dilution, there are no interactions between components and the activity equals the concentration. Nonideality in real solutions at higher concentrations causes a divergence between the values of activity and concentration. The ratio of the activity to the concentration is called the *activity coefficient*, γ; that is,

$$\gamma = \frac{\text{activity}}{\text{concentration}} \qquad (3.25)$$

Depending on the units used to express concentration we can have either a *molal* activity coefficient, γ_m, a *molar* activity coefficient, γ_c, or, if mole fractions are used, a *rational* activity coefficient, γ_x.

In order to be able to express the activity of a particular component numerically, it is necessary to define a reference state in which the activity is arbitrarily unity. The activity of a particular component is then the ratio of its value in a given solution to that in the reference state. For the solvent, the reference state is invariably taken to be the pure liquid and, if this is at a pressure of 1 atmosphere and at a definite temperature, it is also the *standard state*. Since the mole fraction as well as the activity is unity: $\gamma_x = 1$.

Several choices are available in defining the standard state of the solute. If the solute is a liquid which is miscible with the solvent (as, for example, in a benzene–toluene mixture), then the standard state is again the pure liquid. Several different standard states have been used for solutions of solutes of limited solubility. In developing a relationship between drug activity and thermodynamic activity, the pure substance has been used as the standard state. The activity of the drug in solution was then taken to be the ratio of its concentration to its saturation solubility. The use of a pure substance as the standard state is of course of limited value since a different state is used for each compound. A more feasible approach is to use the infinitely dilute solution of the compound as the reference state. Since the activity equals the concentration in such solutions, however, it is not equal to unity as it should be for a standard state. This difficulty is overcome by defining the standard state as a hypothetical solution of unit concentration possessing, at the same time, the properties of an infinitely dilute solution. Some workers[4] have chosen to define the standard state in terms of an alkane solvent rather than water; one advantage of this solvent is the absence of specific solute–solvent interactions in the reference state which would be highly sensitive to molecular structure.

3.3.2 Activity of ionised drugs

A large proportion of the drugs that are administered in aqueous solution are salts which, on dissociation, behave as electrolytes. Simple salts such as ephedrine hydrochloride ($C_6H_5CH(OH)CH(NHCH_3)CH_3HCl$) are $1:1$ (or uni-univalent) electrolytes; that is, on dissociation each mole yields one cation, $C_6H_5CH(OH)CH(N^+H_2CH_3)CH_3$, and one anion, Cl^-. Other salts are more complex in their ionisation behaviour; for example, ephedrine sulfate is a $1:2$ electrolyte, each mole giving two moles of the cation and one mole of SO_4^{2-} ions.

The activity of each ion is the product of its activity coefficient and its concentration, that is

$$a_+ = \gamma_+ m_+ \quad \text{and} \quad a_- = \gamma_- m_-$$

The anion and cation may each have a different ionic activity in solution and it is not possible to determine individual ionic activities experimentally. It is therefore necessary to use combined terms, for example the combined activity term is the *mean ionic activity*, $a_\pm$. Similarly, we have the *mean ion activity coefficient*, $\gamma_\pm$, and the *mean ionic molality*, $m_\pm$. The relationship between the mean ionic parameters is then

$$\gamma_\pm = \frac{a_\pm}{m_\pm}$$

More details of these combined terms are given in Box 3.4.

Values of the mean ion activity coefficient may be determined experimentally using several methods, including electromotive force measurement, solubility determinations and colligative properties. It is possible, however, to calculate $\gamma_\pm$ in very dilute solution

using a theoretical method based on the Debye–Hückel theory. In this theory each ion is considered to be surrounded by an 'atmosphere' in which there is a slight excess of ions of opposite charge. The electrostatic energy due to this effect is related to the chemical potential of the ion to give a limiting expression for dilute solutions

$$-\log \gamma_\pm = z_+ z_- A \sqrt{I} \tag{3.36}$$

where z_+ and z_- are the valencies of the ions, A is a constant whose value is determined by the dielectric constant of the solvent and the temperature ($A = 0.509$ in water at 298 K), and I is the total ionic strength defined by

$$I = \tfrac{1}{2}\Sigma(mz^2) = \tfrac{1}{2}(m_1 z_1^2 + m_2 z_2^2 + \cdots) \tag{3.37}$$

where the summation is continued over all the different species in solution. It can readily be shown from equation (3.37) that for a $1:1$ electrolyte the ionic strength is equal to its molality; for a $1:2$ electrolyte $I = 3m$; and for a $2:2$ electrolyte, $I = 4m$.

The Debye–Hückel expression as given by equation (3.36) is valid only in dilute solution ($I < 0.02$ mol kg^{-1}). At higher concentrations a modified expression has been proposed:

$$\log \gamma_\pm = \frac{-A z_+ z_- \sqrt{I}}{1 + a_i \beta \sqrt{I}} \tag{3.38}$$

where a_i is the mean distance of approach of the ions or the mean effective ionic diameter, and β is a constant whose value depends on the solvent and temperature. As an approximation, the product $a_i \beta$ may be taken to be unity, thus simplifying the equation. Equation (3.38) is valid for I less than 0.1 mol kg^{-1}

• •

EXAMPLE 3.2 Calculation of mean ionic activity coefficient

Calculate: (a) the mean ionic activity coefficient and the mean ionic activity of a 0.002 mol kg^{-1} aqueous solution of ephedrine sulfate; (b) the mean ionic activity coefficient of an aqueous solution containing 0.002 mol kg^{-1} ephedrine sulfate and 0.01 mol kg^{-1} sodium chloride. Both solutions are at 25°C.

Answer

(a) Ephedrine sulfate is a $1:2$ electrolyte and hence the ionic strength is given by equation (3.37) as

$$I = \tfrac{1}{2}[(0.002 \times 2 \times 1^2) + (0.002 \times 2^2)]$$
$$= 0.006 \text{ mol kg}^{-1}$$

From the Debye–Hückel equation (equation 3.36),

$$-\log \gamma_\pm = 0.509 \times 1 \times 2 \times \sqrt{0.006}$$
$$\log \gamma_\pm = -0.0789$$
$$\gamma_\pm = 0.834$$

The mean ionic activity may be calculated from equation (3.35):

$$a_\pm = 0.834 \times 0.002 \times (2^2 \times 1)^{1/3}$$
$$= 0.00265$$

(b) Ionic strength of 0.01 mol kg^{-1} NaCl $= \tfrac{1}{2}(0.01 \times 1^2) + (0.01 \times 1^2) = 0.01$ mol kg^{-1}.

Total ionic strength $= 0.006 + 0.01 = 0.016$

$$-\log \gamma_\pm = 0.509 \times 2 \times \sqrt{0.016}$$
$$\log \gamma_\pm = -0.1288$$
$$\gamma_\pm = 0.743$$

··

Box 3.4 Mean ionic parameters

In general, we will consider a strong electrolyte which dissociates according to

$$C_{v+}A_{v-} \rightarrow v_+ C^{z+} + v_- A^{z-}$$

where v_+ is the number of cations, C^{z+}, of valence $z+$, and v_- is the number of anions, A^{z-}, of valence $z-$.

The activity, a, of the electrolyte is then

$$a = a_+^{v+} a_-^{v-} = a_\pm^v \quad (3.26)$$

where $v = v_+ + v_-$.

In the simple case of a solution of the $1:1$ electrolyte sodium chloride, the activity will be

$$a = a_{Na}^+ \times a_{Cl}^- = a_\pm^2$$

whereas for morphine sulfate, which is a $1:2$ electrolyte,

$$a = a_{morph^+}^2 \times a_{SO_4^{2-}} = a_\pm^3$$

Similarly, we may also define a mean ion activity coefficient, $\gamma_\pm$, in terms of the individual ionic activity coefficients γ_+ and γ_-:

$$\gamma_\pm^v = \gamma_+^{v+} \gamma_-^{v-} \quad (3.27)$$

or

$$\gamma_\pm = (\gamma_+^{v+} \gamma_-^{v-})^{1/v} \quad (3.28)$$

For a $1:1$ electrolyte equation (3.28) reduces to

$$\gamma_\pm = (\gamma_+ \gamma_-)^{1/2} \quad (3.29)$$

Finally, we define a *mean ionic molality*, $m_\pm$, as

$$m_\pm^v = m_+^{v+} m_-^{v-} \quad (3.30)$$

or

$$m_\pm = (m_+^{v+} m_-^{v-})^{1/v} \quad (3.31)$$

For a $1:1$ electrolyte, equation (3.31) reduces to

$$m_\pm = (m_+ m_-)^{1/2} = m \quad (3.32)$$

that is, mean ionic molality may be equated with the molality of the solution.

The activity of each ion is the product of its activity coefficient and its concentration

$$a_+ = \gamma_+ m_+ \quad \text{and} \quad a_- = \gamma_- m_-$$

so that

$$\gamma_+ = \frac{a_+}{m_+} \quad \text{and} \quad \gamma_- = \frac{a_-}{m_-}$$

Expressed as the mean ionic parameters, we have

$$\gamma_\pm = \frac{a_\pm}{m_\pm} \quad (3.33)$$

Substituting for $m_\pm$ from equation (3.31) gives

$$\gamma_\pm = \frac{a_\pm}{(m_+^{v+} m_-^{v-})^{1/v}} \quad (3.34)$$

This equation applies in any solution, whether the ions are added together, as a single salt, or separately as a mixture of salts. For a solution of a single salt of molality m:

$$m_+ = v_+ m \quad \text{and} \quad m_- = v_- m$$

Equation (3.34) reduces to

$$\gamma_\pm = \frac{a_\pm}{m(v_+^{v+} v_-^{v-})^{1/v}} \quad (3.35)$$

For example, for morphine sulfate, $v_+ = 2$, $v_- = 1$, and thus

$$\gamma_\pm = \frac{a_\pm}{(2^2 \times 1)^{1/3} m} = \frac{a_\pm}{4^{1/3} m}$$

3.3.3   Solvent activity

Although the phrase 'activity of a solution' usually refers to the activity of the *solute* in the solution as in the preceding section, we also can refer to the activity of the *solvent*. Experimentally, solvent activity a_1 may be determined as the ratio of the vapour pressure p_1 of the solvent in a solution to that of the pure solvent $p_1^\ominus$, that is

$$a_1 = \frac{p_1}{p_1^\ominus} = \gamma_1 x_1 \qquad (3.39)$$

where γ_1 is the solvent activity coefficient and x_1 is the mole fraction of solvent.

The relationship between the activities of the components of the solution is expressed by the Gibbs–Duhem equation

$$x_1 \, d(\ln a_1) + x_2 \, d(\ln a_2) = 0 \qquad (3.40)$$

which provides a way of determining the activity of the solute from measurements of vapour pressure.

Water activity and bacterial growth

When the aqueous solution in the environment of a microorganism is concentrated by the addition of solutes such as sucrose, the consequences for microbial growth result mainly from the change in water activity a_w. Every microorganism has a limiting a_w below which it will not grow. The minimum a_w levels for growth of human bacterial pathogens such as streptococci, *Klebsiella*, *Escherichia coli*, *Corynebacterium*, *Clostridium perfringens* and other clostridia, and *Pseudomonas* is 0.91.[5] *Staphylococcus aureus* can proliferate at an a_w as low as 0.86. Figure 3.2 shows the influence of a_w, adjusted by the addition of sucrose, on the growth rate of this microorganism at 35°C and pH 7.0. The control medium, with a water

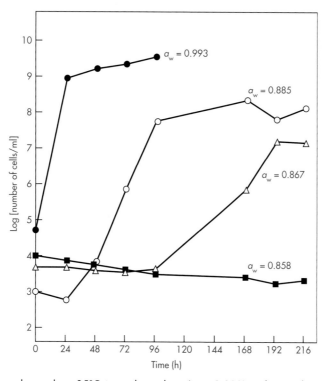

Figure 3.2 Staphylococcal growth at 35°C in medium alone ($a_w = 0.993$) and in media with a_w values lowered by additional sucrose.

Reproduced from J. Chirife, G. Scarmato and C. Herszage, *Lancet*, **319**, 560–561 (1982) with permission.

activity value of $a_w = 0.993$, supported rapid growth of the test organism. Reduction of a_w of the medium by addition of sucrose progressively increased generation times and lag periods and lowered the peak cell counts. Complete growth inhibition was achieved at an a_w of 0.858 (195 g sucrose per 100 g water) with cell numbers declining slowly throughout the incubation period.

The results reported in this study explain why the old remedy of treating infected wounds with sugar, honey or molasses is successful. When the wound is filled with sugar, the sugar dissolves in the tissue water, creating an environment of low a_w, which inhibits bacterial growth. However, the difference in water activity between the tissue and the concentrated sugar solution causes migration of water out of the tissue, hence diluting the sugar and raising a_w. Further sugar must then be added to the wound to maintain growth inhibition. Sugar may be applied as a paste with a consistency appropriate to the wound characteristics; thick sugar paste is suitable for cavities with wide openings, a thinner paste with the consistency of thin honey being more suitable for instillation into cavities with small openings.

An *in vitro* study has been reported[6] of the efficacy of such pastes, and also of those prepared using xylose as an alternative to sucrose, in inhibiting the growth of bacteria commonly present in infected wounds. Polyethylene glycol was added to the pastes as a lubricant and hydrogen peroxide was included in the formulation as a preservative. To simulate the dilution that the pastes invariably experience as a result of fluid being drawn into the wound, serum was added to the formulations in varying amounts. Figure 3.3 illustrates the effects of these sucrose pastes on the colony-forming ability of *Proteus mirabilis* and shows the reduction in efficiency of the pastes as a result of dilution and the consequent increase of their water activity (see Fig. 3.4). It is clear that *P. mirabilis* was susceptible to the antibacterial activity of the pastes, even when they were diluted by 50%. It was reported that although a_w may not be maintained at less

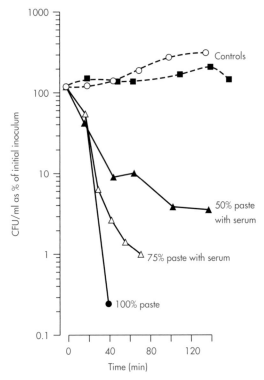

Figure 3.3   The effects of sucrose pastes diluted with serum on the colony-forming ability of *P. mirabilis*.
Reproduced from reference 6 with permission.

than 0.86 (the critical level for inhibition of growth of *S. aureus*) for more than 3 hours after packing of the wound, nevertheless clinical experience had shown that twice-daily dressing was adequate to remove infected slough from dirty wounds within a few days.

3.3.4   Chemical potential

Properties such as volume, enthalpy, free energy and entropy, which depend on the quantity of substance, are called *extensive* properties. In contrast, properties such as temperature, density and refractive index, which are independent of the amount of material, are referred to as *intensive* properties. The quantity denoting the rate of increase in the magnitude of an extensive property with increase in the number of moles of a substance added to the system at constant temperature

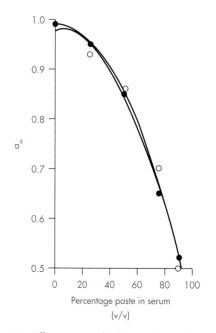

y-axis: a_w
x-axis ticks: 0, 20, 40, 60, 80, 100
y-axis ticks: 0.5, 0.6, 0.7, 0.8, 0.9, 1.0

Percentage paste in serum
(v/v)

Figure 3.4 Effects on a_w of adding xylose (solid symbols) and sucrose paste (open symbols) to serum.
Reproduced from reference 6 with permission.

and pressure is termed a *partial molar quantity*. Such quantities are distinguished by a bar above the symbol for the particular property. For example,

$$\left(\frac{\partial V}{\partial n_2}\right)_{T,P,n_1} = \bar{V}_2 \qquad (3.41)$$

Note the use of the symbol ∂ to denote a partial change which, in this case, occurs under conditions of constant temperature, pressure and number of moles of solvent (denoted by the subscripts outside the brackets).

In practical terms the partial molar volume, $\bar{V}$, represents the change in the total volume of a large amount of solution when one additional mole of solute is added – it is the effective volume of 1 mole of solute in solution.

Of particular interest is the partial molar free energy, $\bar{G}$, which is also referred to as the *chemical potential*, μ, and is defined for component 2 in a binary system by

$$\left(\frac{\partial G}{\partial n_2}\right)_{T,P,n_1} = \bar{G}_2 = \mu_2 \qquad (3.42)$$

Partial molar quantities are of importance in the consideration of open systems, that is those involving transference of matter as well as energy. For an open system involving two components

$$dG = \left(\frac{\partial G}{\partial T}\right)_{P,n_1,n_2} dT + \left(\frac{\partial G}{\partial P}\right)_{T,n_1,n_2} dP$$
$$+ \left(\frac{\partial G}{\partial n_1}\right)_{T,P,n_2} dn_1 + \left(\frac{\partial G}{\partial n_2}\right)_{T,P,n_1} dn_2 \qquad (3.43)$$

At constant temperature and pressure equation (3.43) reduces to

$$dG = \mu_1 \, dn_1 + \mu_2 \, dn_2 \qquad (3.44)$$
$$\therefore G = \int dG = \mu_1 n_1 + \mu_2 n_2 \qquad (3.45)$$

The chemical potential therefore represents the contribution per mole of each component to the total free energy. It is the effective free energy per mole of each component in the mixture and is always less than the free energy of the pure substance.

It can readily be shown (see Box 3.5) that the chemical potential of a component in a two-phase system (for example, oil and water), at equilibrium at a fixed temperature and pressure, is identical in both phases. Because of the need for equality of chemical potential at equilibrium, a substance in a system which is not at equilibrium will have a tendency to diffuse spontaneously from a phase in which it has a high chemical potential to another in which it has a low chemical potential. In this respect the chemical *potential* resembles electrical *potential*; hence its name is an apt description of its nature.

Chemical potential of a component in solution

Where the component of the solution is a *non-electrolyte*, its chemical potential in dilute solution at a molality m, can be calculated from

$$\mu_2 = \mu^\ominus + RT \ln m$$

where

$$\mu^\ominus = \mu_2^\ominus + RT \ln M_1 - RT \ln 1000$$

and M_1 = molecular weight of the solvent.

Cl⁻). In practical terms, this means that a 1 molal solution of NaCl will have (approximately) twice the osmolality (osmotic pressure) as a 1 molal solution of glucose.

According to the definition, $\xi_m = \Pi/\Pi'$. The value of Π' may be obtained from equation (3.59) by noting that for an ideal unionised substance $v = \phi = 1$, and since m is also unity, equation (3.59) becomes

$$\Pi' = \left(\frac{RT}{\overline{V}_1}\right)\frac{M_1}{1000}$$

Thus

$$\xi_m = vm\phi \qquad (3.60)$$

••

EXAMPLE 3.3   Calculation of osmolality

A 0.90% w/w solution of sodium chloride (mol. wt. = 58.5) has an osmotic coefficient of 0.928. Calculate the osmolality of the solution.

Answer
Osmolality is given by equation (3.60) as

$$\xi_m = vm\phi$$

so

$$\xi_m = 2 \times \frac{9.0}{58.5} \times 0.928 = 286 \text{ mosmol kg}^{-1}$$

••

Pharmaceutical labelling regulations sometimes require a statement of the osmolarity; for example, the USP 27 requires that sodium chloride injection should be labelled in this way. *Osmolarity* is defined as the mass of solute which, when dissolved in 1 litre of solution, will exert an osmotic pressure equal to that exerted by 1 mole of an ideal unionised substance dissolved in 1 litre of solution. The relationship between osmolality and osmolarity has been discussed by Streng *et al.*[7]

Table 3.1 lists the osmolalities of commonly used intravenous fluids.

3.4.3   Clinical relevance of osmotic effects

Osmotic effects are particularly important from a physiological viewpoint since bio-

Table 3.1   Tonicities (osmolalities) of intravenous fluids

Solution	Tonicity (mosmol kg⁻¹)
Vamin 9	700
Vamin 9 Glucose	1350
Vamin 14	1145
Vamin 14 Electrolyte-free	810
Vamin 18 Electrolyte-free	1130
Vaminolact	510
Vitrimix KV	1130
Intralipid 10% Novum	300
Intralipid 20%	350
Intralipid 30%	310
Intrafusin 22	1400
Hyperamine 30	1450
Gelofusine	279[a]
Hyperamine 30	1450
Lipofundin MCT/LCT 10%	345[a]
Lipofundin MCT/LCT 20%	380[a]
Nutriflex 32	1400[a]
Nutriflex 48	2300[a]
Nutriflex 70	2100[a]
Sodium Bicarbonate Intravenous Infusion BP	
8.4% w/v	2000[a]
4.2% w/v	1000[a]

[a] Osmolarity (mosmol dm⁻³).

logical membranes, notably the red blood cell membrane, behave in a manner similar to that of semipermeable membranes. Consequently, when red blood cells are immersed in a solution of greater osmotic pressure than that of their contents, they shrink as water passes out of the cells in an attempt to reduce the chemical potential gradient across the cell membrane. Conversely, on placing the cells in an aqueous environment of lower osmotic pressure, the cells swell as water enters and eventually lysis may occur. It is an important consideration, therefore, to ensure that the *effective* osmotic pressure of a solution for injection is approximately the same as that of blood serum. This effective osmotic pressure, which is termed the *tonicity*, is not always identical to the osmolality because it is concerned only with those solutes in solution that can exert an effect on the passage of water through the biological membrane. Solutions that have the same tonicity as blood serum are said to be *isotonic* with blood. Solutions with a higher tonicity are *hypertonic* and those with a lower tonicity are termed *hypotonic* solutions. Similarly, in order to avoid discomfort on administration of solutions to the delicate membranes of the body, such as the eyes, these solutions are made isotonic with the relevant tissues.

The osmotic pressures of many of the products of Table 3.1 are in excess of that of plasma (291 mosmol dm^{-3}). It is generally recommended that any fluid with an osmotic pressure above 550 mosmol dm^{-3} should not be infused rapidly as this would increase the incidence of venous damage. The rapid infusion of marginally hypertonic solutions (in the range 300–500 mosmol dm^{-3}) would appear to be clinically practicable; the higher the osmotic pressure of the solution within this range, the slower should be its rate of infusion to avoid damage. Patients with centrally inserted lines are not normally affected by limits on tonicity as infusion is normally slow and dilution is rapid.

Certain oral medications commonly used in the intensive care of premature infants have very high osmolalities. The high tonicity of enteral feedings has been implicated as a cause of necrotising enterocolitis (NEC). A higher frequency of gastrointestinal illness including

NEC has been reported[8] among premature infants fed undiluted calcium lactate than among those fed no supplemental calcium or calcium lactate eluted with water or formula. White and Harkavy[9] have discussed a similar case of the development of NEC following medication with calcium glubionate elixir. These authors have measured osmolalities of several medications by freezing point depression and compared these with the osmolalities of analogous intravenous (i.v.) preparations (see Table 3.2). Except in the case of digoxin, the osmolalities of the i.v. preparations were very much lower than those of the corresponding oral preparations despite the fact that the i.v. preparations contained at least as much drug per millilitre as did the oral forms. This striking difference may be attributed to the additives, such as ethyl alcohol, sorbitol and propylene glycol, which make a large contribution to the osmolalities of the oral preparations. The vehicle for the i.v. digoxin consists of 40% propylene glycol and 10% ethyl alcohol with calculated osmolalities of 5260 and 2174 mosmol kg^{-1} respectively, thus explaining the unusually high osmolality of this i.v. preparation. These authors have recommended that extreme caution should be exercised in the administration of these oral preparations and perhaps any medication in a

Table 3.2 Measured and calculated osmolalities of drugs[a]

Drug (route)	Concentration of drug	Mean measured osmolality (mosmol kg^{-1})	Calculated available milliosmoles in 1 kg of drug preparation[b]
Theophylline elixir (oral)	80 mg/15 cm^3	>3000	4980
Aminophylline (i.v.)	25 mg cm^{-3}	116	200
Calcium glubionate (oral)	115 mg/5 cm^3	>3000	2270
Calcium gluceptate (i.v.)	90 mg/5 cm^3	507	950
Digoxin elixir	25 mg dm^{-3}	>3000	4420
Digoxin (i.v.)	100 mg dm^{-3}	>3000	9620
Dexamethasone elixir (oral)	0.5 mg/5 cm^3	>3000	3980
Dexamethasone sodium phosphate (i.v.)	4 mg cm^{-3}	284	312

[a] Reproduced from reference 9.

[b] This would be the osmolality of the drug if the activity coefficient were equal to 1 in the full-strength preparation. The osmolalities of serial dilutions of the drug were plotted against the concentrations of the solution, and a least-squares regression line was drawn. The value for the osmolality of the full-strength solution was then estimated from the line. This is the 'calculated available milliosmoles'.

syrup or elixir form when the infant is at risk from necrotising enterocolitis. In some cases the osmolality of the elixir is so high that even mixing with infant formula does not reduce the osmolality to a tolerable level. For example, when a clinically appropriate dose of dexamethasone elixir was mixed in volumes of formula appropriate for a single feeding for a 1500 g infant, the osmolalities of the mixes increased by at least 300% compared to formula alone (see Table 3.3).

Volatile anaesthetics

The aqueous solubilities of several volatile anaesthetics can be related to the osmolarity of the solution.[10] The inverse relationship between solubility (expressed as the liquid/gas partition coefficient) of those anaesthetics and the osmolarity is shown in Table 3.4.

These findings have practical applications for the clinician. Although changes in serum osmolarity within the physiological range (209–305 mosmol dm^{-3}) have only a small effect on the liquid/gas partition coefficient, changes in the serum osmolarity and the concentration of serum constituents at the extremes of the physiological range may significantly decrease the liquid/gas partition coefficient. For example, the blood/gas partition coefficient of isoflurane decreases significantly after an infusion of mannitol. This may be attributed to both a transient increase in the osmolarity of the blood and a more prolonged decrease in the concentration of serum constituents caused by the influx of water due to the osmotic gradient.

Rehydration solutions

An interesting application of the osmotic effect has been in the design of rehydration solutions. During the day the body moves many litres of fluid from the blood into the

Table 3.3 Osmolalities of drug–infant formula mixtures[a]

Drug (dose)	Volume of drug (cm^3) + volume of formula (cm^3)	Mean measured osmolality (mosmol kg^{-1})
Infant formula	–	292
Theophylline elixir, 1 mg kg^{-1}	0.3 + 15	392
	0.3 + 30	339
Calcium glubionate syrup, 0.5 mmol kg^{-1}	0.5 + 15	378
	0.5 + 30	330
Digoxin elixir, 5 μg kg^{-1}	0.15 + 15	347
	0.15 + 30	322
Dexamethasone elixir, 0.25 mg kg^{-1}	3.8 + 15	1149
	3.8 + 30	791

[a] Reproduced from reference 9.

Table 3.4 Liquid/gas partition coefficients of anaesthetics in four aqueous solutions at 37°C[a]

Solution	Osmolarity (mosmol dm^{-3})	Partition coefficient			
		Isoflurane	Enflurane	Halothane	Methoxyflurane
Distilled H$_2$O	0	0.626 ± 0.05	0.754 ± 0.06	0.859 ± 0.02	4.33 ± 0.5
Normal saline	308	0.590 ± 0.01	0.713 ± 0.01	0.825 ± 0.02	4.22 ± 0.30
Isotonic heparin (1000 U cm^{-3})	308	0.593 ± 0.01	0.715 ± 0.01	–	4.08 ± 0.22
Mannitol (20%)	1098	0.476 ± 0.023	0.575 ± 0.024	0.747 ± 0.03	3.38 ± 0.14

[a] Reproduced from reference 10.

intestine and back again. The inflow of water into the intestine, which aids the breakdown of food, is an osmotic effect arising from the secretion of Cl^- ions by the crypt cells of the intestinal lining (see section 9.2.2) into the intestine. Nutrients from the food are taken up by the villus cells in the lining of the small intestine. The villus cells also absorb Na^+ ions, which they pump out into the extracellular spaces, from where they return to the circulation. As a consequence of this flow of Na^+, water and other ions follow by osmotic flow and hence are also transferred to the blood. This normal functioning is disrupted by diarrhoea-causing microorganisms which either increase the Cl^--secreting activity of the crypt cells or impair the absorption of Na^+ by the villus cells, or both. Consequently, the fluid that is normally returned to the blood across the intestinal wall is lost in watery stool. If untreated, diarrhoea can eventually lead to a severe decline in the volume of the blood, the circulation may become dangerously slow, and death may result.

Oral rehydration therapy
Treatment of dehydration by oral rehydration therapy (ORT) is based on the discovery that the diarrhoea-causing organisms do not usually interfere with the carrier systems which bring sodium and glucose simultaneously into the villus cells from the intestinal cavity. This 'co-transport' system only operates when both sodium and glucose are present. The principle behind ORT is that if glucose is mixed into an electrolyte solution it activates the co-transport system, causing electrolyte and then water to pass through the intestinal wall and to enter the blood, so minimising the dehydration.

ORT requires administration to the patient of small volumes of fluid throughout the day (to prevent vomiting); it does not reduce the duration or severity of the diarrhoea, it simply replaces lost fluid and electrolytes. Let us examine, using the principles of the osmotic effect, two possible methods by which the process of fluid uptake from the intestine might be speeded up. It might seem reasonable to suggest that more glucose should be added to the formulation in an attempt to

enhance the co-transport system. If this is done, however, the osmolarity of the glucose will become greater than that of normal blood, and water would now flow from the blood to the intestine and so exacerbate the problem. An alternative is to substitute starches for simple glucose in the ORT. When these polymer molecules are broken down in the intestinal lumen they release many hundreds of glucose molecules, which are immediately taken up by the co-transport system and removed from the lumen. The effect is therefore as if a high concentration of glucose were administered, but because osmotic pressure is a *colligative* property (dependent on the *number* of molecules rather than the mass of substance), there is no associated problem of a high osmolarity when starches are used. The process is summarised in Fig. 3.5. A similar effect is achieved by the addition of proteins, since there is also a co-transport mechanism whereby amino acids (released on breakdown of the proteins in the intestine) and Na^+ ions are simultaneously taken up by the villus cells.

This process of increasing water uptake from the intestine has an added appeal since the source of the starch and protein can be cereals, beans and rice, which are likely to be available in the parts of the world where problems arising from diarrhoea are most prevalent. Food-based ORT offers additional advantages: it can be made at home from low-cost ingredients and can be cooked, which kills the pathogens in water.

3.4.4 Preparation of isotonic solution

Since osmotic pressure is not a readily measurable quantity, it is usual to make use of the relationship between the colligative properties and to calculate the osmotic pressure from a more easily measured property such as the freezing point depression. In so doing, however, it is important to realise that the red blood cell membrane is not a perfect semipermeable membrane and allows through small molecules such as urea and ammonium chloride. Therefore, although the quantity of each substance required for an isotonic

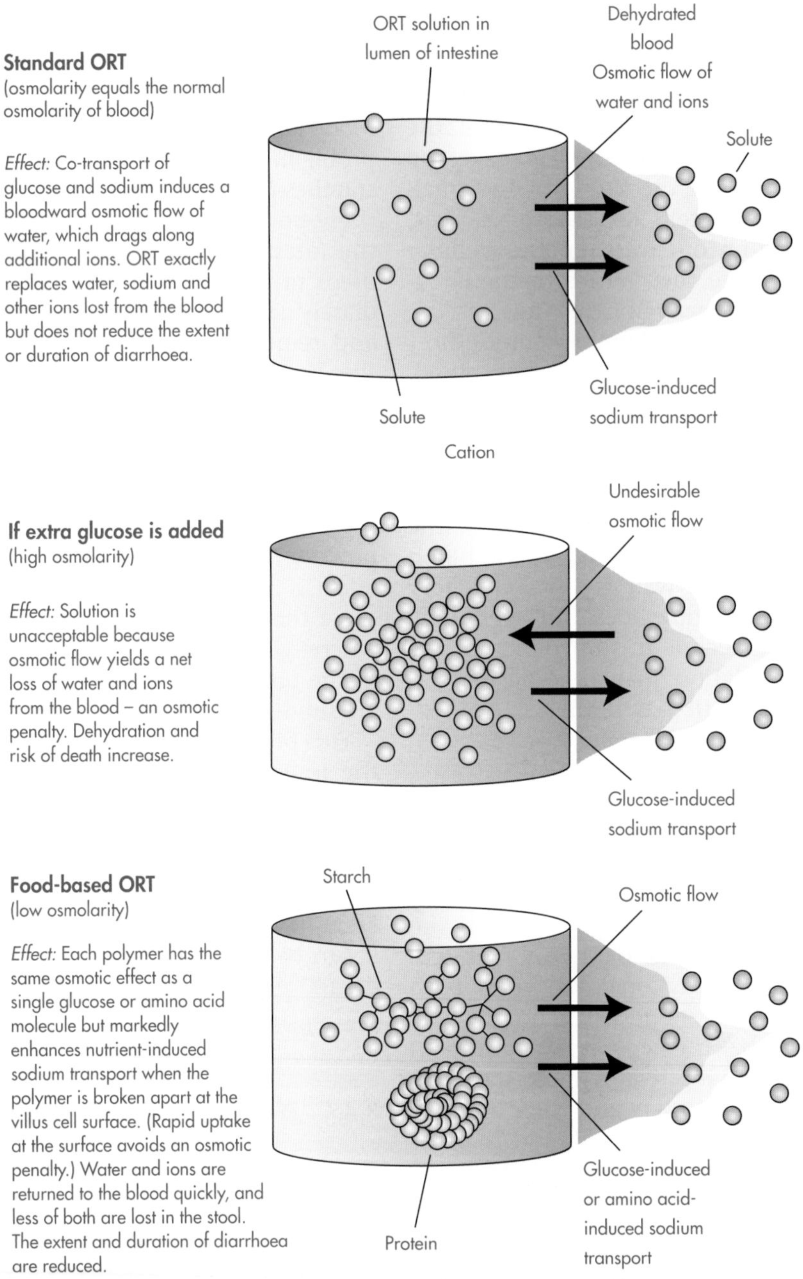
Standard ORT
(osmolarity equals the normal osmolarity of blood)
Effect: Co-transport of glucose and sodium induces a bloodward osmotic flow of water, which drags along additional ions. ORT exactly replaces water, sodium and other ions lost from the blood but does not reduce the extent or duration of diarrhoea.
ORT solution in lumen of intestine
Dehydrated blood
Osmotic flow of water and ions
Solute
Solute
Glucose-induced sodium transport
Cation
If extra glucose is added
(high osmolarity)
Effect: Solution is unacceptable because osmotic flow yields a net loss of water and ions from the blood – an osmotic penalty. Dehydration and risk of death increase.
Undesirable osmotic flow
Glucose-induced sodium transport
Food-based ORT
(low osmolarity)
Effect: Each polymer has the same osmotic effect as a single glucose or amino acid molecule but markedly enhances nutrient-induced sodium transport when the polymer is broken apart at the villus cell surface. (Rapid uptake at the surface avoids an osmotic penalty.) Water and ions are returned to the blood quickly, and less of both are lost in the stool. The extent and duration of diarrhoea are reduced.
Starch
Osmotic flow
Protein
Glucose-induced or amino acid-induced sodium transport

Figure 3.5 How osmosis affects the performance of solutions used in oral rehydration therapy (ORT).

solution may be calculated from freezing point depression values, these solutions may cause cell lysis when administered.

It has been shown that a solution which is isotonic with blood has a freezing point depression, ΔT_f, of 0.52°C. One has therefore to adjust the freezing point of the drug solution to this value to give an isotonic solution. Freezing point depressions for a series of compounds are given in reference texts[1,11] and it is a simple matter to calculate the concentration required for isotonicity from these values. For example, a 1% NaCl solution has a freezing point depression of 0.576°C. The percentage concentration of NaCl required to make isotonic saline solution is therefore $(0.52/0.576) \times 1.0 = 0.90\%$ w/v.

With a solution of a drug, it is not of course possible to alter the drug concentration in this manner, and an adjusting substance must be added to achieve isotonicity. The quantity of adjusting substance can be calculated as shown in Box 3.7

Box 3.7 Preparation of isotonic solutions

If the drug concentration is x g per 100 cm³ solution, then

ΔT_f for drug solution $= x \times (\Delta T_f$ of 1% drug solution$) = a$

Similarly, if w is the weight in grams of adjusting substance to be added to 100 cm³ of drug solution to achieve isotonicity, then

ΔT_f for adjusting solution

$\quad = w \times (\Delta T_f$ of 1% adjusting substance$)$

$\quad = w \times b$

For an isotonic solution,

$a + (w \times b) = 0.52$

$\therefore \quad w = \dfrac{0.52 - a}{b}$ (3.61)

EXAMPLE 3.4 Isotonic solutions

Calculate the amount of sodium chloride which should be added to 50 cm³ of a 0.5% w/v solution of lidocaine hydrochloride to make a solution isotonic with blood serum.

Answer
From reference lists, the values of b for sodium chloride and lidocaine hydrochloride are 0.576°C and 0.130°C, respectively.
From equation (3.61) we have

$a = 0.5 \times 0.130 = 0.065$

Therefore,

$w = \dfrac{0.52 - 0.065}{0.576} = 0.790$ g

Therefore, the weight of sodium chloride to be added to 50 cm³ of solution is 0.395 g.

3.5 Ionisation of drugs in solution

Many drugs are either weak organic acids (for example, acetylsalicylic acid [aspirin]) or weak organic bases (for example, procaine), or their salts (for example, ephedrine hydrochloride). The degree to which these drugs are ionised in solution is highly dependent on the pH. The exceptions to this general statement are the nonelectrolytes, such as the steroids, and the quaternary ammonium compounds, which are completely ionised at all pH values and in this respect behave as strong electrolytes. The extent of ionisation of a drug has an important effect on its absorption, distribution and elimination and there are many examples of the alteration of pH to change these properties. The pH of urine may be adjusted (for example by administration of ammonium chloride or sodium bicarbonate) in cases of overdosing with amfetamines, barbiturates, narcotics and salicylates, to ensure that these drugs are completely ionised and hence readily excreted. Conversely, the pH of the urine may be altered to prevent ionisation of a drug in cases where reabsorption is required for therapeutic reasons. Sulfonamide crystalluria may also be avoided by making the urine alkaline. An understanding of the relationship between pH and drug ionisation is of use in the prediction of the causes of precipitation in admixtures, in the calculation of the solubility of drugs and in the attainment of optimum bioavailability by maintaining a certain ratio of ionised to unionised drug. Table 3.5 shows the nominal pH values of some body fluids and sites, which are useful in the prediction of the percentage ionisation of drugs *in vivo*.

3.5.1 Dissociation of weakly acidic and basic drugs and their salts

According to the Lowry–Brønsted theory of acids and bases, an acid is a substance which

Table 3.5 Nominal pH values of some body fluids and sites[a]

Site	Nominal pH
Aqueous humour	7.21
Blood, arterial	7.40
Blood, venous	7.39
Blood, maternal umbilical	7.25
Cerebrospinal fluid	7.35
Duodenum	5.5
Faeces[b]	7.15
Ileum, distal	8.0
Intestine, microsurface	5.3
Lacrimal fluid (tears)	7.4
Milk, breast	7.0
Muscle, skeletal[c]	6.0
Nasal secretions	6.0
Prostatic fluid	6.45
Saliva	6.4
Semen	7.2
Stomach	1.5
Sweat	5.4
Urine, female	5.8
Urine, male	5.7
Vaginal secretions, premenopause	4.5
Vaginal secretions, postmenopause	7.0

[a] Reproduced from D. W. Newton and R. B. Kluza, *Drug Intell. Clin. Pharm.*, 12, 547 (1978).

[b] Value for normal soft, formed stools, hard stools tend to be more alkaline, whereas watery, unformed stools are acidic.

[c] Studies conducted intracellularly in the rat.

will donate a proton and a base is a substance which will accept a proton. Thus the dissociation of acetylsalicylic acid, a weak acid, could be represented as in Scheme 3.1. In this equilibrium, acetylsalicylic acid acts as an acid, because it donates a proton, and the acetylsalicylate ion acts as a base, because it accepts a proton to yield an acid. An acid and base represented by such an equilibrium is said to be a *conjugate acid–base pair*.

Scheme 3.1 is not a realistic expression, however, since protons are too reactive to exist independently and are rapidly taken up by the solvent. The proton-accepting entity, by the Lowry–Brønsted definition, is a base, and the product formed when the proton has been accepted by the solvent is an acid. Thus a second acid–base equilibrium occurs when the solvent accepts the proton, and this may be represented by

$$H_2O + H^+ \rightleftharpoons H_3O^+$$

The overall equation on summing these equations is shown in Scheme 3.2, or, in general,

$$HA + H_2O \rightleftharpoons A^- + H_3O^+$$

By similar reasoning, the dissociation of benzocaine, a weak base, may be represented by the equilibrium

$$NH_2C_6H_5COOC_2H_5 + H_2O$$
$$\text{base 1} \qquad\qquad \text{acid 2}$$

$$\rightleftharpoons NH_3^+C_6H_5COOC_2H_5 + OH^-$$
$$\text{acid 1} \qquad\qquad \text{base 2}$$

or, in general,

$$B + H_2O \rightleftharpoons BH^+ + OH^-$$

Comparison of the two general equations shows that H_2O can act as either an acid or a base. Such solvents are called *amphiprotic* solvents.

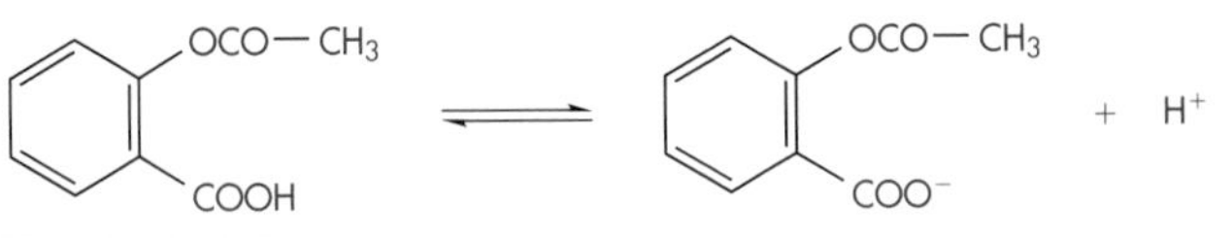

Scheme 3.1

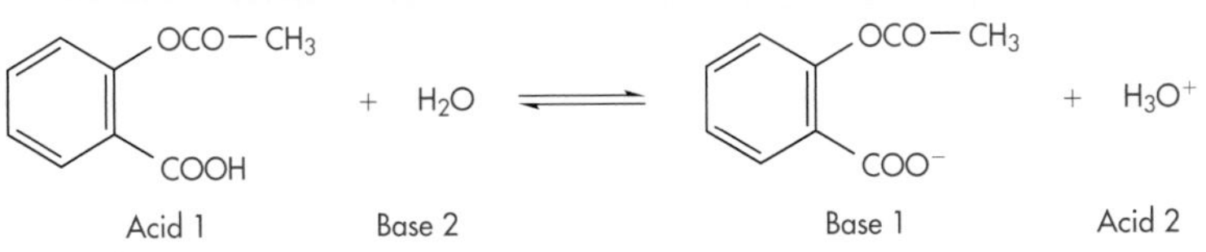

Scheme 3.2

Salts of weak acids or bases are essentially completely ionised in solution. For example, ephedrine hydrochloride (salt of the weak base ephedrine, and the strong acid HCl) exists in aqueous solution in the form of the conjugate acid of the weak base, $C_6H_5CH(OH)CH(CH_3)N^+H_2CH_3$, together with its Cl^- counterions. In a similar manner, when sodium salicylate (salt of the weak acid salicylic acid, and the strong base NaOH) is dissolved in water, it ionises almost entirely into the conjugate base of salicylic acid, $HOC_6H_5COO^-$, and Na^+ ions.

The conjugate acids and bases formed in this way are, of course, subject to acid–base equilibria described by the general equations above.

3.5.2 The effect of pH on the ionisation of weakly acidic or basic drugs and their salts

If the ionisation of a weak acid is represented as described above, we may express an equilibrium constant as follows:

$$K_a = \frac{a_{H_3O^+} \times a_{A^-}}{a_{HA}} \qquad (3.62)$$

Assuming the activity coefficients approach unity in dilute solution, the activities may be replaced by concentrations:

$$K_a = \frac{[H_3O^+][A^-]}{[HA]} \qquad (3.63)$$

K_a is variously referred to as the *ionisation constant*, *dissociation constant*, or *acidity constant* for the weak acid. The negative logarithm of K_a is referred to as pK_a, just as the negative logarithm of the hydrogen ion concentration is called the pH. Thus

$$pK_a = -\log K_a \qquad (3.64)$$

Similarly, the *dissociation constant* or *basicity constant* for a weak base is

$$K_b = \frac{a_{OH^-} \times a_{BH^+}}{a_B} \approx \frac{[OH^-][BH^+]}{[B]} \qquad (3.65)$$

and

$$pK_b = -\log K_b \qquad (3.66)$$

The pK_a and pK_b values provide a convenient means of comparing the strengths of weak acids and bases. The lower the pK_a, the stronger the acid; the lower the pK_b, the stronger is the base. The pK_a values of a series of drugs are given in Table 3.6. pK_a and pK_b values of conjugate acid–base pairs are linked

---

Box 3.8 The degree of ionisation of weak acids and bases

Weak acids

Taking logarithms of the expression for the dissociation constant of a weak acid (equation 3.63)

$$-\log K_a = -\log [H_3O^+] - \log \frac{[A^-]}{[HA]}$$

which can be rearranged to

$$pH = pK_a + \log \frac{[A^-]}{[HA]} \qquad (3.70)$$

Equation (3.70) may itself be rearranged to facilitate the direct determination of the molar percentage ionisation as follows:

$$[HA] = [A^-] \text{ antilog}(pK_a - pH)$$

Therefore,

$$\text{percentage ionisation} = \frac{[A^-]}{[HA] + [A^-]} \times 100$$

$$\text{percentage ionisation} = \frac{100}{1 + \text{antilog}(pK_a - pH)} \qquad (3.71)$$

Weak bases

An analogous series of equations for the percentage ionisation of a weak base may be derived as follows. Taking logarithms of equation (3.65) and rearranging gives

$$-\log K_b = -\log [OH^-] - \log \frac{[BH^+]}{[B]}$$

Therefore,

$$pH = pK_w - pK_b - \log \frac{[BH^+]}{[B]} \qquad (3.72)$$

Rearranging to facilitate calculation of the percentage ionisation leads to

$$\text{percentage ionisation} = \frac{100}{1 + \text{antilog}(pH - pK_w + pK_b)} \qquad (3.73)$$

Table 3.6   pK_a values of some medicinal compounds[a]

Compound	pK_a		Compound	pK_a	
	Acid	Base		Acid	Base
Acebutolol	–	9.2	Diamorphine	–	7.6
Acetazolamide	–	7.2, 9.0	Diazepam	–	3.4
Acetylsalicylic acid	3.5	–	Diclofenac	4.0	–
Aciclovir	–	2.3, 9.3	Diethylpropion	–	8.7
Adrenaline	9.9	8.5	Diltiazem	–	8.0
Adriamycin	–	8.2	Diphenhydramine	–	9.1
Allopurinol	9.4 (10.2)[b]	–	Disopyramide	–	–
Alphaprodine	–	8.7	Dithranol	–	9.4
Alprenolol	–	9.6	Doxepin	–	8.0
Amikacin	–	8.1	Doxorubicin	–	8.2, 10.2
p-Aminobenzoic acid	4.9	2.4	Doxycycline	7.7	3.4, 9.3
Aminophylline	–	5.0	Enalapril	–	5.5
Amitriptyline	–	9.4	Enoxacin	6.3	8.6
Amiodarone	–	6.6	Ergometrine	–	6.8
Amoxicillin	2.4, 7.4, 9.6	–	Ergotamine	–	6.4
Ampicillin	2.5	7.2	Erythromycin	–	8.8
Apomorphine	8.9	7.0	Famotidine	–	6.8
Atenolol	–	9.6	Fenoprofen	4.5	
Ascorbic acid	4.2, 11.6	–	Flucloxacillin	2.7	–
Atropine	–	9.9	Flufenamic acid	3.9	–
Azapropazone	<1.8	6.6	Flumequine	6.5	–
Azathioprine	8.2	–	Fluorouracil	8.0, 13.0	–
Benzylpenicillin	2.8	–	Fluphenazine	–	3.9, 8.1
Benzocaine	–	2.8	Flurazepam	8.2	1.9
Bupivacaine	–	8.1	Flurbiprofen	4.3	–
Captopril	3.5	–	Furosemide	3.9	–
Cefadroxil	7.6	2.7	Glibenclamide	5.3	–
Cefalexin	7.1	2.3	Guanethidine	–	11.9
Cefaclor	7.2	2.7	Guanoxan	–	12.3
Celiprolol	–	9.7	Haloperidol	–	8.3
Cetirizine	2.9	2.2, 8.0	Hexobarbital	8.3	–
Chlorambucil	4.5 (4.9)[b]	2.5	Hydralazine	–	0.5, 7.1
Chloramphenicol	–	5.5	Ibuprofen	4.4	–
Chlorcyclizine	–	8.2	Imipramine	–	9.5
Chlordiazepoxide	–	4.8	Indometacin	4.5	–
Chloroquine	–	8.1, 9.9	Isoniazid	2.0, 3.9	–
Chlorothiazide	6.5	9.5	Ketoprofen	4.0	–
Chlorphenamine	–	9.0	Labetalol	7.4	9.4
Chlorpromazine	–	9.3	Levodopa	2.3, 9.7, 13.4	–
Chlorpropamide	–	4.9	Lidocaine	–	7.94 (26°C),
Chlorprothixene	–	8.8			7.55 (36°C)
Cimetidine	–	6.8	Lincomycin	–	7.5
Cinchocaine	–	8.3	Maprotiline	–	10.2
Clindamycin	–	7.5	Meclofenamic acid	4.0	–
Cocaine	–	8.5	Metoprolol	–	9.7
Codeine	–	8.2	Methadone	–	8.3
Cyclopentolate	–	7.9	Methotrexate	3.8, 4.8	5.6
Daunomycin	–	8.2	Metronidazole	–	2.5
Desipramine	–	10.2	Minocycline	7.8	2.8, 5.0, 9.5
Dextromethorphan	–	8.3			*continued*

Table 3.6 (continued)

Compound	pK$_a$ Acid	pK$_a$ Base	Compound	pK$_a$ Acid	pK$_a$ Base
Minoxidil	–	4.6	Prazocin	–	6.5
Morphine	8.0 (phenol)	9.6 (amine)	Procaine	–	8.8
Nadolol	–	9.7	Prochlorperazine	–	3.7, 8.1
Nafcillin	2.7	–	Promazine	–	9.4
Nalidixic acid	6.4	–	Promethazine	–	9.1
Nalorphine	–	7.8	Propranolol	–	9.5
Naloxone	–	7.9	Quinidine	–	4.2, 8.3
Naltrexone	9.5	8.1	Quinine	–	4.2, 8.8
Naproxen	4.2	–	Ranitidine	–	2.7, 8.2
Nitrofurantoin	–	7.2	Sotalol	8.3	9.8
Nitrazepam	10.8	3.2 (3.4)[b]	Sulfadiazine	6.5	2.0
Norfloxacin	6.2	8.6	Sulfaguanidine	12.1	2.8
Nortriptyline	–	9.7	Sulfamerazine	7.1	2.3
Novobiocin	4.3, 9.1	–	Sulfathiazole	7.1	2.4
Ofloxacin	6.1	8.3	Tamoxifen	–	8.9
Oxolinic acid	6.6	–	Temazepam	–	1.6
Oxprenolol	–	9.5	Tenoxicam	1.1	5.3
Oxycodone	–	8.9	Terfenadine	–	9.5
Oxytetracycline	7.3	3.3, 9.1	Tetracaine	–	8.4
Pentazocine	–	8.8	Tetracycline	7.7	3.3, 9.5
Pethidine	–	8.7	Theophylline	8.6	3.5
Phenazocine	–	8.5	Thiopental	7.5	–
Phenytoin	8.3	–	Timolol	–	9.2 (8.8)[b]
Physostigmine	–	2.0, 8.1	Tolbutamide	5.3	–
Pilocarpine	–	1.6, 7.1	Triflupromazine	–	9.2
Pindolol	–	8.8	Trimethoprin	–	7.2
Piperazine	–	5.6, 9.8	Valproate	5.0	–
Piroxicam	2.3	–	Verapamil	–	8.8
Polymyxin B	–	8.9	Warfarin	5.1	–

[a] For a more complete list see: D. W. Newton and R. B. Kluza, *Drug Intell. Clin. Pharm.*, 12, 547 (1978); G. C. Raymond and J. L. Born, *Drug Intell. Clin. Pharm.*, 20, 683 (1986); D. B. Jack, *Handbook of Clinical Pharmacokinetic Data*, Macmillan, London, 1992; *The Pharmaceutical Codex* 12th edn, Pharmaceutical Press, London, 1994.
[b] Values in parentheses represent alternative values from the literature.

by the expression

$$pK_a + pK_b = pK_w \qquad (3.67)$$

where pK$_w$ is the negative logarithm of the dissociation constant for water, K_w. K_w is derived from consideration of the equilibrium

$$H_2O + H_2O \rightleftharpoons H_3O^+ + OH^-$$

where one molecule of water is behaving as the weak acid or base and the other is behaving as the solvent. Then

$$K = \frac{a_{H_3O^+} \times a_{OH^-}}{a_{H_2O}^2} \approx \frac{[H_3O^+][OH^-]}{[H_2O]^2} \qquad (3.68)$$

The concentration of molecular water is considered to be virtually constant for dilute aqueous solutions. Therefore

$$K_w = [H_3O^+][OH^-] \qquad (3.69)$$

where the dissociation constant for water (*the ionic product*) now incorporates the term for molecular water and has the values given in Table 3.7.

Table 3.7	Ionic product for water	
Temperature (°C)	$K_w \times 10^{14}$	pK_w
0	0.1139	14.94
10	0.2920	14.53
20	0.6809	14.17
25	1.008	14.00
30	1.469	13.83
40	2.919	13.54
50	5.474	13.26
60	9.614	13.02
70	15.1	12.82
80	23.4	12.63

When the pH of an aqueous solution of the weakly acidic or basic drug approaches the pK_a or pK_b, there is a very pronounced change in the ionisation of that drug. An expression that enables predictions of the pH dependence of the degree of ionisation to be made can be derived as shown in Box 3.8. The influence of pH on the percentage ionisation may be determined for drugs of known pK_a using Table 3.8.

....

EXAMPLE 3.5 Calculation of percentage ionisation

Calculate the percentage of cocaine existing as the free base in a solution of cocaine hydrochloride at pH 4.5, and at pH 8.0. The pK_b of cocaine is 5.6.

Answer

From equation (3.73):
At pH 4.5:

percentage ionisation

$$= \frac{100}{1 + \text{antilog}(4.5 - 14.0 + 5.6)}$$

$$= \frac{100}{1.000126}$$

$$= 99.99\%$$

Thus the percentage existing as cocaine base = 0.01%.

At pH 8.0:

percentage ionisation

$$= \frac{100}{1 + \text{antilog}(8.0 - 14.0 + 5.6)}$$

$$= \frac{100}{1.398}$$

$$= 71.53\%$$

Thus the percentage existing as cocaine base = 28.47%

....

If we carry out calculations such as those of Example 3.5 over the whole pH range for both acidic and basic drugs, we arrive at the graphs shown in Fig. 3.6. Notice from this figure that

• The basic drug is virtually completely ionised at pH values up to 2 units below its pK_a, and virtually completely unionised at pH values greater than 2 units above its pK_a.

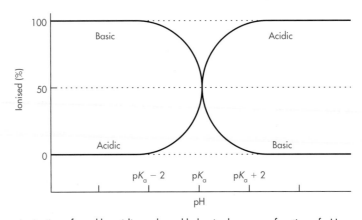

Figure 3.6   Percentage ionisation of weakly acidic and weakly basic drugs as a function of pH.

Table 3.8 Percentage ionisation of anionic and cationic compounds as a function of pH

pH − pK$_a$	At pH above pK$_a$		pK$_a$ − pH	At pH below pK$_a$	
	If anionic	If cationic		If anionic	If cationic
6.0	99.999 90	0.000 099 9	0.1	44.27	55.73
5.0	99.999 00	0.000 999 9	0.2	38.68	61.32
4.0	99.990 0	0.009 999 0	0.3	33.39	66.61
–	–	–	0.4	28.47	71.53
–	–	–	0.5	24.03	75.97
3.5	99.968	0.031 6	–	–	–
3.4	99.960	0.039 8	–	–	–
3.3	99.950	0.050 1	0.6	20.07	79.93
3.2	99.937	0.063 0	0.7	16.63	83.37
3.1	99.921	0.079 4	0.8	13.70	86.30
–	–	–	0.9	11.19	88.81
–	–	–	1.0	9.09	90.91
3.0	99.90	0.099 9	–	–	–
2.9	99.87	0.125 7	–	–	–
2.8	99.84	0.158 2	1.1	7.36	92.64
2.7	99.80	0.199 1	1.2	5.93	94.07
2.6	99.75	0.250 5	1.3	4.77	95.23
–	–	–	1.4	3.83	96.17
–	–	–	1.5	3.07	96.93
2.5	99.68	0.315 2	–	–	–
2.4	99.60	0.396 6	–	–	–
2.3	99.50	0.498 7	1.6	2.450	97.55
2.2	99.37	0.627 0	1.7	1.956	98.04
2.1	99.21	0.787 9	1.8	1.560	98.44
–	–	–	1.9	1.243	98.76
–	–	–	2.0	0.990	99.01
2.0	99.01	0.990	–	–	–
1.9	98.76	1.243	–	–	–
1.8	98.44	1.560	2.1	0.787 9	99.21
1.7	98.04	1.956	2.2	0.627 0	99.37
1.6	97.55	2.450	2.3	0.498 7	99.50
–	–	–	2.4	0.396 6	99.60
–	–	–	2.5	0.315 2	99.68
1.5	96.93	3.07	–	–	–
1.4	96.17	3.83	–	–	–
1.3	95.23	4.77	2.6	0.250 5	99.75
1.2	94.07	5.93	2.7	0.199 1	99.80
1.1	92.64	7.36	2.8	0.158 2	99.84
			2.9	0.125 7	99.87
1.0	90.91	9.09	3.0	0.099 9	99.90
0.9	88.81	11.19	–	–	–
0.8	86.30	13.70	3.1	0.079 4	99.921
0.7	83.37	16.63	3.2	0.063 0	99.937
0.6	79.93	20.07	3.3	0.050 1	99.950
–	–	–	3.4	0.039 8	99.960
0.5	75.97	24.03	3.5	0.031 6	99.968
0.4	71.53	28.47	–	–	–
0.3	66.61	33.39	4.0	0.009 999 0	99.990 0
0.2	61.32	38.68	5.0	0.000 999 9	99.999 00
0.1	55.73	44.27	6.0	0.000 099 9	99.999 90
0	50.00	50.00	–	–	–

- The acidic drug is virtually completely unionised at pH values up to 2 units below its pK_a and virtually completely ionised at pH values greater than 2 units above its pK_a.
- Both acidic and basic drugs are exactly 50% ionised at their pK_a values.

3.5.3 Ionisation of amphoteric drugs

Ampholytes (amphoteric electrolytes) can function as either weak acids or weak bases in aqueous solution and have pK_a values corresponding to the ionisation of each group. They may be conveniently divided into two categories – ordinary ampholytes and zwitterionic ampholytes – depending on the relative acidity of the two ionisable groups.[12, 13]

Ordinary ampholytes

In this category of ampholytes, the pK_a of the acidic group, pK_a^{acidic}, is higher than that of the basic group, pK_a^{basic}, and consequently the first group that loses its proton as the pH is increased is the basic group. Table 3.6 includes several examples of this type of ampholyte. We will consider, as a simple example, the ionisation of *m*-aminophenol (**I**), which has $pK_a^{acidic} = 9.8$ and $pK_a^{basic} = 4.4$.

The steps of the ionisation on increasing pH are shown in the following equilibria:

$$NH_3^+C_6H_4OH \rightleftharpoons NH_2C_6H_4OH \rightleftharpoons NH_2C_6H_5O^-$$

This compound can exist as a cation, as an unionised form, or as an anion depending on the pH of the solution, but because the difference between pK_a^{acidic} and pK_a^{basic} is >2, there will be no simultaneous ionisation of the two groups and the distribution of the species will be as shown in Fig. 3.7. The ionisation pattern will become more complex, however, with drugs in which the difference in pK_a of the two

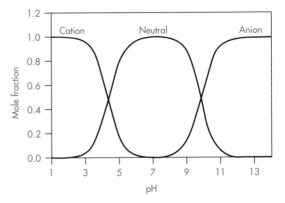

Figure 3.7 Distribution of ionic species for the ordinary ampholyte *m*-aminophenol.
Redrawn from A. Pagliara, P.-A. Carrupt, G. Caron, P. Gaillard and B. Testa, *Chem. Rev.*, 97, 3385 (1997).

groups is much smaller because of overlapping of the two equilibria.

Zwitterionic ampholytes

This group of ampholytes is characterised by the relation $pK_a^{acidic} < pK_a^{basic}$. The most common examples of zwitterionic ampholytes are the amino acids, peptides and proteins. There are essentially two types of zwitterionic electrolyte depending on the difference between the pK_a^{acidic} and pK_a^{basic} values, ΔpK_a.

Large ΔpK_a. The simplest type to consider is that of compounds having two widely separated pK_a values, for example glycine. The pK_a values of the carboxylate and amino groups on glycine are 2.34 and 9.6, respectively and the changes in ionisation as the pH is increased are described by the following equilibria:

$$HOOCCH_2NH_3^+ \rightleftharpoons {}^-OOCCH_2NH_3^+ \rightleftharpoons {}^-OOCCH_2NH_2$$

Over the pH range 3–9, glycine exists in solution predominantly in the form $^-OOCCH_2NH_3^+$ Such a structure, having both positive and negative charges on the same molecule, is referred to as a zwitterion and can react both as an acid,

$$^-OOCCH_2NH_3^+ + H_2O \rightleftharpoons {}^-OOCCH_2NH_2 + H_3O^+$$

or as a base,

$$^-OOCCH_2NH_3^+ + H_2O \rightleftharpoons HOOCCH_2NH_3^+ + OH^-$$

Structure I *m*-Aminophenol

This compound can exist as a cation, as a zwitterion, or as an anion depending on the pH of the solution. The two pK_a values of glycine are >2 pH units apart and hence the distribution of the ionic species will be similar to that shown in Fig. 3.7.

At a particular pH, known as the *isoelectric pH* or *isoelectric point*, pH_i, the effective net charge on the molecule is zero. pH_i can be calculated from

$$pH_i = \frac{pK_a^{acidic} + pK_a^{basic}}{2}$$

Small ΔpK_a. In cases where the two pK_a values are $\ll 2$ pH units apart there is overlap of the ionisation of the acidic and basic groups, with the result that the zwitterionic electrolyte can exist in four different electrical states – the cation, the unionised form, the zwitterion, and the anion (Scheme 3.3).

In Scheme 3.3, $(ABH)^{\pm}$ is the zwitterion and, although possessing both positive and negative charges, is essentially neutral. The unionised form, (ABH), is of course also neutral and can be regarded as a tautomer of the zwitterion. Although only two dissociation constants K_a^{acidic} and K_a^{basic} (*macrodissociation constants*) can be determined experimentally, each of these is composed of individual *microdissociation constants* because of simultaneous ionisation of the two groups (see section 3.5.5). These microdissociation constants represent equilibria between the cation and zwitterion, the anion and the zwitterion, the cation and the unionised form, and the anion and the unionised form. At pH_i, the unionised form and the zwitterion always coexist, but the ratio of the concentrations of each will vary depending on the relative magnitude of the microdissociation constants. The distribution of the ionic species for labetalol which has $pK_a^{acidic} = 7.4$ and $K_a^{basic} = 9.4$ is shown in Fig. 3.8.

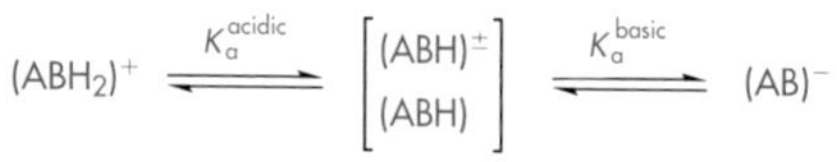

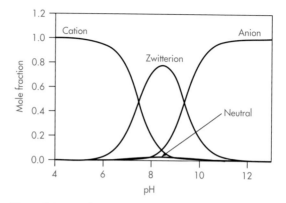

Figure 3.8 Distribution of ionic species for the zwitterionic ampholyte labetalol.

Redrawn from A. Pagliara, P.-A. Carrupt, G. Caron, P. Gaillard and B. Testa, *Chem. Rev.*, 97, 3385 (1997).

Examples of zwitterionic drugs with both large and small ΔpK_a values are given in Box 3.9; others can be noted in Table 3.6.

3.5.4 Ionisation of polyprotic drugs

In the examples we have considered so far, the acidic drugs have donated a single proton. There are several acids, for example citric, phosphoric and tartaric acids, that are capable of donating more than one proton; these compounds are referred to as *polyprotic* or *polybasic* acids. Similarly, a polyprotic base is one capable of accepting two or more protons. Many examples of both types of polyprotic drugs can be found in Table 3.6, including the polybasic acids amoxicillin and fluorourocil, and the polyacidic bases pilocarpine, doxorubicin and aciclovir. Each stage of the dissociation may be represented by an equilibrium expression and hence each stage has a distinct pK_a or pK_b value. The dissociation of phosphoric acid, for example, occurs in three stages; thus:

$$H_3PO_4 + H_2O$$
$$\rightleftharpoons H_2PO_4^- + H_3O^+ \qquad K_1 = 7.5 \times 10^{-3}$$
$$H_2PO_4^- + H_2O$$
$$\rightleftharpoons HPO_4^{2-} + H_3O^+ \qquad K_2 = 6.2 \times 10^{-8}$$
$$HPO_4^{2-} + H_2O$$
$$\rightleftharpoons PO_4^{3-} + H_3O^+ \qquad K_3 = 2.1 \times 10^{-13}$$

$$(ABH_2)^+ \xrightleftharpoons{K_a^{acidic}} \begin{bmatrix} (ABH)^{\pm} \\ (ABH) \end{bmatrix} \xrightleftharpoons{K_a^{basic}} (AB)^-$$

Scheme 3.3

Box 3.9 Chemical structures and pK_a values of some zwitterionic drugs

---

Zwitterions with a large ΔpK_a

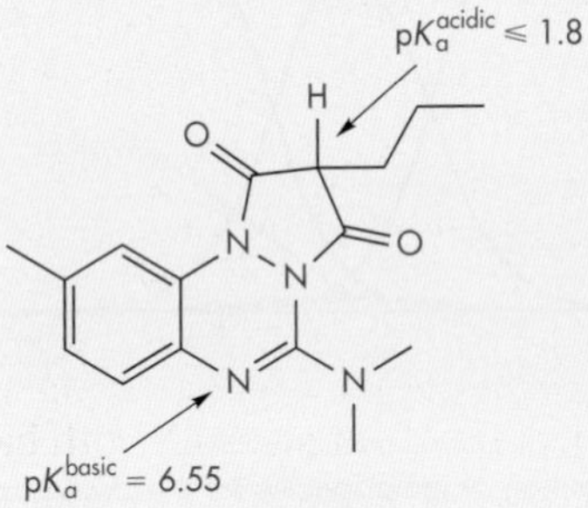

pK_a^{acidic} ⩽ 1.8

pK_a^{basic} = 6.55

Azapropazone

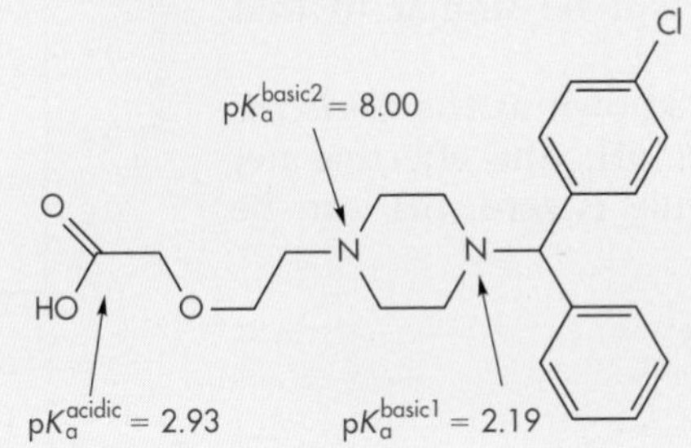

pK_a^{basic2} = 8.00

pK_a^{acidic} = 2.93

pK_a^{basic1} = 2.19

Cetirizine

Zwitterions with a small ΔpK_a

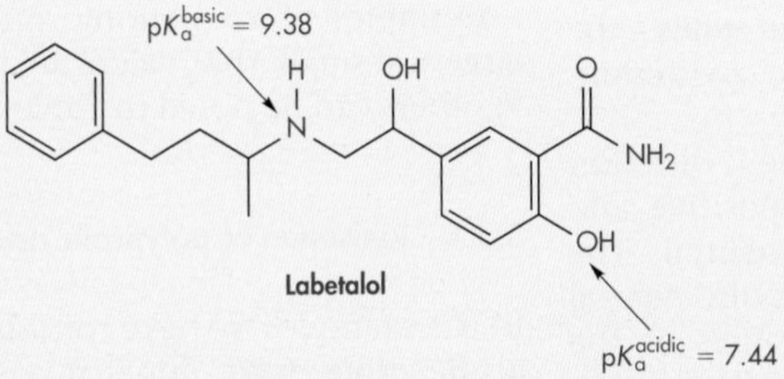

pK_a^{basic} = 9.38

Labetalol

pK_a^{acidic} = 7.44

pK_a^{acidic} = 1.07

pK_a^{basic} = 5.34

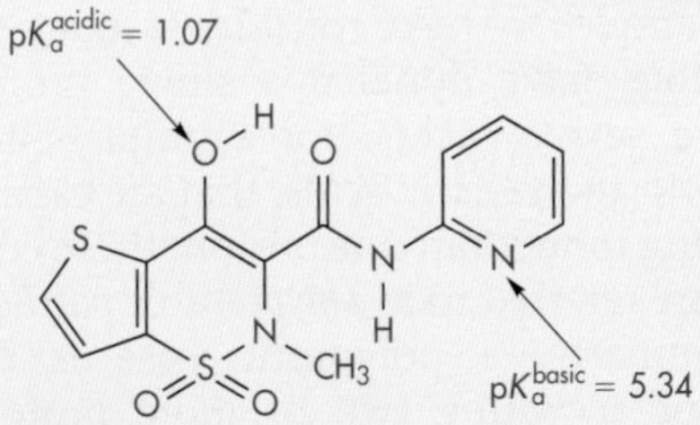

Tenoxicam

(Reproduced from reference 12.)

3.5.5 Microdissociation constants

The experimentally determined dissociation constants for the various stages of dissociation of polyprotic and zwitterionic drugs are referred to as macroscopic values. However, it is not always easy to assign macroscopic dissociation constants to the ionisation of specific groups of the molecule, particularly when the pK_a values are close together, as discussed in section 3.5.4. The diprotic drug morphine has macroscopic pK_a values of 8.3 and 9.5, arising from ionisation of amino and phenolic

groups. Experience suggests that the first pK_a value is probably associated with the ionisation of the amino group and the second with that of the phenolic group; but it is not possible to assign the values of these groups unequivocally and for a more complete picture of the dissociation it is necessary to take into account all possible ways in which the molecule may be ionised and all the possible species present in solution. We may represent the most highly protonated form of morphine, $^+$HMOH, as +O, where the ' + ' refers to the protonated amino group and the

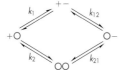

Scheme 3.4

O refers to the uncharged phenolic group. Dissociation of the amino proton only produces an uncharged form MOH, represented by OO, while dissociation of the phenolic proton gives a zwitterion $^+$HMO$^-$, represented by '+−'. The completely dissociated form MO$^-$ is represented as O−. The entire dissociation scheme is given in Scheme 3.4.

The constants K_1, K_2, K_{12} and K_{21} are termed microdissociation constants and are defined by

$$k_1 = \frac{[+-][H_3O^+]}{[+O]} \qquad k_2 = \frac{[OO][H_3O^+]}{[+O]}$$

$$k_{12} = \frac{[O-][H_3O^+]}{[+-]} \qquad k_{21} = \frac{[O-][H_3O^+]}{[OO]}$$

The micro- and macrodissociation constants are related by the following expressions:

$$K_1 = k_1 + k_2 \tag{3.74}$$

$$\frac{1}{K_2} = \frac{1}{k_{12}} + \frac{1}{k_{21}} \tag{3.75}$$

and

$$K_1 K_2 = k_1 k_{12} = k_2 k_{21} \tag{3.76}$$

Various methods have been proposed whereby the microdissociation constants for the morphine system may be evaluated.[14] Other drugs for which microdissociation constants have been derived include the tetracyclines,[15] doxorubicin,[16] cephalosporin,[17] dopamine[18] and the group of drugs shown in Box 3.9.[13]

3.5.6 pK$_a$ values of proteins

The pK$_a$ values of ionisable groups in proteins and other macromolecules can be significantly different from those of the corresponding groups when they are isolated in solution. The shifts in pK$_a$ values between native and denatured states or between bound and free forms of a complex can cause changes in binding constants or stability of the protein due to pH effects. For example, the acid denaturation of proteins may be a consequence of anomalous shifts of the pK$_a$ values of a small number of amino acids in the native protein.[19] Several possible causes of such shifts have been proposed. They may arise from interactions among ionisable groups on the protein molecule; for example, an acidic group will have its pK$_a$ lowered by interactions with basic groups. Other suggested cases of shifts of pK$_a$ include hydrogen-bonding interactions with nonionisable groups and the degree of exposure to the bulk solvent; for example, an acidic group will have its pK$_a$ increased if it is fully or partially removed from solvent, but the effect may be reversed by strong hydrogen-bonding interactions with other groups.

The calculation of pK$_a$ values of protein molecules thus requires a detailed consideration of the environment of each ionisable group, and is consequently highly complex. An additional complication is that a protein with N ionisable residues has 2^N possible ionisation states; the extent of the problem is apparent when it is realised that a moderately sized protein may contain as many as 50 ionisable groups.

3.5.7 Calculation of the pH of drug solutions

We have considered above the effect on the ionisation of a drug of buffering the solution at given pH values. When these weakly acidic or basic drugs are dissolved in water they will, of course, develop a pH value in their own right. In this section we examine how the pH of drug solutions of known concentration can be simply calculated from a knowledge of the pK$_a$ of the drug. We will consider the way in which one of these expressions may be derived from the expression for the ionisation in solution; the derivation of the other expressions follows a similar route and you may wish to derive these for yourselves.

Weakly acidic drugs

We saw above that the dissociation of these types of drugs may be represented by equation (3.63). We can now express the concentrations of each of the species in terms of the degree of dissociation, α, which is a number with a value between 0 (no dissociation) and 1 (complete dissociation):

$$HA + H_2O \rightleftharpoons A^- + H_3O^+$$
$$(1 - \alpha)c \qquad \alpha c \qquad \alpha c$$

where c is the initial concentration of the weakly acidic drug in mol dm^{-3}.

Because the drugs are weak acids, α will be very small and hence the term $(1 - \alpha)$ can be approximated to 1. We may therefore write

$$K_a = \frac{\alpha^2 c^2}{(1 - \alpha)c} \approx \alpha^2 c \qquad (3.77)$$

Therefore,

$$\alpha^2 = \left(\frac{K_a}{c}\right)^{1/2}$$

To introduce pH into the discussion we note that

$$\alpha c = [H_3O^+] = [H^+]$$
$$\therefore \ [H^+] = (K_a c)^{1/2}$$
$$\therefore \ -\log[H^+] = -\tfrac{1}{2}\log K_a - \tfrac{1}{2}\log c$$
$$pH = \tfrac{1}{2}pK_a - \tfrac{1}{2}\log c \qquad (3.78)$$

We now have an expression which enables us to calculate the pH of any concentration of the weakly acidic drug provided that its pK_a value is known.

• •

EXAMPLE 3.6 Calculation of the pH of a weak acid

Calculate the pH of a 50 mg cm^{-3} solution of ascorbic acid (mol. wt = 176.1; $pK_a = 4.17$).

Answer
For a weakly acidic drug,

$$pH = \tfrac{1}{2}pK_a - \tfrac{1}{2}\log c$$
$$c = 50 \ \text{mg cm}^{-3} = 50 \ \text{g dm}^{-3}$$
$$= 0.2839 \ \text{mol dm}^{-3}$$
$$\therefore \ pH = 2.09 + 0.273 = 2.36$$

• •

Weakly basic drugs

We can show by a similar derivation to that above that the pH of aqueous solutions of weakly basic drugs will be given by

$$pH = \tfrac{1}{2}pK_w + \tfrac{1}{2}pK_a + \tfrac{1}{2}\log c \qquad (3.79)$$

• •

EXAMPLE 3.7 Calculation of the pH of a weakly basic drug

Calculate the pH of a saturated solution of codeine monohydrate (mol. wt. = 317.4) given that its $pK_a = 8.2$ and its solubility at room temperature is 1 g in 120 cm^3 water.

Answer
Codeine is a weakly basic drug and hence its pH will be given by

$$pH = \tfrac{1}{2}pK_w + \tfrac{1}{2}pK_a + \tfrac{1}{2}\log c$$

where $c = 1 \ \text{g}$ in $120 \ \text{cm}^3 = 8.33 \ \text{g dm}^{-3} = 0.02633 \ \text{mol dm}^{-3}$.

$$\therefore \ pH = 7.0 + 4.1 - 0.790 = 10.31$$

• •

Drug salts

Because of the limited solubility of many weak acids and weak bases in water, drugs of these types are commonly used as their salts; for example, sodium salicylate is the salt of a weak acid (salicylic acid) and a strong base (sodium hydroxide). The pH of a solution of this type of salt is given by

$$pH = \tfrac{1}{2}pK_w + \tfrac{1}{2}pK_a + \tfrac{1}{2}\log c \qquad (3.80)$$

Alternatively, a salt may be formed between a weak base and a strong acid; for example, ephedrine hydrochloride is the salt of ephedrine and hydrochloric acid. Solutions of such drugs have a pH given by

$$pH = \tfrac{1}{2}pK_a - \tfrac{1}{2}\log c \qquad (3.81)$$

Finally, a salt may be produced by the combination of a weak base and a weak acid, as in the case of codeine phosphate. Solutions of such drugs have a pH given by

$$pH = \tfrac{1}{2}pK_w + \tfrac{1}{2}pK_a - \tfrac{1}{2}pK_b \qquad (3.82)$$

Notice that this equation does not include a concentration term and hence the pH is independent of concentration for such drugs.

● ●

EXAMPLE 3.8 Calculation of the pH of drug salts

Calculate the pH of the following solutions

(a) 5% oxycodone hydrochloride (pK_a = 8.9, mol. wt. = 405.9).
(b) 600 mg of benzylpenicillin sodium (pK_a = 2.76, mol. wt. = 356.4) in 2 cm^3 of water for injection.
(c) 100 mg cm^{-3} chlorphenamine maleate (mol. wt. = 390.8) in water for injection (pK_b chlorphenamine = 5.0, pK_a maleic acid = 1.9).

Answer

(a) Oxycodone hydrochloride is the salt of a weak base and a strong acid, hence

$$pH = \tfrac{1}{2}pK_a - \tfrac{1}{2}\log c$$

where c = 50 g dm^{-3} = 0.1232 mol dm^{-3}.

$$\therefore \;\; pH = 4.45 + 0.45 = 4.90$$

(b) Benzylpenicillin sodium is the salt of a weak acid and a strong base, hence

$$pH = \tfrac{1}{2}pK_w + \tfrac{1}{2}pK_a + \tfrac{1}{2}\log c$$

where c = 600 mg in 2 cm^3 = 0.842 mol dm^{-3}.

$$\therefore \;\; pH = 7.00 + 1.38 - 0.037 = 8.34$$

(c) Chlorphenamine maleate is the salt of a weak acid and a weak base, hence

$$pH = \tfrac{1}{2}pK_w + \tfrac{1}{2}pK_a - \tfrac{1}{2}pK_b$$
$$\therefore \;\; pH = 7.00 + 0.95 - 2.5 = 5.45$$

● ●

3.5.8 Preparation of buffer solutions

A mixture of a weak acid and its salt (that is, a conjugate base), or a weak base and its conjugate acid, has the ability to reduce the large changes in pH which would otherwise result from the addition of small amounts of acid or alkali to the solution. The reason for the buffering action of a weak acid HA and its ionised salt (for example, NaA) is that the A$^-$ ions from the salt combine with the added H$^+$ ions, removing them from solution as undissociated weak acid:

$$A^- + H_3O^+ \rightleftharpoons H_2O + HA$$

Added OH$^-$ ions are removed by combination with the weak acid to form undissociated water molecules:

$$HA + OH^- \rightleftharpoons H_2O + A^-$$

The buffering action of a mixture of a weak base and its salt arises from the removal of H$^+$ ions by the base B to form the salt and removal of OH$^-$ ions by the salt to form undissociated water:

$$B + H_3O^+ \rightleftharpoons H_2O + BH^+$$
$$BH^+ + OH^- \rightleftharpoons H_2O + B$$

The concentration of buffer components required to maintain a solution at the required pH may be calculated using equation (3.70). Since the acid is weak and therefore only very slightly ionised, the term [HA] in this equation may be equated with the total acid concentration. Similarly, the free A$^-$ ions in solution may be considered to originate entirely from the salt and the term [A$^-$] may be replaced by the salt concentration.

Equation (3.70) now becomes

$$pH = pK_a + \log \frac{[\text{salt}]}{[\text{acid}]} \tag{3.83}$$

By similar reasoning, equation (3.72) may be modified to facilitate the calculation of the pH of a solution of a weak base and its salt, giving

$$pH = pK_w - pK_b + \log \frac{[\text{base}]}{[\text{salt}]} \tag{3.84}$$

Equations (3.83) and (3.84) are often referred to as the *Henderson–Hasselbalch equations*.

● ●

EXAMPLE 3.9 Buffer solutions

Calculate the amount of sodium acetate to be added to 100 cm^3 of a 0.1 mol dm^{-3} acetic acid solution to prepare a buffer of pH 5.20.

Answer

The pK_a of acetic acid is 4.76. Substitution in equation (3.83) gives

$$5.20 = 4.76 + \log \frac{[\text{salt}]}{[\text{acid}]}$$

The molar ratio of [salt]/[acid] is 2.754. Since 100 cm^3 of 0.1 mol dm^{-3} acetic acid contains 0.01 mol, we would require 0.027 54 mol of sodium acetate (2.258 g), ignoring dilution effects.

• •

Equations (3.83) and (3.84) are also useful in calculating the change in pH which results from the addition of a specific amount of acid or alkali to a given buffer solution, as seen from the following calculation in Example 3.10.

• •

EXAMPLE 3.10 Calculation of the pH change in buffer solutions

Calculate the change in pH following the addition of 10 cm^3 of 0.1 mol dm^{-3} NaOH to the buffer solution described in Example 3.9.

Answer

The added 10 cm^3 of 0.1 mol dm^{-3} NaOH (equivalent to 0.002 mol) combines with 0.001 mol of acetic acid to produce 0.001 mol of sodium acetate. Reapplying equation (3.83) using the revised salt and acid concentrations gives

$$pH = 4.76 + \log \frac{(0.02754 + 0.001)}{(0.01 - 0.001)} = 5.26$$

The pH of the buffer has been increased by only 0.06 units following the addition of the alkali.

• •

Buffer capacity

The effectiveness of a buffer in reducing changes in pH is expressed as the buffer capacity, β. The buffer capacity is defined by the ratio

$$\beta = \frac{dc}{d(\text{pH})} \tag{3.85}$$

where dc is the number of moles of alkali (or acid) needed to change the pH of 1 dm^3 of solution by an amount d(pH). If the addition of 1 mole of alkali to 1 dm^3 of buffer solution produces a pH change of 1 unit, the buffer capacity is unity.

Equation (3.70) may be rewritten in the form

$$pH = pK_a + \frac{1}{2.303} \ln \left[\frac{c}{c_0 - c} \right] \tag{3.86}$$

where c_0 is the total initial buffer concentration and c is the amount of alkali added. Rearrangement and subsequent differentiation yield

$$c = \frac{c_0}{1 + \exp[-2.303(\text{pH} - pK_a)]} \tag{3.87}$$

Therefore,

$$\beta = \frac{dc}{d(\text{pH})} = \frac{2.303\, c_0 \exp[2.303\,(\text{pH} - pK_a)]}{1 + \exp[2.303 \exp(\text{pH} - pK_a)]^2} \tag{3.88}$$

$$\beta = \frac{2.303\, c_0\, K_a\, [\text{H}_3\text{O}^+]}{([\text{H}_3\text{O}^+] + K_a)^2} \tag{3.89}$$

• •

EXAMPLE 3.11 Calculation of buffer capacity

Calculate the buffer capacity of the acetic acid–acetate buffer of Example 3.9 at pH 4.0.

Answer

The total amount of buffer components in 100 cm^3 of solution = 0.01 + 0.027 54 = 0.037 54 moles. Therefore,

$$c_0 = 0.3754 \text{ mol dm}^{-3}$$

pK_a of acetic acid = 4.76. Therefore,

$$K_a = 1.75 \times 10^{-5}$$

The pH of the solution = 4.0. Therefore,

$$[\text{H}_3\text{O}^+] = 10^{-4}$$

Substituting in equation (3.89),

$$\beta = \frac{2.303 \times 0.3754 \times 1.75 \times 10^{-5} \times 10^{-4}}{(10^{-4} + 1.75 \times 10^{-5})^2}$$

$$= 0.1096$$

The buffer capacity of the acetic acid–acetate buffer is 0.1096 mol dm^{-3} per pH unit.

• •

Figure 3.9 shows the variation of buffer capacity with pH for the acetic acid–acetate buffer used in the numerical examples above ($c_0 = 0.3754$ mol dm^{-3}) as calculated from equation (3.89). It should be noted that β is at a maximum when pH = pK_a (that is, at pH 4.76). When selecting a weak acid for the preparation of a buffer solution, therefore, the chosen acid should have a pK_a as close as possible to the pH required. Substituting pH = pK_a into equation (3.89) gives the useful result that the maximum buffer capacity is $\beta_{max} = 0.576c_0$, where c_0 is the total buffer concentration.

Buffer solutions are widely used in pharmacy to adjust the pH of aqueous solutions to that required for maximum stability or that needed for optimum physiological effect. Solutions for application to delicate tissues, particularly the eye, should also be formulated at a pH not too far removed from that of the appropriate tissue fluid, as otherwise irritation may be caused on administration. The pH of tears lies between 7 and 8, with an average value of 7.4. Fortunately, the buffer capacity of tears is high and, provided that the solutions to be administered have a low buffer capacity, a reasonably wide range of pH may be tolerated, although there is a difference in the irritability of the various ionic species that are commonly used as buffer components. The pH of blood is maintained at about 7.4 by primary buffer components in the plasma (carbonic acid–carbonate and the acid–sodium salts of phosphoric acid) and secondary buffer components (oxyhaemoglobin–haemoglobin and acid–potassium salts of phosphoric acid) in the erythrocytes. Values of 0.025 and 0.039 mol dm^{-3} per pH unit have been quoted for the buffer capacity of whole blood. Parenteral solutions are not normally buffered, or alternatively are buffered at a very low capacity, since the buffers of the blood are usually capable of bringing them within a tolerable pH range.

Universal buffers

We have seen from Fig. 3.9 that the buffer capacity is at a maximum at a pH equal to the pK_a of the weak acid used in the formulation of the buffer system and decreases appreciably as the pH extends more than one unit either side of this value. If, instead of a single weak monobasic acid, a suitable mixture of polybasic and monobasic acids is used, it is possible to produce a buffer which is effective over a wide pH range. Such solutions are referred to as *universal buffers*. A typical example is a mixture of citric acid (p$K_{a1} = 3.06$, p$K_{a2} = 4.78$, p$K_{a3} = 5.40$), Na$_2$HPO$_4$ (pK_a of conjugate acid H$_2$PO$_4^- = 7.2$), diethylbarbituric acid (p$K_{a1} = 7.43$) and boric acid (p$K_{a1} = 9.24$). Because of the wide range of pK_a values involved, each associated with a maximum buffer capacity, this buffer is effective over a correspondingly wide pH range (pH 2.4–12).

3.6 Diffusion of drugs in solution

Diffusion is the process by which a concentration difference is reduced by a spontaneous flow of matter. Consider the simplest case of a solution containing a single solute. The solute will spontaneously diffuse from a region of high concentration to one of low concentration. Strictly speaking, the driving force for

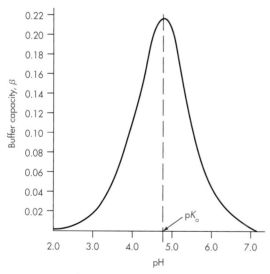

Figure 3.9 Buffer capacity of acetic acid–acetate buffer (initial concentration = 0.3754 mol dm^{-3}) as a function of pH.

diffusion is the gradient of chemical potential, but it is more usual to think of the diffusion of solutes in terms of the gradient of their concentration. Imagine the solution to be divided into volume elements. Although no individual solute particle in a particular volume element shows a preference for motion in any particular direction, a definite fraction of the molecules in this element may be considered to be moving in, say, the x direction. In an adjacent volume element, the same fraction may be moving in the reverse direction. If the concentration in the first volume element is greater than that in the second, the overall effect is that more particles are leaving the first element for the second and hence there is a net flow of solute in the x direction, the direction of decreasing concentration. The expression which relates the flow of material to the concentration gradient (dc/dx) is referred to as *Fick's first law*:

$$J = -D \frac{dc}{dx} \quad (3.90)$$

where J is the flux of a component across a plane of unit area and D is the diffusion coefficient (or diffusivity). The negative sign indicates that the flux is in the direction of decreasing concentration. J is in mol m^{-2} s^{-1}, c is in mol m^{-3} and x is in metres; therefore, the units of D are m^2 s^{-1}.

The relationship between the radius, a, of the diffusing molecule and its diffusion coefficient (assuming spherical particles or molecules) is given by the *Stokes–Einstein equation* as

$$D = \frac{RT}{6\pi\eta a N_A} \quad (3.91)$$

Table 3.9 shows diffusion coefficients of some *p*-hydroxybenzoate (paraben) preservatives and typical proteins in aqueous solution. Although the trend for a decrease of D with increase of molecular size (as predicted by equation 3.91) is clearly seen from the data of this table, it is also clear that other factors, such as branching of the *p*-hydroxybenzoate molecules (as with the isoalkyl derivatives) and the shape of the protein molecules, also affect the diffusion coefficients. The diffusion

Table 3.9   Effect of molecular weight on diffusion coefficient (25°C) in aqueous media

Compound	Molecular weight	D (10^{-10} m^2 s^{-1})
p-Hydroxybenzoates[a]		
Methyl hydroxybenzoate	152.2	8.44
Ethyl hydroxybenzoate	166.2	7.48
n-Propyl hydroxybenzoate	180.2	6.81
Isopropyl hydroxybenzoate	180.2	6.94
n-Butyl hydroxybenzoate	194.2	6.31
Isobutyl hydroxybenzoate	194.2	6.40
n-Amyl hydroxybenzoate	208.2	5.70
Proteins[b]		
Cytochrome c (horse)	12 400	1.28
Lysozyme (chicken)	14 400	0.95
Trypsin (bovine)	24 000	1.10
Albumin (bovine)	66 000	0.46

[a] From reference 20.
[b] From reference 21; see also Chapter 11 for further values of therapeutic peptides and proteins.

coefficients of more complex molecules such as proteins will also be affected by the shape of the molecule, more asymmetric molecules having a greater resistance to flow.

The diffusional properties of a drug have relevance in pharmaceutical systems in a consideration of such processes as the dissolution of the drug and transport through artificial (e.g. polymer) or biological membranes. Diffusion in tissues such as the skin or in tumours is a process which relies on the same criteria as discussed above, even though the diffusion takes place in complex media.

Summary

- We have looked at the meaning of some of the terms commonly used in thermodynamics and how these are interrelated in the three laws of thermodynamics. In particular, we have seen that:

  - *Entropy* is a measure of the disorder or chaos of a system and that processes, such as the melting of a crystal, which result in an increased disorder are accompanied by an increase in entropy. Since spontaneous processes always produce more disordered systems, it follows that the entropy change for these processes is always positive.

- During a spontaneous change at constant temperature and pressure, there is a decrease in the *free energy* until the system reaches an equilibrium state, when the free energy change becomes zero. The free energy is therefore a measure of the useful work that a system can do; when the system has reached equilibrium it has used up its free energy and consequently no longer has the ability to do any further work; thus *all spontaneous processes are irreversible.*

- There is a simple relationship between free energy change and the equilibrium constant for a reaction from which an equation has been derived for the change of equilibrium constant with temperature.

- If there are no interactions between the components of a solution (ideal solution) then the *activity* equals the concentration; in real solutions the ratio of the activity to the concentration is called the *activity coefficient.*

- The *chemical potential* is the effective free energy per mole of each component of a solution. In general, the chemical potential of a component is identical in all phases of a system at equilibrium at a fixed temperature and pressure.

- Parenteral solutions should be of approximately the same tonicity as blood serum; the amount of adjusting substance which must be added to a formulation to achieve isotonicity can be calculated using the freezing point depressions of the drug and the adjusting substance.

- The strengths of weakly acidic or basic drugs may be expressed by their pK_a and pK_b values; the lower the pK_a the stronger is the acid; the lower the pK_b the stronger is the base. Acidic drugs are completely unionised at pH values up to 2 units below their pK_a and completely ionised at pH values greater than 2 units above their pK_a. Conversely, basic drugs are completely ionised at pH values up to 2 units below their pK_a and completely unionised when the pH is more than 2 units above their pK_a. Both types of drug are exactly 50% ionised at their pK_a values. Some drugs can donate or accept more than one proton and so may have several pK_a values; other drugs can behave as both acids and bases, i.e. they are amphoteric drugs. The pH of aqueous solutions of each of these types of drug and their salts can be calculated from their pK_a and the concentration of the drug.

- A solution of a weak acid and its salt (conjugate base) or a weak base and its conjugate acid acts as a buffer solution. The quantities of buffer components required to prepare buffers solutions of known pH can be calculated from the *Henderson–Hasselbalch equation.* The buffering capacity of a buffer solution is maximum at the pK_a of the weak acid component of the buffer. Universal buffers are mixtures of polybasic and monobasic acids that are effective over a wide range of pH.

- The drug molecules in solution will spontaneously diffuse from a region of high chemical potential to one of low chemical potential; the rate of diffusion may be calculated from *Fick's law.*

References

1. *The Pharmaceutical Codex*, 12th edn, The Pharmaceutical Press, London, 1994

2. P. W. Atkins. *Physical Chemistry*, 7th edn, Oxford University Press, 2001

3. D. J. Shaw and H. E. Avery. *Physical Chemistry*, Macmillan Education Limited, London, 1994

4. J. H. Rytting, S. S. Davis and T. Higuchi. Suggested thermodynamic standard state for comparing drug molecules in structure–activity studies. *J. Pharm. Sci.*, 61, 816–8 (1972)

5. J. H. B. Christian. In *Water Activity: Influences on Food Quality* (ed. L. B. Rockland and G. F. Stewart), Academic Press, New York, 1981, p. 825

6. U. Ambrose, K. Middleton and D. Seal. *In vitro* studies of water activity and bacterial growth inhibition of sucrose–polyethylene glycol 400– hydrogen peroxide and xylose–polyethylene glycol 400– hydrogen peroxide pastes used to treat infected wounds. *Antimicrob. Agents Chemother.*, 35, 1799–803 (1991)

7. W. H. Streng, H. E. Huber and J. T. Carstensen. Relationship between osmolality and osmolarity. *J. Pharm. Sci.*, 67, 384–6 (1978)

8. D. M. Willis, J. Chabot, I. C. Radde and G. W. Chance. Unsuspected hyperosmolality of oral solutions contributing to necrotizing enterocolitis in very-low-birth-weight infants. *Pediatrics*, 60, 535–8 (1977)

9. K. C. White and K. L. Harkavy. Hypertonic formula resulting from added oral medications. *Am. J. Dis. Child.*, 136, 931–3 (1982)

10. J. Lerman, M. M. Willis, G. A. Gregory and E. I. Eger. Osmolarity determines the solubility of anesthetics in aqueous solutions at 37°C. *Anesthesiology*, 59, 554–8 (1983)

11. *The Merck Index*, 12th edn, Merck, Rahway, NJ, 1996

12. A. Pagliara, P.-A. Carrupt, G. Caron, *et al.* Lipophilicity profiles of ampholytes. *Chem. Rev.*, 97, 3385–400 (1997)

13. G. Bouchard, A. Pagliara, P.-A. Carrupt, *et al.* Theoretical and experimental exploration of the lipophilicity of zwitterionic drugs in 1,2-dichloroethane/water system. *Pharm. Res.*, 19, 1150–9 (2002)

14. P. J. Niebergall, R. L. Schnaare and E. T. Sugita. Spectral determination of microdissociation constants. *J. Pharm. Sci.*, 61, 232 (1972)

15. L. J. Leeson, J. E. Krueger and R. A. Nash. Structural assignment of the second and third acidity constants of tetracycline antibiotics. *Tetrahedron Lett.*, 18, 1155–60 (1963)

16. R. J. Sturgeon and S. G. Schulman. Electronic absorption spectra and protolytic equilibriums of doxorubicin: direct spectrophotometric determination of microconstants. *J. Pharm. Sci.*, 66, 958–61 (1977)

17. W. H. Streng, H. E. Huber, J. L. DeYoung and M. A. Zoglio. Ionization constants of cephalosporin zwitterionic compounds. *J. Pharm. Sci.*, 65, 1034 (1976); 66, 1357 (1977)

18. T. Ishimitsu, S. Hirose and H. Sakurai. Microscopic acid dissociation constants of 3,4-dihydroxyphenethylamine (dopamine). *Chem. Pharm. Bull.*, 26, 74–8 (1978)

19. B. Honig and A. Nicholls. Classical electrostatics in biology and chemistry. *Science*, 268, 1144–9 (1995)

20. T. Seki, M. Okamoto, O. Hosoya and K. Juni. Measurement of diffusion coefficients of parabens by the chromatographic broadening method. *J. Pharm. Sci. Technol., Jpn.* 60, 114–7 (2000)

21. N. Baden and M. Terazima. A novel method for measurement of diffusion coefficients of proteins and DNA in solution. *Chem. Phys. Lett.*, 393, 539–45 (2004)

4

Drug stability

Many drugs are susceptible to some form of chemical decomposition when formulated in either liquid or even solid dosage forms. Such degradation not only leads to a loss of potency of the drug but may, in some cases, cause changes in the physical appearance of the dosage forms, for example, discoloration following the photochemical decomposition of the drug.

In this chapter we will identify those classes of drugs which are particularly susceptible to chemical breakdown and examine some of the precautions which can be taken to minimise the loss of activity. It is important to be able to determine a time interval over which the drug retains sufficient potency for it to be used. Usually the shelf-life is assumed to be the time taken for the concentration of the drug to be reduced to 95% of its value when originally prepared. To be able to make shelf-life predictions we should first understand the kinetics of the decomposition process. We will look at how reactions can be classified into various 'orders', and how we can calculate the rate constant for a reaction under a given set of environmental conditions. Methods for accelerating the drug breakdown using elevated temperatures will be examined and we will see how it is possible to estimate the stability of the drug for the required storage conditions from these measurements. Although such experiments cannot replace the rigorous stability testing procedures on the product in the form in which it is finally to be marketed, they do lead to considerable saving of time at the product development stage when it is necessary to identify rapidly a formulation in which the stability is at an acceptable level.

4.1 The chemical decomposition of drugs

In this section we examine various ways in which drugs in both liquid and solid formulations can lose their activity, so that we can be aware of those chemical groups which, when present in drug molecules, can cause stability problems. We will later see how to prevent or minimise the chemical breakdown for each type of decomposition process. Although each decomposition scheme is considered separately, it should be noted that with some drug molecules more than one type of decomposition may be occurring at the same time; this, of course, complicates the analysis of the system.

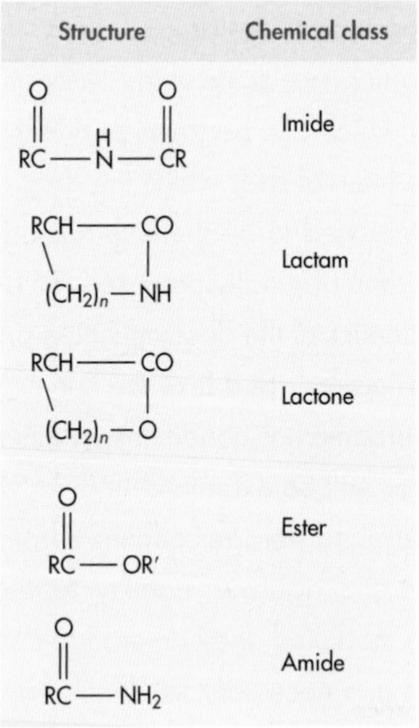

Structure	Chemical class
$RC \overset{O}{\underset{}{\parallel}} - \overset{H}{\underset{}{N}} - \overset{O}{\underset{}{\parallel}} CR$	Imide
$RCH - CO$ \ | $(CH_2)_n - NH$	Lactam
$RCH - CO$ \ | $(CH_2)_n - O$	Lactone
$RC \overset{O}{\underset{}{\parallel}} - OR'$	Ester
$RC \overset{O}{\underset{}{\parallel}} - NH_2$	Amide

Scheme 4.1 Examples of chemical groups susceptible to hydrolysis.

4.1.1 Hydrolysis

Drugs susceptible to hydrolytic degradation

How can we tell whether a drug is likely to be susceptible to this type of degradation? If the drug is a derivative of carboxylic acid or contains functional groups based on this moiety, for example an ester, amide, lactone, lactam, imide or carbamate (see Scheme 4.1), then we are dealing with a drug which is liable to undergo hydrolytic degradation. We will consider some examples.

Drugs that contain ester linkages include acetylsalicylic acid (aspirin), physostigmine, methyldopa, tetracaine and procaine. Ester hydrolysis is usually a bimolecular reaction involving acyl–oxygen cleavage. For example, the hydrolysis of procaine is shown in Scheme 4.2.

The hydrolysis of amides involves the cleavage of the amide linkage as for example, in the breakdown of the local anaesthetic cinchocaine (Scheme 4.3).

This type of link is also found in drugs such as chloramphenicol, ergometrine and benzylpenicillin sodium.

Finally, as examples of lactam ring hydrolysis we can consider the decomposition of nitrazepam and chlordiazepoxide, which is discussed in more detail later (section 4.2.7). Other drugs, apart from the benzodiazepines, which are susceptible to hydrolysis include the penicillins and cephalosporins.

Controlling drug hydrolysis in solution

Optimisation of formulation

Hydrolysis is frequently catalysed by hydrogen ions (specific acid-catalysis) or hydroxyl ions (specific base-catalysis) and also by other acidic

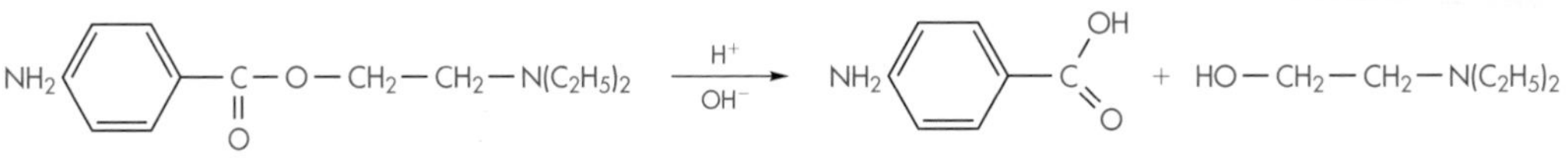

Scheme 4.2 Hydrolysis of the ester group of procaine.

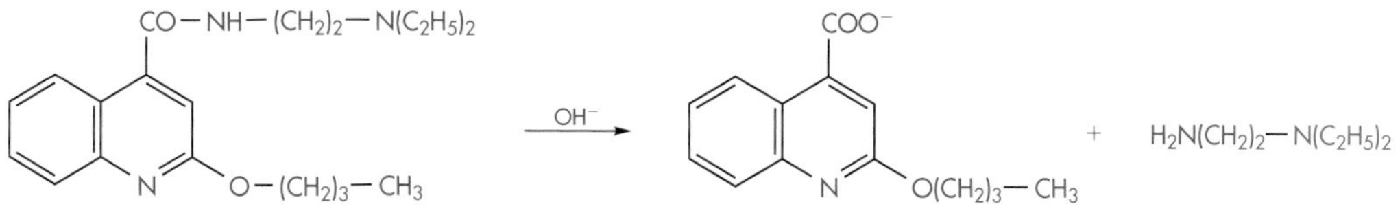

Scheme 4.3 Hydrolysis of the amide linkage of cinchocaine.

or basic species that are commonly encountered as components of buffers. This latter type of catalysis is referred to as general acid–base catalysis. Both types of catalysis will be dealt with in greater depth in section 4.4.1. Several methods are available to stabilise a solution of a drug which is susceptible to acid–base catalysed hydrolysis. The usual method is to determine the pH of maximum stability from kinetic experiments at a range of pH values and to formulate the product at this pH (section 4.4.1). Alteration of the dielectric constant by the addition of nonaqueous solvents such as alcohol, glycerin or propylene glycol may in many cases reduce hydrolysis (section 4.4.1).

Since only that portion of the drug which is in solution will be hydrolysed, it is possible to suppress degradation by making the drug less soluble. The stability of penicillin in procaine–penicillin suspensions was significantly increased by reducing its solubility by using additives such as citrates, dextrose, sorbitol and gluconate. Adding a compound that forms a complex with the drug can increase stability. The addition of caffeine to aqueous solutions of benzocaine, procaine and tetracaine was shown to decrease the base-catalysed hydrolysis of these local anaesthetics in this way. In many cases solubilisation of a drug by surfactants protects against hydrolysis, as discussed in section 4.4.1.

Modification of chemical structure of drug
The control of drug stability by modifying chemical structure using appropriate substituents has been suggested for drugs for which such a modification does not reduce therapeutic efficacy. The *Hammett linear free energy relationship* for the effect of substituents on the rates of aromatic side-chain reactions, such as the hydrolysis of esters, is given by

$$\log k = \log k_0 + \sigma\rho \qquad (4.1)$$

where k and k_0 are the rate constants for the reaction of the substituted and unsubstituted compounds, respectively, σ is the Hammett substituent constant (which is determined by the nature of the substituents and is independent of the reaction), and ρ is the reaction constant, which is dependent on the reaction, the conditions of reaction and the nature of the side-chains undergoing reaction. Thus, a plot of $\log k$ against the Hammett constant (values are readily available in the literature[1]) is linear if this relationship is obeyed, with a slope of ρ. This concept has been used, for example, in the production of the best substituents for allylbarbituric acids to obtain optimum stability.[2]

4.1.2 Oxidation[3]

After hydrolysis, oxidation is the next most common pathway for drug breakdown. However, whereas the hydrolytic degradation of drugs has been thoroughly studied, their oxidative degradation has received comparatively little attention. Indeed, in cases where simultaneous hydrolytic and oxidative degradation can occur, the oxidative process has usually been eliminated by storage under anaerobic conditions without an investigation of the oxidative mechanism.

Oxidation processes

Oxidation involves the removal of an electropositive atom, radical or electron, or the addition of an electronegative atom or radical. Oxidative degradation can occur by *autoxidation*, in which reaction is uncatalysed and proceeds quite slowly under the influence of molecular oxygen, or may involve *chain processes* consisting of three concurrent reactions – initiation, propagation and termination. Initiation can be via free radicals formed from organic compounds by the action of light, heat or transition metals such as copper and iron which are present in trace amounts in almost every buffer. The propagation stage of the reaction involves the combination of molecular oxygen with the free radical $R^{\bullet}$ to form a peroxy radical $ROO^{\bullet}$, which then removes H from a molecule of the organic compound to form a hydroperoxide, ROOH, and in so doing creates a new free radical (Scheme 4.4).

The reaction proceeds until the free radicals are destroyed by inhibitors or by side-reactions which eventually break the chain. The rancid odour which is a characteristic of oxidised fats and oils is due to aldehydes, ketones and short-chain fatty acids which are the breakdown products of the hydroperoxides. Peroxides (ROOR') and hydroperoxides (ROOH) are photolabile, breaking down to hydroxyl ($HO^{\bullet}$) and/or alkoxyl ($RO^{\bullet}$) radicals, which are themselves highly oxidising species. The presence of residual peroxides in polyoxyethylene glycols (PEGs) is a cause for concern when these excipients are used in formulation, as for example in the case of fenprostalene.[4]

Drugs susceptible to oxidation

We will consider some examples of drugs and excipients that are subject to oxidative degradation owing to the possession of functional groups that are particularly sensitive to oxidation.

Steroids and sterols represent an important class of drugs that are subject to oxidative degradation through the possession of carbon–carbon double bonds (alkene moieties) to which peroxyl radicals can readily add. Similarly, *polyunsaturated fatty acids*, commonly used in drug formulations, are particularly susceptible to oxidation and care must be exercised to minimise degradation in formulations containing high concentrations of, for example, vegetable oils.[5] For drugs, such as the cholesterol-lowering agent *simvastatin* (**I**), that contain conjugated double bonds, addition of peroxyl radicals may lead to the formation of polymeric peroxides (simvastatin polymerises up to a pentamer[6]), cleavage of which produces epoxides which may further degrade into aldehydes or ketones.

Polyene antibiotics, such as amphotericin B (**II**) which contains seven conjugated double bonds (heptaene moiety), are subject to attack by peroxyl radicals, leading to aggregation and loss of activity.[7]

The oxidation of *phenothiazines* to the sulfoxide involves two single-electron transfer reactions involving a radical cation intermediate as shown in Scheme 4.5. The sulfoxide is subsequently formed by reaction of the cation with water.

The ether group in drugs such as *econazole nitrate* (**III**) and *miconazole nitrate* (**IV**) is susceptible to oxidation. The process involves removal of hydrogen from the C–H bonds in the α-position to the oxygen to produce radicals, which further degrade to α-hydroperoxides and eventually to aldehydes, ketones, alcohols and carboxylic acids.

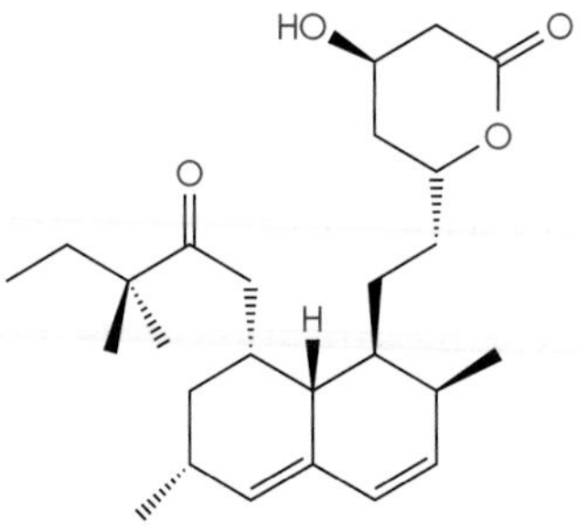

Initiation: $X^{\bullet} + RH \longrightarrow R^{\bullet} + XH$

Propagation: $R^{\bullet} + O_2 \longrightarrow ROO^{\bullet}$

$ROO^{\bullet} + RH \longrightarrow ROOH + R^{\bullet}$

Termination: $ROO^{\bullet} + ROO^{\bullet} \longrightarrow$ stable product

$ROO^{\bullet} + R^{\bullet} \longrightarrow$ stable product

$R^{\bullet} + R^{\bullet} \longrightarrow$ stable product

Scheme 4.4 Simplified oxidation scheme involving a chain process.

Structure I Simvastatin

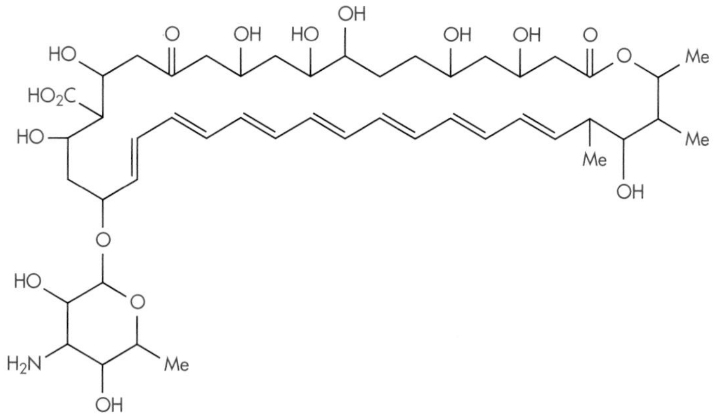

Structure II Amphotericin B

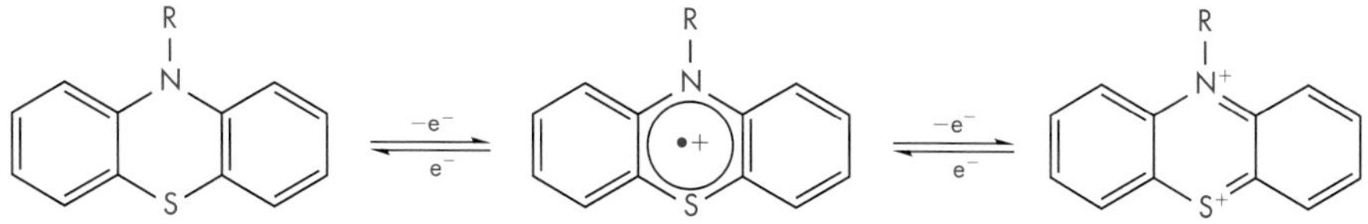

Scheme 4.5   Oxidation of phenothiazines.

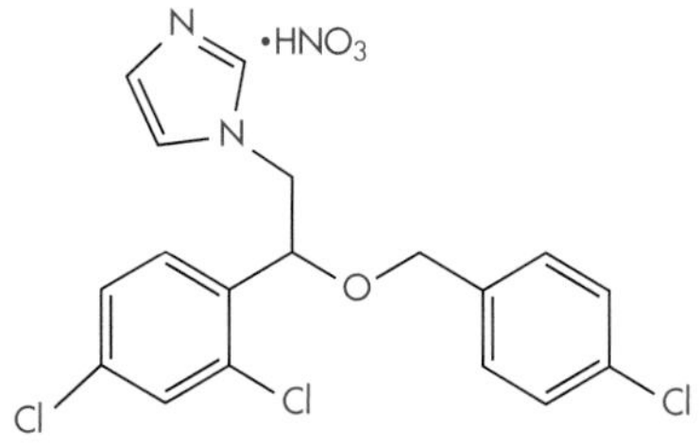

Structure III Econazole nitrate

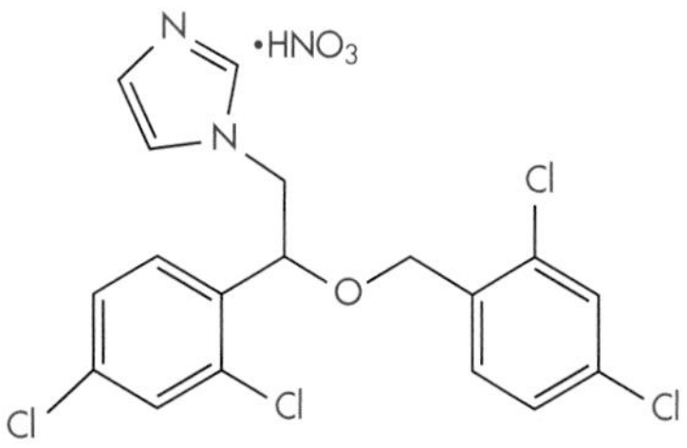

Structure IV Miconazole nitrate

Stabilisation against oxidation

Various precautions should be taken during manufacture and storage to minimise oxidation. The oxygen in pharmaceutical containers should be replaced with nitrogen or carbon dioxide; contact of the drug with heavy-metal ions such as iron, cobalt or nickel, which catalyse oxidation, should be avoided; and storage should be at reduced temperatures.

Antioxidants

It is very difficult to remove all of the oxygen from a container and even traces of oxygen are sufficient to initiate the oxidation chain. The propagation of the chain reaction may be prevented or delayed by adding low concentrations of compounds that act as inhibitors. Such compounds are called *antioxidants* and interrupt the propagation by interaction with the free radical. The antioxidant free radical so formed is not sufficiently reactive to maintain the chain reaction and is eventually annihilated. The structures of some commonly used antioxidants are given in Scheme 4.6. Reducing agents such as sodium metabisulfite may also be added to formulations to prevent oxidation. These compounds are more readily oxidised than the drug and so protect it from

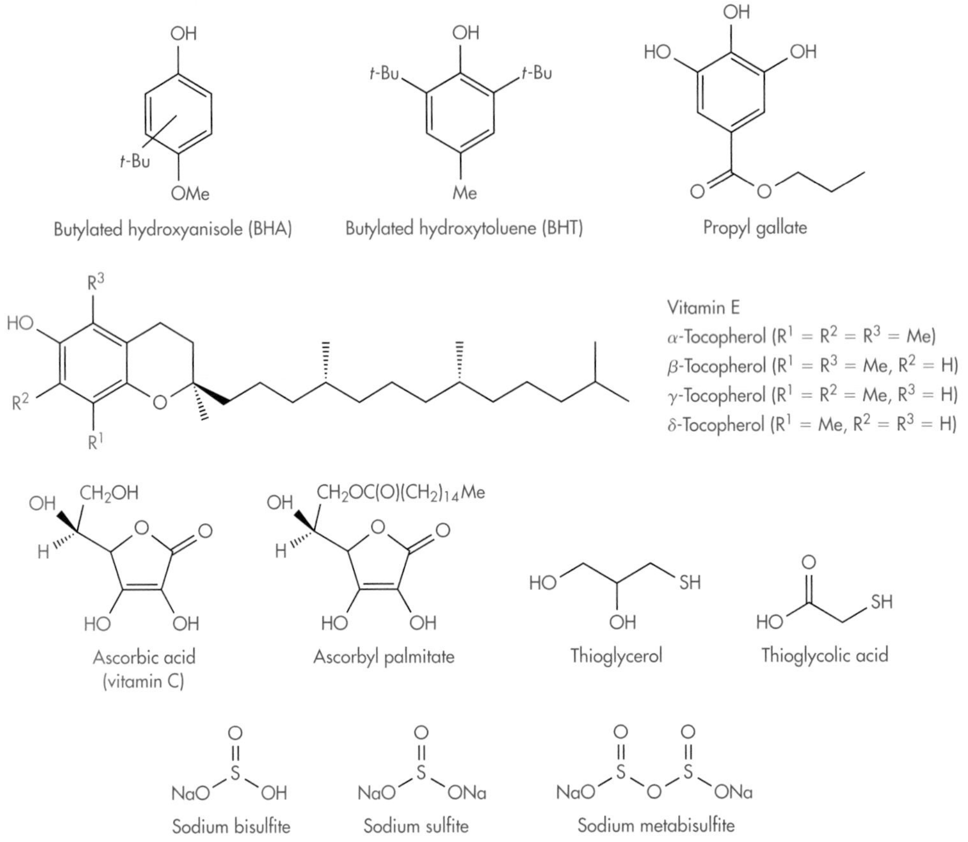

Butylated hydroxyanisole (BHA)   Butylated hydroxytoluene (BHT)   Propyl gallate

Vitamin E
α-Tocopherol ($R^1 = R^2 = R^3 = Me$)
β-Tocopherol ($R^1 = R^3 = Me, R^2 = H$)
γ-Tocopherol ($R^1 = R^2 = Me, R^3 = H$)
δ-Tocopherol ($R^1 = Me, R^2 = R^3 = H$)

Ascorbic acid   Ascorbyl palmitate   Thioglycerol   Thioglycolic acid
(vitamin C)

Sodium bisulfite   Sodium sulfite   Sodium metabisulfite

Scheme 4.6   Structures of some common antioxidants.

oxidation. Oxidation is catalysed by unprotonated amines such as aminophylline, and hence admixture of susceptible drugs with such compounds should be avoided.

4.1.3 Isomerisation

Isomerisation is the process of conversion of a drug into its optical or geometric isomers. Since the various isomers of a drug are frequently of different activity, such a conversion may be regarded as a form of degradation, often resulting in a serious loss of therapeutic activity. For example, the appreciable loss of activity of solutions of adrenaline at low pH has been attributed to *racemisation* – the conversion of the therapeutically active form, in this case the levorotary form, into its less-active isomer.

In acidic conditions the tetracyclines undergo epimerisation at carbon atom 4 to form an equilibrium mixture of tetracycline and the epimer, 4-epi-tetracycline (Scheme 4.7). The 4-epi-tetracycline is toxic and its content in medicines is restricted to not more than 3%. The epimerisation follows the kinetics of a first-order reversible reaction (see equation (4.24)). The degradation rate is pH-dependent (maximum epimerisation occurring

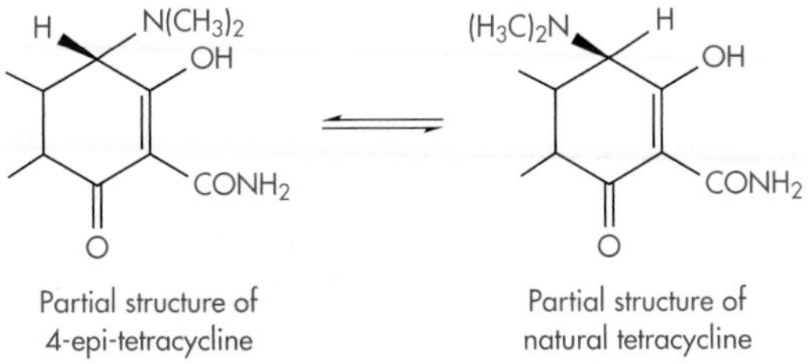

Partial structure of   Partial structure of
4-epi-tetracycline   natural tetracycline

Scheme 4.7   Epimerisation of tetracyclines.

at pH 3.2) and is also catalysed by phosphate and citrate ions.

Cephalosporin esters are widely used as intermediates in cephalosporin synthesis and as prodrugs for oral administration of parenteral cephalosporins. These esters undergo reversible base-catalysed isomerisation according to the mechanism shown in Scheme 4.8. A proton in the 2-position is abstracted by a base (B) and the resulting carbanion can be reprotonated in the 4-postion, giving a Δ^2-ester. On hydrolysis, Δ^2-cephalosporin esters yield Δ^2-cephalosporins, which are biologically inactive.

Cis–trans isomerisation may be a cause of loss of potency of a drug if the two geometric isomers have different therapeutic activities. Vitamin A (all-*trans*-retinol) is enzymatically oxidised to the aldehyde and then isomerised to yield 11-*cis*-retinal (Scheme 4.9), which has a decreased activity compared with the all-*trans* molecule.

4.1.4 Photochemical decomposition[8]

Many pharmaceutical compounds, including the phenothiazine tranquillizers, hydrocortisone, prednisolone, riboflavin, ascorbic acid and folic acid, degrade when exposed to light. As a result there will be a loss of potency of the drug, often accompanied by changes in the appearance of the product, such as discoloration or formation of a precipitate. Photodecomposition might occur not only during storage but also during use of the

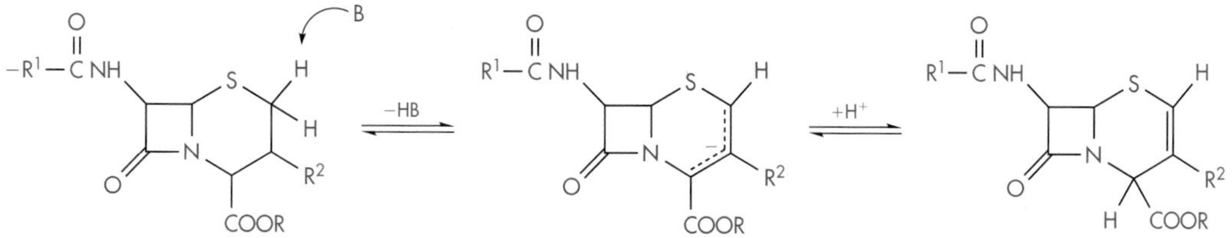

Scheme 4.8 Proposed mechanism for the base-catalysed isomerisation of cephalosporin esters.
Reproduced from W. F. Richter, Y. H. Chong and V. J. Stella, *J. Pharm. Sci.*, 79, 185 (1990).

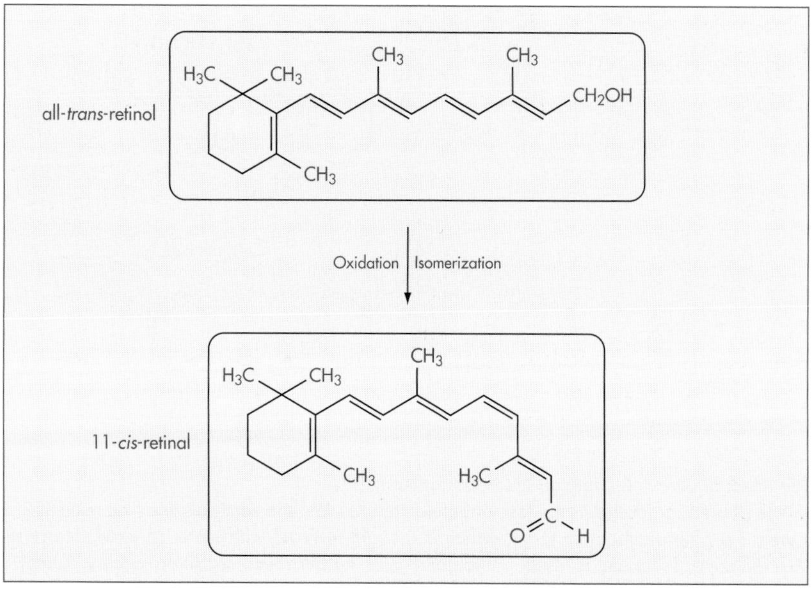

Scheme 4.9 Isomerisation of vitamin A.

product. For example, sunlight is able to penetrate the skin to a sufficient depth to cause photodegradation of drugs circulating in the surface capillaries or in the eyes of patients receiving the drug.

Primary photochemical reaction occurs when the wavelength of the incident light is within the wavelength range of absorption of the drug (usually within the ultraviolet range, unless the drug is coloured), so that the drug molecule itself absorbs radiation and degrades. Photodegradation may also occur with drugs that do not directly absorb the incident radiation, as a consequence of absorption of radiation by excipients in the formulation (*photosensitisers*) which transfer the absorbed energy to the drug, causing it to degrade. In assessing the photostability of a product it is therefore necessary to consider the final formulation rather than simply the drug itself.

The rate of the photodegradation is dependent on the rate at which light is absorbed by the system and also the efficiency of the photochemical process. In formulations that contain low drug concentrations, the primary photochemical reaction follows first-order kinetics; the kinetics are more complicated at higher concentrations and in the solid state because most of the light is then absorbed near the surface of the product.

Although it is difficult to predict which drugs are likely to be prone to photodegradation, there are certain chemical functions that are expected to introduce photoreactivity, including carbonyl, nitroaromatic and N-oxide functions, aryl halides, alkenes, polyenes and sulfides.[9] The mechanisms of photodegradation are of such complexity as to have been fully elucidated in only a few cases. We will consider two examples – chlorpromazine and ketoprofen.

The phenothiazine *chlorpromazine* (CLP) is rapidly decomposed under the action of ultraviolet light, the decomposition being accompanied by discoloration of the solutions (Scheme 4.10).

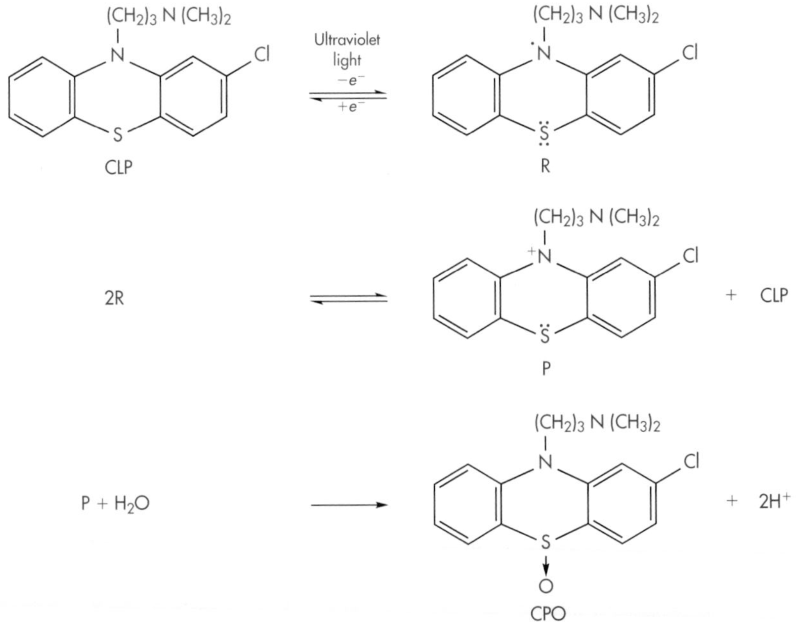

Scheme 4.10 The effect of ultraviolet light on chlorpromazine (CLP).

The first step of the photodegradation is the loss of an electron to yield the semiquinone free radical R. Further stages in the degradation yield the phenazathonium ion P, which is thought to react with water to yield chlorpromazine sulfoxide (CPO). The chlorpromazine sulfoxide is itself photolabile and further decomposition occurs. Other products of the photooxidation include chlorpromazine N-oxide and hydroxychlorpromazine.

Reproduced from F. H. Merkle and C. A. Discher, *J. Pharm. Sci.*, 53, 620 (1964).

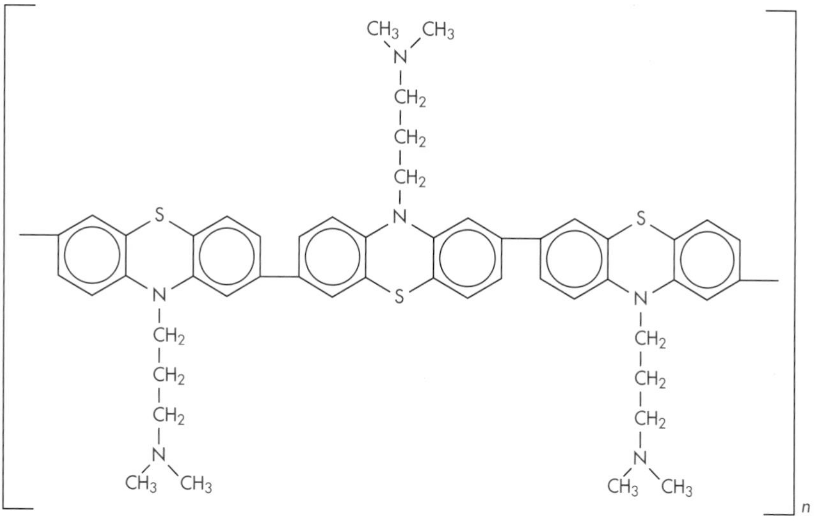

Structure V Polymer produced by the ultraviolet irradiation of chlorpromazine under anaerobic conditions

Chlorpromazine behaves differently towards ultraviolet irradiation under anaerobic conditions. A polymerisation process has been proposed[10] which involves the liberation of HCl in its initial stages. The polymer (V) was isolated, and upon intracutaneous injection it produced a bluish-purple discoloration typical of that observed in some patients receiving prolonged chlorpromazine medication. It was suggested that the skin irritation that accompanies the discoloration may be a result of the liberation of HCl during photodecomposition.

The photodegradation of *ketoprofen* can involve decarboxylation to form an intermediate which then undergoes reduction, or dimerisation of the ketoprofen itself as illustrated in Scheme 4.11.

Stabilisation against photochemical decomposition

Pharmaceutical products can be adequately

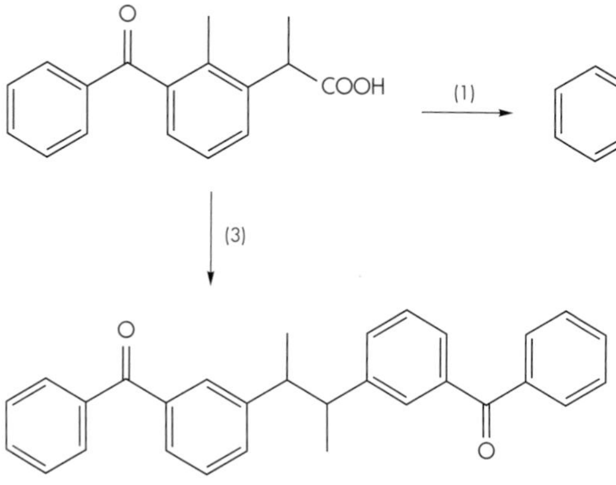

Scheme 4.11 Photodegradation of ketoprofen.
    Photodegradation of ketoprofen by decarboxylation (reaction 1) and subsequent reduction (reaction 2), and also by dimerisation of the ketoprofen (reaction 3).
Reproduced from H. H. Tønnesen, *Int. J. Pharm.*, 225, 1 (2001).

protected from photoinduced decomposition by the use of coloured glass containers and storage in the dark. Amber glass excludes light of wavelength <470 nm and so affords considerable protection of compounds sensitive to ultraviolet light. Coating tablets with a polymer film containing ultraviolet absorbers has been suggested as an additional method for protection from light. In this respect, a film coating of vinyl acetate containing oxybenzone as an ultraviolet absorber has been shown[11] to be effective in minimising the discoloration and photolytic degradation of sulfasomidine tablets.

4.1.5 Polymerisation

Polymerisation is the process by which two or more identical drug molecules combine together to form a complex molecule. It has been demonstrated that a polymerisation process occurs during the storage of concentrated aqueous solutions of aminopenicillins, such as ampicillin sodium. The reactive β-lactam bond of the ampicillin molecule is opened by reaction with the side-chain of a second ampicillin molecule and a dimer is

formed (Scheme 4.12). The process can continue to form higher polymers. Such polymeric substances have been shown to be highly antigenic in animals and they are considered to play a part in eliciting pencilloyl-specific allergic reactions to ampicillin in humans. The dimerising tendency of the aminopenicillins increases with the increase in the basicity of the side-chain group, the order, in terms of increasing rates, being cyclacillin $\ll$ ampicillin < epicillin < amoxycillin.

The hydrate of formaldehyde, $HOCH_2OH$, may under certain conditions polymerise in aqueous solution to form paraformaldehyde, $HOCH_2(OCH_2)_nOCH_2OH$, which appears as a white deposit in the solution. The polymerisation may be prevented by adding to the solution 10–15% of methanol.

4.2 Kinetics of chemical decomposition in solution

Before we can predict the shelf-life of a dosage form it is essential to determine the kinetics of the breakdown of the drug under carefully controlled conditions. Unfortunately, drug

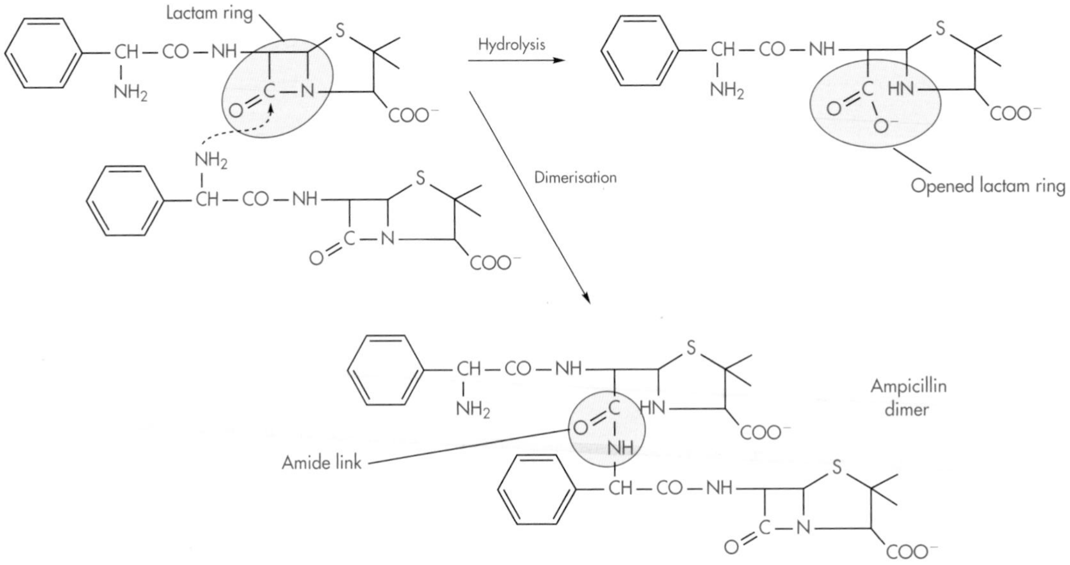

Scheme 4.12 Dimerisation and hydrolysis of ampicillin.
Reproduced from H. Bundgaard, *Acta Pharm. Suec.*, 13, 9 (1976).

decomposition often does not follow simple reaction schemes and in this section we will look not only at the traditional ways of classifying reactions, but also at some of the complications which can arise with pharmaceutical preparations, which confuse this simple classification.

4.2.1 Classifying reactions: the order of reaction

Reactions are classified according to number of reacting species whose concentration determines the rate at which the reaction occurs, i.e. the *order of reaction*. We will concentrate mainly on *zero-order* reactions, in which the breakdown rate is independent of the concentration of any of the reactants; *first-order* reactions, in which the reaction rate is determined by one concentration term, and *second-order* reactions, in which the rate is determined by the concentrations of two reacting species.

Experimentally we can monitor the rate of breakdown of the drug either by its decrease in concentration with time or alternatively by the rate of appearance of one of the breakdown products. If we represent the initial concentration of drug A as a mol dm^{-3} and if we find experimentally that x mol dm^{-3} of the drug has reacted in time t, then the amount of drug remaining at a time t is $(a - x)$ mol dm^{-3} and the rate of reaction is

$$\frac{-d[A]}{dt} = \frac{-d(a-x)}{dt} = dx/dt \qquad (4.2)$$

Notice that the term a is a constant and therefore disappears during differentiation. We will use dx/dt to describe the reaction rate in this section.

If we assume that a typical reaction between a drug molecule A and a reactant B occurs when two molecules are in collision, then we might expect that the number of collisions, and hence the reaction rate, would be proportional to the concentration of the two reacting molecules, i.e.

$$\text{Rate} \propto [A][B]$$

or

$$\frac{dx}{dt} = k[A][B] \qquad (4.3)$$

where the proportionality constant, k, is called the *rate constant*. This is an example of a *second-order* reaction since the order of reaction is the sum of the exponents of the concentration terms in the rate equation. As we will see (section 4.4.1), many hydrolysis reactions are catalysed by H$^+$, OH$^-$ or buffer components and so we can write equation (4.3) as, for example,

$$\frac{dx}{dt} = k_2[A][H^+] \qquad (4.4)$$

k_2 is a second-order rate constant and has units of (concentration)$^{-1}$(time)$^{-1}$, for example (mol dm^{-3})$^{-1}$ min^{-1}. When the solution is buffered at constant pH, [H$^+$] is constant and we can write equation (4.4) as

$$\frac{dx}{dt} = k_1[A] = k_1(a - x) \qquad (4.5)$$

where $k_1 = k_2[H^+]$. Since the rate of reaction now effectively depends on one concentration term it is a *first-order* reaction or, more correctly in this case, a *pseudo first-order* reaction (see section 4.2.3). The majority of decomposition reactions involving drugs fall into this category, either because the species reacting with the drug is maintained constant by buffering or because, as in the case of uncatalysed hydrolysis reactions, the water is in such large excess that any change in its concentration is negligible.

If as well as maintaining a constant amount of water in a reaction, we also maintain a fixed drug concentration, then equation (4.3) becomes

$$\frac{dx}{dt} = k_0 \qquad (4.6)$$

where $k_0 = k_1[A] = k_2[A][B]$.

This type of reaction, which is called a *zero-order* reaction, can often occur in suspensions of poorly soluble drugs. In these systems the suspended drug slowly dissolves as the drug decomposes and so a constant drug concentration in solution is maintained.

We will now examine the ways in which we can determine the rate constants for these three types of reaction.

4.2.2 Zero-order reactions

In this type of reaction the decomposition proceeds at a constant rate and is independent of the concentrations of any of the reactants. The rate equation is given by equation (4.6) as

$$\frac{dx}{dt} = k_0$$

Integration, noting that $x = 0$ at $t = 0$, gives

$$\int_0^x dx = k_0 \int_0^t dt \tag{4.7}$$

i.e.

$$x = k_0 t \tag{4.8}$$

A plot of the amount remaining (as ordinate) against time (as abscissa) is linear with a slope of k_0 (concentration·time^{-1}).

Many decomposition reactions in the solid phase (section 4.3) or in suspensions apparently follow zero-order kinetics. Figure 4.1 shows the hydrolysis of a suspension of acetylsalicylic acid.

4.2.3 First-order reactions

The rate of first-order reactions is determined by one concentration term and may be written using equation (4.5) as

$$\frac{dx}{dt} = k_1(a - x)$$

Since $x = 0$ at the start of the measurements (that is, when $t = 0$)

$$\int_0^x \frac{dx}{(a - x)} = k_1 \int_0^t dt \tag{4.9}$$

$$k_1 = \frac{2.303}{t} \log \frac{a}{a - x} \tag{4.10}$$

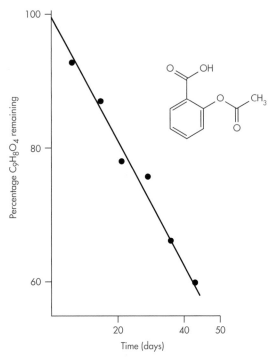

Figure 4.1 Hydrolysis of a suspension of acetylsalicylic acid at 34°C.

Reproduced from K. C. James, *J. Pharm. Pharmacol.*, 10, 363 (1958) with permission.

Or, rearranging into a linear form,

$$t = \frac{2.303}{k_1} \log a - \frac{2.303}{k_1} \log(a - x) \tag{4.11}$$

According to equation (4.11), a plot of the logarithm of the amount of drug remaining (as ordinate) as a function of time (as abscissa) is linear if the decomposition follows first-order kinetics. The first-order rate constant may be obtained from the slope of the plot (slope = $-k_1/2.303$). k_1 has the dimensions of time^{-1}.

The time taken for half of the reactant to decompose is referred to as the *half-life* of the reaction, $t_{0.5}$. An expression for $t_{0.5}$ for a first-order reaction may be derived from equation (4.10), noting that when $t = t_{0.5}$, $x = a/2$:

$$t_{0.5} = \frac{2.303}{k_1} \log \frac{a}{a/2} \tag{4.12}$$

Thus,

$$t_{0.5} = \frac{2.303}{k_1} \log 2 = \frac{0.693}{k_1} \tag{4.13}$$

The half-life is therefore independent of the initial concentration of reactants.

Even in the case of a reaction involving more than one reacting species, the rate may still follow first-order kinetics. The most common example of this occurs when one of the reactants is in such a large excess that any change in its concentration is negligible compared with changes in the concentration of the other reactants. This type of reaction is termed a pseudo first-order reaction. Such reactions are often met in stability studies of drugs that hydrolyse in solution, the water being in such excess that changes in its concentration are negligible and hence the rate of reaction is dependent solely on the drug concentration.

• •

EXAMPLE 4.1 Calculation of first-order rate constant and half-life

The following data were obtained for the hydrolysis of homatropine in 0.226 mol dm^{-3} HCl at 90°C:

Percentage homatropine remaining	93.4	85.2	75.9	63.1	52.5	41.8
Time (h)	1.38	3.0	6.0	8.6	12	17

Show that the hydrolysis follows first-order kinetics and calculate (a) the rate constant, and (b) the half-life.

Answer
(a) The reaction will be first-order if a plot of the logarithm of the amount of homatropine remaining against time is linear.

Log percentage remaining	1.97	1.93	1.88	1.80	1.72	1.62
Time(h)	1.38	3.0	6.0	8.6	12	17

Figure 4.2 shows a linear plot with a slope = $-(1.96 - 1.55)/(20 - 2) = -2.278 \times 10^{-2}$ h^{-1}

$$\text{Slope} = -k_1/2.303$$

Therefore,

$$k_1 = 5.25 \times 10^{-2} \text{ h}^{-1}$$

(b) From equation (4.13)

$$t_{0.5} = 0.693/k_1 = 13.2 \text{ h}$$

The half-life of the reaction is 13.2 h.

• •

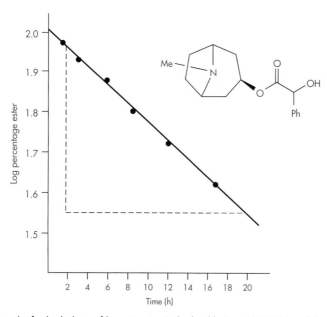

Figure 4.2 First-order plot for hydrolysis of homatropine in hydrochloric acid (0.226 mol dm^{-3}) at 90°C.
Data from M. H. Krasowska, S. Schytt Larsen and K. Ilver, *Dansk. Tidsskr. Farm.*, 42, 170 (1968) with permission.

4.2.4 Second-order reactions

The rate of a second-order reaction is determined by the concentrations of two reacting species. The general rate equation is given by equation (4.3) as

$$\frac{\mathrm{d}x}{\mathrm{d}t} = k_2[A][B] \tag{4.14}$$

If the initial concentrations of reactants A and B are a and b, respectively, equation (4.14) may be written

$$\frac{\mathrm{d}x}{\mathrm{d}t} = k_2(a - x)(b - x) \tag{4.15}$$

where x is the amount of A and B decomposed in time t. Integration of equation (4.15) by the method of partial fractions yields

$$k_2 = \frac{2.303}{t(a - b)} \log \frac{b(a - x)}{a(b - x)} \tag{4.16}$$

Rearranging into a linear form suitable for plotting gives

$$t = \frac{2.303}{k_2(a - b)} = \log \frac{b}{a} + \frac{2.303}{k_2(a - b)} \log \frac{(a - x)}{(b - x)} \tag{4.17}$$

k_2 can then be obtained from the slope, $2.303/k_2(a - b)$, of a plot of t (as ordinate) against $\log[(a - x)/(b - x)]$ (as abscissa).

Examination of equation (4.17) shows that the second-order rate constant is dependent on the units used to express concentration; the units of k_2 are concentration^{-1} time^{-1}.

For reactions in which both concentration terms refer to the same reactant we may write

$$\frac{-\mathrm{d}[A]}{\mathrm{d}t} = k_2[A]^2 \tag{4.18}$$

and

$$\frac{\mathrm{d}x}{\mathrm{d}t} = k_2(a - x)^2 \tag{4.19}$$

A similar equation applies to second-order reactions in which the initial concentrations of the two reactants are the same.

Integration of equation (4.19) between the limits of t from 0 to t and of x from 0 to x

yields

$$t = \frac{1}{k_2}\left[\frac{1}{a - x} - \frac{1}{a}\right] = \frac{x}{k_2 a(a - x)} \tag{4.20}$$

from which it is seen that a plot of t (ordinate) against $x/a(a - x)$ (abscissa) yields a linear plot of slope $1/k_2$.

The half-life of a reaction which follows equation (4.20) is given by

$$t_{0.5} = \frac{1}{k_2 a} \tag{4.21}$$

Unlike $t_{0.5}$ for the first-order reactions, the half-life of the second-order reaction is dependent on the initial concentration of reactants. It is not possible to derive a simple expression for the half-life of a second-order reaction with unequal initial concentrations.

4.2.5 Third-order reactions

Third-order reactions are only rarely encountered in drug stability studies involving, as they do, the simultaneous collision of three reactant molecules. The overall rate of ampicillin breakdown by simultaneous hydrolysis and polymerisation may be represented by an equation of the form

$$\frac{-\mathrm{d}[A]}{\mathrm{d}t} = k_a[A] + k_b[A]^2 + k_c[A]^3 \tag{4.22}$$

where k_a, k_b and k_c are the pH-dependent apparent rate constant for hydrolysis, uncatalysed polymerisation and the general acid–base-catalysed polymerisation of ampicillin, respectively.[12] As seen from equation (4.22) the decomposition rate shows both second-order and third-order dependency on the total ampicillin concentration [A].

4.2.6 Determination of the order of reaction

The most obvious method of determining the order of a reaction is to determine the amount of drug decomposed after various intervals and to substitute the data into the integrated equations for zero-, first- and second-order reactions. The equation giving the most consistent value of k for a series of time intervals is that corresponding most closely to the order of the reaction. Alternatively, the data may be displayed graphically according to the linear equations for the various orders of reactions until a straight-line plot is obtained. Thus, for example, if the data yield a linear graph when plotted as t against $\log(a - x)$ the reaction is then taken to be first-order.

Fitting data to the standard rate equations may, however, produce misleading results if a fractional order of reaction applies. An alternative method of determining the order of reaction, which avoids this problem, is based on equation (4.23):

$$\log t_{0.5} = \log\left[\frac{2^{n-1} - 1}{k(n-1)}\right] + (1 - n) \log C_0$$

$$(4.23)$$

The half-life of the reaction is determined for a series of initial drug concentrations, C_0, and the order, n, is calculated from the slope of plots of $\log t_{0.5}$ as a function of $\log C_0$.

• •

EXAMPLE 4.2 Determination of the order of reaction

The kinetics of decomposition of a drug in aqueous solution were studied using a series of solutions of different initial drug concentrations, C_0. For each solution the time taken for half the drug to decompose (that is, $t_{0.5}$) was determined with the following results:

C_0 (mol dm^{-3})	4.625	1.698	0.724	0.288
$t_{0.5}$ (min)	87.17	240.1	563.0	1414.4

Determine the order of reaction and calculate the rate constant.

Answer

Application of equation (4.23) requires values for $\log C_0$ and $\log t_{0.5}$; thus

$\log C_0$	0.665	0.230	-0.140	-0.540
$\log t_{0.5}$	1.94	2.38	2.75	3.15

A plot of $\log t_{0.5}$ against $\log C_0$ is linear (Fig. 4.3) with slope $(1 - n) = -1.01$. Hence $n = 2.01$, i.e. the reaction is second-order.

The intercept of the graph (that is, the value of $\log t_{0.5}$ at $\log C_0 = 0$) is 2.60. Thus, from equation (4.23),

$$\log[(2 - 1)/k] = 2.60$$

and

$$k = 2.51 \times 10^{-3} \text{ (mol dm}^{-3})^{-1} \text{ min}^{-1}$$

• •

4.2.7 Complex reactions

There are many examples of drugs in which decomposition occurs simultaneously by two or more pathways, or involves a sequence of decomposition steps or a reversible reaction. Indeed, the degradative pathways of some drugs include examples of each of these types of complex reactions. Modification of the rate equations is necessary whenever such reactions are encountered.

Reversible reactions

Treatment of the kinetics of a reversible reaction involves two rate constants; one, k_f, to describe the rate of the forward reaction and the other, k_r, to describe the rate of the reverse reaction. For the simplest example in which both of these reactions are first-order, that is

$$A \underset{k_r}{\overset{k_f}{\rightleftharpoons}} B$$

the rate of decomposition of reactant is

$$\frac{-d[A]}{dt} = k_f[A] - k_r[B] \qquad (4.24)$$

The integrated form of the rate equation is

$$t = \frac{2.303}{k_f + k_r} \log \frac{A_0 - A_{eq}}{A - A_{eq}} \qquad (4.25)$$

where A_0, A and A_{eq} represent the initial concentration, the concentration at time t and the equilibrium concentration of reactant A, respectively. Equation (4.25) indicates that a plot of t (as ordinate) against $\log[(A_0 - A_{eq})/(A - A_{eq})]$ should be linear with a slope of $2.303/(k_f + k_r)$. k_f and k_r may be calculated

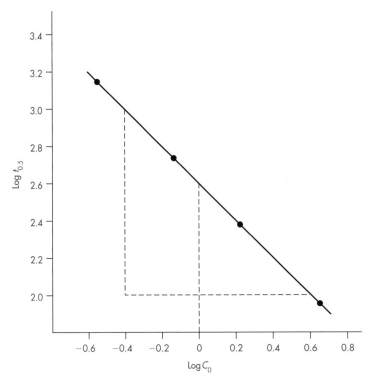

Figure 4.2 Example 4.2: plot of log of half-life ($t_{0.5}$) against log of initial drug concentration (C_0).

separately if the equilibrium constant K is also determined, since

$$K = \frac{B_{eq}}{A_{eq}} = \frac{1 - A_{eq}}{A_{eq}} = \frac{k_f}{k_r} \qquad (4.26)$$

where B_{eq} is the equilibrium concentration of product B.

The epimerisation of tetracycline (see section 4.1.3) is an example of a first-order reversible decomposition reaction.

Parallel reactions

The decomposition of many drugs involves two or more pathways, the preferred route of reaction being dependent on reaction condition. Nitrazepam (**VI**) decomposes in two pseudo first-order parallel reactions giving different breakdown products in solution and in the solid state, as illustrated in Scheme 4.13. Decomposition of nitrazepam tablets in the presence of moisture will occur by both routes, the ratio of the two products being dependent on the amount of water present.

In other cases decomposition may occur simultaneously by two different processes, as in the simultaneous hydrolysis and epimerisation of pilocarpine (see Example 4.3).

The overall rate equation for a parallel reaction is the sum of the constants for each pathway. For example, for a decomposition of a drug X involving two pathways, each of which is first-order,

the rate equation is

$$\frac{-d[X]}{dt} = (k_A + k_B)[X] = k_{exp}[X] \qquad (4.27)$$

where k_A and k_B are the rate constants for the formation of A and B, respectively, and k_{exp} is the experimentally determined rate constant. Values of the rate constants k_A and k_B may be evaluated separately by determining the ratio R of the concentration of products formed by

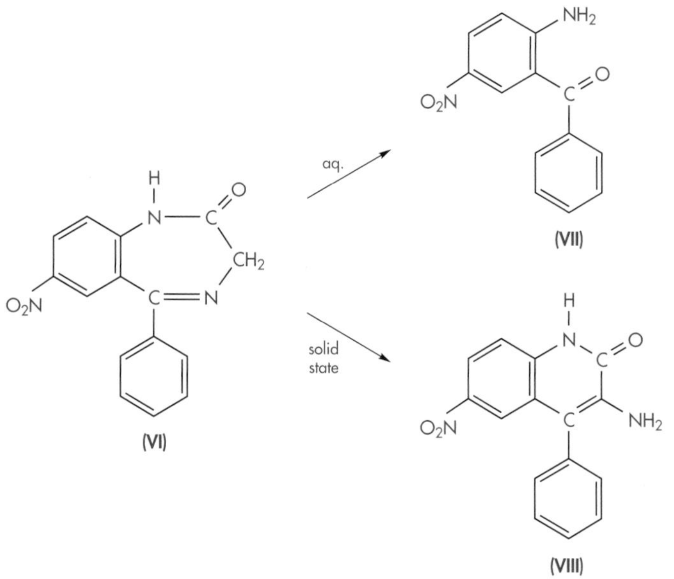

Scheme 4.13 Simplified decomposition scheme for nitrazepam (**VI**) in the solid state and aqueous solution. The main decomposition product is 2-amino-5-nitrobenzophenone (**VII**) in aqueous solution and 3-amino-6-nitro-4-phenyl-2(1H)-quinolone (**VIII**) in the solid state.
Reproduced from W. Meyer, S. Erbe and R. Voigt, *Pharmazie*, 27, 32 (1972).

each reaction:

$$R = \frac{[A]}{[B]} = \frac{k_A}{k_B} \qquad (4.28)$$

Since

$$k_{exp} = k_A + k_B \qquad (4.29)$$

$$k_{exp} = k_A + \frac{k_B}{R} \qquad (4.30)$$

Solving for k_A gives

$$k_A = k_{exp} \frac{R}{(R+1)} \qquad (4.31)$$

Similarly,

$$k_B = \frac{k_{exp}}{(R+1)} \qquad (4.32)$$

• •

EXAMPLE 4.3 Calculation of rate constants of parallel reactions

Pilocarpine has been shown to undergo simultaneous hydrolysis and epimerisation in aqueous solution. The experimentally determined rate constant, k_{exp}, at 25°C is 6.96×10^2 (mol dm^{-3})$^{-1}$ h^{-1}. Analysis has shown that at equilibrium the percentage of the epimerised form of pilocarpine (isopilocarpine) at 25°C is 20.6%. Calculate the rate constants for hydrolysis, k_H, and epimerisation, k_E.

Answer

The ratio R of pilocarpine to isopilocarpine is

$$R = 79.38/20.62 = 3.85$$

From equation (4.31),

$$k_H = (6.96 \times 10^2)(3.85/4.85)$$

i.e.

$$k_H = 5.48 \times 10^2 \text{ (mol dm}^{-3})^{-1} \text{ h}^{-1}$$

From equation (4.32),

$$k_E = (6.96 \times 10^2)/4.85$$

i.e.

$$k_E = 1.44 \times 10^2 \text{ (mol dm}^{-3})^{-1} \text{ h}^{-1}$$

Thus the rate constants for hydrolysis and epimerisation are 5.48×10^2 and 1.44×10^2 (mol dm^{-3})$^{-1}$ h^{-1}, respectively.

• •

Consecutive reactions

The simplest example of a consecutive reaction is that described by a sequence

$$A \xrightarrow{k_A} B \xrightarrow{k_B} C$$

where each step is a nonreversible first-order reaction. The hydrolysis of chlordiazepoxide follows a first-order decomposition scheme similar to that described in this equation (Scheme 4.14).

The rate of decomposition of A is

$$\frac{-d[A]}{dt} = k_A[A] \qquad (4.33)$$

The rate of change of concentration of B is

$$\frac{d[B]}{dt} = k_A[A] - k_B[B] \qquad (4.34)$$

and that of C is

$$\frac{d[C]}{dt} = k_B[B] \qquad (4.35)$$

Integration of the rate equation (4.33) yields

$$[A] = [A]_0 e^{-k_A t} \qquad (4.36)$$

Substitution of equation (4.36) into equation (4.34) gives

$$\frac{d[B]}{dt} = k_A[A]_0 e^{-k_A t} - k_B[B] \qquad (4.37)$$

which upon integration gives

$$[B] = \frac{k_A[A]_0}{(k_B - k_A)} [e^{-k_A t} - e^{-k_B t}] \qquad (4.38)$$

Since, at any time,

$$[A]_0 = [A] + [B] + [C] \qquad (4.39)$$

then

$$[C] = [A]_0 - [A] - [B]$$
$$= [A]_0 \times \left[1 + \frac{1}{k_A - k_B} (k_B e^{-k_A t} - k_A e^{-k_B t}) \right] \qquad (4.40)$$

Equations (4.36), (4.37) and (4.38) may be used to estimate the rate constants k_A and k_B and also the concentration of the breakdown product C.

4.3 Solid dosage forms: kinetics of chemical decomposition

In spite of the importance of solid dosage forms, there have been relatively few attempts to evaluate the detailed kinetics of decomposition. Most of the earlier work was carried out with the sole objective of predicting stability, and data were treated using the rate equations derived for reaction in solution. More recently, the mechanisms that were developed to describe the kinetics of decomposition of pure solids have been applied to pharmaceutical systems and some rationalisation of decomposition behaviour has been possible. A comprehensive account of this topic has been presented by Carstensen[13, 14] on which the following summary is based.

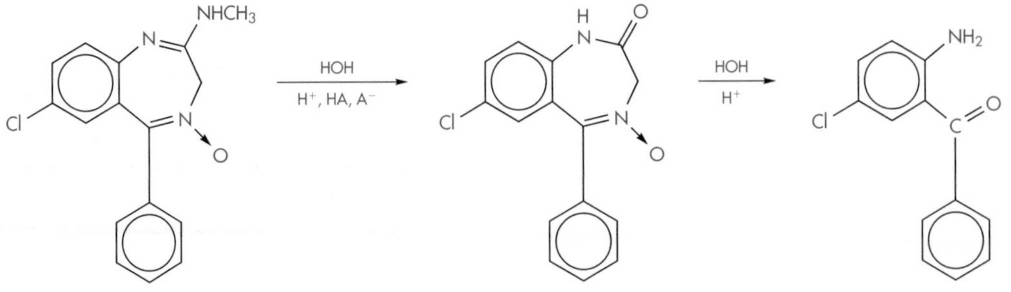

Scheme 4.14 Decomposition scheme for chlordiazepoxide. The neutral or cationic chlordiazepoxide (**IX** or **IXH+**) is transformed to the lactam (**X**) and, finally, in acidic solutions, to the yellow benzophenone (**XI**).
Reproduced from H. V. Maudling et al., J. Pharm. Sci., 64, 278 (1975).

It is convenient to divide single component systems into two categories: those solids that decompose to a solid product and a gas, and those that decompose to give a liquid and a gas.

Solids that decompose to give a solid and a gas

An example of this category is *p*-aminosalicylic acid, which decomposes to a solid (*p*-aminophenol) and a gas (carbon dioxide):

$$NH_2C_6H_3(OH)COOH \rightarrow$$
$$NH_2C_6H_4OH + CO_2$$

The decomposition curves which result from such a reaction show either (a) an initial rapid decomposition followed by a more gradual decomposition rate, or (b) an initial lag period, giving a sigmoidal appearance. The shape produced by (a) can usually be accounted for by *topochemical* (or contracting geometry) reactions and that produced in (*b*) by *nucleation* theories.

The model used in the treatment of topochemical decomposition is that of a cylinder or sphere (Fig. 4.4), in which it is assumed that the radius of the intact chemical substance decreases linearly with time. For the contracting cylinder model, the mole fraction *x* decomposed at time *t* is given by

$$(1 - x)^{1/2} = 1 - \frac{k}{r_0}t \tag{4.41}$$

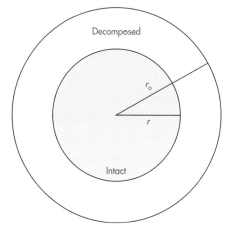

Figure 4.4 Model of a sphere or a cylinder used in theoretical treatment of topochemical reactions.
Reproduced from J. T. Carstensen, *J. Pharm. Sci.*, **63**, 1 (1974).

For the contracting sphere model,

$$(1 - x)^{1/3} = 1 - \frac{k}{r_0}t \tag{4.42}$$

There are a few pharmaceutical examples of compounds that decompose by topochemical reaction. Thus, the decomposition of aspirin at elevated temperatures has been shown to conform to equation (4.41) (Fig. 4.5).

A similarity between equations (4.41) and (4.42) and the first-order rate equations was pointed out by Carstensen,[13] who suggested that this similarity might account for the fact that many decompositions in solid dosage forms appear to follow first-order kinetics.

The sigmoidal decomposition curves can be interpreted using the Prout and Tompkins model. This model assumes that the decomposition is governed by the formation and growth of active nuclei which occur on the surface as well as inside the crystals. The formation of product molecules sets up further strains in the crystal since the surface array of product molecules has a different unit cell from the original substance. The strains are relieved by the formation of cracks. Reaction takes place at the mouth of these cracks owing to lattice imperfections and spreads down into the crevices. Decomposition on these surfaces produces further cracking and so the chain reaction spreads.

The equation proposed to describe decomposition by this process is of the form

$$\ln\left[\frac{x}{(1-x)}\right] = \frac{k}{r_0}t + C \tag{4.43}$$

where *C* is a lag-time term.

The decomposition curves of *p*-aminosalicylic acid are sigmoidal (see Fig. 4.6) and linear plots are produced when the data are plotted according to equation (4.43). Stability measurements made inadvertently in the lag periods of this type of decomposition would suggest zero-order kinetics.

Solids that decompose to give a liquid and a gas

An example of a solid in this category is *p*-aminobenzoic acid, which decomposes into aniline and carbon dioxide. Decomposition

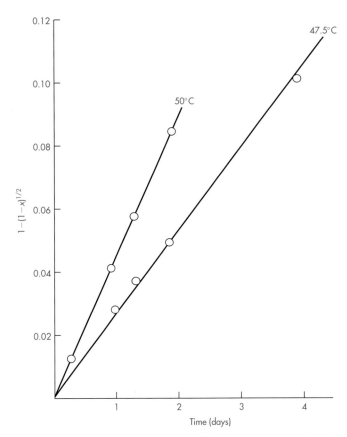

Figure 4.5   Decomposition of aspirin at elevated temperatures in tablets containing sodium bicarbonate plotted according to equation (4.41).

Reproduced from E. Nelson *et al.*, *J. Pharm. Sci.*, 63, 755 (1974) with permission.

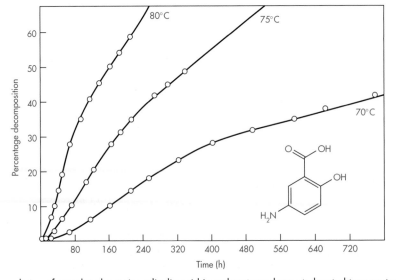

Figure 4.6   Degradation of powdered *p*-aminosalicylic acid in a dry atmosphere at elevated temperatures.

Reproduced from S. S. Kornblum and B. J. Sciarrone, *J. Pharm. Sci.*, 53, 935 (1964) with permission.

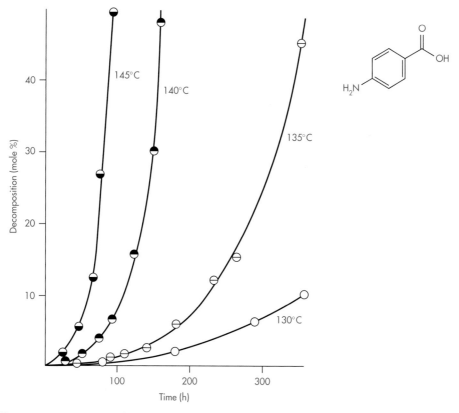

Figure 4.7 Decomposition curves of p-aminobenzoic acid.
Reproduced from J. T. Carstensen and M. N. Musa, J. Pharm. Sci., 61, 1113 (1972).

causes a layer of liquid to form around the solid which dissolves the solid. The decomposition curves show an initial lag period (Fig. 4.7), which corresponds to the establishment of the liquid layer. Beyond this region, the plot represents the first-order decomposition of the solid in solution in its liquid decomposition products. There are thus two rate constants, that for the initial decomposition of the solid itself, and that for the decomposition of the solid in solution.

4.4 Factors influencing drug stability

Before we can suggest ways in which we might prevent the decomposition of drugs, we should first consider the various factors that accelerate the decomposition processes. For convenience we will consider liquid and solid dosage forms separately, although, as we will see, there are similarities in the influence of several factors on drug breakdown in both.

4.4.1 Liquid dosage forms

pH

pH is perhaps the most important parameter which affects the hydrolysis rate of drugs in liquid formulations; it is certainly the one which has been most widely examined.

Studying the influence of pH on degradation rate is not as simple as might at first be imagined. If the hydrolysis rate of the drug in a series of solutions buffered to the required pH is measured and the hydrolytic rate constant is then plotted as a function of pH, a pH–rate profile will be produced, but this will almost certainly be influenced by the buffers used to prepare the solutions. It is probable that a different pH–rate profile would be obtained using a different buffer. To understand why this should be, we have to consider not only the catalytic effect of hydrogen and hydroxyl ions, which is called *specific acid–base catalysis*, but also the possible accelerating effect of the components of the buffer system, which we refer to as *general acid–base catalysis*. These two types of acid–base catalysis can be combined together in a general expression as follows:

$$k_{obs} = k_0 + k_{H^+}[H^+] + k_{OH^-}[OH^-]$$
$$+ k_{HX}[HX] + k_{X^-}[X^-] \qquad (4.44)$$

In this equation, k_{obs} is the experimentally determined hydrolytic rate constant, k_0 is the uncatalysed or solvent catalysed rate constant, k_{H^+} and k_{OH^-} are the specific acid- and base-catalysis rate constants respectively, k_{HX} and k_{X^-} are the general acid- and base-catalysis rate constants respectively, and [HX] and [X$^-$] denote the concentrations of protonated and unprotonated forms of the buffer.

For a complete evaluation of the stability of the drug, we need to evaluate the catalytic coefficients for specific acid and base catalysis and also to determine the catalytic coefficients of possible buffers which we might wish to use in the formulation.

First we will examine how to achieve a buffer-independent pH–rate profile, since this will show us at which pH the stability is greatest. By way of illustration we can consider a specific example of a stability study which has been reported for the antihypertensive vasodilator ciclosidomine. Experiments carried out at constant temperature and constant ionic strength using a series of different buffers over the pH range 3–6 produced the graphs shown in Fig. 4.8. These plots show that an increase of buffer concentration, particularly at pH 3, had a marked effect on the hydrolysis rate. The effect of the phosphate buffer on this system became less pronounced with increase of pH and was found to have a negligible effect above pH 7.5.

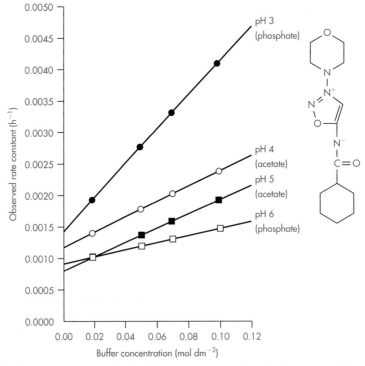

Figure 4.8   Effect of buffer concentration on the hydrolytic rate constant for ciclosidomine at 60°C as a function of pH.
Reproduced from C. F. Carney, *J. Pharm. Sci.*, **76**, 393 (1987) with permission.

To remove the influence of the buffer, the reaction rate should be measured at a series of buffer concentrations at each pH and the data extrapolated back to zero concentration as shown in Fig. 4.8. If these extrapolated rate constants are plotted as a function of pH, the required buffer-independent pH–rate profile will be obtained. Figure 4.9 illustrates the simple type of pH–rate profile which is obtained with codeine sulfate.

As we can see from Fig. 4.9, this drug is very stable in unbuffered solution over a wide pH range but degrades relatively rapidly in the presence of strong acids or bases. Since the influence of buffer components has been removed, this plot allows us to calculate the rate constants for specific acid and base catalysis. Removing the terms for the effect of buffer from equation (4.44), we have

$$k_{obs} = k_0 + k_{H^+}[H^+] + k_{OH^-}[OH^-] \qquad (4.45)$$

and consequently a plot of measured rate constant k_{obs} against the hydrogen ion concentration $[H^+]$ at low pH will have a gradient equal to the rate constant for acid catalysis. Similarly, of course, if we plot k_{obs} against

[OH⁻] at high pH, the gradient will be the rate constant for base-catalysed hydrolysis. Example 4.4 illustrates the calculation of these catalytic coefficients.

• •

EXAMPLE 4.4 Calculation of rate constants for base-catalysed hydrolysis

The following data were obtained for the hydrolytic rate constant, k_{obs} of codeine sulfate in aqueous buffer-free solution at 80°C

$10^7 k_{obs}$ (s⁻¹)	5.50	4.40	2.30	1.25	0.70
pH	11.63	11.53	11.23	10.93	10.63

Determine graphically (a) the catalytic coefficient for base-catalysis, k_{OH^-}, and also (b) the coefficient for solvent catalysis, k_0.

Answer
At high pH,

$$k_{obs} = k_0 + k_{OH^-}[OH^-]$$

where $[OH^-]$ is calculated from

$$p[OH^-] = -\log[OH^-] = 12.63 - pH$$

(Note: $pK_w = 12.63$ at 80°C.)

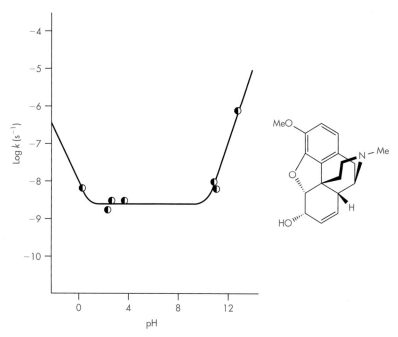

Figure 4.9 Log rate–pH profile for the degradation of codeine sulfate in buffer-free solutions at 60°C.
Reproduced from M. F. Powell, *J. Pharm. Sci.*, 75, 901 (1986) with permission.

A plot of k_{obs} against $[OH^-]$ has a gradient of k_{OH^-} and an intercept of k_0.

From a graph of the above data,

$$k_0 = 2.0 \times 10^{-8}\,s^{-1}$$

$$k_{OH^-} = 5.2 \times 10^{-6}(mol\,dm^{-3})^{-1}\,s^{-1}$$

• •

The degradation of codeine is particularly susceptible to the effects of buffers. Its hydrolysis rate in $0.05\,mol\,dm^{-3}$ phosphate buffer at pH 7 is almost 20 times faster than in unbuffered solution at this pH, so this is a good drug to use as an example of the determination of the influence of buffer components on the breakdown rate.

In phosphate buffers of neutral pH, the major buffer species are $H_2PO_4^-$ and HPO_4^{2-}, either of which may act as a catalyst for codeine degradation. To find out which of these is the stronger catalyst, we can treat the experimental data in the following way. In neutral pH solutions we can write the following expression for the observed rate constant,

$$k_{obs} = k_0 + k_{H_2PO_4^-}[H_2PO_4^-] + k_{HPO_4^{2-}}[HPO_4^{2-}]$$
(4.46)

or

$$k_{obs} = k_0 + k'B_T$$

where $k_{H_2PO_4^-}$ and $k_{HPO_4^{2-}}$ are the rate constants for catalysis by $H_2PO_4^-$ and HPO_4^{2-} ions respectively, and B_T is the total concentration of phosphate buffer. Notice that the terms for specific acid- and base-catalysis have little effect at this pH and we need not consider them in this treatment.

From equation (4.46), a plot of k_{obs} against B_T will have an intercept k_0 and a gradient k'. To find values for the catalytic coefficients, we rearrange the equation into the following linear form:

$$k' = \frac{(k_{obs} - k_0)}{B_T} = \frac{k_{H_2PO_4^-}[H_2PO_4^-]}{B_T}$$
$$+ k_{HPO_4^{2-}}\left(\frac{B_T - [H_2PO_4^-]}{B_T}\right)$$
(4.47)

We can now see that a second plot of the apparent rate constant k' against the fraction of the acid buffer component present, i.e.

$[H_2PO_4^-/B_T]$, will have an intercept at $[H_2PO_4^-/B_T] = 0$ equal to $k_{HPO_4^{2-}}$. Furthermore, the k' value at $[H_2PO_4^-/B_T] = 1$ is the other catalytic coefficient, $k_{H_2PO_4^-}$.

• •

EXAMPLE 4.5 Calculation of the catalytic coefficients for buffer species

The following data were obtained for the hydrolytic rate constant k of codeine sulfate at 100°C in phosphate buffers of varying total concentration B_T at pH values of 6 and 8:

B_T (mol dm^{-3})	0.03	0.06	0.09	0.12
$10^7 k$ (s^{-1}) at pH 6	6.1	11.2	16.3	21.4
$10^7 k$ (s^{-1}) at pH 8	12.9	25.0	37.0	49.0

If the fraction of $[H_2PO_4^-]$ present in buffer solutions at pH 6 is 0.74 and at pH 8 is 0.23, determine graphically the catalytic coefficients for the buffer species (a) $H_2PO_4^-$ and (b) HPO_4^{2-}.

Answer

From equation (4.46), a plot of k_{obs} against B_T has an intercept k_0 and a gradient k'. Therefore plot k_{obs} against B_T from the given data at each pH and measure the gradient of the graph.

From the graph:

$$k' \text{ at pH 6} = 1.7 \times 10^{-5}\,(mol\,dm^{-3})^{-1}\,s^{-1}$$
$$k' \text{ at pH 8} = 4.0 \times 10^{-5}\,(mol\,dm^{-3})^{-1}\,s^{-1}$$

From equation (4.47), a plot of k' against the fraction of acidic buffer component, $[H_2PO_4^-]/B_T$, has an intercept of $k_{HPO_4^{2-}}$. Also when $[H_2PO_4^-]/B_T = 1$,

$$k' = k_{H_2PO_4^-}$$

From the graph:

$$k_{HPO_4^{2-}} = 5.1 \times 10^{-5}\,(mol\,dm^{-3})^{-1}\,s^{-1}$$
$$k_{H_2PO_4^-} = 0.5 \times 10^{-5}\,(mol\,dm^{-3})^{-1}\,s^{-1}$$

• •

The relationship between the ability of a buffer component to catalyse hydrolysis, denoted by the catalytic coefficient, k, and its dissociation constant, K, may be expressed by the Brønsted catalysis law as

$$k_A = aK_A^\alpha \quad \text{for a weak acid}$$
(4.48)

and

$$k_B = bK_B^\beta \quad \text{for a weak base} \qquad (4.49)$$

where a, b, α and β are constants characteristic of the solvent and temperature. α and β are positive and vary between 0 and 1.

In our treatment of the degradation of codeine sulfate we have not yet considered any effect which changes in its ionisation might have on its stability. Codeine has a pK_a of 8.2 at 25°C and so its ionisation state will change over the pH range 6–10. With this particular drug, the stability was not affected by any such changes. This is not the case with many drugs, however, and complex pH–rate profiles are often produced because of the differing susceptibility of the unionised and ionised forms of the drug molecule to hydrolysis.

By way of illustration we will look at the case of the hydrolysis of mecillinam (**XII**), which is an antimicrobially active amidopenicillamic acid. This amphoteric drug can exist as a cation, which we can write as MH_2^+, as a zwitterion $MH^\pm$ or as an anion M^-. Figure 4.10 shows the pH–rate profile at zero buffer concentration. The reason this plot is so much more complex than that of codeine sulfate is that each of the species present in solution can undergo specific acid–base catalysis to varying extents and so each contributes to the overall profile shown in Fig. 4.10.

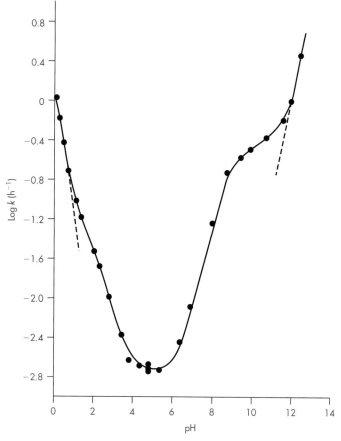

Figure 4.10 Log k–pH profile for the degradation of mecillinam in aqueous solution at 35°C (ionic strength = 0.5 mol kg^{-1}), where k is the apparent first-order rate constant for degradation in buffer-free solutions or in buffers showing no effect on rate of degradation.

Reproduced from C. Larsen and H. Bundgaard, *Arch Pharm. Chem.*, 5, 66 (1977).

Structure XII Mecillinam

The various reactions which are thought to occur are

$$MH_2^+ + H^+ \xrightarrow{k_H} \text{products} \qquad 1$$

$$MH^\pm + H^+ \xrightarrow{k'_H} \text{products} \qquad 2$$

$$MH^\pm + H_2O \xrightarrow{k_0} \text{products} \qquad 3$$

$$MH^\pm + OH^- \xrightarrow{k_{OH}} \text{products} \qquad 4$$

$$M^- + OH^- \xrightarrow{k'_{OH}} \text{products} \qquad 5 \quad (4.50)$$

The part of the pH–rate profile at very low pH (below pH 1.5) is given entirely by reaction (1). This is because the mecillinam exists as the cation MH_2^+, the hydrolysis of which will be acid-catalysed over this pH range. The shoulder in the pH–rate profile at around pH 2 coincides approximately with the first pK_a value of mecillinam and indicates an increased acid-catalysis of the zwitterion relative to the cationic species. The decrease of hydrolysis rate constant with increasing pH up to pH 4 can be explained by assuming that both reactions (1) and (2) are occurring. We can see from Fig. 4.10 that the hydrolysis rate is almost constant between pH 4 and 6, and this suggests that the hydrolysis is water-catalysed (reaction 3) over this pH region. The hydrolysis rate now starts to increase with increasing pH, which indicates that base-catalysis is now the dominating factor. Between pH 6.5 and the pK_a for ionisation of the amidino side-chains ($pK_{a2} = 8.79$), it is reaction (4) which describes the hydrolysis rate. The plot changes slope at around pH 8 because it is affected by the changes which are occurring in the state of ionisation of the amidino side-chain. Above pH 12, the mecillinam exists in solution as the anion and this final part of the graph is described entirely by the base-catalysis of this species (reaction 5).

Even though we may not always be able to explain the pH–rate profile as completely as we can for mecillinam, we can still, of course, choose the pH at which to buffer the drug solution for maximum stability. In the case of mecillinam this would be between pH 4 and 6.

We should also note that the *oxidative degradation* of some drugs in solution may be pH-dependent; for example, the oxidation of prednisolone is base-catalysed. Similarly, the oxidation of morphine occurs more rapidly in alkaline or neutral solution than in acid solution. The reason for this may be the effect of pH on the oxidation–reduction potential, E_0, of the drug.

The *photodegradation* of several drugs is also pH-dependent. For example, the photochemical decomposition of the benzodiazepine derivative midazolam (**XIII**) increases with pH,[15] and ciprofloxacin (**XIV**) is most sensitive to photodegradation at slightly basic pH where the drug is in zwitterionic form, the stability increasing when the pH is lowered to 3–4[16] (Fig. 4.11).

Temperature

Increase in temperature usually causes a very pronounced increase in the hydrolysis rate of

Structure XIII Midazolam

Structure XIV Ciprofloxacin

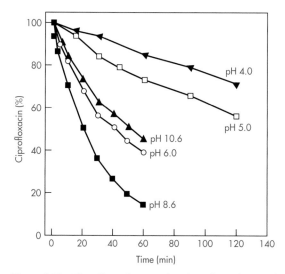

Figure 4.11 The effect of pH on the photodegradation of ciprofloxacin. Radiation source: mercury lamp at wavelength of 313 nm.

Reproduced from K. Torniainen, S. Tammilehto and V. Ulvi, *Int. J. Pharm.*, 132, 53 (1996).

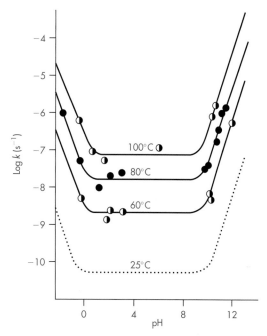

Figure 4.12 Log rate–pH profiles for the degradation of codeine sulfate in buffer-free solutions at several temperatures. The dashed line is the log rate–pH profile calculated from the Arrhenius equation.

Reproduced from M. F. Powell, *J. Pharm. Sci.*, 75, 901 (1986).

drugs in solution, a fact which is used to good effect in the experimental studies of drug stability described above. Such studies are usually carried out at high temperatures, say 60 or 80°C, because the hydrolysis rate is greater at these temperatures and can therefore be measured more easily. Of course, if a formulation has to be heat sterilized then its stability will, in any case, have to be measured at elevated temperatures. Figure 4.12 shows the pH–rate profiles for the degradation of codeine sulfate at several temperatures and also the calculated values at 25°C. We will now see how these calculated values can be obtained.

The equation which describes the effect of temperature on decomposition, and which shows us how to calculate the rate of breakdown at room temperature from measurements at much higher temperatures, is the *Arrhenius equation*.

$$\log k = \log A - \frac{E_a}{2.303RT} \tag{4.51}$$

In this equation, E_a is the activation energy, that is the energy barrier which has to be overcome if reaction is going to occur when two

reactant molecules collide. A is the frequency factor and this is assumed to be independent of temperature for a given reaction. R is the gas constant (8.314 J mol^{-1} K^{-1}) and T is the temperature in kelvins. We can see from equation (4.51) that a plot of the log of the rate constant k against the reciprocal of the temperature should be linear with a gradient of $-E_a/2.303R$. Therefore, assuming that there is not a change in the order of the reaction as the temperature is changed, we can extrapolate plots of log k against $1/T$ to any required temperature and so determine the rate of breakdown at that temperature. We can also, of course, calculate the activation energy from the gradient of this plot. Figure 4.13 shows Arrhenius plots for the breakdown of the drug ciclosidomine at several pH values.

When it is clear from stability determinations that a drug is particularly unstable at room temperature, then of course it will need to be labelled with instructions to store in a cool place. This is the case, for example, with

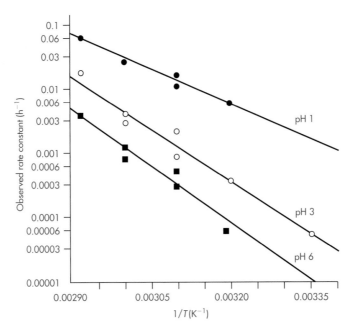

Figure 4.13 Arrhenius plots for the hydrolysis of ciclosidomine in buffer solutions at several pH values.
Reproduced from C. F. Carney, *J. Pharm. Sci.*, 76, 393 (1987).

injections of penicillin, insulin, oxytocin and vasopressin.

• •

EXAMPLE 4.6 Calculation using the Arrhenius equation

The following values were determined for the specific acid-catalytic constants k_{H^+} for an anti-inflammatory drug:

Temp (°C)	95	90	85	75	65
$10^3 k_{H^+}$ (mol dm^{-3})$^{-1}$ s^{-1}	8.15	4.85	2.76	1.02	0.29

Determine graphically (a) the rate constant for acid-catalysis at 25°C, (b) the activation energy.

Answer

According to the Arrhenius equation, a plot of $\log k$ against $1/T$ has a gradient of $-E_a/2.303R$. From the graph:

(a) At $1/T = 3.356 \times 10^{-3}$ K^{-1}, $\log k = -5.85$. Therefore, k at 25°C $= 1.41 \times 10^{-6}$ (mol dm^{-3})$^{-1}$ s^{-1}.
(b) Gradient $= -5.91 \times 10^3$ K. Therefore $E_a = 113$ kJ mol^{-1}.

• •

Ionic strength

We often need to add electrolytes to drug solutions, for example to control their tonicity. Consequently we must pay particular attention to any effect they may have on stability. In fact, the stability experiments that we considered earlier in this section should all be carried out at constant electrolyte concentration to avoid any confusion arising from possible differences in electrolyte effects between different systems.

The equation which describes the influence of electrolyte on the rate constant is the *Brønsted–Bjerrum equation*,

$$\log k = \log k_0 + 2A z_A z_B \mu^{1/2} \qquad (4.52)$$

In this equation, z_A and z_B are the charge numbers of the two interacting ions and A is a constant for a given solvent and temperature (see equation 3.36). μ is the ionic strength of the solution, which we can calculate from

$$\mu = \tfrac{1}{2} \Sigma (mz^2) = \tfrac{1}{2}(m_A z_A^2 + m_B z_B^2 + \cdots) \quad (4.53)$$

For example, if we have a monovalent drug ion of concentration 0.01 mol kg^{-1} in the presence of 0.001 mol kg^{-1} of Ca^{2+} ions then the ionic strength of the solution will be

$$\mu = \tfrac{1}{2}[(0.01 \times 1^2) + (0.001 \times 2^2)]$$
$$= 0.007 \text{ mol kg}^{-1}$$

If the drug ion and the electrolyte ion are both monovalent, then the ionic strength will be equal to the total molality of the solution.

We can see from equation (4.52) that if we determine the rate constant of a reaction in the presence of a series of different concentrations of the same electrolyte and plot log k against $\mu^{1/2}$, then the plot should be linear with an intercept of log k_0 and a gradient of $2Az_A z_B$. This is frequently found to be the case even in solutions of high ionic strength, although equation (4.52) is strictly valid only for ionic strengths of less than 0.01 mol kg^{-1}. At higher ionic strengths (up to about 0.1 mol kg^{-1}) it is preferable to use a modified form of the Brønsted–Bjerrum equation in which we plot log k against $\mu^{1/2}/(1 + \mu^{1/2})$:

$$\log k = \log k_0 + 2Az_A z_B \left[\frac{\mu^{1/2}}{(1 + \mu^{1/2})} \right] \quad (4.54)$$

Figure 4.14 shows the degradation of phentolamine hydrochloride at two different pH values plotted according to equation (4.54). The gradients of these plots should be proportional to the product of the charge carried by the reactive species. Whether the gradient is positive or negative depends on the reaction involved. Reactions between ions of similar charge, for example the acid-catalysed hydrolysis of a cationic drug ion, will produce plots of positive slope (i.e. the reaction rate will be increased by electrolyte addition), whereas the base-catalysed hydrolysis of positively charged drug species will produce negative gradients. Investigations of the influence of ionic strength on reaction rate may therefore be used to provide confirmation of the type of reaction which is occurring. For example, the gradients of the two plots of Fig. 4.14 are 0.260 and –1.759 at pH 3.1 and 7.2 respectively. Since the value of $2A$ at 90°C is 1.174, we can calculate values of the product $z_A z_B$ as 0.221 and 1.498 at pH 3.1 and 7.2 respectively. These values are not integers as they should be if the reactions involved were simple acid- and base-catalysed reactions. This has been explained by suggesting complex reactions between the buffer species and the phentolamine at each pH.

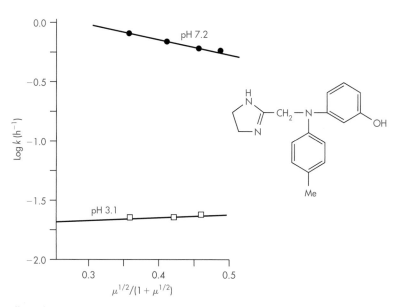

Figure 4.14 The effect of ionic strength, μ, on the hydrolytic rate constant, k, for phentolamine hydrochloride in buffer solutions of pH 3.1 and 7.2 at 90°C.

EXAMPLE 4.7 Calculation using the Brønsted–Bjerrum equation

The following values of the rate constant, k, were obtained at 60°C for the hydrolysis of penicillin in phosphate buffer at pH 8.8 in a series of solutions of varying ionic strength, μ:

$k (h^{-1})$	0.078	0.068	0.056	0.049
μ (mol kg^{-1})	0.49	0.38	0.27	0.20

Plot the data in accordance with the modified Brønsted-Bjerrum equation (equation (4.54)) and determine the gradient of the plot. Comment on whether this value would be expected for the acid-catalysis of the protonated penicillin ion. (Note: Assume a value of unity for A at this temperature.)

Answer
The gradient of the plot of $\log k$ against $\mu^{1/2}/(1 + \mu^{1/2})$ is +2.0. As expected for a reaction between ions of like charge (acid and protonated penicillin ion), the gradient is positive.

Solvent effects

Since we are considering the hydrolysis of drugs it might seem that an obvious way to reduce the breakdown would be to replace some or all of the water in the system with a solvent such as alcohol or propylene glycol. As we will see in this section, however, this is effective only in certain systems and in others it can, in fact, increase the rate of breakdown. The equation that allows us to predict the effect of the solvent on the hydrolysis rate is

$$\log k = \log k_{\varepsilon = \infty} - \frac{Kz_A z_B}{\varepsilon} \qquad (4.55)$$

In this equation, K is a constant for a given system at a given temperature. We can see that a plot of $\log k$ as a function of the reciprocal of the dielectric constant, ε, of the solvent should be linear with a gradient of magnitude $Kz_A z_B$ and an intercept equal to the logarithm of the rate constant in a theoretical solvent of infinite dielectric constant. If the charges on the drug ion and the interacting species are the same, then we can see that the gradient of the line will be negative. In this case, if we replace the water with a solvent of lower dielectric constant then we will achieve the desired effect of reducing the reaction rate. If the drug ion and the interacting ion are of opposite signs, however, then the slope will be positive and the choice of a nonpolar solvent will only result in an increase of decomposition.

Oxygen

Since molecular oxygen is involved in many oxidation schemes, we could use oxygen as a challenge to find out whether a particular drug is likely to be affected by oxidative breakdown. We would do this by storing solutions of the drug in ampoules purged with oxygen and then comparing their rate of breakdown with similar solutions stored under nitrogen. Formulations that are shown to be susceptible to oxidation can be stabilized by replacing the oxygen in the storage containers with nitrogen or carbon dioxide, by avoiding contact with heavy metal ions, and by adding antioxidants (see section 4.1.2).

Light

Photolabile drugs are usually stored in containers which exclude ultraviolet light, since exposure to light in this wavelength range is the most usual cause of photodegradation (see section 4.1.4) Amber glass is particularly effective in this respect because it excludes light of wavelength of less than about 470 nm. As an added precaution, it is always advisable to store photolabile drugs in the dark.

Surfactants

As might be expected, the presence of surfactants in micellar form has a modifying effect on the rate of hydrolysis of drugs. The magnitude of the effect depends on the difference in the rate constant when the drug is in aqueous solution and when it is solubilised within the micelle, and also on the extent of solubilisation. Thus,

$$k_{obs} = k_m f_m + k_w f_w \qquad (4.56)$$

where k_{obs}, k_m and k_w are the observed, micellar and aqueous rate constants, respectively, and f_m and f_w are the fractions of drug associated with the micelles and aqueous phase, respectively. The value of k_m is dependent on the location of the drug within the micelle. A solubilisate may be incorporated into the micelle in a variety of locations. Nonpolar compounds are thought to be solubilised within the lipophilic core and, as such, are likely to be more effectively removed from the attacking species than those compounds that are located close to the micellar surface. Where the drug is located near to the micellar surface, and therefore still susceptible to attack, the ionic nature of the surfactant is an important influence on decomposition rate. For base-catalysed hydrolysis, solubilisation into anionic micelles affords an effective stabilisation due to repulsion of OH^- by the micelles. Conversely, solubilisation into cationic micelles might be expected to cause an enhanced base-catalysed hydrolysis.

Many drugs associate to form micelles in aqueous solution (see section 6.3) and several studies have been reported of the effect of this self-association on stability. In micellar solutions of benzylpenicillin (500 000 units cm^{-3}) the apparent rate of the hydrogen-ion-catalysed degradation was increased twofold, but that of water- and hydroxide-ion-catalysed hydrolysis was decreased twofold to threefold.[17] Consequently, the pH profile was shifted to higher pH values and the pH of minimum degradation was found to be 7.0 compared to 6.5 for monomeric solution (8000 units cm^{-3}). When compared at the respective pH–rate profile minima, micellar benzylpenicillin was reported to be 2.5 times as stable as the monomeric solutions under conditions of constant pH and ionic strength.

or cream base used in the formulation. Hydrocortisone in a series of commercially available bases exhibits maximum decomposition in polyethylene glycol base.[18, 19] The reported shelf-life was only 6 months in this base, which makes manufacture on a commercial basis an unreasonable proposition, considering the length of time involved in distribution of the drug from wholesaler to patient.

Not only should possible stability problems be borne in mind in the choice of ointment base at the formulation stage, but also similar care should be exercised if the ointment is diluted at a later stage. Such dilution is, unfortunately, common practice in cases where the practitioner wishes to reduce the potency of highly active topical preparations, particularly steroids. The pharmaceutical and biopharmaceutical dangers of this procedure have been stressed.[20] Of particular interest here are the problems of drug stability which can occur through the use of unsuitable diluents. An example has been cited of the dilution of betamethasone valerate cream with a cream base having a neutral to alkaline pH. Under such conditions, conversion of the 17-ester to the less-active betamethasone 21-ester can occur. Similarly, diluents containing oxidising agents could cause chemical degradation of fluocinolone acetate to less-active compounds.

Incorporation of drugs into gel structures frequently leads to a change in their stability, such as increased degradation of benzylpenicillin sodium in hydrogels of various natural and semisynthetic polymers.[21] At pH 6 in Carbopol hydrogels, the percentage of undecomposed pilocarpine at equilibrium is a simple function of the apparent viscosity of the medium.[22] The rate constant for degradation was not, however, significantly affected by changes in viscosity. Little influence of viscosity on the rate of oxidation of ascorbic acid in solutions of gels of Polysorbate 80 has been noted.[23]

4.4.2 Semisolid dosage forms

The chemical stability of active ingredients incorporated into ointments or creams is frequently dependent on the nature of the ointment

4.4.3 Solid dosage forms

Moisture

Water-soluble drugs present in a solid dosage form will dissolve in any moisture which has adsorbed on the solid surface. The drug will now be in an aqueous environment and its decomposition could be influenced by many of the factors which we have already discussed when dealing with liquid dosage forms. For example, decomposition could now occur by hydrolytic cleavage of ester or amide linkages in the drug molecule and hence will be affected by the pH of the adsorbed moisture film. It is not surprising, therefore, that moisture is considered to be one of the most important factors that must be controlled in order to minimise decomposition.

We can get an idea of the extent to which moisture adsorption affects stability from the results shown in Fig. 4.15. We can see from this figure that an increase in the water vapour pressure (and therefore an increase in the amount of moisture associated with the drug) greatly increases the percentage decomposition at any given time. The problem is even more pronounced with drugs which are hygroscopic or which decompose to give hygroscopic products. In such cases it is worth trying to prepare a less hygroscopic salt of the drug.

In all cases it is important to minimise access of moisture during manufacture and storage. The correct selection of packaging is obviously important, although this is not as straightforward as you might at first think. For example, tablets containing a water-labile drug were found to be more stable in a water-permeable blister package at 50°C than in a sealed glass bottle and yet the situation was reversed at room temperature and 70% relative humidity.[24] The reason for this behaviour was attributed to the loss of considerable amounts of water through the film at 50°C, so improving stability, and the reverse diffusion at room temperature, so decreasing stability.

Excipients

One of the main ways in which the excipients of the solid dosage form can affect the degradation of drugs is by increasing the moisture content of the preparation. Excipients such as starch and povidone have particularly high water contents (povidone contains about 28% equilibrium moisture at 75% relative humidity). However, whether this high moisture

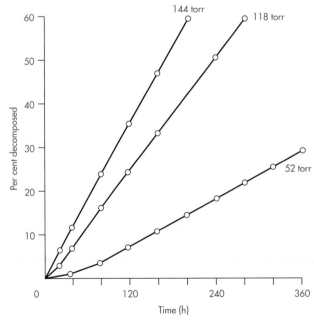

Figure 4.15 The effect of water vapour pressure on the decomposition of aminosalicylic acid.
Reproduced from S. S. Kornblum and B. J. Sciarrone, *J. Pharm. Sci.*, 53, 935 (1964).

level has an effect on stability depends on how strongly it is bound and whether the moisture can come into contact with the drug. Magnesium trisilicate causes increased hydrolysis of aspirin in tablet form because, it is thought, of its high water content.

Many examples of the effects of tablet excipients on drug decompositions are reported in the pharmaceutical literature. Chemical interaction between components in solid dosage forms may lead to increased decomposition. Replacement of the phenacetin in compound codeine and APC tablets by paracetamol in NHS formulations in Australia in the 1960s (because of the undesirable side-effects of phenacetin), led to an unexpected decreased stability of the tablets. The cause was later attributed to a transacetylation reaction between aspirin and paracetamol and also a possible direct hydrolysis of the paracetamol (Scheme 4.15).

Figure 4.16 shows the increased generation of free salicylic acid at 37°C in the tablets containing paracetamol. It is interesting to note from this figure the effect on stability of tablet excipients. Addition of 1% talc caused only a minimal increase in the decomposition, while 0.5% magnesium stearate increased the breakdown rate dramatically.

Other studies on the influence of tablet excipients on drug decomposition have identified problems with stearate salts and it has been suggested that these salts should be avoided as tablet lubricants if the active component is subject to hydroxide-ion-catalysed degradation. The degradative effect of the alkali stearates is inhibited in the presence of malic, hexamic or maleic acids owing, it is thought, to competition for the lubricant cation between the drug and the additive acid.

The base used in the formulation of suppositories can often affect the rate of decomposition of the active ingredients. Aspirin decomposes in several polyoxyethylene glycols which are often incorporated into suppository bases.[25] Degradation was shown to be due in part to transesterification, giving the decomposition products salicylic acid and acetylated polyethylene glycol. The rate of decomposition, which followed pseudo first-order kinetics, was considerably greater than when a fatty base such as cocoa butter was used.[26] Analysis of commercial batches of 100 mg indometacin–polyethylene glycol

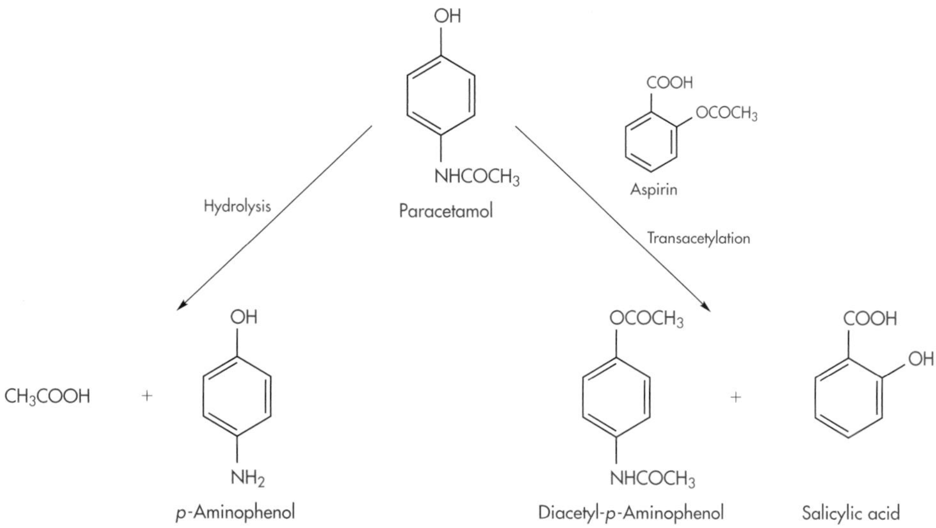

Scheme 4.15 Reactions showing the postulated transacetylation between aspirin and paracetamol and the direct hydrolysis of paracetamol.
Reproduced from B. G. Boggianno et al., Aust. J. Pharm., 51, S14 (1970).

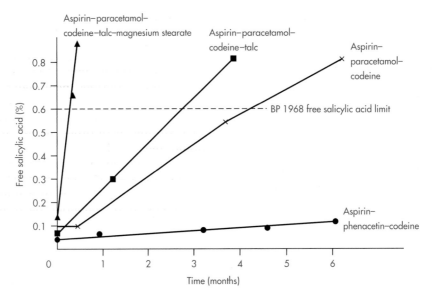

Figure 4.16 Development of free salicylic acid in aspirin–paracetamol–codeine and aspirin–phenacetin–codeine tablets at 37°C.
Reproduced from B. G. Boggianno et al., Aust. J. Pharm., 51, S14 (1970).

suppositories[27] showed that approximately 2%, 3.5% and 4.5% of the original amount of indometacin was esterified with polyoxyethylene glycol 300 (**XV**) after storage times of 1, 2 and 3 years, respectively.

Excipients present in tablet formulations can have an impact on the photostability of the product, the effect arising in many cases from impurities present in the excipients.[8] For example, free radical reactions involving phenolic impurities in tablet binding agents such as povidone, disintegrants such as crospovidone and viscosity-modifying agents such as alginates can lead to photodegradation. Similarly, coloured products may be formed by the reaction of aldehydes formed during spray-drying or autoclaving of lactose with primary amine groups in the product.

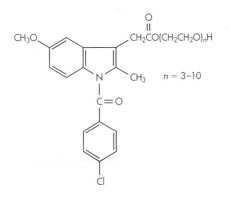

Structure XV Polyethylene glycol esters of indometacin identified in stored suppositories (n = number of ethylene oxide units)

Temperature

The effect of temperature change on the stability of solid dosage forms can be complicated for many possible reasons. The drug or one of the excipients may, for example, melt or change its polymorphic form as temperature is increased, or it may contain loosely bound water which is lost at higher temperatures. We should also remember that the relative humidity will change with temperature and so we must take care to keep this at a constant value.

Despite these possible complications, many authors have found that the effect of temperature on decomposition rate can be described by an Arrhenius-type equation; i.e. plots of log k against $1/T$ are linear. This then enables the stability to be predicted at room temperature from measurements made at elevated temperatures. Also, of course, we can calculate an apparent activation energy, E_a, from the gradient of the plots, but we must remember that this does not have the same meaning as the activation energy for reactions in solution. The E_a value in the solid state is affected, for example, by changes not only in the solubility of the drug in the moisture layer but also in the intrinsic rate of reaction. We cannot, however, use the Arrhenius equation in cases where decomposition shows an approach to equilibrium. Examples of such systems include vitamin A in gelatin beadlets and vitamin E in lactose base tablets. In these cases we can often use the van't Hoff equation to describe the effect of temperature on breakdown. We determine the equilibrium concentrations of products and reactants at a series of temperatures and then plot the logarithm of the equilibrium constant K against the reciprocal of the temperature (see Fig. 4.17) according to the equation

$$\ln K = \frac{-\Delta H}{RT} + \text{constant} \qquad (4.57)$$

Light and oxygen

We have examined above the stability problems which arise with drugs which are susceptible to photodecomposition or oxidation. We will not reconsider them here but merely re-emphasise that we should take all the necessary precautions to exclude light or oxygen when storing these drugs. In this respect we should remember that water contains dissolved oxygen and so the presence of moisture on the surface of solid preparations may increase the oxidation of susceptible drugs; such drugs must, therefore, be stored under dry conditions.

4.5 Stability testing and prediction of shelf-life

It is clearly most important to be able to ensure that a particular formulation when packaged in a specific container will remain within its physical, chemical, microbiological, therapeutic and toxicological specifications

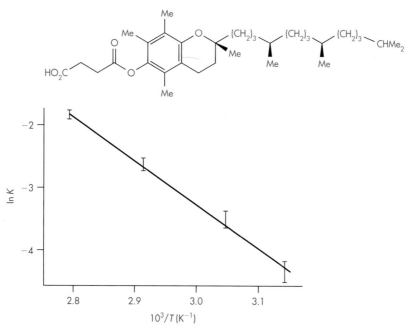

Figure 4.17 Van't Hoff plot for vitamin E succinate decomposition in lactose base tablets.
Reproduced from J. T. Carstensen *et al., J. Pharm. Sci.,* *57,* 23 (1968) with permission.

on storage for a specified time. In order to make such an assurance, we obviously need to conduct a rigorous stability testing programme on the product in the form that is finally to be marketed. Since the testing period can be as long as two years, it has become essential to devise a more rapid technique which can be used during product development to speed up the identification of the most suitable formulation. In this section we shall examine ways of predicting the chemical stability of a formulation during preformulation studies using accelerated storage tests. We will not be considering the toxicological or microbiological studies or the determination of physical stability, all of which are essential elements in the overall stability testing of the formulation but which are outside the scope of this chapter. Although most of this section will be concerned with the prediction of the effect of temperature on drug decomposition, other environmental factors will also be briefly considered.

4.5.1 Effect of temperature on stability

We have already considered the basic method of accelerating the chemical decomposition by raising the temperature of the preparations. We will briefly reconsider essential steps in the process. The order of reaction can be determined by plotting stability data at several elevated temperatures according to the equations relating decomposition to time for each of the orders of reaction, until linear plots are obtained. We can now calculate values of rate constant at each temperature from the gradient of these plots, and plot the logarithm of k against reciprocal temperature according to the Arrhenius equation:

$$\log k = \log A - \frac{E_a}{2.303RT} \qquad (4.58)$$

The required value of k can be interpolated from this plot at room temperature, and the activation energy E_a can be calculated from the gradient, which is $-E_a/2.303R$. Values of E_a are usually within the range 50–96 kJ mol^{-1}.

A convenient, approximate method which is useful for estimation of decomposition rates at room temperature makes use of the ratio of rate constants at room temperature (T_1) and at a higher temperature (T_2). If we subtract the Arrhenius equations at temperatures T_1 and T_2, assuming that the log A term is the same at each temperature, we obtain

$$\log\left[\frac{k_2}{k_1}\right] = -\frac{E_a}{2.303R}\left[\frac{1}{T_2} - \frac{1}{T_1}\right] \qquad (4.59)$$

or

$$\log\left[\frac{k_2}{k_1}\right] = \frac{E_a(T_2 - T_1)}{2.303RT_2T_1} \qquad (4.60)$$

We must, of course, have a value of E_a in order to be able to use these equations for the calculation of the room temperature rate constant k_1. If we only require a rough estimation of k_1 then we can assume a mid-range value of E_a, say 75 kJ mol^{-1}, for these calculations.

• •

EXAMPLE 4.8 Application of the Arrhenius equation

The first-order rate constant for the hydrolysis of sulfacetamide at 120°C is 9×10^{-6} s^{-1} and the activation energy is 94 kJ mol^{-1}. Calculate the rate constant at 25°C.

Answer
Using equation (4.60) with an E_a value of 94 kJ mol^{-1} we have

$$\log\left[\frac{k_{120}}{k_{25}}\right] = \frac{94 \times 10^3 \times (393 - 298)}{2.303 \times 8.314 \times (393 \times 298)}$$

$$= 3.98$$

Removing the logarithms, $k_{120}/k_{25} = 9.55 \times 10^3$. Therefore, $k_{25} = 9 \times 10^{-6}/9.55 \times 10^3 = 9.4 \times 10^{-10}$ s^{-1}.

• •

An alternative method of data treatment is to plot the logarithm of the half-life $t_{0.5}$ as a function of reciprocal temperature. From equation (4.13), $t_{0.5} = 0.693/k$. Therefore,

$$\log k = \log 0.693 - \log t_{0.5} \qquad (4.61)$$

and substituting into equation (4.51) gives

$$\log t_{0.5} = \log 0.693 - \log A + (E_a/2.303RT) \qquad (4.62)$$

Once the rate constant is known at the required storage temperature, it is a simple matter to calculate a shelf-life for the product based on an acceptable degree of decomposition. The equations which we can use for 10% loss of activity are obtained by substituting $x = 0.1a$ in the zero- and first-order equations (equations 4.8 and 4.10), giving

$$t_{0.9} = 0.1\frac{[D]_0}{k_0} \quad \text{(zero order)} \quad (4.63)$$

and

$$t_{0.9} = \frac{0.105}{k_1} \quad \text{(first order)} \quad (4.64)$$

where $[D]_0$ is the initial concentration of drug. Although $t_{0.9}$ is usually used as an estimate of shelf-life, other percentage decompositions may be required, for example when the decomposition products produce discoloration or have undesirable side-effects. The required equations for these may be derived by substituting in the relevant rate equations.

• •

EXAMPLE 4.9 Calculation of shelf-life

The initial concentration of active principle in an aqueous preparation was 5.0×10^{-3} g cm^{-3}. After 20 months the concentration was shown by analysis to be 4.2×10^{-3} g cm^{-3}. The drug is known to be ineffective after it has decomposed to 70% of its original concentration. Assuming that decomposition follows first-order kinetics, calculate the expiry date of the drug preparation.

Answer
Substituting into the first-order equation (equation 4.10)

$k = (2.303/20)\log[(5 \times 10^{-3})/(4.2 \times 10^{-3})]$
$k = 8.719 \times 10^{-3}$ month^{-1}

70% of the initial concentration = 3.5×10^{-3} g cm^{-3}

$t = (2.303/8.719 \times 10^{-3})$
$\quad \times \log[(5 \times 10^{-3})/(3.5 \times 10^{-3})]$
$t = 40.9$ months

The expiry date is thus 40.9 months after initial preparation.

• •

Although accelerated storage testing based on the use of the Arrhenius equation has resulted in a very significant saving of time, it still involves the time-consuming step of the initial determination of the order of reaction for the decomposition. While most investigators have emphasised the need for a knowledge of the exact kinetic pathway of degradation, some have bypassed this initial step by assuming a particular decomposition model. At less than 10% degradation and within the limits of experimental error involved in stability studies, it is not possible to distinguish between zero-, first- or simple second-order kinetics using curve-fitting techniques; consequently, the assumption of first-order kinetics for any decomposition reaction should involve minimum error. In fact, it was shown that there was a linear relationship between the logarithm of $t_{0.9}$ (the time taken for the concentration of the reactant to decompose to 90% of its original value) and the reciprocal temperature, which was independent of the order of reaction for the decomposition of a series of drugs.[28] On the basis of these findings it was suggested that the use of such linear plots to determine $t_{0.9}$ at the required temperature would provide a rapid, and yet sufficiently accurate, means of studying decomposition rate during the development stage.

Even with the modifications suggested above, the method of stability testing based on the Arrhenius equation is still time-consuming, involving as it does the separate determination of rate constants at a series of elevated temperatures. Experimental techniques have been developed[29, 30] which enable the decomposition rate to be determined from a single experiment. Such methods involve raising the temperature of the product in accordance with a predetermined temperature–time programme and are consequently referred to as nonisothermal stability studies.

Any suitable temperature–time programme may be used. In the method of Rogers[25] the rise of temperature was programmed so that the reciprocal of the temperature varied logarithmically with time according to

$$\frac{1}{T_0} - \frac{1}{T_t} = 2.303b \log(1 + t) \quad (4.65)$$

where T_0 and T_t are the temperatures at zero time and at time t, respectively, and b is any suitable proportionality constant. Applying the Arrhenius equation at both temperatures and subtracting gives

$$\log k_t = \log k_0 + \frac{E_a}{2.303R}\left(\frac{1}{T_0} - \frac{1}{T_t}\right) \quad (4.66)$$

Substituting equation (4.65) into equation (4.66) gives

$$\log k_t = \log k_0 + \frac{E_a b}{R} \log(1 + t) \quad (4.67)$$

Therefore,

$$k_t = k_0(1 + t)^{E_a b/R} \quad (4.68)$$

For first-order reactions $-dc/dt = kc$, where c is concentration. Substituting for k from equation (4.68) and integrating gives

$$-\int_{c_0}^{c_t} \frac{dc}{c} = k_0 \int_0^t (1 + t)^{E_a b/R}\, dt \quad (4.69)$$

where c_0 and c_t are the concentrations at zero time and at time t, respectively.

Therefore,

$$\log f(c) = \log k_0 - \log\left(1 + \frac{E_a b}{R}\right) + \left(1 + \frac{E_a b}{R}\right)$$
$$\times \log(1 + t) + \log\left[1 - \left(\frac{k_0}{k_t}\right)^{1 + R/E_a b}\right] \quad (4.70)$$

where

$$f(c) = 2.303 \log \frac{c_0}{c_t} \quad (4.71)$$

A similar equation applies to second-order reactions with

$$\log f(c) = \frac{2.303}{a_0 - b_0} \log \frac{a_t}{b_t} + \frac{2.303}{a_0 - b_0} \log \frac{b_0}{a_0} \quad (4.72)$$

where a_0 and b_0 are the concentrations of the reactants at the beginning of the experiment, and a_t and b_t are their concentrations at time t. The value of the final term of equation (4.70) rapidly tends to zero as k_t becomes greater than k_0. Thus a graph of $\log f(c)$ against $\log(1 + t)$ will be linear from that time after which k_0 is negligible in comparison with k_t. The slope of the line is $(1 + E_a b/R)$, enabling E_a to be determined. The rate constant k_0 may then be calculated from the intercept when $\log(1 + t) = 0$, which is equal to $\log k_0 - \log(1 + E_a b/R)$. The rate constant at any other temperature may be calculated from k_0 and E_a.

• •

EXAMPLE 4.10 Accelerated storage testing using temperature–time programme

In a study of the first-order decomposition of riboflavin in 0.05 mol dm^{-3} NaOH using accelerated storage techniques, the temperature was programmed to rise from 12.5 to 55°C using a programme constant, b, of 2.171×10^{-4} K^{-1}. The initial concentration, c_0, of riboflavin was 10^{-4} mol dm^{-3}, and the concentration c_t remaining at time t was as follows:

t (h)	0.585	0.996	1.512	2.163	2.982	4.013	5.312	6.946
$10^5 c_t$ (mol dm^{-3})	9.881	9.763	9.532	9.109	8.371	6.902	4.931	2.435

Calculate the activation energy and the rate constant at 20°C.

Answer

For first-order reactions the data are plotted according to equations (4.70) and (4.71).

t	$\log(1 + t)$	$\log[2.303 \log(c_0/c_t)]$
0.585	0.2	−1.94
0.996	0.3	−1.62
1.512	0.4	−1.32
2.163	0.5	−1.03
2.982	0.6	−0.75
4.013	0.7	−0.43
5.321	0.8	−0.15
6.946	0.9	+0.15

A plot of $\log[2.303 \log(c_0/c_t)]$ against $\log(1 + t)$ is linear (see Fig. 4.18) with a slope of 2.95. From equation (4.70),

$$\text{Slope} = 1 + \frac{E_a b}{R}$$

Therefore,

$$E_a = (1.95 \times 8.314)/(2.171 \times 10^{-4})$$
$$= 74.68 \text{ kJ mol}^{-1}$$

Intercept at $\log(1 + t) = 0$ is -2.55. From equation (4.70),

$$\text{Intercept} = \log k_0 - \log\left[1 + \frac{E_a b}{R}\right]$$

where the final term on the right of equation (4.70) is neglected.

Therefore,

$$\log k_0 = -2.55 + \log 2.95 = -2.08$$

and

$$k_0 = 0.0083 \text{ h}^{-1}$$

That is, the rate constant at temperature T_0 (12.5°C) is 0.0083 h^{-1}.

The rate constant at 20°C may then be calculated from the Arrhenius equation in the form of equation (4.66):

$$\log k_t = -2.08 + [74\,680/(2.303 \times 8.314)]$$
$$\times [(1/285.5) - (1/293)]$$
$$= -2.08 + 0.3497 = -1.730$$

and

$$k_t = 1.86 \times 10^{-2} \text{ h}^{-1}$$

The rate constant at 20°C is thus 0.0186 h^{-1}.

• •

The advantages of this method over the conventional method of stability testing are that (a) the data required to calculate the stability are obtained in a single one-day experiment rather than from a series of experiments which may last for several weeks; (b) no preliminary experiments are required to determine the optimum temperatures for the accelerated storage test; and (c) the linearity of the plot of $\log f(c)$ against $\log(1 + t)$ confirms that

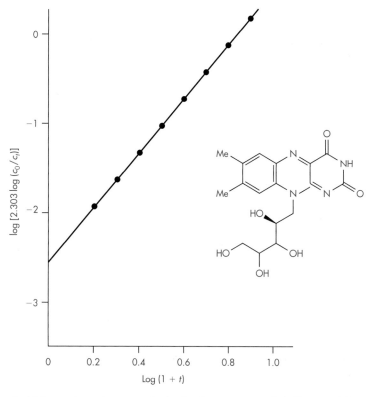

Figure 4.18 Example 4.10: accelerated storage plot for the decomposition of riboflavin in 0.05 mol dm^{-3} NaOH using data from reference 29.

the correct order of reaction has been assumed.

Several improvements on the original non-isothermal stability testing methods have been suggested. Rather than subjecting the drug formulation to a predetermined fixed time–temperature profile, the temperature may be changed during the course of the experiment at a rate consistent with the analytical results from the experiment.[30] The resultant time–temperature data are fitted to a polynomial expression of sufficient degree to describe the changes. This relationship and the experimental data are then combined and utilised to compute a series of degradation pathways corresponding to a series of values of activation energy. The curves are matched with the experimental analytical data to obtain the correct activation energy for the reaction. Using this activation energy and the analytical data, the reaction rate and stability may be calculated. Computational procedures whereby the activation energy and frequency factor of the Arrhenius equation may be determined from simple nonisothermal experiments with a fixed temperature–time profile have been described.[31, 32]

An improvement in the design of stability tests which avoids the difficulties inherent in the nonlinear curve-fitting procedures outlined above has been suggested.[33] The experimental procedure involves changing the temperature of the samples being studied until degradation is rapid enough to proceed at a convenient rate for isothermal studies to be carried out. The analytical information obtained during the nonisothermal and isothermal portions of the experiment is utilised in calculating the activation energy and determining the order of reaction and the reaction rate and predicting stability at any required temperature.

Although accelerated storage testing has proved invaluable in the development of stable formulations, it is important that we consider some of the limitations of this technique. We must take care that the order of reaction is not different at the higher temperatures from that which occurs at room temperature. There are several cases where this might be so. For example, with complex

decomposition processes involving parallel or consecutive reactions, there may be a change in the relative contributions of the component reactions as the temperature is increased.

Suspensions

One complication which arises when we are carrying out stability testing of suspensions is the changes in the solubility of the suspended drug with increase in temperature. With suspensions, the concentration of the drug in solution usually remains constant because, as the decomposition reaction proceeds, more of the drug dissolves to keep the solution saturated. As we have seen, this situation usually leads to zero-order release kinetics. If the actual decomposition of dissolved drug is first-order, then we can express the decrease of concentration, c, with time, t, as

$$-\frac{dc}{dt} = k_0 \qquad (4.73)$$

where $k_0 = k_1 S$ and S is the solubility of the drug.

The problem that arises with these systems is that an increase of temperature causes not only the usual increase in rate constant but also an increase in solubility. Application of the Arrhenius equation to the data involves the measurement of the changes in solubility of the drug over the temperature range involved. An alternative method which does not necessitate the determination of solubility uses the relationship between solubility and temperature:

$$\log S = -\frac{\Delta H_f}{2.303RT} + \text{constant} \qquad (4.74)$$

Since $k_0 = k_1 S$,

$$\log k_0 = \log k_1 + \log S$$

If we substitute for $\log k_1$, using the Arrhenius equation, we obtain

$$\log k_0 = \frac{(-E_a + \Delta H_f)}{2.303RT} + \text{constant} \qquad (4.75)$$

where ΔH_f is the molar heat of fusion. You can now see that we can plot $\log k_0$ against $1/T$

and extrapolate to give a room temperature value of k_0. It is important that we remember that this treatment assumes that drug degradation in solution follows first-order kinetics and that the kinetics are not limited by the dissolution rate.

Solid state

The main problems arising in stability testing of solid dosage forms are[24] (a) that the analytical results tend to have more scatter because tablets and capsules are distinct dosage units rather than the true aliquots encountered with stability studies on drugs in solution, and (b) that these dosage forms are heterogeneous systems often involving a gas phase (air and water vapour), a liquid phase (adsorbed moisture) and the solid phase itself. The compositions of all of these phases can vary during an experiment.

The first of these problems can be overcome by ensuring uniformity of the dosage form before commencing the stability studies. The problems arising from the heterogeneity are more difficult to overcome. The main complicating factor is associated with the presence of moisture. As we have seen in section 4.4.3, moisture can have a significant effect on the kinetics of decomposition and this may produce many experimental problems during stability testing. For example, with gelatin capsules the water in the capsule shell must equilibrate with that in the formulation and surrounding air and this may require an appreciable time. The prediction of stability is difficult in solid dosage forms in which there is chemical interaction between components, or chemical equilibrium phenomena. In fact, the data for stability studies involving the latter are often plotted using a van't Hoff plot rather than an Arrhenius plot.

To reduce some of these problems, particularly those associated with moisture, during stability testing, the following have been suggested:[24] (a) the use of tightly sealed containers, except where the effect of packaging is to be investigated; (b) that the amount of water present in the dosage form should be determined, preferably at each storage

temperature; and (c) that a separate, sealed ampoule should be taken for each assay point and water determination, thus avoiding disturbance of water equilibrium on opening the container.

As has been discussed above, we can often use the Arrhenius equation to predict stability in the solid state, even though the kinetics of breakdown are different from those in solution. The exception to this is when equilibrium reactions occur, in which case we can often use the van't Hoff equation (equation 4.57) to predict room-temperature stability.

4.5.2 Other environmental factors affecting stability

Light

Photostability testing of drug substances usually involves the initial stress testing of the drug to determine its overall photostability and the identification of any degradation products. In this process the sample is irradiated at all absorbing wavelengths using a broad-spectrum light source. Those drugs or formulations which are shown to be photosensitive are then subjected to more formal photostability testing in which they are challenged with light of wavelength comparable to that to which the formulations are exposed in practical situations. During their shelf-life it is most likely that the products will be exposed to fluorescent light, direct daylight and daylight filtered through window glass, and the stability testing procedures are designed to cover these possibilities. A specific protocol for testing the photostability of new drugs and products is described in the ICH Guideline.[34]

Oxygen

The stability of an oxidisable drug in a liquid dosage form is generally a function of the efficiency of any antioxidant included in the formulation. Exaggeration of the effect of oxygen on stability may be achieved by an increase in the partial pressure of oxygen in the system. It is not often easy, however, to make decisions on what would be the normal access of oxygen during storage and a meaningful extrapolation of the acquired data may be difficult.

Moisture content

The stability of solid dosage forms is usually very susceptible to the moisture content of the atmosphere in the container in which they are stored (see section 4.4.3) A linear relationship between log k and the water vapour pressure for vitamin A palmitate beadlets in sugar-coated tablets has been found.[35] Similarly, a linear relationship between the logarithm of the rate constant for the decomposition of nitrazepam in the solid state and the relative humidity has been established (Fig. 4.19). The need for consideration of the effect of moisture on stability has been stressed by Carstensen,[13] who stated that stability programmes should always include samples that have been artificially stressed by addition of moisture. One purpose of a stability programme should be to define the stability of the dosage form as a function of moisture content.

4.5.3   Protocol for stability testing

A recently agreed stability-testing requirement for a Registration Application within the three areas of the EC, Japan and the USA exemplifies the core stability data package required for new drug substances and associated drug products.[36] Under this agreement, information on stability generated in any one of these three areas which meets the appropriate requirements of this guideline is mutually acceptable in both of the other two areas. The following summarises some of the main points of the guideline as it affects the stability testing of both drug substances and drug products; the original document should of course be consulted if a more detailed account is required.

Drug substances

Stability information from accelerated and long-term testing is required to be provided on at least three batches manufactured to a minimum of pilot plant scale by the same synthetic route and using a method of manufacture and

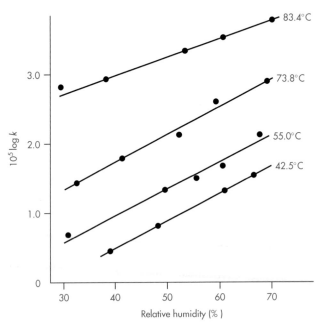

Figure 4.19 Logarithm of the nitrazepam decomposition constant, k, as a function of relative humidity at various temperatures.
Reproduced from D. Genton and U. W. Kesselring, J. Pharm. Sci., 66, 676 (1977) with permission.

procedure that simulates the final process to be used on a manufacturing scale. In this context, 'pilot plant scale' is taken to mean a minimum scale of one tenth that of the full production process. The containers to be used in the long-term evaluation should be the same as, or simulate, the actual packaging used for storage and distribution. The overall quality of the batches of drug substance subjected to stability testing should be representative of both the quality of the material used in preclinical and clinical studies and the quality of material to be made on a manufacturing scale.

The testing should be designed to cover those features susceptible to change during storage and likely to influence quality, safety and/or efficacy, including, as necessary, the physical, chemical and microbiological characteristics. The length of the studies and the storage conditions should be sufficient to cover storage, shipment and subsequent use. The specifications for the long-term testing are a temperature of 25 ± 2°C and 60 ± 5% relative humidity (RH) for a period of 12 months. For accelerated testing the temperature is specified as 40 ± 2°C and RH as 75 ± 5% for a period of 6 months. Other storage conditions are allowable if justified; in particular, temperature-sensitive drugs should be stored at a lower temperature, which then becomes the designated long-term testing temperature. The 6-month accelerated testing should then be carried out at a temperature at least 15°C above this designated temperature together with the relative humidity appropriate to that temperature. Where 'significant change' occurs during the 6-month accelerated storage testing, additional testing at an intermediate temperature (such as 30 ± 2°C/60% ± 5% RH) should be conducted for drug substances to be used in the manufacture of dosage forms tested for long-term stability at 25°C/60% RH. 'Significant change' at 40°C/75% RH or 30°C/60% RH is defined as failure to meet the specification.

The long-term testing is required to be continued for a sufficient period beyond 12 months to cover all appropriate re-test periods. The frequency of testing should be

sufficient to establish the stability characteristics of the drug substance; under the long-term conditions this will normally be every 3 months over the first year, every 6 months over the second year and then annually.

Drug product

The design of the stability programme for the finished product is based on the knowledge of the behaviour and properties of the drug substance and the experience gained from clinical formulation studies and from stability studies on the drug substance. Stability information from long-term and accelerated testing is required to be presented on three batches of the same formulation and dosage form in the containers and closure proposed for marketing. Two of the three batches should be at least pilot scale; the third batch may be smaller, for example 25 000–50 000 tablets or capsules for solid dosage forms. Data on laboratory-scale batches are not acceptable as primary stability information. It is stipulated that the manufacturing process to be used should meaningfully simulate that which would be applied to large-scale batches for marketing and should provide product of the same quality intended for marketing, and meeting the same quality specification as to be applied for release of material. Where possible, batches of the finished product should be manufactured using identifiably different batches of drug substance.

As with the stability testing of drug substance, the testing of the product should cover those features susceptible to change during storage and likely to influence quality, safety and/or efficacy. The range of testing should cover not only chemical and biological stability but also loss of preservative, physical properties and characteristics, organoleptic properties and, where required, microbiological attributes. The conditions and time periods for long-term and accelerated storage testing are the same as those outlined above for drug substances but with special considerations arising from the nature of the drug product. If it is necessary to store the product at a lower temperature because of its heat sensitivity, then consideration should be given to any physical or chemical change in the product which might occur at this temperature; for example, suspensions or emulsions may sediment or cream, while oils and semi-solid preparations may show an increased viscosity. Storage under conditions of high relative humidity applies particularly to solid dosage forms. For products such as solutions and suspensions contained in packs designed to provide a permanent barrier to water loss, specific storage under conditions of high RH is not necessary, but the same range of temperatures should be applied. It is recognised that low RH (10–20%) can adversely affect products packed in semipermeable containers such as solutions in plastic bags and nose drops in small plastic containers, and consideration should be given to appropriate testing under such conditions.

In the case of drug products, 'significant change' at the accelerated condition is defined as

- A 5% potency loss from the initial assay value of a batch
- Any specified degradant exceeding its specification limit
- The product exceeding its pH limits
- Dissolution exceeding the specification limits for 12 capsules or tablets
- Failure to meet specifications for appearance and physical properties, e.g. colour, phase separation, resuspendability, delivery per actuation, caking and hardness

If significant change occurs at 40°C/75% RH then it is necessary to submit a minimum of 6 months' data from an ongoing one-year study at 30°C/60% RH using the same criteria for 'significant change'.

Summary

- The most common cause of degradation of drugs in aqueous systems is *hydrolysis* and the most susceptible drugs are those containing ester, amide, lactone, lactam, imide or carbamate groups. Hydrolysis can be controlled by adjusting the pH to that of maximum stability or in some cases by the addition of nonaqueous solvents.
- Oxidative degradation is a problem with drugs possessing carbon–carbon double bonds such as the steroids, polyunsaturated fatty acids and polyene antibiotics. Such drugs can be stabilised by replacing the oxygen in the system with inert gases such as nitrogen; by avoiding contact with metals such as iron, cobalt and nickel, and by adding antioxidants or reducing agents to the solution. Some oxidative degradations are pH-dependent and can be stabilised by buffering the system.
- Loss of activity of solutions of some drugs such as the tetracyclines can occur because of epimerisation of the drug molecule, while others such as vitamin A lose activity because of geometrical isomerisation.
- Photochemical decomposition can be a problem with drugs such as the phenothiazine tranquillisers and can cause discoloration of the solution and loss of activity. Such systems have to be stored in amber glass containers, which remove the ultraviolet components of light.
- Reactions can be classified according to their order of reaction; the breakdown of drugs in the majority of preparations in which the drug is dissolved in aqueous solution follows first-order or pseudo first-order kinetics. There are, however, many cases of drugs in which decomposition occurs simultaneously by two or more pathways (parallel reactions), or involves a sequence of decomposition steps (consecutive reactions) or a reversible reaction.
- The hydrolysis rate of drugs in liquid dosage forms is strongly influenced by the pH of the solution and can be catalysed not only by H^+ and OH^- ions (specific acid–base catalysis) but also by the components of the buffer used (general acid–base catalysis). We have looked at the ways in which the effect of the buffer components can be removed so that the pH of maximum stability of the solution can be determined from the pH–rate profile and the rate constants for specific acid–base catalysis can be calculated.

- Temperature increase usually causes a pronounced increase of hydrolytic degradation. We have seen how to calculate the hydrolytic rate constant at room temperature from data at elevated temperatures using the Arrhenius equation.
- The addition of electrolyte can increase the hydrolysis rate if the reaction involves the interaction of the drug ion with an ion of similar charge. Similarly, a change of solvent to one of lower dielectric constant will stabilise only this type of system but not one involving the reaction between ions of opposite sign.
- In solid dosage forms containing drugs that are susceptible to hydrolysis, decomposition of the drug can occur if moisture is allowed to adsorb on the surface of the dosage form. Careful selection of packaging is important to reduce this possibility. Drug which dissolves in this surface layer will be affected by many of the factors which influence the decomposition of drugs in aqueous solution. Excipients of the solid dosage form can affect the drug breakdown by increasing the moisture content of the dosage form.
- Temperature increase causes an increase in the rate of breakdown of drugs in solid dosage forms, which can often be described by the Arrhenius equation, although the effect of temperature change is usually far more complicated than for liquid formulations. This equation cannot be used for systems that show an approach to equilibrium. The van't Hoff equation is often useful to describe the effect of temperature on the decomposition of these systems.
- In liquid formulations the shelf-life of a formulation can be estimated by application of the Arrhenius equation. The protocol for stability testing of drug substances and drug products has been discussed.

References

1. P. R. Wells. Linear free energy relationships. *Chem. Rev.*, 63, 171–219 (1963)

2. J. T. Cartensen, E. G. Serenson and J. J. Vance. Use of Hammett graphs in stability programs. *J. Pharm. Sci.*, 53, 1547–8 (1964)

3. S. W. Hovorka and C. Schöneich. Oxidative degradation of pharmaceuticals: theory, mechanisms and inhibition. *J. Pharm. Sci.*, 90, 253–69 (2001)

4. D. M. Johnson and W. F. Taylor. Degradation of fenprostalene in polyethylene glycol 400 solution. *J. Pharm. Sci.*, 73, 1414–7 (1984)

5. L. Halbaut, C. Barbé, M. Aróztegui and C. de la Torre. Oxidative stability of semi-solid excipient mixtures with corn oil and its implication in the degradation of vitamin A. *Int. J. Pharm.*, 147, 31–40 (1997)

6. G. B. Smith, L. DiMichele, L. F. Colwell, *et al.* Autooxidation of simvastatin. *Tetrahedron*, 49, 4447–62 (1993)

7. M. T. Lamy-Freund, V. F. N. Ferreira, A. Faljoni-Alário and S. Schreier. Effect of aggregation on the kinetics of autoxidation of the polyene antibiotic amphotericin B. *J. Pharm. Sci.*, 82, 162–6 (1993)

8. H. H. Tønnesen. Formulation and stability testing of photolabile drugs. *Int. J. Pharm.*, 225, 1–14 (2001)

9. J. V. Greenhill and M. A. McLelland. Photodecomposition of drugs. *Prog. Med. Chem.*, 27, 51–121 (1990)

10. C. L. Huang and F. L. Sands. Effect of ultraviolet irradiation on chlorpromazine. II. Anaerobic condition. *J. Pharm. Sci.*, 56, 259–64 (1967)

11. Y. Matsuda, H. Inouye and R. Nakanishi. Stabilization of sulfisomidine tablets by use of film coating containing UV absorber: Protection of coloration and photolytic degradation from exaggerated light. *J. Pharm. Sci.*, 67, 196–201 (1978)

12. H. Bundgaard. Polymerization of penicillins: kinetics and mechanism of di- and polymerization of ampicillin in aqueous solution. *Acta Pharm. Suec.*, 13, 9–26 (1976)

13. J. T. Carstensen. Stability of solids and solid dosage forms. *J. Pharm. Sci.*, 63, 1–14 (1974)

14. J. T. Carstensen. *Drug Stability. Principles and Practices* 2nd edn, Marcel Dekker, New York, 1995

15. R. Andersin and S. Tammilehto. Photochemical decomposition of midazolam. IV. Study of pH-dependent stability by high-performance liquid chromatography. *Int. J. Pharm.*, 123, 229–35 (1995)

16. K. Torniainen, S. Tammilehto and V. Ulvi. The effect of pH, buffer type and drug concentration on the photodegradation of ciprofloxacin. *Int. J. Pharm.*, 132, 53–61 (1996)

17. J. T. H. Ong and H. B. Kostenbauder. Effect of self-association on rate of penicillin G degradation in concentrated aqueous solutions. *J. Pharm. Sci.*, 64, 1378–80 (1975)

18. A. E. Allen and V. Das Gupta. Stability of hydrocortisone in polyethylene glycol ointment base. *J. Pharm. Sci.*, 63, 107–9 (1974)

19. V. Das Gupta. Effect of vehicles and other active ingredients on stability of hydrocortisone. *J. Pharm. Sci.*, 67, 299–302 (1978)

20. M. J. Busse. Dangers of dilution of topical steroids. *Pharm. J.*, 220, 25 (1978)

21. E. Ullmann, K. Thoma and G. Zelfel. The stability of sodium penicillin G in the presence of ionic surfactants, organic gel formers, and preservatives. *Pharm. Acta. Helv.*, 38, 577–86 (1963)

22. B. Testa and J. C. Etter. Hydrolysis of pilocarpine in Carbopol hydrogels. *Can. J. Pharm. Sci.*, 10, 16–20 (1975)

23. R. I. Poust and J. C. Colaizzi. Copper-catalyzed oxidation of ascorbic acid in gels and aqueous solutions of polysorbate 80. *J. Pharm. Sci.*, 57, 2119–25 (1968)

24. J. Tingstad and J. Dudzinski. Preformulation studies. II. Stability of drug substances in solid pharmaceutical systems. *J. Pharm. Sci.*, 62, 1856–60 (1973)

25. H. W. Jun, C. W. Whitworth and L. A. Luzzi. Decomposition of aspirin in polyethylene glycols. *J. Pharm. Sci.*, 61, 1160–2 (1972)

26. C. W. Whitworth, L. A. Luzzi, B. B. Thompson and H. W. Jun. Stability of aspirin in liquid and semi-solid bases. II. Effect of fatty additives on stability in a polyethylene glycol base. *J. Pharm. Sci.*, 62, 1372–4 (1973)

27. R. Ekman, L. Liponkoski and P. Kahela. Formation of indomethacin esters in polyethylene glycol suppositories. *Acta Pharm. Suec.*, 19, 241–6 (1982)

28. A. K. Amirjahed. Simplified method to study stability of pharmaceutical preparations. *J. Pharm. Sci.*, 66, 785 (1977)

29. A. R. Rogers. An accelerated storage test with pro-grammed temperature rise. *J. Pharm. Pharmacol.*, 15, 101T (1963)

30. H. V. Maudling and M. A. Zoglio. Flexible non-isothermal stability studies. *J. Pharm. Sci.*, 59, 333–7 (1970)

31. B. W. Madsen, R. A. Anderson, D. Herbison-Evans and W. Sneddon. Integral approach to noniso-thermal estimation of activation energies. *J. Pharm. Sci.*, 63, 777–81 (1974)

32. A. I. Kay and T. H. Simon. Use of an analog com-puter to simulate and interpret data obtained from linear nonisothermal stability studies. *J. Pharm. Sci.*, 60, 205–8 (1971)

33. M. A. Zoglio, H. V. Maudling, W. H. Streng and W. C. Vincek. Nonisothermal kinetic studies III: rapid nonisothermal-isothermal method for stability prediction. *J. Pharm. Sci.*, 64, 1381 (1975)

34. ICH Harmonised Tripartite Guideline. Q1B: Photostability Testing of New Drug Substances and Products. *Federal Register*, 62, 27115 (1997)

35. L. Lachman. Physical and chemical stability testing of tablet dosage forms. *J. Pharm. Sci.*, 54, 1519–26 (1965)

36. Stability testing of new drug substances and products (ICH), MCA EuroDirect Publication No. 3335/92.

5

The solubility of drugs

There are many reasons why it is vital to understand the way in which drugs dissolve in solution and the factors that maintain solubility or cause drugs to come out of solution, that is, to precipitate. These include the facts that:

- Many drugs are formulated as solutions or are added in powder or solution form to the liquids, such as infusion fluids, in which they must remain in solution for a given period.
- In whatever way drugs are presented to the body, they must usually be in a molecularly dispersed form (that is in solution) before they can be absorbed across biological membranes*.
- The solution process will precede absorption unless the drug is administered as a solution, but even solutions may precipitate in the stomach contents or in blood, and the precipitated drug will then have to re-dissolve before being absorbed.
- Drugs of low aqueous solubility (e.g. Taxol) frequently present problems in relation to their formulation and bioavailability.

---

* In section 9.2.1 we discuss the special circumstances under which microparticulate materials can be taken up by specialised cells in the gut and, by way of the lymphatic circulation, reach the liver and blood and other organs. It may be that very insoluble colloidal drug suspensions are absorbed by this route also.

In this chapter we will consider the factors controlling the solubility of drugs in solution, in particular the nature of the drug molecule and the crystalline form in which it exists, its hydrophobicity, its shape, its surface area, its state of ionisation, the influence of pH of the medium and the importance of the pK_a of the drug. The equation linking solubility to solution pH and drug pK_a (equation 5.11) is possibly one of the most important in this book. Experimental methods of measurement of solubility are essential in drug development, as is the ability to predict the solubility of a drug from a knowledge of its chemical structure, recognising hydrophilic and hydrophobic groups and their influence on solubility. How additives such as salts, cosolvents, surfactants and other agents can affect the solubility of a drug should to an extent be predictable from the theory, bearing in mind the complexity of many formulations.

Pharmaceutical solutions might appear to be extremely simple systems, but it is in the solution state that degradation takes place most rapidly, and the solubilisation of poorly soluble compounds is often very difficult. It is ideal if a drug can be formulated as a simple stable aqueous solution when required for injection, but resort to additives such as water-miscible solvents and surfactants, hydrotropes and cyclodextrins to increase the water solubility of the drug complicates the formulation. Here we deal with simple solutions. Some of the special problems related to peptide and protein solubility are discussed in Chapter 11.

Aqueous solvents are the most common in pharmaceutical and, of course, in biological systems, so this chapter is concerned mainly with solutions of aqueous and mixed aqueous solvents, such as alcohol–water mixtures. The solution of drugs in nonaqueous media (such as oils) is also considered because of the many pharmaceutical applications of nonaqueous solutions and formulations such as oil-in-water emulsions, and because of the need to understand the process of the transport of drugs across biological and artificial membranes, which are effectively structured non-aqueous phases. A primary factor in passive membrane transport is the relative solubility of the drug in an aqueous medium and in the lipid cell membrane, the relative affinities being quantified in the partition coefficient of the compound, a topic discussed at the end of this chapter.

5.1 Definitions

A *solution* can be defined as a system in which molecules of a solute (such as a drug or protein) are dissolved in a solvent vehicle. When a solution contains a solute at the limit of its solubility at any given temperature and pressure, it is said to be *saturated*. If the solubility limit is exceeded, solid particles of solute may be present and the solution phase will be in equilibrium with the solid, although under certain circumstances *supersaturated solutions* may be prepared, where the drug exists in solution above its normal solubility limit.

The maximum *equilibrium solubility* of a drug in a given medium is of practical pharmaceutical interest because it dictates the *rate of solution (dissolution)* of the drug (the rate at which the drug dissolves from the solid state). The higher the solubility, the more rapid is the rate of solution when no chemical reaction is involved.

5.1.1 Expressions of solubility

The solubility of a solute in a solvent can be expressed quantitatively in several ways (see Chapter 3, section 3.1). Other less-specific forms of noting solubility include parts per parts of solvent (for example, parts per million, ppm). The British Pharmacopoeia and other chemical and pharmaceutical compendia frequently use this form and also the expressions 'insoluble', 'very highly soluble' and 'soluble'. These are imprecise and often not very helpful. For quantitative work specific concentration terms must be used.

Most substances have at least some degree of solubility in water and while they may appear to be 'insoluble' by a qualitative test, their solubility can be measured and quoted precisely. In aqueous media at pH 10, chlorpromazine base has a solubility of 8×10^{-6} mol dm^{-3}, that is it is very slightly soluble, but it might be considered to be 'insoluble' if judged visually by the lack of disappearance of solid placed in a test-tube of water.

5.2 Factors influencing solubility

Progress has been made in ways of predicting the solubility of solutes in aqueous media, both from estimates of their molecular surface area and from the nature of the key chemical groups in the parent structure. The importance of the surface area becomes clear if we think of the processes involved in the dissolution of a crystal (Fig. 5.1). The process can be considered in three stages:

1 A solute (drug) molecule is 'removed' from its crystal.
2 A cavity for the molecule is created in the solvent.
3 The solute molecule is inserted into this cavity.

Placing the solute molecule in the solvent cavity requires a number of solute–solvent contacts; the larger the solute molecule, the more contacts are created. If the surface area of the solute molecule is A, the solute–solvent interface increases by $\sigma_{12}A$, where σ_{12} is the interfacial tension between the solvent (subscript 1) and the solute (subscript 2). σ is a parameter not readily obtained for solid interfaces on the molecular scale, but reasonable estimates can be made from knowledge of the interfacial tensions of molecules at normal interfaces.[1–5]

The number of solvent molecules which can pack around the solute molecule is considered in calculations of the thermodynamic properties of the solution. The molecular surface area of the solute is therefore the key parameter and good correlations can be obtained between aqueous solubility and this parameter.[4, 5]

Of course, most drugs are not simple nonpolar hydrocarbons and we have to consider polar molecules and weak organic electrolytes. The term w_{12} in Fig. 5.1, a measure of solute–solvent interactions, has to be further divided to take into account the interactions involving the nonpolar part and the polar portion of the solute. The molecular surface area of each portion can be considered separately: the greater the area of the hydrophilic portion relative to the hydrophobic portion, the greater is the aqueous solubility. For a hydrophobic molecule of area A, the free energy change in placing the solute in the solvent cavity is $-\sigma_{12}A$. Indeed, it can be shown that the reversible work of solution is $(w_{11} + w_{22} - 2w_{12})A$.

Implicit in this derivation is the assumption that the solution formed is dilute, so that solute–solute interactions are unimportant. The success of the molecular area approach is evidenced by the fact that equations can be

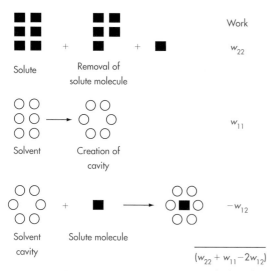

Work

w_{22}

Solute   Removal of solute molecule

w_{11}

Solvent   Creation of cavity

$-w_{12}$

Solvent cavity   Solute molecule

$(w_{22} + w_{11} - 2w_{12})$

Figure 5.1 Diagrammatic representation of the three processes involved in the dissolution of a crystalline solute: the expression for the work involved is $w_{22} + w_{11} - 2w_{12}$ (solute–solvent interaction in the last stage is $-2w_{12}$ as bonds are made with one solute and two solvent molecules).

written to relate solubility to surface area. For example, equation (5.1) has been shown to hold for a range of 55 compounds (some of which are listed in Table 5.1):

$$\ln S = -4.3A + 11.78 \qquad (5.1)$$

where S is the *molal* (not molar) solubility, and A is the total surface area in nm^2.

The compounds in Table 5.1 are liquids, so the process of dissolution is simpler than that outlined in Fig. 5.1.

5.2.1 Structural features and aqueous solubility

Shape

Interactions between nonpolar groups and water were discussed above, where the importance of both size and shape was indicated. Chain branching of hydrophobic groups influences aqueous solubility, as shown by the solubilities of a series of straight and branched-chain alcohols in Table 5.2.

What other predictors of solubility might there be? The *boiling point* of liquids and the *melting point* of solids are useful in that both reflect the strengths of interactions between the molecules in the pure liquid or the solid state. Boiling point correlates with total surface area, and in a large enough range of compounds we can detect the trend of decreasing aqueous solubility with increasing boiling point (see data in Table 5.2).

As boiling points of liquids and melting points of solids are indicators of molecular cohesion, these can be useful indicators of trends in a series of similar compounds. There are other empirical correlations that are useful. Melting points, even of compounds which form nonideal solutions, can be used as a guide to the order of solubility in a closely related series of compounds, as can be seen in the properties of sulfonamide derivatives listed in Table 5.3. Such correlations depend on the relatively greater importance of w_{22} in the solution process in these compounds.

Substituents

The influence of substituents on the solubility of molecules in water can be due to their effect on the properties of the solid or liquid (for example, on its molecular cohesion) or to the effect of the substituent on its interaction with water molecules. It is not easy to predict what effect a particular substituent will have on crystal properties, but as a guide to the solvent interactions, substituents can be classified as either hydrophobic or hydrophilic, depending on their polarity (see Table 5.4). The position of the substituent on the molecule can influence its effect, however. This can be seen in the aqueous solubilities of o-, m- and p-dihydroxy-benzenes; as expected, all are much greater than that of benzene, but they are not the same, being 4, 9 and 0.6 mol dm^{-3}, respectively. The relatively low solubility of the *para* compound is due to the greater stability of its crystalline state. The melting points of the derivatives indicate that is so, as they are 105°C, 111°C, and 170°C, respectively. In the case of the *ortho*

Table 5.1 Experimental aqueous solubilities, boiling points, surface areas and predicted aqueous solubilities[a]

Compound	Solubility (mol kg^{-1})	Surface area (nm^2)	Boiling point (°C)	Predicted solubilities (mol kg^{-1})
1-Butanol	1.006	2.721	117.7	0.821
1-Pentanol	2.5×10^{-1}	3.039	137.8	2.09×10^{-1}
1-Hexanol	6.1×10^{-2}	3.357	157	5.32×10^{-2}
1-Heptanol	1.55×10^{-2}	3.675	176.3	1.36×10^{-2}
Cyclohexanol	3.83×10^{-1}	2.905	161	4.3×10^{-1}
1-Nonanol	1×10^{-3}	4.312	213.1	0.88×10^{-3}

[a] Reproduced from reference 1.

Table 5.2 Solubilities of pentanol isomers in water[a]

Compound	Solubility (molality, m)	Surface area (nm^2)	Boiling point $(°C)$	Structure
n-Pentanol	2.6×10^{-1}	3.039	137.8	
3-Methyl-1-butanol	3.11×10^{-1}	2.914	131.2	
2-Methyl-1-butanol	3.47×10^{-1}	2.894	128.7	
2-Pentanol	5.3×10^{-1}	2.959	119.0	
3-Pentanol	6.15×10^{-1}	2.935	115.3	
3-Methyl-2-butanol	6.67×10^{-1}	2.843	111.5	
2-Methyl-2-butanol	1.403	2.825	102.0	

[a] Reproduced from reference 1.

Table 5.3 Correlation between melting points of sulfonamide derivatives and aqueous solubility

Compound	Melting point $(°C)$	Solubility
Sulfadiazine	253	1 g in 13 dm^3 $(0.077 \text{ g dm}^{-3})$
Sulfamerazine	236	1 g in 5 dm^3 (0.20 g dm^{-3})
Sulfapyridine	192	1 g in 3.5 dm^3 (0.29 g dm^{-3})
Sulfathiazole	174	1 g in 1.7 dm^3 (0.59 g dm^{-3})

Table 5.4 Substituent group classification

Substituent	Classification
$-CH_3$	Hydrophobic
$-CH_2-$	Hydrophobic
$-Cl, -Br, -F$	Hydrophobic
$-N(CH_3)_2$	Hydrophobic
$-SCH_3$	Hydrophobic
$-OCH_2CH_3$	Hydrophobic
$-OCH_3$	Slightly hydrophilic
$-NO_2$	Slightly hydrophilic
$-CHO$	Hydrophilic
$-COOH$	Slightly hydrophilic
$-COO^-$	Very hydrophilic
$-NH_2$	Hydrophilic
$-NH_3^+$	Very hydrophilic
$-OH$	Very hydrophilic

derivative, the possibility of intramolecular hydrogen bonding in aqueous solution, decreasing the ability of the OH group to interact with water, may explain why its solubility is lower than that of its *meta* analogue.

One can best illustrate the use of the information in Table 5.4 by considering the solu-bility of a series of substituted acetanilides, data for which are provided in Table 5.5. The strong hydrophilic characteristics of polar groups capable of hydrogen bonding with

Table 5.5 The effect of substituents on solubility of acetanilide derivatives in water

Derivative	X	Solubility ($mg\ dm^{-3}$)
NHCOCH$_3$	H	6.38
	Methyl	1.05
	Ethoxyl	0.93
	Hydroxyl	13.9
	Nitro	15.98
	Aceto	9.87

water molecules are evident. The presence of hydroxyl groups can therefore markedly change the solubility characteristics of a compound; phenol, for example, is 100 times more soluble in water than is benzene. In the case of phenol, where there is considerable hydrogen-bonding capability, the solute–solvent interaction (w_{12}) outweighs other factors (such as w_{22} or w_{11}) in the solution process. But, as we have discovered, the position of any substituent on the parent molecule will affect its contribution to solubility.

Table 5.6 The effect of substituents on solubility of acetanilide derivatives in water[a]

Structure	Compound	Solubility ($\mu g\ cm^{-3}$)
(I)	Estradiol (I)	5
(II)	Ethinylestradiol (II)	10
(III)	Estradiol benzoate (III)	0.4
(IV)	Testosterone (IV)	24
	Testosterone propionate	0.4
(V)	Methyltestosterone (V)	32

continued

Table 5.6   *(continued)*

Structure	Compound	Solubility (μg cm^{-3})
(VI)	Prednisolone (VI)	215
(VII)	Prednisone (VII) Prednisone acetate	115 23
(VIII)	Cortisone (VIII)	230
(IX)	Dexamethasone (IX)	84
(X)	Betamethasone (X)	58

continued

Table 5.6 (continued)

Structure	Compound	Solubility ($\mu g\ cm^{-3}$)
(XI)	Progesterone (XI)	9
(XII)	Hydrocortisone (XII)	285

[a] Reproduced from reference 6.

Steroid solubility

The steroids as a group tend to be poorly soluble in water. Their complex structure makes prediction of solubility somewhat difficult, but one can generally rationalise, *post hoc*, the solubility values of related steroids. Table 5.6 gives solubility data for 14 steroids. As examples, the substitution of an ethinyl group has conferred increased solubility on the estradiol molecule, as would be expected. Estradiol benzoate with its 3-OH substituent is much less soluble than the parent estradiol because of the loss of the hydroxyl and its substitution with a hydrophobic group. The same relationships are seen in testosterone and testosterone propionate. As both estradiol benzoate and testosterone propionate are oil soluble, they are used as solutions in castor oil and sesame oil for intramuscular and subcutaneous injection (see Chapter 9).

Methyltestosterone might be expected to be less soluble in water than is testosterone, but in fact it is not; this demonstrates again the importance of crystal properties in determining solubility. The methyl compound is more soluble because of the smaller heat of fusion of this derivative, hence the solid state more readily 'disintegrates' in the solvent.

Dexamethasone and betamethasone are isomeric fluorinated derivatives of methylprednisolone, but their solubilities are not identical, which might be a crystal property or a solution property. A simpler example of differences in isomeric solubility is that of the *o*-, *m*-, and *p*-dihydroxybenzenes referred to above. A steric argument may be applied to the case of dexamethasone, water molecules being less able to move close to the 17-OH group than in the case of betamethasone.

5.2.2 Hydration and solvation

The way in which solute molecules interact with the water molecules of the solvent is crucial to determining their affinity for the solvent. Ionic groups and electrolytes interact avidly with the polar water molecules, but nonelectrolytes also do not leave the structure of water unchanged, nor even do nonpolar groups and molecules such as the hydrocarbons.

Hydration of nonelectrolytes

Solvation is the general term used to describe the process of binding of solvent to solute molecules. If the solvent is water, the process is *hydration*. In a solution of sucrose (**XIII**), six water molecules are bound to each sucrose molecule with such avidity that water and sucrose move as a unit in solution, and the extent of hydration can therefore be measured by hydrodynamic techniques.

Chemically very similar molecules such as mannitol (**XIV**), sorbitol (**XV**) and inositol have very different affinities for water. The solubility of sorbitol in water is about 3.5 times that of mannitol.

Most favourable hydration occurs when there is an equatorial –OH group on pyranose sugars.[7] This is thought to be due to the compatibility of the equatorial –OH with the organised structure of water in bulk. Axial

Structure **XIII** Sucrose

Structure **XIV** Mannitol

Structure **XV** Sorbitol

hydroxyl groups cannot bond onto the water 'lattice' without causing it to distort considerably. This may be one explanation of the difference, although differences in the lattice energies of the crystals may also contribute.

Hydration of ionic species: water structure breakers and structure makers

The study of ionic solvation is complicated but is relevant in pharmaceutics because of the effect ions have on the solubility of other species. The forces between cations and water molecules are so strong that the cations may retain a layer of water molecules in their crystals. The effect of ions on water structure is complex and variable. All ions in water possess a layer of tightly bound water – the water molecules being directionally orientated. Four water molecules are in the bound layer of most monovalent, monatomic ions. The firmly held layer can be regarded as being in a 'frozen' condition around a positive ion. The water molecules could be orientated with all the hydrogen atoms of the water molecules pointing outwards (see Fig. 5.2). Because of this and because their orientation depends on the ion size, they cannot all participate in the normal tetrahedral arrangements of bulk water (see Section 6.3.1). For this to be feasible, two of the water molecules must be orientated with the hydrogens of the water molecules pointing in towards the ion. Inevitably, then, with cations and many small anions there tends to be a layer of water around the bound layer which is *less ordered* than bulk water (Fig. 5.2). Such ions, which include all the alkali and halide ions except Li^+ and F^-, are called

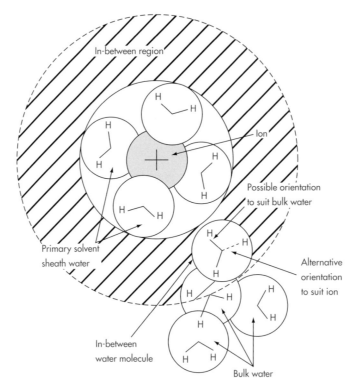

Figure 5.2 Schematic diagram to indicate that, in the (hatched) region between the primary solvated ion and bulk water, the orientation of the 'in-between' water molecules must be a compromise between that which suits the ion (oxygen-facing ion) and that which suits the bulk water (hydrogen-facing ion).
Reproduced from J. O'M. Bockris and A. K. N. Reddy, *Modern Electrochemistry*, vol. 1, MacDonald, London, 1970, with permission.

structure breakers. The size of the ion is important, as the surface area of the ion determines the constraints on the polarised water molecules. Many polyvalent ions, for example Al^{3+}, increase the structured nature of water beyond the immediate hydration layer, and are therefore *structure makers*.

Hydration numbers

Hydration numbers (the number of water molecules in the primary hydration layer) can be determined by various physical techniques (for example, compressibility) and the values obtained tend to differ depending on the method used. The overall total action of the ion on water may be replaced conceptually by a strong binding between the ion and some effective number (solvation number) of solvent molecules; this effective number may well be almost zero in the case of large ions

such as iodide, caesium and tetraalkylammonium ions. The solvation numbers decrease with increase of ionic radius because the ionic force field diminishes with increasing radius, and consequently water molecules are less inclined to be abstracted from their position in bulk water.

Hydrophobic hydration

Water is associated in a dynamic manner with nonpolar groups, but only in rare cases (where crystalline clathrates can be formed) is this water able to be isolated along with the hydrophobic groups. The phrase 'hydrophobic hydration' is used to describe this layer of water. The motion of water molecules is slowed down in the vicinity of nonpolar groups. Hydrophobic groups induce structure formation in water, hence the negative entropy $(-\Delta S)$ of their dissolution in water and the positive entropy ($+\Delta S$) gained on their removal. In the discussion of hydrophobic bonding (Section 6.3.1) and nonpolar interactions, this special relationship between water and hydrocarbon chains is elaborated.

The solubility of inorganic materials in water

While a minority of therapeutic agents are inorganic electrolytes, it is nevertheless pertinent to consider the manner of their interaction with water. Electrolytes are, of necessity, components of replacement fluids, injections and eye drops and many other formulations. An increasing number of metal-containing compounds are used in diagnosis and therapy, some of which have interesting solution behaviour.

First consider the simpler salts. What determines the solubility of a salt such as sodium chloride and its solubility in relation to, say, silver chloride? The solubility of NaCl is in excess of 5 mol dm^{-3} while the solubility of AgCl is 500 000 times less. The heats of solution ($\Delta H_{\text{solution}}$) are 62.8 kJ mol^{-1} for silver chloride and 4.2 kJ mol^{-1} for sodium chloride, suggesting a substantial difference either in the crystal properties or in the interaction of the ions with water. In fact the very great strength of the silver chloride crystal is due to the high polarisability of the silver ion. The heat of solution of an ionic solute can be written as

$$\Delta H_{\text{solution}} = \Delta H_{\text{sublimation}} - \Delta H_{\text{hydration}} \quad (5.2)$$

Conceptually, the solid salt (sodium chloride, for instance) is converted to the gaseous (g) state, $Na^+(g) + Cl^-(g)$, and each unit is then hydrated to form the species $Na^+(aq)$ and $Cl^-(aq)$. If the heat of hydration is sufficient to provide the energy needed to overcome the lattice forces, the salt will be freely soluble at a given temperature and the ions will readily dislodge from the crystal lattice. If the partial molal enthalpy of solution of the substance is positive, the solubility will increase with increasing temperature; if it is negative the solubility will decrease, in agreement with Le Chatelier's principle.

5.2.3 The effect of simple additives on solubility

Solubility products

For poorly soluble materials such as silver chloride and barium sulfate the concept of the solubility product can be used. The following equilibrium exists in solution between crystalline silver chloride $AgCl_c$ and ions in solution:

$$AgCl_c \rightleftharpoons Ag^+ + Cl^- \quad (5.3)$$

An equilibrium constant K can be defined as

$$K = \frac{[Ag^+][Cl^-]}{[AgCl_c]} \quad (5.4)$$

Strictly, K should be written in terms of thermodynamic activities and not concentrations, but activities can be replaced by concentrations (denoted by square brackets) because of the low solubilities involved (see section 3.3.1). At saturation the concentration of the crystalline silver chloride $[AgCl_c]$ is essentially constant and the solubility product, K_{sp}, may therefore be written:

$$K_{sp} = [Ag^+][Cl^-] \quad (5.5)$$

The solubility product is useful for evaluating the influence of other species on the solubility of salts of low aqueous solubility. Some values of solubility products are quoted in Table 5.7.

Additives may either increase or decrease the solubility of a solute in a given solvent. The effect that they have will depend on several factors:

- The effect the additive has on the structure of water
- The interaction of the additive with the solute
- The interaction of the additive with the solvent

Table 5.7 Solubility products of some inorganic salts

Compound	K_{sp} (mol^2 dm^{-6})
AgCl	1.25×10^{-10}
Al(OH)$_3$	7.7×10^{-13}
BaSO$_4$	1.0×10^{-10}

Salting in and salting out

Salts that increase solubility are said to *salt in* the solute and those that decrease solubility *salt out* the solute.

The effect of a solute additive on the solubility of another solute may be quantified by the Setschenow equation:

$$\log \frac{S}{S_a} = kc_a \qquad (5.6)$$

where S_a is the solubility in the presence of an additive, S is the solubility in its absence, c_a is the concentration of additive, and k is the salting coefficient. The sign of k is positive when the activity coefficient is increased; it is negative if the activity coefficient is decreased by the additive. The Setschenow equation frequently holds up to additive concentrations of 1 mol dm^{-3}, a measure of the sensitivity of the activity coefficient of the solute towards the salt.

Hydrotropy

Several salts with large anions or cations which are themselves very soluble in water result in salting in, i.e. solubilisation of nonelectrolytes. Sodium benzoate and sodium *p*-toluenesulfonate are good examples of such agents and are referred to as *hydrotropic salts*; the increase in the solubility of other solutes is known as *hydrotropy*. Values of k (in $(\text{mol dm}^{-3})^{-1}$) for three salts added to benzoic acid in aqueous solution are 0.17 for NaCl; 0.14 for KCl; and −0.22 for sodium benzoate. That is, NaCl and KCl decrease the solubility of benzoic acid, and sodium benzoate increases it.

5.2.4   The effect of pH on the solubility of ionisable drugs

pH is one of the primary influences on the solubility of most drugs that contain ionisable groups. As the great majority of drugs are organic electrolytes, there are four parameters which determine their solubility:

- Their degree of ionisation

- Their molecular size
- Interactions of substituent groups with solvent
- Their crystal properties

In this section consideration is given to the solubility of weak electrolytes and the influence of pH on aqueous solubility, important in both formulation and dissolution of drugs *in vivo*, and ultimately and importantly their biological activity.

Acidic drugs

The object of this section is to obtain an equation to relate drug solubility to the pH of the solution and to the pK_a of the drug.

Acidic drugs such as the nonsteroidal anti-inflammatory agents, are less soluble in acidic solutions than in alkaline solutions because the predominant undissociated species cannot interact with water molecules to the same extent as the ionised form, which is readily hydrated.

If we represent the drug as HA and the total saturation solubility of the drug as S, and if S_0 is the solubility of the undissociated species HA, it is clear that the total solubility is the sum of the solubility of the unionised and ionised species, that is

$$S = S_0 + (\text{concentration of ionised species})$$

The dissociation of the acid in water can be written

$$HA + H_2O \rightleftharpoons H_3O^+ + A^- \qquad (5.7)$$

and the dissociation constant K_a is given by

$$K_a = \frac{[H_3O^+][A^-]}{[HA]} \qquad (5.8)$$

Rearranging and substituting S_0 for [HA] gives

$$\frac{K_a}{[H_3O^+]} = \frac{[A^-]}{S_0} \qquad (5.9)$$

but as $[A^-] = S - S_0$,

$$\frac{K_a}{[H_3O^+]} = \frac{S - S_0}{S_0} \qquad (5.10)$$

Taking logarithms,

$$pH - pK_a = \log\left(\frac{S - S_0}{S_0}\right) \quad (5.11)$$

Hence the solubility of the drug at any pH can be calculated provided pK_a and S_0 are known.

Examples of the use of equation (5.11) to calculate the effect of pH on the solubility of acidic drugs are given below.

- -

EXAMPLE 5.1

What is the pH below which sulfadiazine ($pK_a = 6.48$) will begin to precipitate in an infusion fluid, when the initial molar concentration of sulfadiazine sodium is 4×10^{-2} mol dm^{-3} and the solubility of sulfadiazine is 3.07×10^{-4} mol dm^{-3}?

Answer

The pH below which the drug will precipitate is calculated using equation (5.11):

$$pH = 6.48 + \log\frac{(4.00 \times 10^{-2}) - (3.07 \times 10^{-4})}{3.07 \times 10^{-4}}$$

$$= 8.60$$

- -

EXAMPLE 5.2

What is the solubility of benzylpenicillin G at a pH sufficiently low to allow only the nondissociated form of the drug to be present?

The pK_a of benzylpenicillin G is 2.76 and the solubility of the drug at pH 8.0 is 0.174 mol dm^{-3}. (From R. E. Notari, *Biopharmaceutics and Pharmacokinetics*, 2nd edn, Marcel Dekker, New York, 1978.)

Answer

If only the undissociated form is present at low pH then we need to find S_0. This can be obtained from the information given using equation (5.11):

$$pH - pK_a = \log\left(\frac{S - S_0}{S_0}\right)$$

Therefore,

$$8.0 - 2.76 = \log\left(\frac{0.174 - S_0}{S_0}\right)$$

$$5.24 = \log\left(\frac{0.174 - S_0}{S_0}\right)$$

Therefore, $S_0 = 1 \times 10^{-6}$ mol dm^{-3}.

- -

Basic drugs

Basic drugs such as ranitidine are more soluble in acidic solutions, where the ionised form of the drug is predominant. If S_0 is the solubility of an undissociated base, RNH_2, the expression for the solubility (S) as a function of pH can be obtained as follows.

In water:

$$RNH_2 + H_2O \rightleftharpoons RNH_3^+ + OH^- \quad (5.12)$$

Therefore,

$$K_b = \frac{[RNH_3^+][OH^-]}{[RNH_2]} \quad (5.13)$$

That is

$$\frac{K_b}{[OH^-]} = \frac{[H^+]}{K_a} = \frac{S - S_0}{S_0} \quad (5.14)$$

Taking logarithms,

$$pK_a - pH = \log\left(\frac{S - S_0}{S_0}\right) \quad (5.15)$$

or

$$pH - pK_a = \log\left(\frac{S_0}{S - S_0}\right) \quad (5.16)$$

Solubility–pH profiles of a basic drug (chlorpromazine) and an acidic drug (indometacin) and values for the more complex profile of the amphoteric drug oxytetracycline are plotted in Fig. 5.3.

Despite the widespread use of this approach to predict the pH dependence of drug solubility, it should be noted that a recent study of the accuracy of equation (5.15) in predicting the solubility of a series of cationic drugs as a function of pH in divalent buffer systems

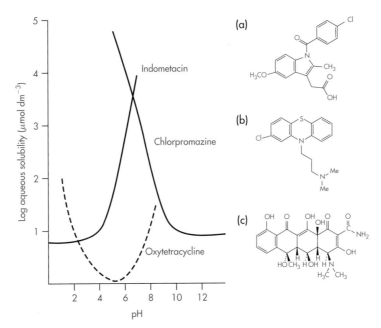

Figure 5.3 Solubility of (a) indometacin, (b) chlorpromazine and (c) oxytetracycline as a function of pH, plotted as logarithm of the solubility.

mimicking the intestinal fluid highlighted some limitations of this equation and the authors cautioned against its uncritical use.[8]

• •

EXAMPLE 5.3

A drug is found to have the following saturation solubilities at room temperature:

pH	S (μmol dm^{-3})
7.4	205.0
9.0	10.0
10.0	5.5
12.0	5.0

What type of compound is it likely to be and what is its pK_a?

Answer

As the solubility decreases with increasing pH, the compound is a base. At pH 12 the solubility quoted is likely to be the solubility of the unprotonated species, that is, S_0. Using the figures given, we can apply equation (5.15) at each of the other pH values:

$$pK_a = pH + \log\left(\frac{S - S_0}{S_0}\right)$$

$$= 7.4 + \log\frac{200}{5}$$

$$= 7.4 + \log 40 = 7.4 + 1.602 = 9.0$$

$$pK_a = 9.0 + \log\frac{10 - 5}{5} = 9.0 + \log 1 = 9.0$$

$$pK_a = 10.0 + \log\frac{5.5 - 5}{5} = 10.0 + \log 0.1 = 9.0$$

The drug has a pK_a value of 9.0 and is thus likely to be an amine.

• •

Amphoteric drugs

Several drugs and amino acids, peptides and proteins are amphoteric, displaying both basic and acidic characteristics. Frequently encountered drugs in this category are the sulfonamides and the tetracyclines. If, for simplicity, one were to use a generalised structure for an amphoteric compound

$$\begin{array}{c} R - X - COOH \\ | \\ NH_2 \end{array}$$

and if the solution equilibrium between the species is written down, we would obtain, as before, equations relating solubility to pH. The equilibria can be written as

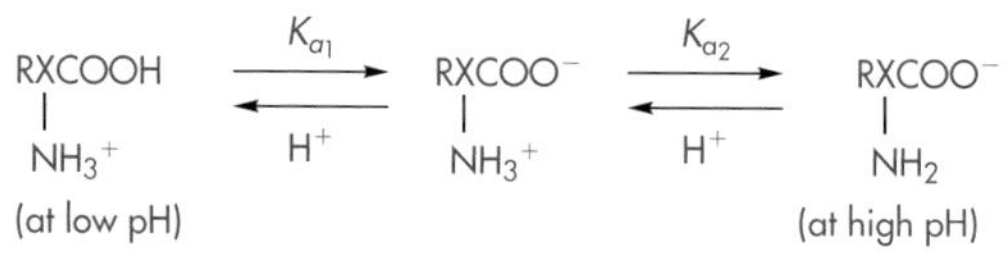

RXCOOH $\xrightleftharpoons[H^+]{K_{a_1}}$ RXCOO$^-$ $\xrightleftharpoons[H^+]{K_{a_2}}$ RXCOO$^-$
| | |
NH$_3^+$ NH$_3^+$ NH$_2$
(at low pH)   (at high pH)

More simply,

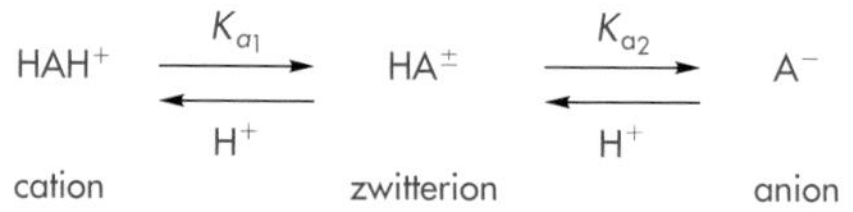

HAH$^+$ $\xrightleftharpoons[H^+]{K_{a_1}}$ HA$^\pm$ $\xrightleftharpoons[H^+]{K_{a_2}}$ A$^-$

cation   zwitterion   anion

The two dissociation constants can be defined in the normal way as

$$K_{a_1} = \frac{[HA^\pm][H^+]}{[HAH^+]} \tag{5.17}$$

and

$$K_{a_2} = \frac{[A^-][H^+]}{[HA^\pm]} \tag{5.18}$$

That is

$$\frac{K_{a_1}}{[H^+]} = \frac{[HA^\pm]}{[HAH^+]} \tag{5.19}$$

and

$$\frac{K_{a_2}}{[H^+]} = \frac{[A^-]}{[HA^\pm]} \tag{5.20}$$

It is observed that the zwitterion has the lowest solubility (see Fig. 5.3 and Table 5.8), which we take to be S_0.

$$\frac{K_{a_1}}{[H^+]} = \frac{S_0}{S - S_0} \tag{5.21}$$

and

$$\frac{K_{a_2}}{[H^+]} = \frac{S - S_0}{S_0} \tag{5.22}$$

Therefore,

$$pH - pK_a = \log\left(\frac{S_0}{S - S_0}\right) \tag{5.23}$$

at pH values below the isoelectric point, and

$$pH - pK_a = \log\left(\frac{S - S_0}{S_0}\right) \tag{5.24}$$

at pH values above the isoelectric point.

Table 5.8 gives solubility data for oxytetracycline (**XVI**) as a function of pH. Oxytetracycline has three pK_a values: $pK_{a1} = 3.27$, $pK_{a2} = 7.32$, and $pK_{a3} = 9.11$, corresponding to the regions 1, 2 and 3 in the structure shown.

The equations for the solubilities of acidic, basic and zwitterionic drugs (equations 5.11, 5.16, 5.23 and 5.24) can all be used to calculate the pH at which a drug will precipitate from solution of a given concentration (or the concentration at which a drug will reach its maximum solubility at a given pH). This is especially important in determining the maximum allowable levels of a drug in infusion fluids or formulations. Some idea of the range of pH values encountered in common infusion fluids is given in Table 5.9. The variation in pH between preparations and within batches of the same infusion fluid (the monograph for Dextrose Infusion BP allows a pH ranging from 3.5 to 5.5) means that the fluids vary considerably in their solvent capacity for weak electrolytes.

Table 5.8 Oxytetracycline: pH dependence of solubility at 20°C[a]

pH	Solubility (g dm^{-3})
1.2	31.4
2	4.6
3	1.4
4	0.85
5	0.5
6	0.7
7	1.1
8	28.0
9	38.6

[a] Data from the *United States Dispensatory*, 25th edn.

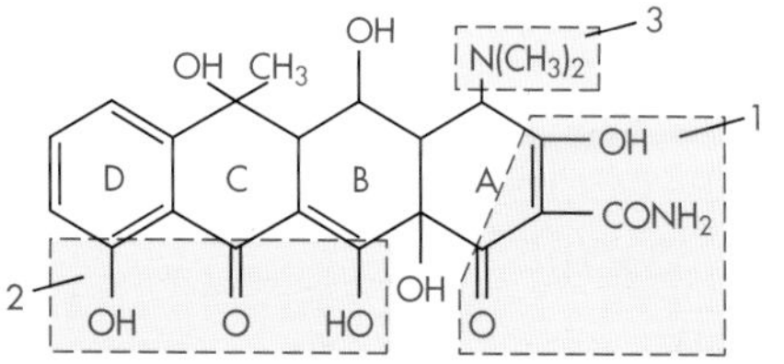

Structure XVI Oxytetracycline

Table 5.9 pH of some parenteral solutions[a]

Solution	pH
5% Dextrose in water (5% D/W)	4.40, 4.70
5% D/W (1 dm^3 containing 2 cm^3 of vitamins)	4.30, 4.38
5% D/W (1 dm^3 containing 100 mg thiamine hydrochloride)	3.90, 3.96
5% D/W (1 dm^3 containing 300 mg thiamine hydrochloride)	3.82, 4.00
5% D/W (1 dm^3 containing 2 cm^3 of vitamins, 200 mg thiamine hydrochloride)	4.15
5% D/W (1 dm^3 containing 4 cm^3 of vitamins, 300 mg thiamine hydrochloride)	4.28
Normal saline	5.35, 5.40
Lactated Ringer's solution (Ringer)	7.01
Ringer (1 dm^3 containing 2 cm^3 of vitamins)	5.50
Ringer (1 dm^3 containing 2 cm^3 of vitamins, 100 mg thiamine hydrochloride)	5.38
Ringer (1 dm^3 containing 2 cm^3 of vitamins, 200 mg thiamine hydrochloride)	5.16

[a] Reproduced from R. L. Tse and M. W. Lee, *J. Am. Med. Ass.*, 215, 642 (1971).

Rule of thumb

From equations (5.11), (5.16), (5.23) and (5.24) it is seen that, as a rough guide, the solubility of drugs with unionised species of low solubility varies by a factor of 10 for each pH unit change. A compilation of the dissociation constants of drugs is given in Table 3.6, p. 78.

• •

EXAMPLE 5.4

Tryptophan has two pK_a values: 2.4 and 9.4. Calculate the solubility of tryptophan at pH 10 and at pH 2, given that the solubility of the compound in neutral solutions is 2×10^{-2} mol dm^{-3}.

Answer

$S_0 = 2 \times 10^{-2}$ mol dm^{-3}. We must use equations (5.23) and (5.24). At pH 2.0,

$$pH - pK_a = \log\left(\frac{S_0}{S - S_0}\right)$$

$$2 - 2.4 = \log\left(\frac{2 \times 10^{-2}}{S - (2 \times 10^{-2})}\right)$$

Rearranging,

$$\log\left(\frac{S - (2 \times 10^{-2})}{2 \times 10^{-2}}\right) = 0.4$$

That is,

$$\frac{S - (2 \times 10^{-2})}{2 \times 10^{-2}} = 2.5118$$

Therefore, $S = (5.02 \times 10^{-2}) + (2 \times 10^{-2}) = 7.02 \times 10^{-2}$ mol dm^{-3}.

At pH 10 (using equation 5.24)

$$10 - 9.4 = \log\left(\frac{S - (2 \times 10^{-2})}{2 \times 10^{-2}}\right)$$

That is,

$$\frac{S - (2 \times 10^{-2})}{2 \times 10^{-2}} = 3.981$$

Therefore, $S = (7.96 \times 10^{-2}) + (2 \times 10^{-2}) = 9.96 \times 10^{-2}$ mol dm^{-3}.

• •

• •

EXAMPLE 5.5

Calculate the pH at which the following drugs will precipitate from solution given the information supplied.

Drug	pK_a	Solubility of unionised species	Concentration of solution
(a) Thioridazine HCl (mol. wt. 407)	9.5	1.5×10^{-6} mol dm^{-3}	0.407% w/v
(b) Oxytetracycline HCl	3.3, 7.3 and 9.1	0.5 g dm^{-3}	1.4 mg cm^{-3}

Answer

(a) We use equation (5.15) or (5.16) to calculate the pH above which thioridazine will precipitate:

$$pH = pK_a + \log\left(\frac{S_0}{S - S_0}\right)$$

The concentration of solution is the saturation solubility at the point of precipitation. 0.407% w/v $= 1 \times 10^{-2}$ mol dm^{-3} = S. $S_0 = 1.5 \times 10^{-6}$ mol dm^{-3}.

$$pH = 9.5 + \log\left(\frac{1.5 \times 10^{-6}}{(1 \times 10^{-2}) - (1.5 \times 10^{-6})}\right)$$

$$= 9.5 + \log\left(\frac{1.5 \times 10^{-6}}{1.0 \times 10^{-2}}\right)$$

$$= 9.5 - 3.284$$

$$= 5.68$$

(b) The concentration of solution is 1.4 mg cm^{-3}, which is 1.4 g dm^{-3}. $S_0 = 0.5$ g dm^{-3}. At pH values below 7, the pH at which S is the maximum solubility is given by

$$pH = pK_a + \log\left(\frac{S_0}{S - S_0}\right)$$

$$= 3.3 + \log(0.556)$$

$$= 3.3 - 0.255$$

$$= 3.05$$

At pH values above 7, the pH at which S is

the maximum value is given by

$$pH = pK_a + \log\left(\frac{S - S_0}{S_0}\right)$$

$$= 7.3 + \log(1.8)$$

$$= 7.3 + 0.255$$

$$= 7.56$$

Thus at pH values between 3.05 and 7.56 the solution containing 1.4 mg cm^{-3} will precipitate.

• •

5.3 Measurement of solubility

A simple turbidimetric method for the determination of the solubility of acids and bases in buffers of different pH can be used.[9] Solutions of the hydrochloride (or other salt) of a basic drug, or the soluble salt of an acidic compound, are prepared in water over a range of concentrations. Portions of each solution are added to buffers of known pH and the turbidity of the solutions is determined in the visible region. Typical results are shown in Fig. 5.4. Below the solubility limit there is no

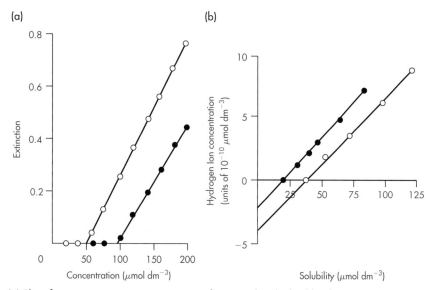

Figure 5.4 (a) Plot of extinction against concentration of amitriptyline hydrochloride at pH 9.78 (O) and pH 9.20 (●).
(b) Relationship between hydrogen ion concentration and solubility of pecazine (●) and amitriptyline (O).
Reproduced from reference 9.

turbidity. As the solubility limit is progressively exceeded, the turbidity rises. The solubility can be determined by extrapolation as shown in Fig. 5.4. Table 5.10 shows results obtained by this method for some phenothiazines and tricyclic antidepressant compounds. Determination of the solubility of weak electrolytes at several pH values provides one method of obtaining the dissociation constant of the drug substance. For basic drugs, equation (5.16) is rearranged to give

$$pH = pK_a + \log\left(\frac{S_0}{S - S_0}\right)$$

S_0, the solubility of the undissociated species (base), is determined at high pH, and S is determined at several different lower pH values. A plot of $\log[S_0/(S - S_0)]$ versus pH will have the pK_a as the intercept on the pH axis.

Alternatively, S may be plotted against $[H^+]$ as in Fig. 5.4(b). Equation (5.14) can be written in the form

$$[H^+] = \left(\frac{K_a S}{S_0}\right) - K_a \qquad (5.25)$$

Plotting data as in Fig. 5.4(b) yields S_0 when the line crosses the x-axis as $[H^+] = 0$ (and $S = S_0$). The intercept on the y-axis gives K_a and the slope of the line is K_a/S_0.

5.4 The solubility parameter

Regular solution theory characterises non-polar solvents in terms of solubility parameter, δ_1, which is defined as

$$\delta_1 = \left(\frac{\Delta U}{V}\right)^{1/2} = \left(\frac{\Delta H - RT}{V}\right)^{1/2} \qquad (5.26)$$

where ΔU is the molar energy and ΔH is the molar heat of vaporisation of the solvent. ΔH is determined by calorimetry at temperatures below the boiling point at constant volume. V is the molar volume of the solvent. The solubility parameter is thus a measure of the intermolecular forces within the solvent and gives us information on the ability of the liquid to act as a solvent. Table 5.11 gives the solubility parameters of some common solvents calculated using equation (5.26).

$\Delta U/V$ is the liquid's *cohesive energy density*, a measure of the attraction of a molecule from its own liquid, which is the energy required to remove it from the liquid and is equal to the energy of vaporisation per unit volume. Because cavities have to be formed in a solvent, by separating other solvent molecules, to accommodate solute molecules (as discussed earlier) the solubility parameter δ_1

Table 5.10 Water solubilities and pK_a values of aminoalkylphenothiazines and related compounds[a]

Structure	Trivial or approved name	pK_a, solubility method	pK_a, Chatten–Harris[b]	Solubility (μmol dm^{-3})	Calculated relative solubility at pH 7.4
R=H; R'=CH₂CH(Me)•NMe₂	Promethazine	9.1	9.1	55	4.5
R=H; R'=[CH₂]₃•NMe₂	Promazine	9.4	–	50	8.0
R=Cl; R'=[CH₂]₃•NMe₂	Chlorpromazine	9.3	9.2	8	1.0
R=CF₃; R'=[CH₂]₃•NMe₂	Triflupromazine	9.2	9.4	5	0.4
R=H; R'=CH₂– (piperidine N-Me)	Pecazine	9.7	–	18	5.0
R=SMe; R'=[CH₂]₂– (piperidine N-Me)	Thioridazine	9.5	9.2	1.5	0.3

[a] Reproduced from reference 9.
[b] Data from L. G. Chatten and L. E. Harris, *Anal. Chem.*, **34**, 1495 (1962).

Table 5.11 Solubility parameters of common solvents

Solvent	δ_1 (cal$^{1/2}$ cm$^{-3/2}$)[a]
Methanol	14.50
Ethanol	12.74
1-Propanol	11.94
2-Propanol	11.56
1-Butanol	11.40
1-Octanol	10.24
Ethyl acetate	8.58
Isoamyl acetate	8.07
Hexane	7.3
Hexadecane	8
Carbon disulfide	10
Membrane (erythrocytes)	10.3 ± 0.40
Cyclohexane	8.2
Benzene	9.2

[a] The solubility parameter is commonly expressed in hildebrand units:
1 hildebrand unit = 1 (cal cm^{-3})$^{1/2}$.
1 cal = 4.18 J.

enables predictions of solubility to be made in a semiquantitative manner, especially in relation to the solubility parameter of the solute, δ_2.

By itself the solubility parameter can explain the behaviour of only a relatively small group of solvents – those with little or no polarity and those unable to participate in hydrogen-bonding interactions. The difference between the solubility parameters expressed as $(\delta_1 - \delta_2)$ will give an indication of solubility relationships.

For solid solutes a hypothetical value of δ_2 can be calculated from $(U/V)^{1/2}$, where U is in this case the lattice energy of the crystal. In a study of the solubility of ion pairs in organic solvents it has been found that the logarithm of the solubility (log S) correlates well with $(\delta_1 - \delta_2)^2$.

5.4.1 Solubility parameters and biological processes

The solubility of small molecules in biological membranes is of importance from pharmacological, physiological and toxicological viewpoints. Biological membranes are not simple solvents – the bilayer has an interior core of hydrocarbon chains about 2.5–3.5 nm thick – and therefore one would not expect simple solution theory to hold. Regular solution theory has been applied to biomembranes to obtain a value of δ_1 for a membrane.[10] From experimental solubility data for anaesthetic gases in erythrocyte ghosts, a mean empirical solubility parameter of 10.3 ± 0.40 for the whole membrane and 8.7 ± 1.03 for membrane lipid was calculated. The values compare with solubility parameters of 7.3 for hexane and 8.0 for hexadecane. The value for the whole membrane (10.3) is very close to the solubility parameter of 1-octanol (10.2), a solvent which is used widely in partition coefficient work to simulate biological lipid phases.

Solubility parameters of drugs (δ_2) have also been correlated with membrane absorption rates in model systems. A reasonable relationship was obtained between δ_2 and a logarithmic absorption term, thus providing one predictive index of absorption. Scott[11] has said of solubility parameters and equations employing them that 'the theory offers a useful initial approach to a very wide area of solutions. Like a small-scale map for a very broad long-distance view of a sub-continent they are unlikely to prove highly accurate when a small area is examined carefully, but they are equally unlikely to prove completely absurd.'

5.5 Solubility in mixed solvents

The device of using mixed solvents is resorted to when drug solubility in one solvent is limited or perhaps when the stability characteristics of soluble salts forbid the use of single solvents. Many pharmaceutical preparations are complex systems. Common water-miscible solvents used in pharmaceutical formulations include glycerol, propylene glycol, ethyl alcohol and polyoxyethylene glycols. As can be imagined, the addition of another component complicates any system and explanations of the often complex solubility patterns are not easy. Only recently has there been any attempt to predict solubility in mixed solvents theoretically, although the solubility parameters of the mixed solvent systems have been used for this purpose for some time. Toxicity considerations are, of course, a constraint on the choice of solvent for products for administration by any route.

Figure 5.5 shows the solubility of phenobarbital in glycerol–water, ethanol–water and ethanol–glycerol mixtures. Phenobarbital dissolves up to 0.12% w/v in water at 25°C. Glycerol, even in high concentrations, does not significantly increase the solubility of the drug. Ethanol is a much more efficient cosolvent than glycerol as it is less polar. Solubility is at a maximum at 90% ethanol in ethanol–water mixtures, and at 80% ethanol in ethanol–glycerol mixtures. It is naive to assume that the drug dissolves in 'pockets' of the cosolvent (for example, ethanol in ethanol–water mixtures), although obviously the affinity of cosolvent for the solute is of importance.

Additives will influence solute–solvent interfacial energies or dissociation of electrolytes through changes in dielectric constant. A reduction in ionisation through a decrease in dielectric constant will favour decreased solubility, but this effect may be counterbalanced by the greater affinity of the undissociated species in the presence of the cosolvent.

5.6 Cyclodextrins as solubilising agents

Solubilisation by surface-active agents is discussed in Chapter 6. Alternatives to micellar solubilisation (or solubilisation in vesicles) include the use of the cyclodextrin family. When the first edition of this book was published in 1981 (and a diagram of a cyclodextrin–drug complex was used to adorn the cover), the use of cyclodextrins was in its infancy. Attention was then focused around α-, β- and γ-cyclodextrins, but a veritable industry has grown up with an array of derivatives which can lend useful new properties to the complexes they form. There is now Encapsin HPB (hydroxypropyl-β-cyclodextrin), which is available commercially for pharmaceutical use. Ten per cent of this cyclodextrin can enhance the solubility of betamethasone 118 times, of diazepam 21 times and of ibuprofen 55 times.

Cyclodextrins (CDs) are enzymatically modified starches. Their glucopyranose units form a ring: α-CD a ring of 6 units; β-CD a ring of 7 units; and γ-CD a ring of 8 units (Table 5.12; Fig. 5.6). The 'ring' is cylindrical, the outer surface being hydrophilic and the internal surface of the cavity being nonpolar. Appropriately sized lipophilic molecules can be accommodated wholly or partially in the complex, in which the host–guest ratio is usually 1 : 1 (Fig. 5.7), although other stoichiometries are possible, one, two or three CD molecules complexing with one or more drug molecules. The dissolution–dissociation–

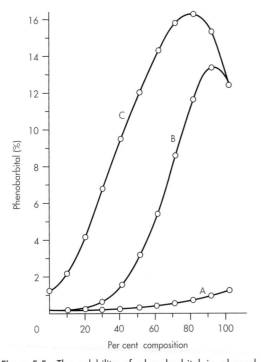

Figure 5.5 The solubility of phenobarbital in glycerol–water, ethanol–water and absolute ethanol–glycerol mixtures as a function of the percentage composition of the mixtures. Abscissa indicates percentage of: A, glycerol in water; B, ethanol in water; C, absolute ethanol in glycerol. Reproduced from G. M. Krause and J. M. Cross, *J. Am. Pharm. Assoc.*, 40, 137, (1951).

Table 5.12 Properties of α, β and γ cyclodextrins[a]

Property	Alpha (α)	Beta (β)	Gamma (γ)
Molecular weight	973	1135	1297
Glucose monomers	6	7	8
Internal cavity diameters (nm)	0.5	0.6	0.8
Water solubility (g/100 cm^3; 25°C)	14.2	1.85	23.2
Surface tension (mN m^{-1})	71	71	71
Melting range (°C)	255–260	255–260	240–245
Water of crystallisation (no. of molecules)	10.2	13–15	8–18
Water in cavity (no. of molecules)	6	11	17

[a] Reproduced from M. E. Brewster, et al. J. Parenter. Sci. Technol., 43, 262 (1989).

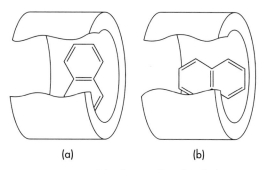

Figure 5.7 Two models of a complex of cyclodextrin with a lipophilic guest compound: (a) equatorial inclusion, (b) axial inclusion.
Reproduced from K. Harata and H. Uedaira, Bull. Chem. Soc. Jpn., 48, 375 (1975).

crystallisation process that can occur on dissolution is illustrated in Fig. 5.8.

Not all cyclodextrins are free of adverse effects; di-O-methyl β-CD, for example, has a strong affinity for cholesterol and is haemolytic. It is also one of the best solubilisers technically.

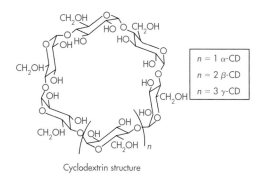

Cyclodextrin structure

n = 1 α-CD	
n = 2 β-CD	
n = 3 γ-CD	

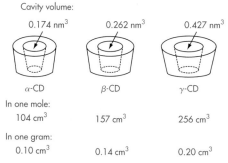

Cavity volume:

0.174 nm^3	0.262 nm^3	0.427 nm^3
α-CD	β-CD	γ-CD

In one mole:

| 104 cm^3 | 157 cm^3 | 256 cm^3 |

In one gram:

| 0.10 cm^3 | 0.14 cm^3 | 0.20 cm^3 |

Figure 5.6 Structures of the α-, β- and γ-cyclodextrins.
Reproduced from J. Szejtli, Pharm. Tech. Int., 3(2), 15 (1991).

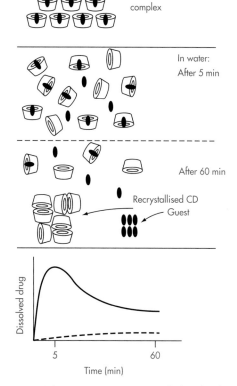

Figure 5.8 Schematic representation of the dissolution–dissociation–recrystallisation process of a cyclodextrin complex with a poorly soluble guest. The complex rapidly dissolves, and a metastable oversaturated solution is obtained. The anomalously high level of dissolved guest drops back but remains higher than the level that can be obtained with noncomplexed drug. Solid curve = complexed drug; broken curve = noncomplexed drug.
Redrawn after J. Szejtli, Pharm. Tech. Int., 3(2), 15 (1991).

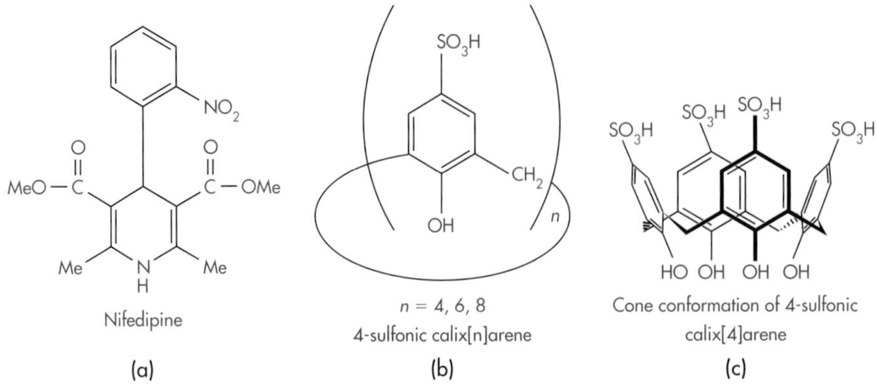

(a)   **(b)**   **(c)**

Figure 5.9 Molecular structures of (a) nifedipine and (b) 4-sulfonic calix[n]arenes. As n increases (4, 6, 8) the cavity size (see (c)) increases from 0.3 nm, through 0.76 nm to 1.16 nm. The solubility increase for nifedipine is greatest with calix[8]arene, being nearly 250% at a concentration of 0.008 mol dm^{-3} and pH of 5.
Reproduced from Yang and de Villiers, *Eur. J. Pharm. Biopharm.*, 58, 629–636 (2004).

The cyclodextrins have obvious uses in parenteral formulations, including use as components of vehicles for peptides and other biologicals (ovine growth hormone, IL-2 and insulin)

Calixarenes

Research continues into other agents, apart from surfactants (which are discussed in Chapter 6), which can enhance the solubility of drugs. The calixarenes are another type of host, existing in a 'cup-shape' in a rigid conformation. The 4-sulfonic calix[n]arenes can form host–guest type interactions with drugs such as nifedipine, a poorly water soluble agent,[12] seen in Fig. 5.9.

5.7 Solubility problems in formulation

5.7.1 Mixtures of acidic and basic compounds

Sometimes a combination formulation requires the admixture of acidic and basic drugs. One example (Septrin infusion) is discussed here.
Because sulfamethoxazole (**XVII**) is a weakly acidic substance and trimethoprim (**XVIII**) is a weakly basic one, for optimal solubility basic and acidic solutions, respectively, are required. In consequence, in an ordinary aqueous

solution sulfamethoxazole and trimethoprim demonstrate a high degree of incompatibility and mutual precipitation occurs on mixing. To optimise mutual dissolution, an aqueous solution which includes 40% propylene glycol is utilised in the formulation of the infusion. This solution, which has a pH between 9.5 and 11.0, allows adequate amounts of both substances to coexist in solution to give the correct ratio of concentration for antibacterial action. On dilution, the infusion becomes less

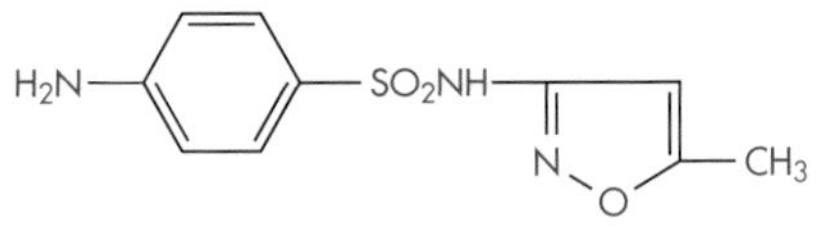

Structure **XVII** Sulfamethoxazole, pK_a = 6.03

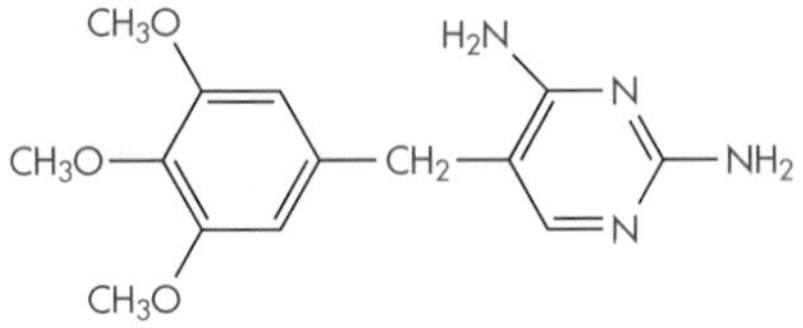

Structure **XVIII** Trimethoprim, pK_a = 7.05

stable and at the recommended 1 in 25 dilution stability is about 7 hours. Owing to incompatibility of the two constituents, their degrees of solubility are sensitive to changes in ionic composition, pH and any drug additives. If there is imbalance in pH or ionic composition, then precipitation of one or other of the components may well occur.

5.7.2   Choice of drug salt to optimise solubility

The choice of a particular salt of a drug for use in formulations may depend on several factors. The solubility of the drug in aqueous media may be markedly dependent on the salt form. The chemical stability rather than the solubility may be a criterion and in many cases this is dependent on the choice of salt, sometimes through a pH effect. Deliberate choice of an insoluble form for use in suspen-

sions is an obvious ploy; the formation of water-soluble entities from poorly soluble acids or bases by the use of hydrophilic counterions is frequently attempted to produce injectable solutions of a drug. Table 5.13 gives some indication of the range of solubilities that can be obtained through the use of different salt forms, in this case of an experimental antimalarial drug (**XIX**).

The large hydrophobic compound **XIX**, even as its hydrochloride salt, is poorly soluble and this is presumably the reason for its poor oral bioavailability. Similar conclusions were drawn several years ago for novobiocin. The acid salt administered at 12.5 mg kg^{-1} to dogs was not absorbed, but the monosodium salt, which is about 300 times as soluble in water, produced plasma levels of 22 μg cm^{-3} after 3 hours. Unfortunately, the sodium salt is unstable in solution. An amorphous form of the acid produced even higher levels of drug than the sodium salt, illustrating the fact that choice of salt and crystalline form of a drug substance may be of critical importance.

Some of the solubility differences obviously arise from differences in the pH of the salt solutions, which in the case of compound **XIX** ranged from 2.4 to 5.8 pH units. This is not atypical. The pH of solutions of salts of a 3-oxyl-1,4-benzodiazepine derivative at 5 mg cm^{-3} ranged from 2.3 for its dihydrochloride, to 4.3 for the maleate, and to 4.8 for the methanesulfonate.

Further examples of the solubility range in drug salts and derivatives are shown in

Structure XIX Compound used in Table 5.13

Table 5.13   Solubilities of salts of an antimalarial drug (**XIX**)[a]

Salt	Melting point (°C)[b]	Solubility (mg cm^{-3})	Saturated solution pH
Free base	215	7–8	–
Hydrochloride	331	32–15	5.8
dl-Lactate	172 (dec)	1800	3.8
l-Lactate	193 (dec)	900	–
2-Hydroxy-1-sulfonate	250 (dec)	620	2.4
Methanesulfonate	290 (dec)	300	5.1
Sulfate	270 (dec)	20	–

[a] Reproduced from S. Agharkar, S. Lindenbaum and T. Higuchi, *J. Pharm. Sci.*, 65, 747 (1976).
[b] (dec) = with decomposition.

Table 5.14. The increase in the solubility on the formation of the hydrochloride is readily attributable in the case of tetracycline to a lowering of the solution pH by the hydrochloride. The common ion effect can, however, produce an unexpected trend in the solubilities of bases in the presence of high concentrations of hydrochloric acid. Increase in Cl^- concentrations will cause the equilibrium between solid and solution forms

$$BH^+Cl^-_{(c)} \overset{K_{sp}}{\rightleftharpoons} (BH^+)_{aq} + (Cl^-)_{aq}$$

to be pushed to the left-hand side, with a resultant decrease in solubility. The solubility of XIX as the hydrochloride decreases from 24×10^{-5} mol dm^{-3} in 1.3 mmol dm^{-3} chloride ion, to 3×10^{-5} mol dm^{-3} in 40 mmol dm^{-3} chloride ion concentration. It should be noted that the stomach contents are rich in chloride ions. The common ion effect will be apparent in many infusion fluids to which drugs may be added, and therefore the effect of pH as well as electrolyte concentrations must be considered.

Consideration of Table 5.14 suggests that the hydrochloride salts of tetracyclines are always more readily dissolved than the base. The situation is more complex than at first appears, however. In dilute HCl at pH 1.2, the free base dissolves more than the hydrochloride, probably owing to the differences in crystallinity. The amount of compound derived from the base in solution decreases with time as the drug is converted to the hydrochloride. At pH 1.6 the rate of solution of the two forms is identical, and at pH 2.1 the hydrochloride has a higher solubility owing to its effect on local pH around the dissolving particles.

Erythromycin (XX) is labile at pH values below pH 4, and hence is unstable in the stomach contents. Erythromycin stearate (the salt of the tertiary aliphatic amine and stearic acid), being less soluble, is not as susceptible to degradation. The salt dissociates in the intestine to yield the free base, which is absorbed. There are differences in the absorption behaviour of the erythromycin salts and differences in toxicity, which may be related to their aqueous solubilities. Erythromycin ethylsuccinate was originally developed for paediatric use because its low water solubility and relative tastelessness were suited to paediatric formulations. The soluble lactobionate is used in intravenous infusions.

5.7.3   Drug solubility and biological activity

There should be a broad correlation between aqueous solubility and indices of biological activity. On the one hand, as drug solubility in aqueous media is inversely related to the

Table 5.14   Aqueous solubilities of tetracycline, erythromycin and chlorhexidine salts

Compound	Solubility in water (mg cm^{-3})
Tetracycline	1.7
Tetracycline hydrochloride	10.9
Tetracycline phosphate	15.9
Erythromycin	2.1
Erythromycin estolate[a]	0.16
Erythromycin stearate	0.33
Erythromycin lactobionate	20
Chlorhexidine	0.08
Chlorhexidine dihydrochloride	0.60
Chlorhexidine digluconate	>700

[a] Lauryl sulfate ester of erythromycin propionate

Structure **XX** Erythromycin

solubility of the agent in biological lipid phases, there will be some relationship between pharmacodynamic activity and drug solubility. On the other, we should expect that drug or drug salt solubility might influence the absorption phase; drugs of very low aqueous solubility will dissolve slowly in the gastro-intestinal tract, and in many cases the rate of dissolution is the rate-controlling step in absorption.

With drugs of low aqueous solubility such as digoxin, chlorpropamide, indometacin, griseofulvin, and many steroids, the physical properties of the drug can influence biological properties. At early stages in a drug's development, pharmacological and toxicological tests are frequently carried out on extemporaneously prepared suspensions whose physical characteristics are not always well defined. This is not good practice as the toxicity of some drugs given by gavage to rats is dependent on the drug species used[13] (Table 5.15). This has been shown to be true with polymorphic forms of the same drug, but in the cases discussed in Table 5.15 different salts of the drugs were used.

There are other examples in which aqueous solubility acts as a rough and ready guide to

Table 5.15 The effect of solubility in water on the toxicity of drugs given by gavage to albino rats[a]

Drug	Salt	Solubility	$LD_{50} \pm SEM$
Benzylpenicillin	Ammonium	<20 mg cm^{-3}	8.4 ± 0.13
Benzylpenicillin	Potassium	>20 mg cm^{-3}	6.7 ± 0.1
Iron	Free metal	Insoluble	98.6 ± 26.7
Iron	Ferrous sulfate	Soluble	0.78
Spiramycin	Free base	Poorly soluble	9.4 ± 0.8
Spiramycin	Adipate	Soluble	4.9 ± 0.2

[a] Modified from reference 13.

absorption characteristics. Of the cardiotonic glycosides digitoxin, digoxin and ouabain, the least water soluble, being the most lipid soluble, is best absorbed. But because of the lipophilicity of digitoxin and digoxin, the rate-limiting step is the rate of solution, which is influenced directly by the solubility of the compounds.

High molecular weight quaternary salts such as bephenium hydroxynaphthoate (**XXI**) and pyrvinium embonate (**XXII**), being quaternary, have low lipid solubility but also have

Structure **XXI** Bephenium hydroxynaphthoate

Structure **XXII** Pyrvinium embonate

low aqueous solubility. They are virtually unabsorbed from the gut and indeed are used in the treatment of worm infestation of the lower bowel.

5.8 Partitioning

Here we discuss the topic of partitioning of a drug or solute between two immiscible phases. One phase might be blood or water and the other a biomembrane, or an oil or a plastic. As many processes (not least the absorption process) depend on the movement of molecules from one phase to another, it is vital that this topic is mastered. Here we will learn of the simple concepts of the partitioning of drugs and the calculation of partition coefficient (P) of the nonionised form of the solute (and its logarithm, log P), as well as the use of the log P concept in determining the relative activities or toxicities of drugs from a knowledge of log P between an oil, most commonly octanol, and water. Where P cannot be measured, calculations of log P can be accomplished.[14, 15] An outline of the methods available is given here.

Drugs, whether in formulations containing more than one phase or in the body, move from one liquid phase to another in ways that depend on their relative concentrations (or chemical potentials) and their affinities for each phase. So a drug will move from the blood into extravascular tissues if it has the appropriate affinity for the cell membrane and the nonblood phase.

The movement of molecules from one phase to another is called *partitioning*. Examples of the process include:

- Drugs partitioning between aqueous phases and lipid biophases
- Preservative molecules in emulsions partitioning between the aqueous and oil phases
- Antibiotics partitioning into microorganisms
- Drugs and preservative molecules partitioning into the plastic of containers or giving sets

Plasticisers will sometimes partition from plastic containers into formulations. It is, therefore, important that the process can be quantified and understood.

5.8.1 Theoretical background

If two immiscible phases are placed in contact, one containing a solute soluble to some extent in both phases, the solute will distribute itself so that when equilibrium is attained no further net transfer of solute takes place, as then the chemical potential of the solute in one phase is equal to its chemical potential in the other phase. If we think of an aqueous (w) and an organic (o) phase, we can write, according to equations (3.49) and (3.52),

$$\mu_w^\ominus + RT \ln a_w = \mu_o^\ominus + RT \ln a_o \qquad (5.27)$$

Rearranging equation (5.27) we obtain

$$\frac{\mu_o^\ominus - \mu_w^\ominus}{RT} = \ln \frac{a_w}{a_o} \qquad (5.28)$$

The term on the left hand side of equation (5.28) is constant at a given temperature and pressure, so it follows that a_w/a_o = constant and, of course a_o/a_w = constant. These constants are the *partition coefficients* or *distribution coefficients*, P. If the solute forms an ideal solution in both solvents, activities can be replaced by concentration, so that

$$P = \frac{C_o}{C_w} \qquad (5.29)$$

P is therefore a measure of the relative affinities of the solute for an aqueous and a nonaqueous or lipid phase. Unless otherwise stated, P is calculated according to the convention in equation (5.29), where the concentration in the nonaqueous (oily) phase is divided by the concentration in the aqueous phase. The greater the value of P, the higher the lipid solubility of the solute.

It has been shown for several systems that the partition coefficient can be approximated by the solubility of the agent in the organic phase divided by its solubility in the aqueous phase, a useful starting point for estimating relative affinities.

In many systems the ionisation of the solute in one or both phases or the association of the solute in one of the solvents complicates the calculation of partition coefficient. As early as 1891, Nernst stressed the fact that the partition coefficient as a function of concentration would be constant only if a single molecular species was involved. If the solute forms aggregates or otherwise self-associates, the following equilibrium between the two phases 1 and 2 occurs when dimerisation occurs in phase 2:

$$\underset{\text{phase 1}}{2A} \rightleftharpoons \underset{\text{phase 2}}{A \cdot A}$$

$$K = \frac{[A]_{\text{phase 2}}}{[A]^2_{\text{phase 1}}}$$

Hence

$$K' = \frac{\sqrt{C_2}}{C_1} \tag{5.30}$$

K' is a constant combining the partition coefficient and the association constant. Table 5.16 illustrates the use of equations (5.29) and (5.30).

Partitioning of ionisable species

Being weak electrolytes many drugs will ionise in at least one phase, usually the aqueous

---

phase. The partition coefficient refers to the distribution of one species, so the assay data of the solute in each phase have to be corrected for ionisation. We can use the convention that C_w is the total concentration of all species in the aqueous phase, C_o is the concentration in the organic phase and C_{ion} is the concentration of ions in the aqueous phase. If we consider the dissociation of a weak acid

$$\underset{(C_w - C_{\text{ion}})}{HA} \rightleftharpoons \underset{C_{\text{ion}}}{H^+} + \underset{C_{\text{ion}}}{A^-}$$

the concentration of the species may be written as shown, and therefore the dissociation constant in the aqueous phase, K_w is given by

$$K_w = \frac{(C_{\text{ion}})^2}{(C_w - C_{\text{ion}})} \tag{5.31}$$

If dimerisation occurs in the organic phase and if K_D is the dissociation constant of dimers into single molecules, we can consider the process in the organic phase to be

$$\underset{\text{organic phase}}{(HA)_2} \rightleftharpoons \underset{\text{acqueous phase}}{2HA}$$

$$K_D = \frac{2(P[C_w - C_{\text{ion}}])^2}{C_o - P(C_w - C_{\text{ion}})} = \frac{2(PN)^2}{C_o - PN} \tag{5.32}$$

where N is $(C_w - C_{\text{ion}})$, that is, the concentration of unionised molecules in water, the species which will distribute into the nonaqueous phase. It is generally accepted that only the nonionised species partitions from the aqueous phase into the nonaqueous phase. Ionised species, being hydrated and highly soluble in the aqueous phase, disfavour the organic phase. Transfer of such a hydrated species involves dehydration. In addition, organic solvents of low polarity do not favour the existence of free ions.

Equation (5.32) can be rearranged to give

$$K_D(C_o - PN) = 2(PN)^2 \tag{5.33}$$

Multiplying by $1/K_D N^2$ and rearranging, we obtain

$$C_o/N^2 = P(1/N) + \text{constant} \tag{5.34}$$

A plot of C_o/N^2 against $1/N$ will yield a straight line with slope P.

Table 5.16 Distribution of two acids between immiscible phases at 25°C[a]

C_1 (mol dm^{-3})[b]	C_2 (mol dm^{-3})[c]	C_2/C_1	$\sqrt{C_2}/C_1$
Succinic acid			
0.191	0.0248	0.130	
0.370	0.0488	0.132	
0.547	0.0736	0.135	
0.749	0.101	0.135	
Benzoic acid			
4.88×10^{-3}	3.64×10^{-2}	7.46	39.06
8.00×10^{-3}	8.59×10^{-2}	10.75	36.63
16.00×10^{-3}	33.8×10^{-2}	21.13	36.36
23.7×10^{-3}	75.3×10^{-2}	31.77	36.63

[a] Reproduced from S. Glasstone and D. Lewis, *Elements of Physical Chemistry*, 2nd edn, Macmillan, 1964.
[b] Aqueous phase concentration.
[c] Nonaqueous phase concentration (succinic acid in ether; benzoic acid in benzene).

If ionisation and its consequences are neglected, an *apparent* partition coefficient, P_{app}, is obtained simply by assay of both phases, which will provide information on how much of the drug is present in each phase, regardless of status. The relationship between the true thermodynamic P and P_{app} is given by the following equations:

For acids:

$$\log P = \log P_{app} - \log\left(\frac{1}{1 + 10^{pH-pK_a}}\right) \quad (5.35)$$

For bases:

$$\log P = \log P_{app} - \log\left(\frac{1}{1 + 10^{pK_a-pH}}\right) \quad (5.36)$$

5.8.2   Free energies of transfer

The standard free energy of transfer of a solute between two phases is given by

$$\Delta G^{\ominus}_{trans} = \mu^{\ominus}_w - \mu^{\ominus}_o = RT \ln P \quad (5.37)$$

In a homologous series, P can be measured and the increase in its value observed for each substituent group (for example, $-CH_2-$). As the chain length of nonpolar aliphatic compounds increases, it has been found that P increases by a factor of 2–4 per methylene group. The substituent contributions to P are additive, so a *substituent constant*, π_X, may be defined as

$$\pi_X = \log P_X - \log P_H \quad (5.38)$$

where P_X is the partition coefficient of the derivative of the parent compound whose partition coefficient is P_H and π_X is the logarithm of the partition coefficient of the function X. For example, π_{Cl} can be obtained by subtracting $\log P_{benzene}$ from $\log P_{chlorobenzene}$.

5.8.3   Octanol as a nonaqueous phase

Octanol is often used as the nonaqueous phase in experiments to measure the partition coefficient of drugs. Its polarity means that water is solubilised to some extent in the octanol phase and thus partitioning is more complex than with an anhydrous solvent, but perhaps its usefulness stems from the fact that biological membranes are also not simple anhydrous lipid phases. While octanol is favoured, other alcohols have also been used. For example, isobutanol has been used to show that the binding of many drugs to serum protein is determined by the hydrophobicity or lipophilicity of the drug, following the relationship

$$\log K = 0.9 \log P_{isobutanol} + \text{constant} \quad (5.39)$$

where K is an equilibrium constant measuring the binding of solute to protein. Transfer of a hydrophobic drug from an aqueous phase to a protein is, of course, a type of partitioning.

The correlation of lipophilicity and biological activity usually involves equations of the type

$$\log \frac{1}{C} = A \log P + \text{constant} \quad (5.40)$$

where C is the concentration required to produce a given pharmacological response.

5.9   Biological activity and partition coefficients: thermodynamic activity and Ferguson's principle

As the site of action of many biologically active species is in lipid components such as membranes, correlations between partition coefficients and biological activity were found early on by investigators of structure–action relationships. For example, a wide range of simple organic compounds can exert qualitatively identical depressant actions (narcosis) on many simple organisms. Lack of any chemical specificity in the compounds tested led to the suggestion that physical, rather than chemical, properties governed the activity of the compounds. Early work by Meyer and Overton related narcotic potency to the oil/water partition coefficient of the compounds concerned, and in a later re-interpretation of the data, it was concluded that narcosis commences when any chemically nonspecific substance has attained a certain molar concentration in the lipids of the cells.

In 1939 Ferguson placed the Overton–Meyer theory on a more quantitative basis by applying thermodynamics to the problem of narcotic action. By expressing compound potency in terms of thermodynamic activity, rather than concentration, he avoided the problem of there being various distribution coefficients between the numerous different phases within the cell, any of which might be the phase in which the drug exerted its pharmacological effects (the biophase). The fact that the narcotic action of a drug remains at a constant level while a critical concentration of drug is applied, decreasing rapidly when administration of the drug is stopped, indicates that an equilibrium exists between some external phase and the biophase.

According to equation (3.49) the chemical potentials in two phases at equilibrium are equal. Thus, from equation (3.52),

$$\mu_A^\ominus + RT \ln a_A = \mu_B^\ominus + RT \ln a_B \qquad (5.41)$$

If the standard states are identical, consequently the activities will be equal in the two phases. The activity of a substance in the biophase at equilibrium is thus identical to the readily determined value in an external phase.

For narcotic agents applied as a vapour, the standard state can be taken to be the saturated vapour, and thus activity $a = p_t/p_s$ where p_t is the partial pressure of the vapour and p_s is the saturated vapour pressure at the same temperature. When the narcotic agent was applied in solution and was also of limited solubility, activity was equated with the ratio S_t/S_0 where S_t is the molar concentration of the narcotic solution and S_0 its limiting solubility; the ratio S_t/S_0 therefore represents proportional saturation. This is in contrast to the normal procedure of taking the standard state as an infinitely dilute solution.

From recalculations of published data and also from measurements of the potency of many different compounds, Ferguson concluded that, within reasonable limits, substances present at approximately the same proportional saturation (that is with the same thermodynamic activity) in a given medium have the same biological potency. For example, Table 5.17 shows that while the bactericidal concentrations against *Bacillus typhosus* vary widely (0.0022–3.89 mol dm^{-3}), the thermodynamic activities vary within a relatively restricted range (0.11–0.76).

As with most physicochemical theories there may be problems in applying the equations to real life. If an attempt is made to correlate hydrophobicity with the *rate* of

Table 5.17   Bactericidal concentrations and activities of organic substances in solution[a]

Substance	Bactericidal concentration (mol dm^{-3}) (S_t)	Solubility at 25°C (mol dm^{-3}) (S_0)	Activity or S_t/S_0
Phenol	0.097	0.90	0.11
o-Cresol	0.039	0.23	0.17
Propionaldehyde	1.08	2.88	0.37
Thymol	0.0022	0.0057	0.38
Acetone	3.89	∞	0.40
Methyl ethyl ketone	1.25	3.13	0.40
Aniline	0.17	0.40	0.44
Cyclohexanol	0.18	0.38	0.47
Resorcinol	3.09	6.08	0.54
Methyl propyl ketone	0.39	0.70	0.56
Butyraldehyde	0.39	0.51	0.76

[a] Reproduced from K. H. Meyer and H. Hemmi, *Biochem. Z.*, 277, 39 (1935).

inhibition of local anaesthetic activity, the answers are complex, i.e. there is not necessarily a clear correlation because (1) molecular size as well as hydrophobicity is a factor in kinetics, (2) membranes are nonhomogeneous and if adsorption occurs at phospholipid head groups there is no way to mimic this with octanol and water; and (3) there is the problem of using equilibrium measurements for kinetic predictions.

5.10 Using log *P*

As we have seen, the value of log *P* is a measure of lipophilicity and, as so many pharmaceutical and biological events are dependent on lipophilic characteristics, the examples where correlations can be found between log *P* and biological indices are legion. A selection of applications of the log *P* concept is discussed here. Table 5.18 provides a sample of log *P* data for a range of pharmaceuticals. The relatively simple *in vitro* measurement of *P* can give an accurate prediction of activity in a complex biological system, provided that the obvious limitations of the simple system are recognised and that the biological activity of the drug depends on its lipophilic nature. Applications of *P* or log *P* come into their own particularly in homologous series or series of closely related compounds, where the influence of substituent groups can be accurately examined.

5.10.1 The relationship between lipophilicity and behaviour of tetracyclines

The lipid solubility of four tetracyclines (minocycline, doxycycline, tetracycline and oxytetracycline) correlates inversely with the mean concentration of antibiotic in plasma and with renal uptake and excretion. Only the more lipophilic minocycline and doxycycline pass across the blood–brain and blood–ocular barriers in detectable concentrations. Table 5.19 gives some of these characteristics of the tetracyclines. These analogues of tetracycline, while active *in vitro* against meningococci, are

Table 5.18 Log *P* values for representative drugs[a]

Drug	log *P*
Acetylsalicylic acid (aspirin)	1.19
Amiodarone	6.7
Benzocaine	1.89
Bupivacaine	3.4
Bromocriptine	6.6
Caffeine	0.01
Chlorpromazine	5.3
Cisapride	3.7
Ciprofloxacin	−1.12
Desipramine	4.0
β-Estradiol	2.69
Glutethimide	1.9
Haloperidol	1.53
Hydrocortisone	4.3
Hyoscine	1.90
Indometacin	3.1
Lidocaine	2.26
Methadone	3.9
Misoprostil	2.9
Nicotinamide	−0.37
Norfloxacin	−1.55
Ondansetron	3.2
Oxytetracycline	−1.12
Pergolide	3.8
Phenytoin	2.5
Physostigmine	2.2
Prednisone	1.46
Sulfadiazine	0.12
Sulfadimethoxine	1.56
Sulfafurazole	1.01
Sulfaguanidine	−1.22
Sulfamerazine	0.13
Sulfanilamide	−1.05
Sulfapyridine	0.90
Sulfathiazole	0.35
Tetracaine	3.56
Thiopental	2.8
Xamoterol	0.5
Zimeldine	2.7

[a] Data from B. J. Herbert and J. G. Dorsey, *Anal. Chem.*, **67**, 744 (1995); J. F. Butterworth and G. R. Strichartz, *Anaesthesiology*, **72**, 711 (1990); D. B. Jack, *Handbook of Clinical Pharmacokinetic Data*, Macmillan, London, 1992.

not of equal value in clinical use; oxytetracycline and doxycycline fail to change the state of 'carriers' of the disease, whereas minocycline has a significant effect. It is thought that the ability to enter the saliva and tears influences the clinical activity, for although saliva does

Table 5.19 Some characteristics of four tetracyclines

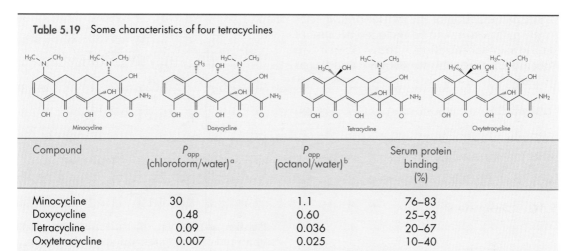

Compound	P_{app} (chloroform/water)[a]	P_{app} (octanol/water)[b]	Serum protein binding (%)
Minocycline	30	1.1	76–83
Doxycycline	0.48	0.60	25–93
Tetracycline	0.09	0.036	20–67
Oxytetracycline	0.007	0.025	10–40

[a] pH 7.4.
[b] pH 7.5.

not usually wet the nasopharynx, tears pass into the nasopharynx as the normal route of drainage from the conjunctival sac.

The pH dependence of partition coefficients of tetracyclines is more complex than for most drugs, as the tetracyclines are amphoteric.

For slightly simpler amphoteric compounds, such as *p*-aminobenzoic acid and sulfonamides, the apparent partition coefficient is maximal at the isoelectric point. Figure 5.10 illustrates the variation with pH of log P_{app} for *p*-aminobenzoic acid and for two sulfonamides.

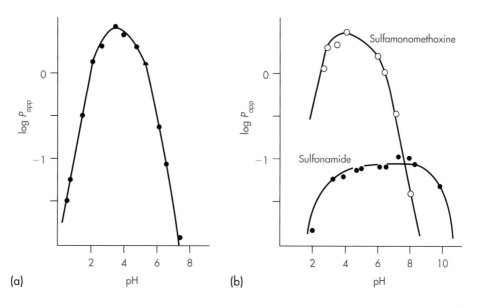

(a)   (b)

Figure 5.10 (a) Variation of log P_{app} with pH for *p*-aminobenzoic acid. (b) Variation of log P_{app} with pH for sulfamonomethoxine and sulfonamide.
Reproduced from H. Terada, *Chem. Pharm. Bull.*, **20**, 765 (1972).

The participation of the zwitterionic species in the partitioning can be excluded because of its low concentration, thus $K_t \rightarrow 0$ in Scheme 5.1. From this we obtain P and P_{app} as follows:

$$P = \frac{[I]_o}{[I]_w} \qquad (5.42)$$

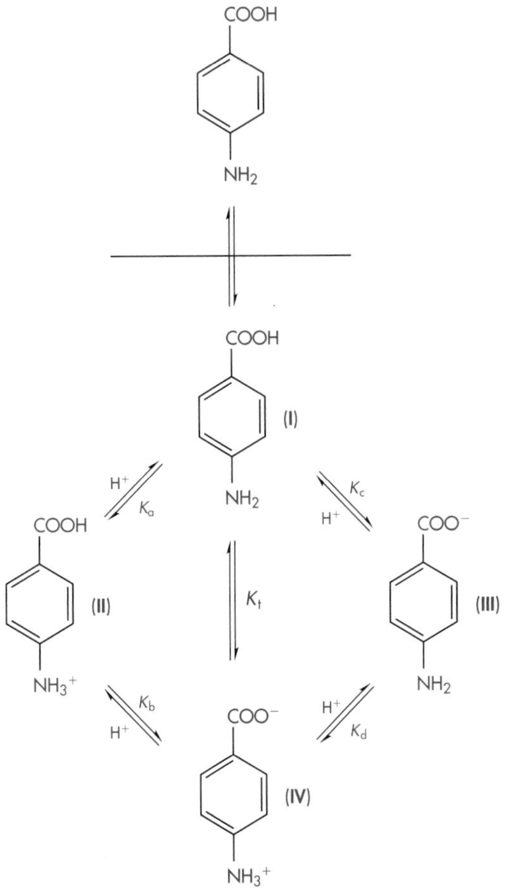

Scheme 5.1 Partitioning of p-aminobenzoic acid. K_a, K_b, K_c and K_d are microdissociation constants for each equilibrium and the relation between them is

$$K_1 = K_a + K_b$$

$$\frac{1}{K_2} = \frac{1}{K_c} + \frac{1}{K_d}$$

$$K_t = \frac{[\text{zwitterion}]}{[\text{neutral form}]} = \frac{K_b}{K_a} = \frac{K_c}{K_d}$$

where K_1 and K_2 are composite or macroscopic acid dissociation constants and K_t is the tautomeric constant between the zwitterionic and neutral forms.

Reproduced from H. Terada, *Chem. Pharm. Bull.*, **20**, 765 (1972).

and

$$P_{app} + \frac{[I]_o}{[II]_w + [I]_w + [IV]_w + [III]_w}$$
$$= P \left[\frac{1}{\dfrac{[H^+]}{K_a} + \dfrac{K_c}{[H^+]} + K_t + 1} \right] \qquad (5.43)$$

If $K_t \rightarrow 0$,

$$P_{app} = P \left[\frac{1}{\dfrac{[H^+]}{K_A} + \dfrac{K_c}{[H^+]} + 1} \right] \qquad (5.44)$$

Passive diffusion of sulfonamides into human red cells is determined by plasma drug binding and lipid solubility. Apparent partition coefficients between chloroform and water at pH 7.4 show an almost linear relation with penetration constant for sulfonamides and a number of other acids. Penetration rates of sulfonamides into the aqueous humour and cerebrospinal fluid also correlate with partition coefficients (Fig. 5.11); moreover, as can be seen from the data in Fig. 5.12, the antibacterial effects of fatty acids and esters towards *B. subtilis* correlate with octanol/water partition coefficients.

There are many quantitative relationships between physiological action and $\log P$ or $\log P_{app}$. A few examples are given here.

Absorption of acidic drugs from the colon may be quantified according to P and pK_a by the equation

$$\log(\text{percentage absorption})$$
$$= 0.156(pK_a - 6.8) - 0.366 \log P + 0.755 \qquad (5.45)$$

Absorption of bases from the small intestine has been similarly treated:

$$\log(\text{percentage absorbed})$$
$$= -0.131(\log P)^2 + 0.362 \log P \qquad (5.46)$$

Local anaesthetic action on peripheral nerves is also proportional to P since the unionised form must diffuse across the continuous cell layer of the perineurium. Once across the perineurium, the molecules ionise and they combine with the receptors in the nerve membrane in their ionised form.

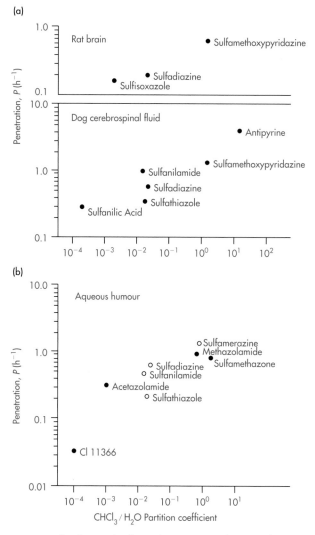

(a)

Penetration, $P (h^{-1})$

Rat brain

Sulfamethoxypyridazine

Sulfadiazine
Sulfisoxazole

Dog cerebrospinal fluid

Antipyrine

Sulfamethoxypyridazine

Sulfanilamide

Sulfadiazine

Sulfathiazole

Sulfanilic Acid

(b)

Penetration, $P (h^{-1})$

Aqueous humour

○ Sulfamerazine
● Methazolamide
Sulfamethazone

○ Sulfadiazine
○ Sulfanilamide   Sulfamethazone

● Acetazolamide

○ Sulfathiazole

● Cl 11366

$CHCl_3 / H_2O$ Partition coefficient

Figure 5.11 (a) Penetration rates of sulfonamides from plasma into rat brain and into canine cerebrospinal fluid. Dog cerebrospinal fluid data from D. P. Rall, *J. Pharm Exp. Ther.*, 125, 185 (1959). (b) Penetration rates of sulfonamides from plasma into aqueous humour for the rabbit (○) and for the rat (●) against partition coefficients (chloroform/water). Data from P. J. Wistrand, *Acta Pharmacol. Toxicol.*, 17, 337 (1960) and A. Sorsby, *Br. J. Ophthalmol.*, 33, 347 (1949).

The toxicity of some agents such as X-ray contrast media and penicillins has also been related to lipophilicity. Rates of entry into the brain of X-ray contrast agents used in cerebral angiography are proportional to P, and P correlates with clinical neurotoxicity. Figure 5.13 shows the positive relationship between toxicity of the penicillins and partition coefficient.

5.10.2 Sorption

Figure 5.14 summarises the physicochemical problems in the use of preservative molecules in formulations. Solubility and partition coefficients of ionised species are determined, as we have seen, by the pH and ionic strength of the system. In this example, partitioning may occur from the aqueous phase to the oily

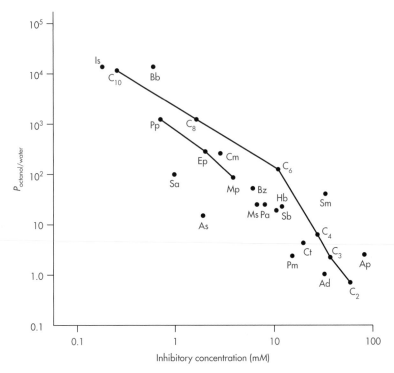

Figure 5.12 Relationship between the partition coefficient (P) and growth inhibitory concentration of a wider range of compounds. The octanol/water partition coefficient of the undissociated compounds is plotted against the concentrations of compounds needed to inhibit growth of *B. subtilis* by 50%.
Reproduced from G. W. Sheu *et al.*, *Antimicrob. Agents Chemother.*, 7, 349 (1975).

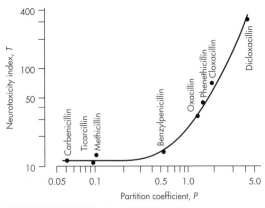

Figure 5.13 Relation of neurotoxicity to the hydrophobic character of various penicillins: the hydrophobic character is measured by the partition coefficient *P* and toxicity by a neurotoxicity index *T*.
Reproduced from T. R. Weihrauch *et al.*, *Arch. Pharmacol. (NS)*, 289, 55 (1975).

phase of an emulsion, to the micellar phase of a surfactant, or to a closure. Adsorption may also occur onto container closures and suspended solid particles.

Permeation of antimicrobial agents into rubber stoppers and other closures is another example of partitioning. Although rubber is an amorphous solid, partitioning between the aqueous phase and rubber depends, as in liquid systems, on the relative affinities of the solute for each phase.

Glyceryl trinitrate, a volatile drug with a chloroform/water partition coefficient of 109, diffuses from simple tablet bases into the walls of plastic bottles and into plastic liners used in packaging tablets. This partitioning can be prevented if there is included in the tablet formulation an agent (such as polyoxyethylene glycol) which complexes with the drug substance, thereby increasing its affinity for the 'tablet phase' – in other words, reducing its

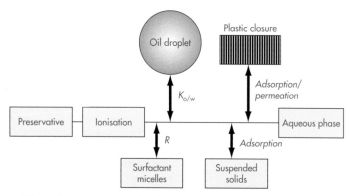

Figure 5.14 The potential fate of preservative molecules in pharmaceutical products. Much depends on the state of ionisation of the molecules. Partitioning into oil droplets or surfactant micelles can occur, as well as adsorption onto suspended solids. Adsorption, sorption or permeation of plastic closures can occur, leaving the less active form in the aqueous phase.

escaping tendency or 'fugacity'. Significant losses of glyceryl trinitrate have been detected when the drug was given as an infusion through plastic giving sets from a plastic reservoir, the absorption (of as much as 50% of the drug) resulting in the necessity to use unusually high doses of the drug.

Some relation has been found between the rate of sorption by poly(vinyl chloride) (PVC) bags of a series of drugs and their hexane/water partition coefficients.[16] Table 5.20 shows the data for sorption of 100 cm^3 PVC infusion bags (equivalent to 11 g of PVC). In the table, P_{app} values have been calculated from

$$P_{app} = \left(\frac{1 - F_\infty}{F_\infty}\right)\frac{W_s}{W_p} \qquad (5.47)$$

where W_s is the weight of solution in contact with a given weight W_p of plastic and F_∞ is the equilibrium fraction of drug remaining in solution. Only the unionised form of the drug is sorbed; the kinetics of the process can be accounted for by considering the diffusion of the molecules in the plastic matrix.

There are concerns over phthalates in medical devices, including diethylhexylphthalate (DEHP), used in medical products made of PVC such as i.v. bags, blood bags and tubing. DEHP can 'leach' out of PVC into liquids such as intravenous fluids, especially in the presence of formulations containing additives such as surfactants, as with Cremophor EL in Taxol. Figure 5.15 illustrates some of the problems that can occur in giving sets.

Table 5.20 Sorption into PVC and partitioning of drugs[a]

Compound	Initial rate of sorption (10^{-2}h^{-1})	Extent of sorption at equilibrium (%)	log P_{app}	log P (hexane/water)
Medazepam	51	85	1.7	2.9
Diazepam	27	90	1.9	0.9
Warfarin (pH 2–4)	22	90	1.9	0.2
Glyceryl trinitrate	20	83	1.6	0.2
Thiopental (pH 4)	6	73	1.4	0.1
Oxazepam	4.6	46	0.9	−0.1
Nitrazepam	4.1	47	0.9	−0.1
Hydrocortisone acetate	0	0	–	−1.2
Pentobarbital (pH 4)	0	0	–	−1.3

[a] Reproduced from reference 16.

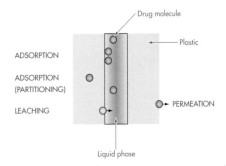

Figure 5.15 Diagram showing opportunities in plastic systems for adsorption of drug molecules, partitioning into and eventually permeation through the plastic. Leaching of molecules from the plastic also may occur.

5.10.3   A chromatographic model for the biophase

Octanol/water partition coefficients, as we have seen, have been useful predictors of biological activity. In spite of this it has been suggested that bulk liquid phases may not be the most appropriate models for a structured biophase such as a biological membrane, and chromatographic stationary phases have been proposed as an alternative because of the structuring of the 'membranous' hydrophobic chains.

5.10.4   Calculating log P from molecular structures

The large number of methods used to calculate log P values have been elegantly reviewed by Leo.[15] The method proposed in 1964 by Fujita, Iwasa and Hansch[17] used values for the 'parent' molecule and values for substituents gathered by analysis of thousands of values of log P for homologous and other series. In this method of 'substituents' log P is considered to be an additive-constitutive free-energy-related property, where one can define Π for substituent X as the difference between the log P values for the parent solute and the compound with the substituent:

$$\Pi_{(X)} = \log P_{(R-X)} - \log P_{(R-H)} \qquad (5.48)$$

By definition $\Pi_{(H)} = 0$. For example,

$$\log P_{NO_2-C_6H_4CH_3} = \log P_{C_6H_6} + \Pi_{NO_2} + \Pi_{CH_3}$$
$$\log P = 2.13 - 0.28 + 0.56 = 2.41$$

against a measured value of 2.45.

The fragmental method developed by Rekker and Mannhold[18] uses the contributions of simple fragments. This may be illustrated by the example:

$$\log P_{C_6H_5OCH_2COOH} =$$
$$= f_{C_6H_5} \pm f_O + f_{CH_2} + f_{COOH} + PE1$$

PE1 being a 'proximity effect,' an adjusting fraction for polar fragments in nonpolar surroundings. So

$$\log P_{C_6H_5OCH_2COOH}$$
$$= 1.866 - 0.433 + 0.53 - 0.954 + 0.861$$
$$= 1.87$$

compared with a measured value of 1.34.

A method based on the surface areas of molecules has also been proposed to obtain measures of log P in a manner analogous to the calculation of solubility.[19] Computer programs for calculation of log P are also in use and are described in detail, in Leo's 1993 review.[15]

5.10.5   Drug distribution into human milk

The distribution of drugs into the milk of breastfeeding mothers is of obvious importance. Nearly all drugs find their way into milk and it is, therefore, useful to be able to predict which of them will achieve high concentrations in milk in relation to their plasma level, defined in one model[20] described below as the milk : plasma (M/P) ratio (see Table 5.21). Three key parameters are the pK_a of the drug, plasma protein binding and the octanol/water partition coefficients of the drugs. Protein binding is the most important single predictor, an increase in M/P ratios generally being found as protein binding decreases.

The two key equations, each with three independent variables, are as follows:

For basic drugs:

$$\ln\left(\frac{M}{P}\right) = 0.025 + 2.28 \ln\left(\frac{M_u}{P_u}\right)$$
$$+ 0.89 \ln f_{u,p} + 0.51 \ln K \qquad (5.49)$$

Table 5.21 Distribution of drugs into milk: the M/P ratio[a, b]

Drug	M/P	Drug	M/P
Acidic drugs		*Neutral drugs*	
Carbenicillin	0.02	Alcohol	0.89
Ethosuximide	0.78	Digoxin	0.55
Ibuprofen	0	Medroxyprogesterone	0.72
Paracetamol	0.76	Norethisterone	0.19
Valproic acid	0.05	Prednisolone	0.13
Basic drugs			
Amitriptyline	0.83		
Atenolol	0.32		
Cimetidine	1.7		
Clonazepam	0.33		
Codeine	2.16		
Lamotrigine	0.4–0.45		
Morphine	2.46		
Verapamil	0.6		
Vigabatrin	0.01–0.05		

[a] Reproduced from reference 20.
[b] M/P = Milk : plasma drug concentration ratio.

For acidic drugs:

$$\ln\left(\frac{M}{P}\right) = -0.405 + 9.36 \ln\left(\frac{M_u}{P_u}\right) \\ - 0.69 \ln f_{u,p} - 1.54 \ln K \quad (5.50)$$

where

M_u/P_u = milk : plasma unbound drug concentration ratio
$f_{u,p}$ = fraction of drug unbound in plasma
$f_{u,m}$ = fraction of drug unbound in milk
P_{app} = apparent partition coefficient at pH 7.2
$K = (0.955/f_{u,m}) + [0.045 P_{app} \text{ (milk/lipid)}]$

Few measurements of $f_{u,m}$ and P_{app} (milk/lipid) have been made, but these parameters can be predicted from $f_{u,p}$ and log P.[21]

It is clear from equations (5.49) and (5.50) that there is a degree of empiricism about these equations which arises in their derivation from the fitting of data sets based on the independent variables. The ratio M_u/P_u can be obtained from the modified Henderson–Hasselbalch equation:

for basic drugs,

$$\frac{M_u}{P_u} = \frac{1 + 10^{(pK_a - pH_m)}}{1 + 10^{(pK_a - pH_p)}} \quad (5.51)$$

and for acidic drugs,

$$\frac{M_u}{P_u} = \frac{1 + 10^{(pH_m - pK_a)}}{1 + 10^{(pH_p - pK_a)}} \quad (5.52)$$

where pH_m and pH_p are the pH values of milk and plasma respectively. Milk has a mean pH of 7.2, slightly lower than that of plasma at 7.4

For neutral drugs the predicted M_u/P_u ratio would be unity, since the distribution of unbound unionised drugs would not be expected to be altered by pH gradients.

Summary

- Definitions of solubility, modes of expression of solubility and means of estimating solubility from the surface area of molecules were some of the key subjects discussed in this chapter.
- Molecular shape factors and substituents on molecules affect solubility, one of the key parameters in a drug substance. Effects such as solvation (or hydration in aqueous media) and the effects of additives on solubility are also dealt with, but perhaps the most important effect of all is that of pH on

the solubility of ionisable drugs. This is treated in detail, and equations for acids, bases and zwitterions are considered. An understanding of pH–solubility relationships is vital to predicting the behaviour of ionic drugs in pharmaceutical formulations and in the body.

- When additives, such as surfactants and cyclodextrins, do not achieve appropriate

levels of practical solubility, we can resort to the use of cosolvents. The relative advantages and disadvantages of these different approaches to formulating a solution have to be considered, but in the last analysis other factors such as stability may determine which is the best approach to achieve a satisfactory solution formulation.

References

1. G. L. Amidon, S. G. Yalkowsky and S. Leung, Solubility of nonelectrolytes in polar solvents. II. Solubility of aliphatic alcohols in water. *J. Pharm. Sci.*, 63, 1858–66 (1974)

2. G. L. Amidon. Theoretical calculation of heats of complexation in carbon tetrachloride. *J. Pharm. Sci.*, 63, 1520–3 (1974)

3. G. L. Amidon, S. G. Yalkowsky, A. T. Anik and S. C. Valvani. Solubility of nonelectrolytes in polar solvents. V. Estimation of the solubility of aliphatic monofunctional compounds in water using a molecular surface area approach. *J. Phys. Chem.*, 79, 2239–46 (1975)

4. R. B. Hermann. Theory of hydrophobic bonding. II. Correlation of hydrocarbon solubility in water with solvent cavity surface area. *J. Phys. Chem.*, 76, 2754–9 (1972)

5. R. B. Hermann. Theory of hydrophobic bonding. I. Solubility of hydrocarbons in water, within the context of the significant structure theory of liquids. *J. Phys. Chem.*, 75, 363–8 (1971)

6. P. Kabasakalian, E. Britt and M. D. Yudis. Solubility of some steroids in water. *J. Pharm. Sci.*, 55, 642 (1966)

7. F. Franks. In *Water Relations of Foods* (ed. R. D. Duckworth), Academic Press, London, 1975

8. C. A. S. Bergstrom, K. Luthman and P. Artursson. Accuracy of calculated pH-dependent aqueous drug solubilities. *Eur. J. Pharm. Sci.*, 22, 387–98 (2004)

9. A. L. Green. Ionisation constants and water solubilities of some aminoalkyl phenothiazine tranquillizers and related compounds. *J. Pharm. Pharmacol.*, 19, 10–16 (1967)

10. L. J. Bennett and K. W. Miller. Application of regular solution theory to biomembranes. *J. Med. Chem.*, 17, 1124–5 (1974)

11. R. S. Scott. Solutions of nonelectrolytes. *Annu. Rev. Phys. Chem.*, 7, 43–66 (1956)

12. W. Yang and M. M. de Villiers. The solubilization of the poorly water soluble drug nifedipine by water soluble 4-sulphonic calix[n]arenes. *Eur. J. Pharm. Biopharm.*, 58, 629–36 (2004)

13. E. Boyd. *Predictive Toxicometrics*, Scientechnica, Bristol, 1972

14. A. J. Leo, C. Hansch and D. Elkins. Partition coefficients and their uses. *Chem. Rev.*, 71, 525–616 (1971)

15. A. J. Leo. Calculating log P_{oct} from structures. *Chem. Rev.*, 93, 1281–306 (1993)

16. L. Illum and H. Bundgaard. Sorption of drugs by plastic infusion bags. *Int. J. Pharm.*, 10, 339–51 (1982)

17. T. Fujita, J. I. Iwasa and C. Hansch. A new substituent constant, π, derived from partition coefficients. *J. Am. Chem. Soc.*, 86, 5175–80 (1964)

18. R. Rekker and R. Mannhold. *Calculations of Drug Lipophilicity*, VCH, Weinheim, 1992

19. P. Broto, G. Moreau and C. Vandycke. Molecular structures: perception, autocorrelation descriptor and SAR studies. Perception of molecules: topological structure and 3-dimensional structure. *Eur. J. Med. Chem.*, 19, 61–5 (1984)

20. H. C. Atkinson and E. J. Begg. Prediction of drug distribution into human milk from physicochemical characteristics. *Clin. Pharmacokinet.*, 18, 151–67 (1990)

21. E. J. Begg, H. C. Atkinson and S. B. Duffull. Prospective evaluation of a model for the prediction of milk : plasma drug concentrations from physicochemical characteristics. *Br. J. Clin. Pharmacol.*, 33, 501–5 (1992)

6

Surfactants

Certain compounds, because of their chemical structure, have a tendency to accumulate at the boundary between two phases. Such compounds are termed *amphiphiles, surface-active agents,* or *surfactants*. The adsorption at the various interfaces between solids, liquids and gases results in changes in the nature of the interface which are of considerable importance in pharmacy. For example, the lowering of the interfacial tension between oil and water phases facilitates emulsion formation; the adsorption of surfactants on the insoluble particles enables these particles to be dispersed in the form of a suspension; and the incorporation of insoluble compounds within micelles of the surfactant can lead to the production of clear solutions.

In this chapter we will see how the surface activity of a molecule is related to its molecular structure and look at the properties of some surfactants which are commonly used in pharmacy. We will examine the nature and properties of films formed when water-soluble surfactants accumulate spontaneously at liquid/air interfaces and when insoluble surfactants are spread over the surface of a liquid to form a monolayer. We will look at some of the factors that influence adsorption onto solid surfaces and how experimental data from adsorption experiments may be analysed to gain information on the process of adsorption. An interesting and useful property of surfactants is that they may form aggregates or *micelles* in aqueous solutions when their concentration exceeds a critical concentration. We will examine why this should be so and some of the factors that influence micelle formation. The ability of micelles to solubilise water-insoluble drugs has obvious pharmaceutical importance and the process of solubilisation and its applications will be examined in some detail.

6.1 Amphipathic compounds

Surface-active compounds are characterised by having two distinct regions in their chemical structure; these are termed *hydrophilic* ('water-liking') and *hydrophobic* ('water-hating') regions. The existence of two such moieties in a molecule is referred to as *amphipathy* and the molecules are consequently often referred to as *amphipathic* molecules.

The hydrophobic portions are usually saturated or unsaturated hydrocarbon chains or, less commonly, heterocyclic or aromatic ring systems. The hydrophilic regions can be anionic, cationic, zwitterionic, or nonionic. Surfactants are generally classified according to the nature of the hydrophilic group. Typical examples are given in Box 6.1.

The zwitterionic or *ampholytic* surfactants shown in Box 6.1 possess both positively and negatively charged groups and can exist as either an anionic or a cationic surfactant depending on the pH of the solution. A typical example is *N*-dodecyl-*N*,*N*-dimethylbetaine $(C_{12}H_{25}N^+(CH_3)_2CH_2COO^-)$.

The dual structure of amphipathic molecules is the unique feature which is responsible for the characteristic behaviour of this type of compound. Thus their surface activity arises from adsorption at the solution/air interface – the means by which the hydrophobic region of the molecule 'escapes' from the hostile aqueous environment by protruding into the vapour phase above. Similarly, adsorption at the interface between aqueous and non-aqueous solutions occurs in such a way that

---

Box 6.1   Classification of surfactants[a]

Anionic

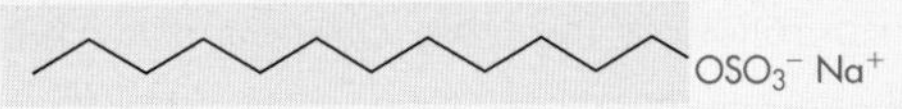

Alkyl sulfate

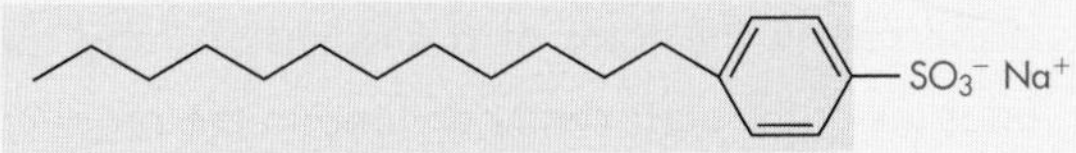

Alkylbenzene sulfonate

Cationic

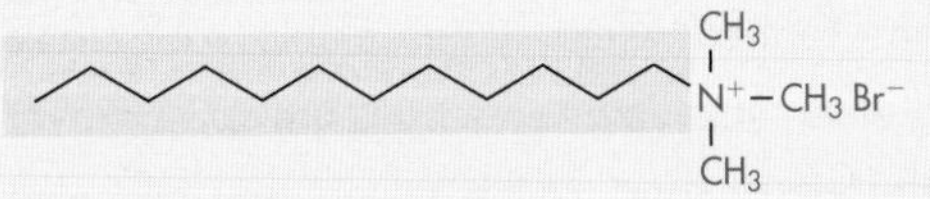

Alkyltrimethylammonium bromide

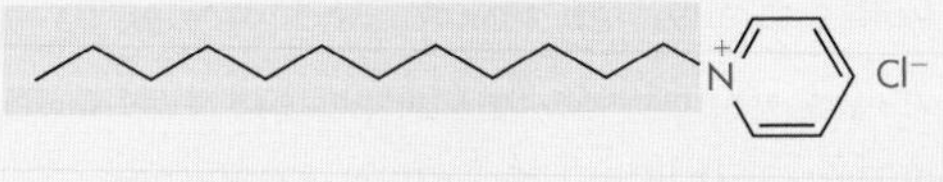

Alkylpyridinium chloride

Zwitterionic

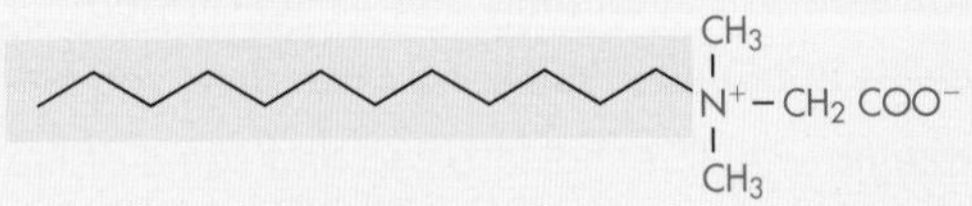

Alkyl betaine

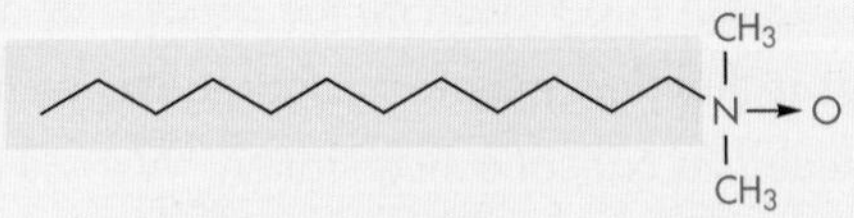

Alkyldimethylamine oxide

Nonionic

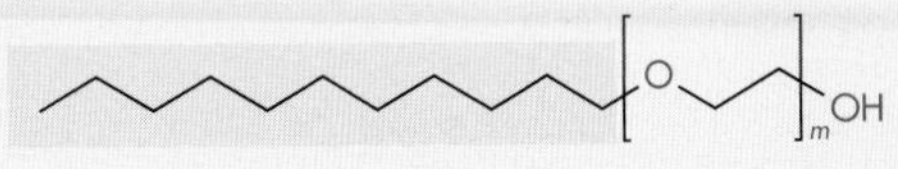

Alcohol ethoxylate

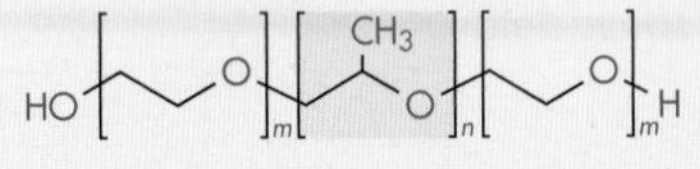

Polyoxyethylene–polyoxypropylene–polyoxyethylene
block copolymer

[a] Hydrophobic areas of the molecules are shaded.

the hydrophobic group is in the solution in the nonaqueous phase, leaving the hydrophilic group in contact with the aqueous solution. Adsorption on hydrophobic solutes such as carbon again represents a means of reduction of the contact between the hydrophobic groups and water and allows the consequent attainment of a minimum-energy state. Perhaps the most striking consequence of the dual structure is micellisation – the formation in solution of aggregates in which the component molecules are usually arranged in a spheroidal structure with the hydrophobic cores shielded from the water by a mantle of hydrophilic groups.

In the following sections we will examine in more detail the various characteristic properties of surfactants which arise as a consequence of their amphipathic nature.

6.2 Surface and interfacial properties of surfactants

6.2.1 Effects of amphiphiles on surface and interfacial tension

The molecules at the surface of a liquid are not completely surrounded by other molecules as they are in the bulk of the liquid. As a result there is a net inward force of attraction exerted on a molecule at the surface from the molecules in the bulk solution, which results in a tendency for the surface to contract.

The contraction of the surface is spontaneous; that is, it is accompanied by a decrease in free energy. The contracted surface thus represents a minimum free energy state and any attempt to expand the surface must involve an increase in the free energy. The surface free energy of a liquid is defined as the work, w, required to increase the surface area A by 1 m^2:

$$w = \gamma \, \Delta A \qquad (6.1)$$

where ΔA is the increase in surface area. γ is also referred to as *surface tension* and in this context is defined as the force acting at right angles to a line 1 m in length along the surface. Surface free energy and surface

tension are numerically equal and both have SI units of N m^{-1}. It is usual, however, to quote values of surface tension in mN m^{-1} (which is numerically equivalent to the cgs unit, dyne cm^{-1}).

A similar imbalance of attractive forces exists at the interface between two immiscible liquids. Table 6.1 lists surface tensions of various liquids and also interfacial tensions at the liquid/water interface. The value of the interfacial tension is generally between those of the surface tensions of the two liquids involved, except where there is interaction between them. Table 6.1 includes several such examples. The interfacial tension at the octanol/water interface is considerably lower than the surface tension of octanol owing to hydrogen bonding between these two liquids.

Amphiphilic molecules in aqueous solution have a tendency to seek out the surface and to orientate themselves in such a way as to remove the hydrophobic group from the aqueous environment and hence achieve a minimum free energy state (see Fig. 6.1). A consequence of the intrusion of surfactant molecules into the surface or interfacial layer is that some of the water molecules are effectively replaced by hydrocarbon or other nonpolar groups. Since the forces of intermolecular attraction between water molecules and nonpolar groups are less than those

Table 6.1 Surface tensions of pure liquids and interfacial tensions against water at 20°C

Substance	Surface tension (mN m^{-1})	Interfacial tension (mN m^{-1})
Water	72	–
Glycerol	63	–
Oleic acid	33	16
Benzene	29	35
Chloroform	27	33
n-Octanol	27	8.5
Carbon tetrachloride	27	45
Castor oil	39	–
Olive oil	36	33
Cottonseed oil	35	–
n-Octane	22	51
Ethyl ether	17	11

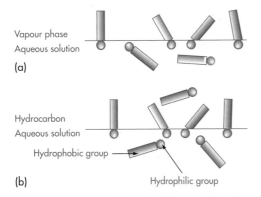

Figure 6.1   Orientation of amphiphiles at (a) solution/vapour interface, and (b) hydrocarbon/solution interface.

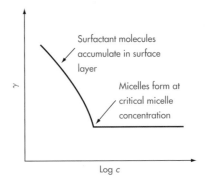

Figure 6.2   Typical plot of the surface tension, γ, against logarithm of surfactant concentration, c.

exerted between two water molecules, the contracting power of the surface is reduced and so therefore is the surface tension. In some cases the interfacial tension between two liquids may be reduced to such a low level (10^{-3} mN m^{-1}) that spontaneous emulsification of the two immiscible liquids is observed. These very low interfacial tensions are of relevance in understanding the formation and stabilisation of emulsions and are dealt with in more detail in Chapter 7.

6.2.2   Change of surface tension with surfactant concentration – the critical micelle concentration

Fig. 6.2 shows a typical plot of surface tension against the logarithm of concentration for a surfactant solution. Appreciable lowering of surface tension is evident even at low concentrations. As the surfactant concentration is increased, the surface tension continues to decrease as the concentration of surfactant molecules at the surface increases. A concentration is reached, however, when the surface layer becomes saturated with surfactant molecules and no further decrease in surface tension is possible. An alternative means of shielding the hydrophobic portion of the amphiphile from the aqueous environment now occurs as the surfactant molecules form small spherical aggregates or *micelles* in the bulk of the solution. The hydrophobic groups

of the surfactants form the core of these aggregates and are protected from contact with water by their hydrophilic groups, which form a shell around them. The concentration of surfactant molecules in the surface layer remains approximately constant in the presence of micelles and hence the γ–log concentration plot becomes almost horizontal. The concentration at which the micelles first form in solution is called the *critical micelle concentration* (cmc) and corresponds to the concentration at which there is an abrupt change of slope of the plot. We will consider the formation and properties of micelles in more detail in section 6.3. At the moment we will concentrate on the region of the γ–log concentration plot below the cmc and see how it is possible to calculate the area occupied by a surfactant molecule at the surface using the Gibbs equation.

6.2.3   Gibbs adsorption equation

It is important to remember that an equilibrium is established between the surfactant molecules at the surface or interface and those remaining in the bulk of the solution. This equilibrium is expressed in terms of the Gibbs equation. In developing this expression it is necessary to imagine a definite boundary between the bulk of the solution and the interfacial layer (see Fig. 6.3). The real system containing the interfacial layer is then compared with this reference system, in which

---

Box 6.2   The Gibbs equation

We can treat the thermodynamics of the surface layer in a similar way to the bulk of the solution. The energy change, dU, accompanying an infinitesimal, reversible change in the system is given by

$$dU = dq_{rev} - dw$$

or

$$dU = T\,dS - dw \qquad (6.2)$$

where dq_{rev} and dw are, respectively, the heat absorbed and the work done during the reversible change (see section 3.1).

For an open system (one in which there is transfer of material between phases) equation (6.2) must be written

$$dU = T\,dS - dw + \Sigma \mu_i\,dn_i \qquad (6.3)$$

where μ_i and n_i are the chemical potential and number of moles respectively of the ith component.

When applying equation (6.3) to the surface layer, the work is that required to increase the area of the surface by an infinitesimal amount, dA, at constant T, P and n. This work is done against the surface tension and is given by equation (6.1) as $dw = \gamma\,dA$.

Thus, equation (6.3) becomes

$$dU^s = T\,dS^s + \gamma\,dA + \Sigma\mu_i\,dn_i^s \qquad (6.4)$$

where the superscript, s, denotes the surface layer.

If the energy, entropy and number of moles of component are allowed to increase from zero to some finite value, equation (6.4) becomes

$$U^s = TS^s + \gamma A + \Sigma\mu_i n_i^s \qquad (6.5)$$

General differentiation of equation (6.5) gives

$$dU^s = T\,dS^s + S^s\,dT + \gamma\,dA + A\,d\gamma$$
$$+ \Sigma\mu_i\,dn_i^s + \Sigma n_i^s\,d\mu_i \qquad (6.6)$$

Comparison with equation (6.4) gives

$$0 = S^s\,dT + \Sigma\,n_i^s\,d\mu_i + A\,d\gamma \qquad (6.7)$$

At constant temperature equation (6.7) becomes

$$d\gamma = -\Sigma\,\Gamma_i\,d\mu_i \qquad (6.8)$$

where $\Gamma_i = n_i^s / A$ and is termed the *surface excess concentration*. Γ_i is the amount of the ith component in the surface phase s, in excess of that which there would have been had the bulk phases a and b extended to the dividing surface without change in composition.

For a two-component system at constant temperature, equation (6.8) reduces to

$$d\gamma = -\Gamma_1\,d\mu_1 - \Gamma_2\,d\mu_2 \qquad (6.9)$$

where subscripts 1 and 2 denote solvent and solute, respectively. The surface excess concentrations are defined relative to an arbitrarily chosen dividing surface. A convenient choice of location of this surface is that at which the surface excess concentration of the solvent, Γ_1, is zero. Indeed, this is the most realistic position since we are now considering the surface layer of adsorbed solute. Equation (6.9) then becomes

$$d\gamma = -\Gamma_2\,d\mu_2 \qquad (6.10)$$

The chemical potential of the solute is given by equation (3.52) as

$$\mu_2 = \mu_2^\ominus + RT\ln a_2$$
$$d\mu_2 = RT\,d(\ln a_2)$$

Substituting in equation (6.10) gives the Gibbs equation:

$$\Gamma_2 = -\frac{1}{RT}\frac{d\gamma}{d(\ln a_2)} = -\frac{a_2}{RT}\frac{d\gamma}{da_2} \qquad (6.11)$$

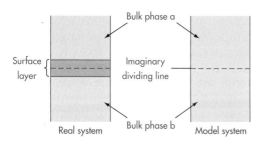

Figure 6.3 Diagrammatic representation of an interface between two bulk phases in the presence of an adsorbed layer.

it is assumed that the properties of the two bulk phases remain unchanged up to the dividing surface. A thermodynamic derivation of the Gibbs equation is provided in Box 6.2

The form of the Gibbs equation applicable to dilute solutions is

$$\Gamma_2 = -\frac{1}{RT}\frac{d\gamma}{d(\ln c)} = -\frac{c}{RT}\frac{d\gamma}{dc} \qquad (6.12)$$

where activity in equation (6.11) has been replaced by concentration, c. Equation (6.12) is the form of the Gibbs equation applicable to the adsorption of nonionic surfactants at the surface of the solution. For ionic surfactants the derivation becomes more complex since consideration must be taken of the adsorption of both surfactant ion and counterion. The general form of the Gibbs equation is then written

$$\Gamma_2 = -\frac{1}{xRT}\frac{d\gamma}{d(\ln c)}$$

$$= -\frac{1}{xRT}\frac{d\gamma}{2.303\, d(\log c)} \quad (6.13)$$

where x has a numerical value varying from 1 (for ionic surfactants in dilute solution or in the presence of excess electrolyte) to 2 (in concentrated solution).

Application of the Gibbs equation to surfactant solutions

The slope of the surface tension against log concentration plot reaches a constant value at concentrations just below the cmc before becoming approximately zero at higher concentrations (Fig. 6.2). The surfactant molecules are closely packed in the surface over this narrow concentration range and we can calculate the area A that each molecule occupies at the surface from

$$A = \frac{1}{N_A \Gamma_2} \quad (6.14)$$

where Γ_2 is the value of surface excess concentration calculated from the Gibbs equation using the value of $d\gamma/d(\ln c)$ just below the cmc and N_A is the Avogadro constant. The calculation is shown in Example 6.1 using surface tension data for the surface-active drug diphenhydramine.

. . . .

EXAMPLE 6.1 Calculation of area per molecule using the Gibbs equation

The slope of a plot of γ against log c just below the cmc for the antihistamine diphenhydramine hydrochloride (see Box 6.3) is -0.0115 N m^{-1} at 30°C. Calculate the area per molecule of this drug at the air/solution inter-

face.

Answer

The surface excess concentration, Γ_2, may be calculated from equation (6.13), assuming a value of $x = 1$:

$$\Gamma_2 = \frac{0.0115}{8.314 \times 303 \times 2.303}$$

$$= 1.982 \times 10^{-6} \text{ mol m}^{-2}$$

Substituting in equation (6.14):

$$A = 1/(6.023 \times 10^{23} \times 1.982 \times 10^{-6})$$

$$= 83.8 \times 10^{-20} \text{ m}^2 \text{ per molecule}$$

The area per molecule of diphenhydramine = 0.84 nm^2.

. . . .

An interesting effect arises when the surfactant is contaminated with surface-active impurities. A pronounced minimum in the surface tension–log c plot is observed at the cmc, which would seem to be an apparent violation of the Gibbs equation, suggesting a desorption (positive $d\gamma/d[\log c]$ value) in the vicinity of the cmc. The minimum in fact arises because of the release below the cmc of the surface-active impurities on the breakup of the surfactant micelles in which they were solubilised.

6.2.4 The influence of the surfactant structure on surface activity

The surface activity of a particular surfactant depends on the balance between its hydrophilic and hydrophobic properties. For the simplest case of a homologous series of surfactants, an increase in the length of the hydrocarbon chain as the series is ascended results in increased surface activity. Conversely, an increase in the hydrophilicity, which for polyoxyethylated nonionic surfactants may be effected by increasing the length of the ethylene oxide chain, results in a decreased surface activity. This latter effect is demonstrated by Fig. 6.4, from which it is noted that lengthening of the hydrophilic

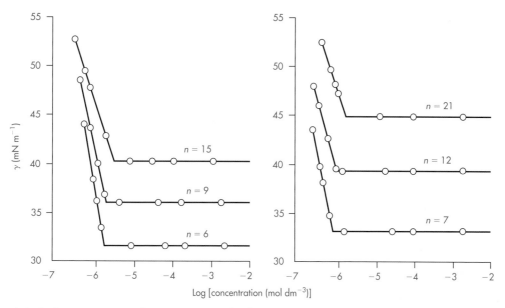

Figure 6.4 Surface tension versus log concentration plots for nonionic surfactants with the general formula $CH_3(CH_2)_{15}$ $(OCH_2CH_2)_nOH$ for a series of ethylene oxide chain lengths, n.
Reproduced from P. H. Elworthy and C. B. Macfarlane, *J. Pharm. Pharmacol.*, 14, 100T (1962) with permission.

chain results in an increase in both the surface tension (decrease of surface activity) and the cmc.

The relationship between hydrocarbon chain length and surface activity is expressed by *Traube's rule*, which states that 'in dilute aqueous solutions of surfactants belonging to any one homologous series, the molar concentrations required to produce equal lowering of the surface tension of water decreases threefold for each additional CH_2 group in the hydrocarbon chain of the solute'. Traube's rule also applies to the interfacial tension at oil/water interfaces.

• •

EXAMPLE 6.2 Use of Traube's rule

The surface tension lowering of an anionic surfactant (mol. wt. = 328) with a hydrocarbon chain length of 16 carbon atoms, is 15 mN m^{-1} at a concentration of 0.0276% w/v. For a surfactant with an identical hydrophilic group and a hydrocarbon chain length of 14 carbon atoms, estimate the percentage concentration that is required to produce an equal lowering of surface tension,

assuming that both concentrations are below the cmc.

Answer
The molar concentration of the first surfactant = 8.415×10^{-4} mol dm^{-3}. Since the second surfactant has two CH_2 groups fewer than the first, the concentration required to produce an equal lowering of surface tension is, according to Traube's rule,

$$8.415 \times 10^{-4} \times 3 \times 3 = 75.74 \times 10^{-4} \text{ mol dm}^{-3}$$

The molecular weight of the second surfactant = $328 - 28 = 300$. Thus, the concentration required = 0.227% w/v.

• •

6.2.5 Surface activity of drugs

The surface activity at the air/solution interface has been reported for a wide variety of drugs.[1,2] This surface activity is a consequence of the amphipathic nature of the drugs. The hydrophobic portions of the drug molecules are in general more complex than those of typical surfactants, often being composed of aromatic or heterocyclic ring systems. Examples of the types of drug that exhibit surface activity are illustrated in Box 6.3. They include the phenothiazine tranquillisers, such as promazine, chlorpromazine and promethazine, and the antidepressants, such as imipramine, amitriptyline and nortriptyline, which have tricyclic hydrophobic moieties; the antihistamines (for example, chlorcyclizine and diphenhydramine) and the antiacetylcholine drugs such as orphenadrine, which are based on a diphenylmethane hydrophobic group; the local anaesthetics (tetracaine, for example);

and several antihistamines, such as brompheniramine and mepyramine, which have a hydrophobic group consisting of a single phenyl ring. Many peptides also have clearly amphipathic structures and adsorb at the air/water interface.

As with typical surfactants, the surface activity depends on the nature of the hydrophobic and hydrophilic portions of the drug molecule. The presence of any substituents on the aromatic ring systems can have an appreciable effect on hydrophobicity. Fig. 6.5 shows the decrease of cmc and increased surface activity

---

Box 6.3   Structures of some surface-active drugs[a]

Antidepressants

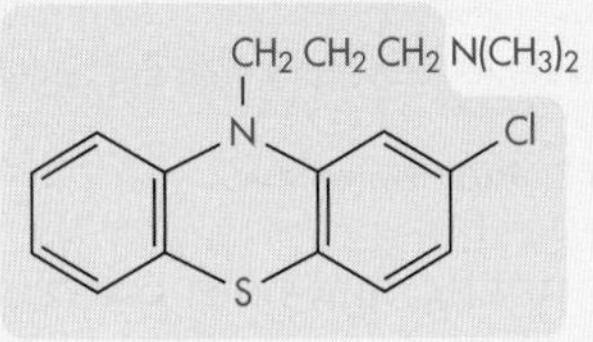

Chlorpromazine

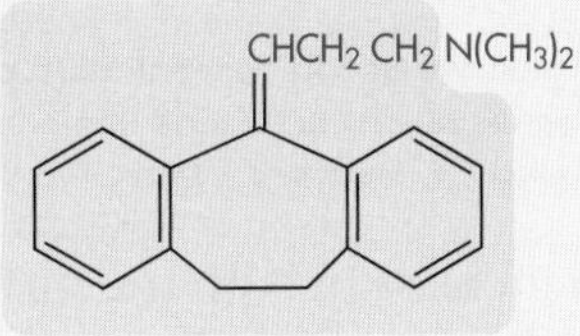

Amitriptyline

Antihistamines

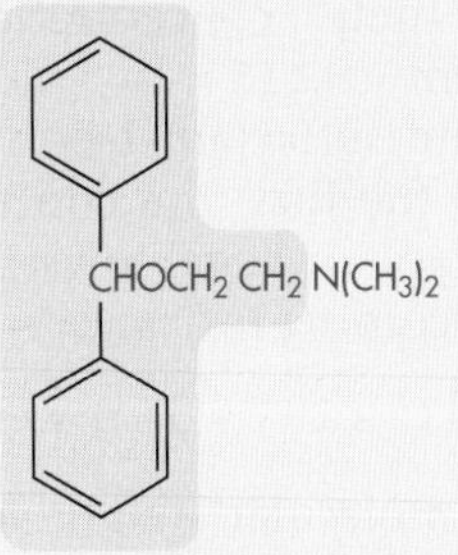

Diphenhydramine

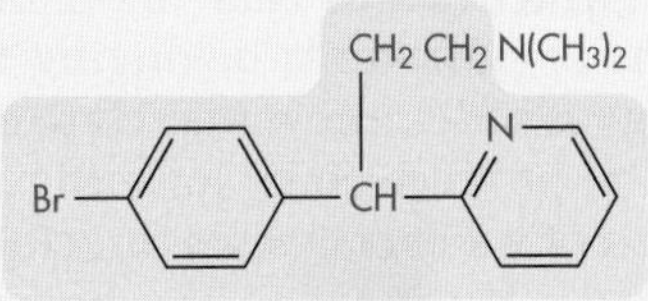

Brompheniramine

Anticholinergic drugs

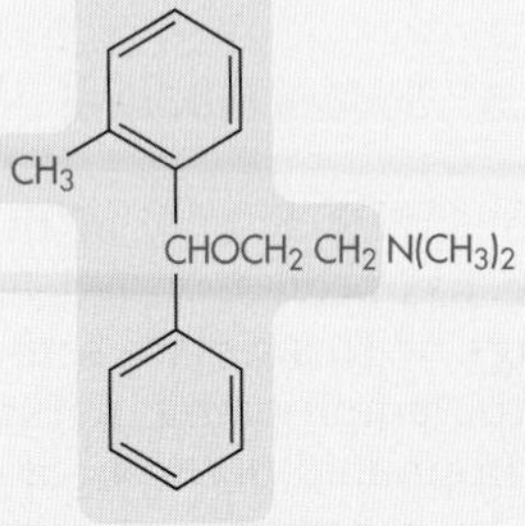

Orphenadrine

Local anaesthetics

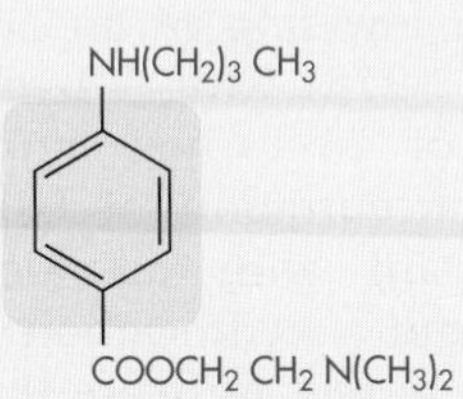

Tetracaine

[a] Hydrophobic areas of the molecules are shaded.

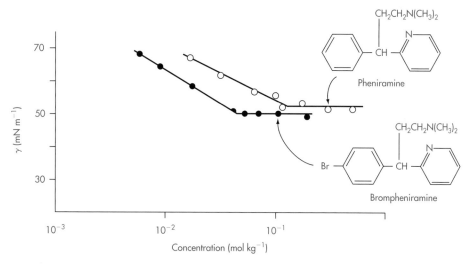

Figure 6.5 Surface tension, γ, as a function of log molal concentration at 30°C showing the increase of hydrophobicity associated with a Br substituent on the phenyl ring of an antihistamine.
Reproduced from D. Attwood and O. K. Udeala, *J. Pharm. Pharmacol.*, 27, 754 (1975) with permission.

that is associated with the Br substituent on the phenyl ring of an antihistaminic drug. Similarly, substitution on the phenothiazine ring systems increases surface activity in the order $CF_3 \gg Cl > H$.

6.2.6 Insoluble monolayers

In section 6.2.4 we examined the case in which the surface of a solution containing an amphiphile became covered with a monomolecular film as a result of spontaneous adsorption from solution. The molecules in such films are in equilibrium with those in the bulk of the solution, i.e. there is a continuous movement of molecules between the surface and the solution below it. If, however, a surfactant has a very long hydrocarbon chain it will be insufficiently water-soluble for a film to be formed in this way. In such cases we can spread a film on the surface of the solution by dissolving the surfactant in a suitable volatile solvent and carefully injecting the solution on to the surface. The *insoluble monolayer* formed by this process contains all of the molecules injected on the surface; there is no equilibrium with the bulk solution because of the low water solubility of the surfactant. Conse-

quently, the number of molecules per unit area of surface is generally known directly.

Although the films are called insoluble films, this is not meant to imply that any insoluble substance will form a stable monolayer; in fact, only two classes of materials will do so. The simpler and larger of the two classes includes the water-insoluble amphiphiles discussed above. Such structures orientate themselves at the water surface in the manner of typical surfactants, with the polar group acting as an anchor and the hydrocarbon chain protruding into the vapour phase. The other class of film-forming compounds includes a range of polymeric materials such as proteins and synthetic polymers. With these compounds a high degree of water insolubility is not so essential and stable films will form, providing there is a favourable free energy of adsorption from the bulk solution.

Experimental study of insoluble films

One of the earliest studies of insoluble films was conducted by Benjamin Franklin in 1765 on a pond in Clapham Common in London. Surprisingly Franklin's experiment was sufficiently controlled to establish that olive oil formed a film of monolayer thickness (quoted as one ten millionth of an inch: approximately 2.5 nm). Figure 6.6 illustrates a commonly used apparatus – the Langmuir trough – for study of monolayers on a laboratory scale.

In its simplest form the apparatus consists of a shallow trough with waxed or Teflon sides (nonwetting), along which a nonwetting barrier may be mechanically moved. In use, the trough is filled completely so as to build up a meniscus above the level of the sides. The surface is swept clean with the movable barrier and any surface impurities are sucked away using a water pump. The film-forming material is dissolved in a suitable volatile solvent and an accurately measured amount, usually about 0.01 cm³, of this solution is carefully distributed onto the surface. The solvent evaporates and leaves a uniformly spread film which can now be compressed using the movable barrier. For each setting of the barrier, a force is applied to a torsion wire attached to the float to maintain the float at a fixed position. This force is a direct measure of the surface pressure, π, of the film, that is, the difference between the surface tension of the clean surface γ_0 and that of the film-covered surface, γ_m:

$$\pi = \gamma_0 - \gamma_m \qquad (6.15)$$

The results are generally presented as graphs of π against the surface area per molecule, A, which is readily calculated from the number of molecules added to the surface and the area enclosed between the float and the barrier as shown by the following example.

• •

EXAMPLE 6.3 *Calculation of the area per molecule in an insoluble monolayer*

When 1 cm³ of a solution containing 8.5 mg per 100 cm³ of stearic acid (mol. wt. = 284.3) dissolved in a volatile organic solvent is placed on the surface of water in a Langmuir trough, the solvent evaporates off, leaving the stearic acid spread over the surface as an insoluble monomolecular film. If the surface area occupied by the film is 400 cm², calculate the area occupied by each molecule of stearic acid in the film.

Answer
1 cm³ of the solution contains 8.5×10^{-5} g of stearic acid = 2.99×10^{-7} mol.

Since 1 mol contains 6×10^{23} (Avogadro constant) molecules, the solution contains

$$2.99 \times 10^{-7} \times 6 \times 10^{23} =$$
$$1.79 \times 10^{17} \text{ molecules}$$

Therefore, the area per molecule of stearic acid in the film is

$$\frac{400 \times 10^{-4}}{1.79 \times 10^{17}} = 2.23 \times 10^{-19} \text{ m}^2$$
$$= 0.22 \text{ nm}^2$$

• •

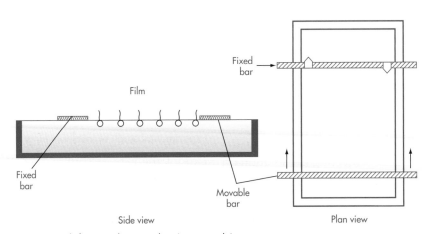

Figure 6.6 Langmuir trough for monolayer studies (not to scale).

Monolayer states

The surface film acts as a two-dimensional analogue to normal matter in that it may exist in different physical states, which in some ways resemble solids, liquids and gases. In this section we shall consider the three different states of monolayers of simple amphiphiles, referred to as solid or condensed, expanded, and gaseous monolayers (see Fig. 6.7).

Solid or condensed state

Figure 6.8 shows the π–A curve for cholesterol, which produces a typical condensed film on an aqueous substrate. The film pressure remains very low at high film areas and rises abruptly when the molecules become tightly packed on compression. Simultaneous electron micrography of the film-covered surface has shown cholesterol clusters or islands which gradually pack more tightly at greater pressures. The film becomes continuous as the pressure is further increased and at such high pressures the molecules are in contact and orientated vertically in the surface as depicted in Fig. 6.8. The extrapolated limiting surface area of 0.39 nm^2 is very close to the cross-sectional area of a cholesterol ring system calculated from molecular models.

Similar films are formed by long-chain fatty acids such as stearic and palmitic acid, for which a limiting surface area of about 0.20 nm^2 is found. This value is very close to the cross-sectional area of the compounds in the bulk crystal as determined by X-ray diffraction.

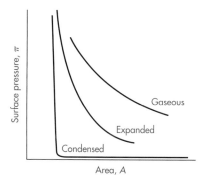

Figure 6.7   Surface pressure, π, versus area per molecule, A, for the three main types of monolayer.

Gaseous monolayers

These films represent the opposite extreme in behaviour to the condensed film. They resemble the gaseous state of three-dimensional matter in that the molecules move around in the film, remaining a sufficiently large distance apart so as to exert very little force on each other. Upon compression, there is a gradual change in the surface pressure, in marked contrast to the behaviour of solid films. It is thought that the molecules in these types of monolayers lie along the surface and this is certainly so with those dibasic esters with terminal polar groups which anchor the molecules flat on the surface. Those steroids in which the polar groups are distributed about the molecule tend to form gaseous films for similar reasons.

Expanded monolayers

Variously named liquid-expanded, expanded or liquid, these monolayers represent intermediate states between gaseous and condensed films. The π–A plots are quite steeply curved and extrapolation to a limiting surface area yields a value which is usually several times greater than the cross-sectional area from molecular models. Films of this type tend to be formed by molecules in which close packing into condensed films is prohibited by bulky side-chains or, as in the case of oleyl alcohol (Fig. 6.9), by a *cis* configuration of the molecule.

Transition between monolayer states

Many simple molecules, rather than exhibiting behaviour exclusively characteristic of one monolayer state, show transitions between one state and another as the film is compressed. Estradiol diacetate, for example (Fig. 6.10), shows typical gaseous behaviour at a large area per molecule, and in this state the molecules are thought to be lying along the surface, as might be expected from the location of the hydrophilic groups on the molecule. As compression is applied, the molecules are gradually pressed closer together until at a molecular surface area of approximately 0.96 nm^2 the molecules begin to stand upright. The film

Condensed monolayer

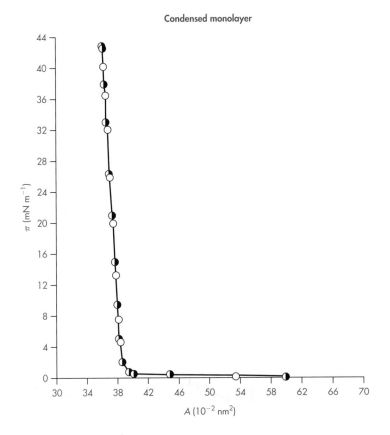

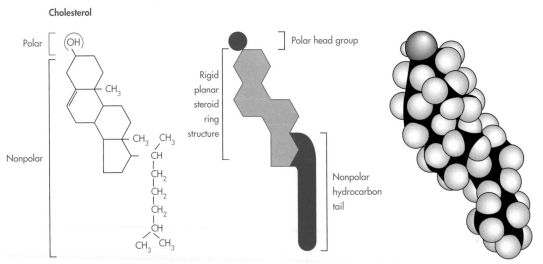

Figure 6.8 Surface pressure, π, versus area per molecule, A, for cholesterol, which shows a typical condensed monolayer, and a schematic drawing of the oriented molecule.

Reproduced from H. E. Reiss, *et al.*, *J. Colloid Interface Sci.*, 57, 396 (1976) with permission.

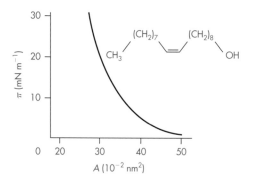

now undergoes a gradual transition to a condensed film as the proportion of upright molecules increases with further compression, until at approximately 0.38 nm² the film is totally in the condensed form.

In some compounds, notably myristic acid, the extent of the gaseous, expanded and condensed regions varies with temperature (Fig. 6.11). There is an analogy between the π–A curves of such compounds and the PV isotherms of three-dimensional gases.

Figure 6.9 Surface pressure, π, versus area per molecule, A, for oleyl alcohol, which forms a typical expanded monolayer.
Reproduced from D. J. Crisp, in *Surface Phenomena in Chemistry and Biology* (ed. J. F. Danielli, K. G. A. Pankhurst and A. C. Riddiford), Pergamon Press, Oxford, 1958, p. 23 with permission.

Polymer monolayers
Monolayers of polymers and proteins lack the characteristic features described in the previous section. Most produce smooth curves, typical of those for gaseous monolayers of amphiphiles.

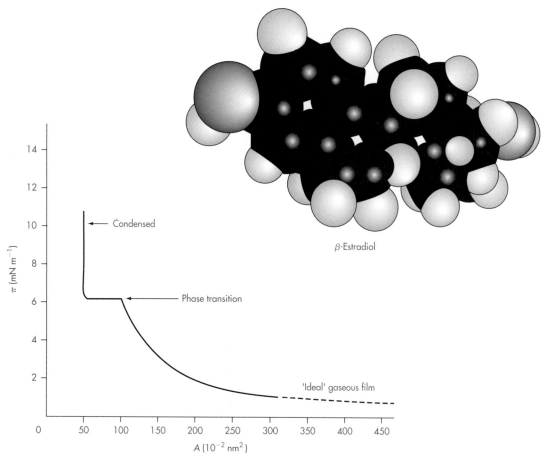

Figure 6.10 Surface pressure, π, versus area per molecule, A, for β-estradiol diacetate, showing a transition from a gaseous to a condensed film on compression.
Reproduced from D. A. Cadenhead and M. C. Philips, *J. Colloid Interface Sci.*, 24, 491 (1967).

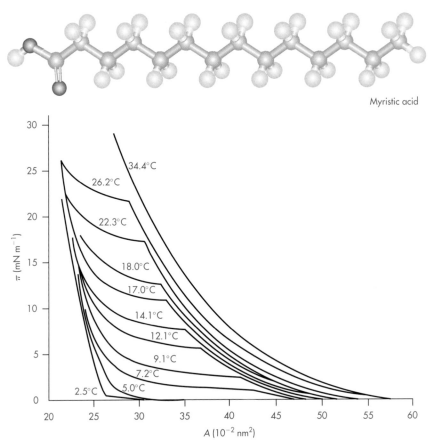

Myristic acid

Figure 6.11   Surface pressure, π, versus area per molecule, A, for myristic acid spread on 0.01 mol dm^{-3} HCl showing a transition from condensed to an expanded film with temperature increase.

6.2.7   Pharmaceutical applications of surface film studies

Study of polymers used as packaging materials and film coatings

Packaging materials must protect the drug without altering in any way the composition of the product. One problem is that of adsorption of constituents, for example, preservatives, from the drug product (see section 6.2.8). The permeability of the packing material to gases or liquids should also be considered, since this may result in deterioration of the product due to oxidation, hydrolysis or loss of volatile ingredients. Monolayers are useful models by which the properties of polymers used as packaging materials can be investigated.

Several methods have been employed in the determination of the resistance of monolayers to evaporation. The evaporation rate may be determined from the increase in mass of a desiccant suspended over the monolayer, or from the loss of weight of a Petri dish containing solution and spread monolayer, under carefully controlled conditions. Such experiments are useful in determining the effect on permeability of incorporation of a plasticiser into the polymer structure.[3]

Polymer monolayers have been used as models to assess the suitability of new polymers and of polymer mixtures as potential enteric and film coatings for solid dosage forms. The effects of substrate pH on the properties of three esters of cellulose, namely, cellulose acetate phthalate (Cellacefate), cellulose acetate butyrate and cellulose acetate stearate have been examined. Monolayers of the butyrate and stearate esters were virtually unaffected by changes of pH of the substrate from 3 to 6.5. Condensed films were formed at both pH values, indicating that disintegration in either the stomach or small intestine would be prevented. Neither of these cellulose esters would therefore be of use as enteric coatings. The phthalate ester, on the other hand, formed a much more condensed monolayer at pH 3 than at pH 6.5 (Fig. 6.12). The conformational changes of this ester suggested its suitability as an enteric coating: the more

tightly packed film at low pH would restrict dissolution in the stomach, whereas the more expanded film at higher pH would allow penetration of water and tablet disintegration in the small intestine where the environmental pH is approximately 6.

Cell membrane models

Phospholipid monolayers provide useful models for studying drug–lipid interactions as we can see from the following recent example[4] which explores the interaction of the phenothiazine drugs trifluoperazine (TFP) and chlorpromazine (CPZ) with the anionic glycerophospholipid dipalmitoylphosphatidylglycerol (DPPG). The surface pressure isotherms of

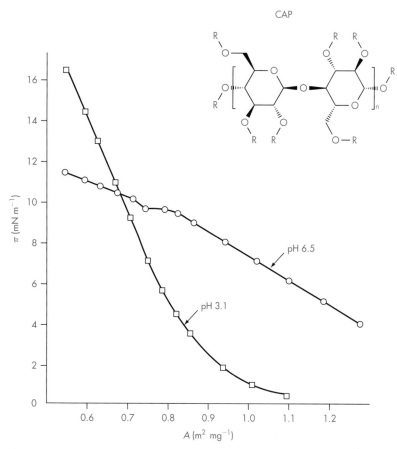

Figure 6.12 Surface pressure, π, versus area per molecule, A, for cellulose acetate phthalate (CAP) spread on an aqueous substrate, showing a more condensed monolayer at a substrate pH of 3 than at pH 6.5.
Reproduced from J. L. Zatz and B. Knowles, *J. Pharm. Sci.*, **57**, 1188 (1970) with permission.

Fig. 6.13 show interesting differences in the interaction of the two drugs with this phospholipid. Incorporation of CPZ expands the monolayer and an additional phase transition appears at higher drug concentrations; at high surface pressures there is little increase in area, suggesting that this drug is being excluded from the interface. TFP also expands the monolayer, although there is no appearance of an additional phase transition; the increase of area per molecule is noted even at high surface pressures, indicating that this drug remains in the monolayer. The considerable expansion of the monolayer observed even at relatively low drug/phospholipid ratios for both systems suggests that phospholipid

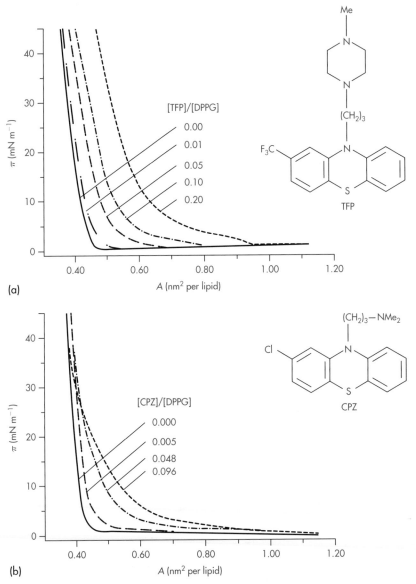

Figure 6.13 Surface pressure isotherms for mixed monolayers of dipalmitoylphosphatidylglycerol (DPPG) and (a) trifluoperazine (TFP) and (b) chlorpromazine (CPZ) for a range of drug/phospholipid molar ratios.
Reproduced from A. A. Hidalgo *et al.*, *Biophys. Chem.*, 109, 85, (2004) with permission.

molecules not in immediate contact with the drug are affected by incorporation of the drug into the monolayer. This 'cooperative effect', which is thought to be a consequence of either a significant reorientation and different packing of the DPPG molecules or a change in their hydration state, may explain why drugs such as these with relatively nonspecific effects on the membrane are highly effective at very low concentrations.

Cholesterol monolayers are also used to model drug–membrane interactions. Figure 6.14 shows the surface pressure–area isotherms for equimolar mixtures of valinomycin (a cyclic peptide), which orientates horizontally at the air/solution interface to give an expanded film, and cholesterol, which orientates vertically to give a solid film. The shape of the mixed isotherm at low and intermediate pressures is similar to that of valinomycin, while the behaviour at high surface pressures is similar to that of cholesterol, suggesting that the valinomycin has been squeezed out of the mixed film. The position of the mixed curve to the left of the calculated average curve suggests some form of interaction between the components which condenses the mixed film.

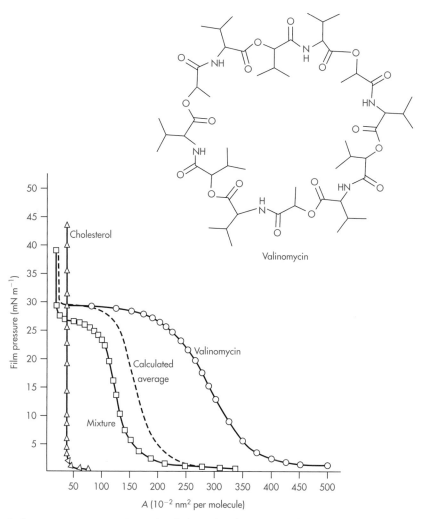

Figure 6.14 Surface pressure–area isotherms for cholesterol, valinomycin and an equimolar mixture of the two.
Reproduced from H. E. Reiss and H. S. Swift, *J. Colloid Interface Sci.*, **64**, 111 (1978) with permission.

6.2.8   Adsorption at the solid/liquid interface

The term *adsorption* is used to describe the process of accumulation at an interface. Adsorption is essentially a surface effect and should be distinguished from *absorption*, which implies the penetration of one component throughout the body of a second. The distinction between the two processes is not always clear-cut, however, and in such cases the noncommittal word *sorption* is sometimes used.

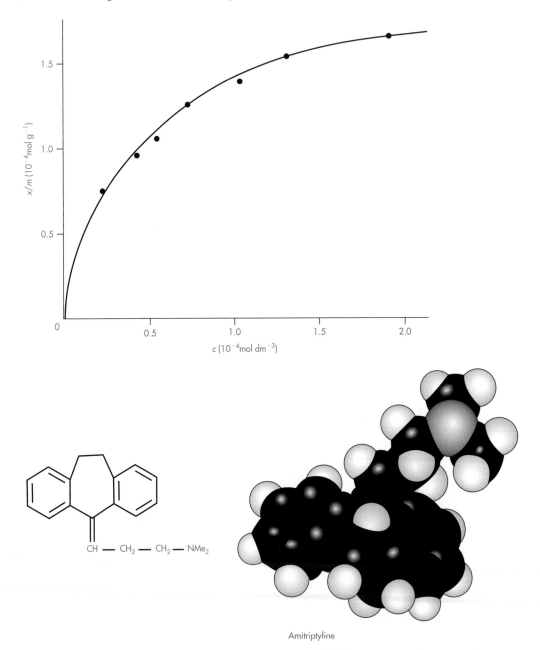

Amitriptyline

Figure 6.15   Langmuir adsorption isotherm of amitriptyline on carbon black from aqueous solution at 30°C.
Reproduced from N. Nambu, S. Sakurai and T. Nagai, *Chem. Pharm. Bull.*, 23 1404 (1975) with permission.

There are two general types of adsorption: physical adsorption, in which the adsorbate is bound to the surface through the weak van der Waals forces, and chemical adsorption or *chemisorption*, which involves the stronger valence forces. Of the two processes, chemisorption is the more specific, and usually involves an ion-exchange process. Frequently both physical and chemical adsorption may be involved in a particular adsorption process. This is the case with the adsorption of toxins in the stomach by attapulgite and kaolin: there is both chemisorption involving cation exchange with the basic groups of the toxins and physical adsorption of the remainder of the molecule.

Adsorption isotherms

The study of adsorption from solution is experimentally straightforward. A known mass of the adsorbent material is shaken with a solution of known concentration at a fixed temperature. The concentration of the supernatant solution is determined by either physical or chemical means and the experiment continued until no further change in the concentration of the supernatant is observed, that is, until equilibrium conditions have been established. Equations originally derived for the adsorption of gases on solids are generally used in the interpretation of the data, the Langmuir and Freundlich equations being the most commonly used.

Langmuir equation
When applied to adsorption from solution, the Langmuir equation becomes

$$\frac{x}{m} = \frac{abc}{1 + bc} \tag{6.16}$$

where x is the amount of solute adsorbed by a weight, m, of adsorbent, c is the concentration of solution at equilibrium, b is a constant related to the enthalpy of adsorption, and a is related to the surface area of the solid. Figure 6.15 shows a typical Langmuir isotherm for the adsorption of the antidepressant drug amitriptyline on carbon black.

Equation (6.16) can be arranged into the linear form

$$\frac{c}{x/m} = \frac{1}{ab} + \frac{c}{a} \tag{6.17}$$

Values of a and b may be determined from the intercept and slope of plots of $c/(x/m)$ against concentration as shown in Example 6.4.

••

EXAMPLE 6.4   Use of the Langmuir equation

Calculate the Langmuir constants for the adsorption of amitriptyline on carbon black using the following data (taken from Fig. 6.15):

$10^3 x/m$ (mol g^{-1})	0.75	0.95	1.10	1.25	1.40	1.55	1.65
$10^4 c$ (mol dm^{-3})	0.25	0.40	0.60	0.70	1.10	1.35	1.95
$10^2 c/(x/m)$ (g dm^{-3})	3.33	4.21	5.45	5.60	7.86	8.71	11.82

Answer
The slope of the plot of $c/(x/m)$ against c (see Fig. 6.16) = 4.88×10^2 g mol^{-1} = $1/a$. Therefore,

$$a = 1/\text{slope} = 2.05 \times 10^{-3} \text{ mol g}^{-1}$$

Intercept = $2.35 \times 10^{-2} = 1/ab$. Therefore,

$$b = 1/(2.35 \times 10^{-2} \times 2.05 \times 10^{-3})$$
$$= 2.07 \times 10^4 \text{ dm}^3 \text{ mol}^{-1}$$

••

The value of a is a measure of the adsorptive capacity of the adsorbent for the particular adsorbate under examination. Table 6.2 gives the adsorptive capacity of carbon black for a series of antidepressant and phenothiazine drugs, arranged in order of decreasing degree of adsorption.

Deviations from the typical Langmuir plot can occur at high concentrations and are then usually attributed to the formation of multi-layers.

Freundlich equation

The Freundlich equation, is generally written

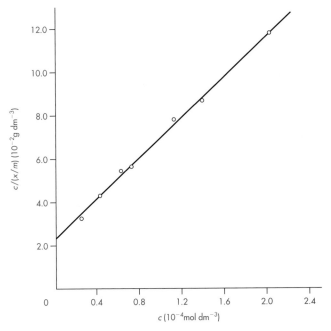

Figure 6.16   Adsorption of amitriptyline by carbon black plotted according to equation (6.17) using the data from Fig. 6.15.

Table 6.2   Langmuir constants a and b in the adsorption of antidepressants and phenothiazines by carbon black[a]

Drug	a $(10^3 \text{ mol kg}^{-1})$	b $(10^{-4} \text{ dm}^3 \text{ mol}^{-1})$
Antidepressants		
Amitriptyline	2.05	2.07
Imipramine	1.80	1.48
Opipramol	1.51	1.77
Desipramine	1.36	4.70
Phenothiazines		
Promazine	1.70	3.36
Chlorpromazine	1.70	4.37
Isothipendyl	1.30	2.23
Chlorpromazine sulfoxide	1.13	3.18

[a] Reproduced from N. Nambu, S. Sakurai and T. Nagai, *Chem. Pharm. Bull.*, **23**, 1404 (1975).

in the form

$$\frac{x}{m} = ac^{1/n} \qquad (6.18)$$

where a and n are constants, the form $1/n$ being used to emphasise that c is raised to a power less than unity. $1/n$ is a dimensionless parameter and is related to the intensity of drug adsorption. Equation (6.18) can be written in a linear form by taking logarithms of both sides, giving

$$\log(x/m) = \log a + (1/n)\log c \qquad (6.19)$$

A plot of $\log(x/m)$ against $\log c$ should be linear, with an intercept of $\log a$ and slope of $1/n$; it is generally assumed that, for systems that obey this equation, adsorption results in the formation of multilayers rather than a single monolayer. Figure 6.17 shows Freundlich isotherms for the adsorption of local anaesthetics on activated carbon; the method of calculating the constants a and $1/n$ from these plots is given in Example 6.5.

• •

EXAMPLE 6.5   Use of the Freundlich equation

The following data refer to the adsorption of tetracaine from aqueous solution at 25°C on to a sample of activated charcoal:

Equilibrium conc. (mg dm⁻³)	0.155	0.468	1.259	2.510	5.370
Amount adsorbed (mg g⁻¹)	202.8	217.8	232.0	243.2	254.7

Show that these data can be represented by the Freundlich isotherm and calculate the constants a and $1/n$.

Answer
Plot a graph of $\log(x/m)$ against $\log c$, noting that the data for the amount adsorbed are given per g of carbon (x/m). This graph is linear, showing that the data can be represented by the Freundlich equation.

At $\log c = 0$, the value of $\log(x/m)$ interpolated from this graph is 2.359. Therefore,

$$a = 229 \text{ mg g}^{-1}$$

The gradient of this plot = 0.065. Therefore,

$$1/n = 0.065$$

• •

Factors affecting adsorption

Solubility of the adsorbate
Solubility is an important factor affecting adsorption. In general, the extent of adsorption of a solute is inversely proportional to its solubility in the solvent from which adsorption

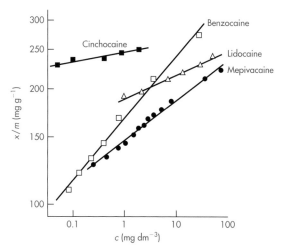

Figure 6.17   Freundlich adsorption isotherms of local anaesthetics on activated carbon at pH 7.0 and 25°C.
Reproduced from I. Abe, H. Kamaya and I. Ueda, *J. Pharm. Sci.*, 79, 354 (1990) with permission.

occurs. This empirical rule is termed *Lundelius's rule*. There are numerous examples of the applicability of this rule; for example, in Lundelius's original work it was noted that the adsorption of iodine onto carbon from CCl_4, $CHCl_3$ and CS_2 was $1 : 2 : 4.5$, respectively. These ratios are close to the inverse ratios for the solubilities of iodine in the respective solvents. The effect of solubility on adsorption might be expected since, in order for adsorption to occur, solute–solvent bonds must first be broken. The greater the solubility, the stronger are these bonds and hence the smaller the extent of adsorption.

For homologous series, adsorption from solution increases as the series is ascended and the molecules become more hydrophobic. There is, for example, a good correlation between the Freundlich adsorption constant, $1/n$ (related to the extent of adsorption) and the molecular weight of the local anaesthetics discussed above (Fig. 6.18). The data for phenobarbital deviated from this linear relationship possibly as a result of the difficulty of adhesion of the phenobarbital molecules to the carbon surface because the barbiturate ring and benzene ring are not aligned in the same plane.

pH

pH affects adsorption for a variety of reasons, the most important from a pharmaceutical viewpoint being its effect on the ionisation and solubility of the adsorbate drug molecule. In general, for simple molecules adsorption increases as the ionisation of the drug is suppressed, the extent of adsorption reaching a maximum when the drug is completely unionised. Figure 6.19 shows that the pH profile for the sorption (this is not a true adsorption process) of benzocaine by nylon 6 powder is indeed almost superimposable on the drug dissociation curve. For amphoteric compounds, adsorption is at a maximum at the isoelectric point, that is, when the compound bears a net charge of zero.

In general, pH and solubility effects act in concert, since the unionised form of most drugs in aqueous solution has a low solubility.

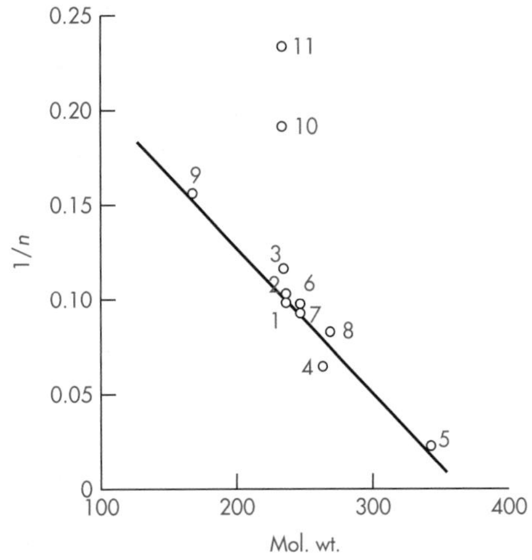

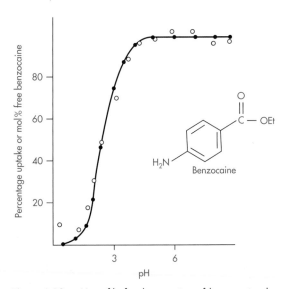

Figure 6.18 Relationship between the Freundlich adsorption constant, $1/n$, and the molecular weight for (1) procaine, pH 7; (2) procaine, pH 11; (3) lidocaine, pH 7; (4) tetracaine, pH 7; (5) cinchocaine, pH 7; (6) mepivacaine, pH 6.6; (7) mepivacaine, pH 8.6; (8) chloroprocaine, pH 7; (9) benzocaine, pH 7; (10) phenobarbital, pH 7; (11) phenobarbital, pH 9.
Reproduced from I. Abe, H. Kamaya and I. Ueda, *J. Pharm. Sci.*, 79, 354 (1990) with permission.

Figure 6.19 pH profile for the sorption of benzocaine by nylon 6 powder from buffered solutions at 30°C and ionic strength 0.5 mol dm^{-3} (O) and the corresponding drug dissociation curve (●).
Reproduced from N. E. Richards and B. J. Meakin, *J. Pharm. Pharmacol.*, 26, 166 (1974) with permission.

Of the two effects, the solubility effect is usually the stronger. Thus, in the adsorption of hyoscine and atropine on magnesium trisilicate it was noted[5] that hyoscine, although in its completely unionised form, was less strongly adsorbed than atropine, which at the pH of the experiment was 50% ionised. The reason for this apparently anomalous result is clear when the solubilities of the two bases are considered. Hyoscine base is freely soluble (1 in 9.5 parts of water at 15°C) compared with atropine base (1 in 400 at 20°C). Even when 50% ionised, atropine is less soluble than hyoscine and consequently is more strongly adsorbed.

Nature of the adsorbent

The physicochemical nature of the adsorbent can have profound effects on the rate and capacity for adsorption. The most important property affecting adsorption is the surface area of the adsorbent; the extent of adsorption is proportional to the specific surface area. Thus the more finely divided or the more porous the solid, the greater will be its adsorptive capacity. Indeed, adsorption studies are frequently used to calculate the surface area of a solid.

Adsorbent–adsorbate interactions are of a complex nature and beyond the scope of this book. Particular adsorbents have affinities for particular adsorbates for a wide variety of reasons. The surfaces of adsorbent clays such as bentonite, attapulgite and kaolin carry cation-exchange sites and such clays have strong affinities for protonated compounds, which they adsorb by an ion-exchange process. In many cases, different parts of the surface of the same adsorbent have different affinities for different types of adsorbents. There is evidence, for example, that anionic materials are adsorbed on the cationic edge of kaolin particles while cationics are adsorbed on the cleavage surface of the particles, which are negatively charged. An example of the differing affinities of a series of adsorbents used as antacids is shown in Fig. 6.20. The adsorptive capacity of a particular adsorbent often depends on the source from which it was prepared and also on its pretreatment.

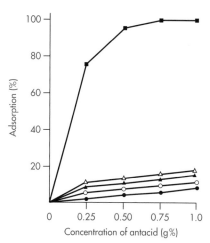

Figure 6.20 Adsorption of digoxin by some antacids at 37 ± 0.1°C: (■) magnesium trisilicate, (△) aluminium hydroxide gel BP (Aludrox was used in the concentration range 2.5–10% v/v), (▲) light magnesium oxide, (○) light magnesium carbonate, (●) calcium carbonate. Initial concentration of the glycoside: 0.25 mg%.
Reproduced from S. A. H. Khalil, *J. Pharm. Pharmacol.*, **26**, 961 (1974) with permission.

Temperature

Since adsorption is generally an exothermic process, an increase in temperature normally leads to a decrease in the amount adsorbed. The changes in enthalpy of adsorption are usually of the order of those for condensation or crystallisation. Thus small variations in temperature tend not to alter the adsorption process to a significant extent.

Some medical and pharmaceutical applications and consequences of adsorption

Adsorption at the solid/liquid interface plays a crucial role in preparative and analytical chromatography, and in heterogeneous catalysis, water purification and solvent recovery. These applications are, however, outside the scope of this book and we will be concerned with examples of the involvement of adsorption in more medical and pharmaceutical situations.

Adsorption of poisons/toxins

The 'universal antidote' for use in reducing the effects of poisoning by the oral route is composed of activated charcoal, magnesium oxide and tannic acid. A more recent use of adsorbents has been in dialysis to reduce toxic concentrations of drugs by passing blood through a haemodialysis membrane over charcoal and other adsorbents. Several drugs are adsorbed effectively by activated charcoal. These include chlorphenamine, dextropropoxyphene hydrochloride, colchicine, phenytoin and aspirin. Some of these are easily recognisable as surface-active molecules (chlorphenamine, dextropropoxyphene) and will be expected to adsorb onto solids. Highly ionised substances of low molecular weight are not well adsorbed, neither are drugs such as tolbutamide that are poorly soluble in acidic media. The formation of a monolayer of drug molecules covering the surface of the charcoal particles through nonpolar interactions is indicated.

The direct application of *in vitro* data for estimating doses of activated charcoal for antidotal purposes may lead to use of inadequate amounts of adsorbent.[6] In an animal study, charcoal : drug ratios of 1 : 1, 2 : 1, 4 : 1 and 8 : 1 reduced absorption of drugs as follows: pentobarbital sodium, 7%, 38%, 62% and 89%; chloroquine phosphate 20%, 30%, 70% and 96%; isoniazid 1.2%, 7.2%, 35% and 80%. Activated charcoal, of course, is not effective in binding all poisons. Biological factors such as gastrointestinal motility, secretions and pH may influence charcoal adsorption. While 5 g of activated charcoal has been said to be capable of binding 8 g of aspirin *in vitro*,[7] 30 g of charcoal *in vivo* was reported to inhibit the gastrointestinal absorption of 3 g of aspirin by only 50%[8]. The surface area of the charcoal is a factor in its effectiveness; charcoal tablets have been found to be approximately half as effective as powdered material.

Taste masking
The intentional adsorption of drugs such as diazepam onto solid substrates should be mentioned, the object being to minimise taste problems. Desorption of the drug *in vivo* is essential but should not occur during the shelf-life of the preparation. Desorption may be a rate-limiting step in absorption. Diazepam adsorbed onto an inorganic colloidal

magnesium aluminium silicate (Veegum) had the same potency in experimental animals as a solution of the drug, but when adsorbed onto microcrystalline cellulose (Avicel) its efficacy was much reduced. Flocculation of the cellulose in the acidic environment of the stomach probably retards the desorption process.

Haemoperfusion
Carbon haemoperfusion is an extracorporeal method of treating cases of severe drug overdoses, and originally involved perfusion of the blood directly over charcoal granules. Although activated charcoal granules were very effective in adsorbing many toxic materials, they were found to give off embolising particles and also to lead to removal of blood platelets. Microencapsulation of activated charcoal granules by coating with biocompatible membranes such as acrylic hydrogels was found to be a successful means of eliminating charcoal embolism and to lead to a much reduced effect on platelet count. *In vitro* tests showed that the coated granules had a reduced adsorption rate although the adsorptive capacity was unchanged.[9] A large proportion of drug overdoses in Great Britain involve barbiturates, and the applicability of carbon haemoperfusion in the treatment of such cases has been demonstrated.[10] Many other drugs taken as overdoses are also present in the plasma at sufficiently high concentration to allow removal by this technique.

Adsorption in drug formulation
Examples of the adsorption of drugs and excipients on to solid surfaces are found in many aspects of drug formulation, some of which, for example the adsorption of surfactants and polymers in the stabilisation of suspensions, are considered elsewhere in this book (see section 7.4). An interesting approach to the improvement of the dissolution rate of poorly water-soluble drugs is to adsorb very small amounts of surfactant on to the drug surface. For example, the adsorption of Pluronic F127 onto the surface of the hydrophobic drug phenylbutazone significantly increased its dissolution rate when compared with untreated material.[11]

In addition to the beneficial use of surfactants in the preparation of formulations, we should also be aware of problems that can arise as a result of inadvertent adsorption occurring both in the manufacture and storage of the product and in its subsequent usage. Problems arising from the adsorption of medicaments by adsorbents such as antacids which may be taken simultaneously by the patient, or which may be present in the same formulation, are discussed in section 10.7. Problems also arise from the adsorption of medicaments onto the container walls. Containers for medicaments, whether glass or plastic, may adsorb a significant quantity of the drug or bacteriostatic or fungistatic agents present in the formulation and thereby affect the potency and possibly the stability of the product. The problem is particularly significant where the drug is highly surface active and present in low concentration. With plastic containers the process is often referred to as sorption rather than adsorption since it often involves significant penetration of the drug into the polymer matrix. Plastics are a large and varied group of materials and their properties are often modified by various additives, such as plasticisers, fillers and stabilisers (see Chapter 8). Such additives may have a pronounced effect on the sorption characteristics of the plastics. The sorption of the fungistatic agent sorbic acid from aqueous solution by plastic cellulose acetate and cellulose triacetate shows an appreciable pH dependence, the sorption declining to zero in the vicinity of the point of maximum ionisation of the sorbic acid. The sorption of local anaesthetics by polyamide and polyethylene depends on the kind of plastic, the reaction conditions and the chemical structure of the drugs. As with sorbic acid, significant sorption was observed only when the drugs were in their unionised forms.

6.3 Micellisation

As the concentration of aqueous solutions of many amphiphilic substances increases, there is a pronounced change in the physical properties of the solution. For example, we have seen in section 6.2.2 that a sharp inflection appears in surface tension plots of surfactant solutions at a critical concentration (the *critical micelle concentration*, cmc) which is attributable to the self-association of the amphiphile into small aggregates called *micelles*. Similar inflection points are observed when other physical properties such as solubility, conductivity, osmotic pressure and light scattering intensity are plotted as a function of concentration (see Fig. 6.21).

The idea that molecules should come together at a critical concentration to form aggregates in solution was quite novel when first proposed by McBain in 1913, but the concept of micellisation has long gained universal acceptance. The micelles are in dynamic equilibrium with free molecules (monomers) in solution; that is, the micelles are continuously breaking down and reforming. It is this fact that distinguishes micellar solutions from other types of colloidal solution and this difference is emphasised by referring to micelle-forming compounds as *association colloids*.

The primary reason for micelle formation is the attainment of a state of minimum free energy. At low concentration, amphiphiles

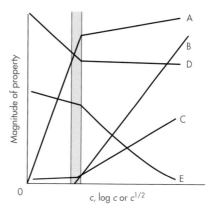

Figure 6.21 Solution properties of an ionic surfactant as a function of concentration, c. A, Osmotic pressure (against c); B, solubility of a water-insoluble solubilisate (against c); C, intensity of light scattered by the solution (against c); D, surface tension (against log c); E, molar conductivity (against $c^{1/2}$).

can achieve an adequate decrease in the overall free energy of the system by accumulation at the surface or interface, in such a way as to remove the hydrophobic group from the aqueous environment. As the concentration is increased, this method of free energy reduction becomes inadequate and the monomers form into micelles. The hydrophobic groups form the core of the micelle and so are shielded from the water.

The free energy change of a system is dependent on changes in both the entropy and enthalpy; that is, $\Delta G = \Delta H - T \Delta S$. For a micellar system at normal temperatures the entropy term is by far the most important in determining the free energy changes ($T \Delta S$ constitutes approximately 90–95% of the ΔG value). Micelle formation entails the transfer of a hydrocarbon chain from an aqueous to a nonaqueous environment (the interior of the micelle). To understand the changes in enthalpy and entropy that accompany this process, we must first consider the structure of water itself.

6.3.1   Water structure and hydrophobic bonding

Water possesses many unique features that distinguish it from other liquids. These arise from the unusual structure of the molecule in which the O and H atoms are arranged at the apices of a triangle (see Fig. 6.22).

Each of the covalent bonds between a hydrogen atom and the oxygen atom of the water molecule involves the pairing of the electron of the hydrogen atom with an electron in the oxygen atom's outer shell of six electrons. This pairing leaves two lone pairs of electrons in the outer-shell, the orbitals of which point to the vertices of an approximately regular tetrahedron formed by the lone pairs and the OH bonds. The resulting tetrahedral structure has two positively charged sites at one side and two negatively charged sites at the other. It will readily attach itself by hydrogen bonds to four neighbouring molecules, two at the negatively charged sites and two at the positively charged sites. In its usual form, ice demonstrates an almost perfect tetrahedral arrangement of bonds with a distance of about 0.276 nm between neighbouring oxygen atoms. There is much unfilled space in the crystal, which accounts for the low density of ice.

When ice melts, a high degree of hydrogen bonding persists in the resulting liquid. In spite of extensive investigation by a variety of techniques such as X-ray diffraction, thermochemical determination, and infrared and Raman spectroscopy, the structural nature of liquid water is still to be completely resolved. There are, broadly speaking, two distinct types of model: those which involve distortion but not breaking of hydrogen bonds, and a second type in which unbonded detached water molecules exist in addition to the hydrogen-bonded structures. Of the former type, the model which is considered to be the most acceptable is one in which all the water molecules continue to be hydrogen-bonded to their four neighbours, but the intermolecular links are bent or stretched to give an irregular framework. Such distorted networks are known to exist in some of the denser forms of ice.

Many proposed structures for water involve mixtures of structured material and free water molecules. One of the most highly developed theories encompasses the so-called 'flickering cluster' concept of water structure. The model is based on the cooperative nature of hydrogen bonding. The formation of one hydrogen bond on a water molecule leaves the molecule more susceptible to further hydrogen bonding, and similarly when one bond breaks there is a tendency for large groups of bonds to break. As a result, clusters of ice-like

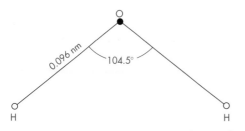

Figure 6.22 Diagram of water molecule showing bond angle and length.

hydrogen-bonded material are imagined to be suspended in a fluid of unbonded water (Fig. 6.23). Because of the continual formation and rupture of hydrogen bonds throughout the liquid, these clusters have only a temporary existence, and are aptly described by the term 'flickering'.

Most of the models proposed for the structure of water, only two of which have been considered here, can account for some, but not all of the physical and thermodynamic anomalies which have been observed with water.

The flickering cluster model can be used to describe possible structural changes that occur when nonpolar and polar solutes are dissolved in water. A nonpolar molecule or portion of a molecule tends to seek out the more ice-like regions within the water. Such regions, as we have seen, contain open structures into which the nonpolar molecules may fit without breaking hydrogen bonds or otherwise disturbing the surrounding ice-like material. In solution, therefore, hydrophobic molecules tend always to be surrounded by structured water. This concept is important in discussing interactions between nonpolar molecules in aqueous solution, such as those that occur in micelle formation. The interaction of hydrocarbons in aqueous solution was first thought to arise simply as consequence of the van der Waals forces between the hydrocarbon molecules. It was later realised, however, that changes in the water structure around the nonpolar groups must play an important role in the formation of bonds between the nonpolar molecules – the so-called *hydrophobic bonds*. In fact the contribution from the van der Waals forces is only about 45% of the total free energy of formation of a hydrophobic bond. When the nonpolar groups approach each other until they are in contact, there will be a decrease in the total number of water molecules in contact with the nonpolar groups. The formation of the hydrophobic bond in this way is thus equivalent to the partial removal of hydrocarbon from an aqueous environment and a consequent loss of the ice-like structuring which always surrounds the hydrophobic molecules. The increase in entropy and decrease in free energy which accompany the loss of structuring make the formation of the hydrophobic bond an energetically favourable process.

There is much experimental evidence to support this explanation for the decrease in ΔG. Thus the enthalpy of micelle formation becomes more negative as the temperature is increased; a fact which was attributed to a reduction in water structure as temperature is increased. Nuclear magnetic resonance (NMR) measurements indicate an increase in the mobility of water protons at the onset of micellisation. The addition of urea, a water-structure-breaking compound, to surfactant solutions leads to an increase of cmc, again indicating the role of water structure in the micellisation process. An alternative explanation of the free energy decrease emphasises the increase in internal freedom of the hydrocarbon chains which occurs when these chains are transferred from the aqueous environment, where their motion is restrained by the hydrogen-bonded water molecules, to the interior of the micelle. It has been suggested that the increased mobility of the hydrocarbon chains, and of course their mutual attraction, constitute the principal hydrophobic factor in micellisation.

6.3.2 Theories of micelle formation

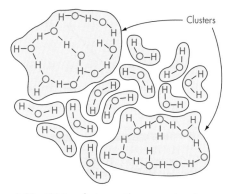

Figure 6.23 Water clusters with unassociated water molecules around them.

Two general approaches have been employed in attempting to describe the process of micellisation. In one of these, the phase separation model, the cmc is assumed to represent the saturation concentration of the unassociated molecules and the micelles are regarded as a distinct phase which separates out at the cmc. In the alternative approach, the micelle and associated monomers are assumed to be in an association–dissociation equilibrium to which the law of mass action may be applied. Neither of these models is rigorously correct, although the mass action approach seems to give a more realistic description of micellisation, and thus will be considered in more detail.

The aggregation process may in its simplest form be described by

$$ND^+ + (N - p)X^- \rightleftharpoons M^{p+} \qquad (6.20)$$

Equation (6.20) represents the formation of a cationic micelle M^{p+} from N surfactant ions D^+ and $(N - p)$ firmly held counterions X^-. Whenever the thermodynamics of a process is under consideration, it is important to define the standard states of the species. In this example, the standard states are such that the mole fractions of the ionic species are unity and the solution properties are those of the infinitely dilute solutions. The equilibrium constant K_m may be written in the usual way

$$K_m = \frac{[M^{p+}]}{[D^+]^N [X^-]^{N-p}} \qquad (6.21)$$

where activity coefficients have been neglected. The analogous equation for nonionic micelles is of a simpler form since counterion terms and charges need not be considered.

$$K_m = \frac{[M]}{[D]^N} \qquad (6.22)$$

Equation (6.21) and (6.22) are important in that they can be used to predict the variation of both monomers and micelles with total solution concentration.

Figure 6.24 shows the result of such a calculation for a model system. It illustrates several important points about the micellisation process. According to the mass action treatment, the monomer concentration decreases very slightly above the cmc: this is a very small

effect (although it can be detected experimentally from surface-tension measurements) and for most purposes it is reasonable to assume that the monomer concentration remains constant at the cmc value. A second point of interest illustrated by the mass action treatment concerns the predicted sharpness of the cmc. It is readily shown by calculations that combinations of low values of N and K_m lead to gradual changes of slope of the cmc region, while larger values for both of these parameters give sharp inflections. The cmc, rather than being an exact concentration, is often a region of concentration over which the solution properties exhibit a gradual change and hence is often difficult to locate exactly.

6.3.3   Micellar structure

Critical packing parameter

The shape of the micelle formed by a particular surfactant is influenced to a large extent by the geometry of the surfactant molecule, as can be seen if we consider the packing of space-filling models of the surfactants. The dimensionless parameter of use in these considerations is called the *critical packing parameter* (CPP) and is defined as

$$CPP = \frac{v}{l_c a}$$

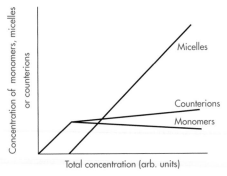

Figure 6.24 Concentration of micelles, monomers and counterions against total concentration (arbitrary units) calculated from equation (6.21) for an aggregation number (N) of 100, micellar equilibrium constant (K_m) of 1, and with 85% of the counterions bound to the micelle.

where v is the volume of one chain, a is the cross-sectional area of the surfactant head group and l_c is the extended length of the surfactant alkyl chain (see Fig. 6.25). This parameter provides a simple geometric characterisation of the surfactant molecule, which is useful when we consider the structure of the aggregate that will be formed in solution. Consideration of the packing of molecules into spheres shows that when $CPP \leqslant 1/3$, which is the case for surfactants having a single hydrophobic chain and a simple ionic or large nonionic head group, a spherical micelle will be formed. Most surfactants of pharmaceutical interest fall into this category. It is easily seen that if we double v by adding a second alkyl chain then the value of CPP will exceed 1/3 and nonspherical structures such as bilayers ($CPP \approx 1$) will form in solution, from which vesicles are formed (see section 6.4.2). One important factor not considered in this simple geometrical model is the interaction between the head groups in the aggregate. The 'effective' cross-sectional area of the

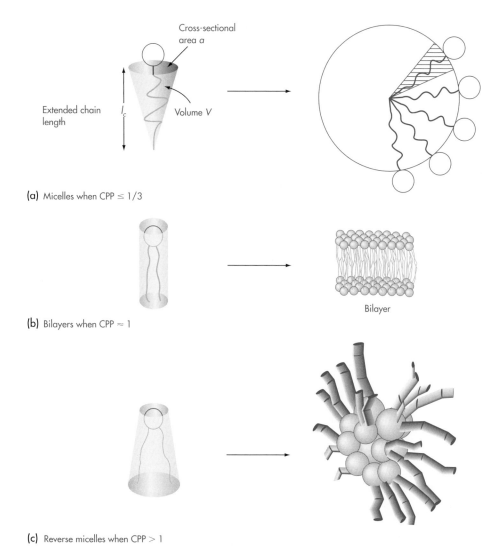

Cross-sectional area a

Extended chain length l_c Volume V

(a) Micelles when $CPP \leq 1/3$

(b) Bilayers when $CPP \approx 1$

Bilayer

(c) Reverse micelles when $CPP > 1$

Figure 6.25 Influence of the critical packing parameter, $CPP = v/(l_c a)$, on the type of aggregate formed by surfactants in solution.

surfactant molecule is strongly influenced by the interaction forces between adjacent head groups in the micelle surface. These forces are decreased by addition of electrolyte, leading to a decrease of a, an increase of the CPP, and a change of shape of the aggregate, as discussed below.

In nonaqueous media, reverse (or inverted) micelles may form, in which the hydrophilic charge groups form the micellar core shielded from the nonaqueous environment by the hydrophobic chains; such structures are generally formed when CPP > 1 (see Fig. 6.25).

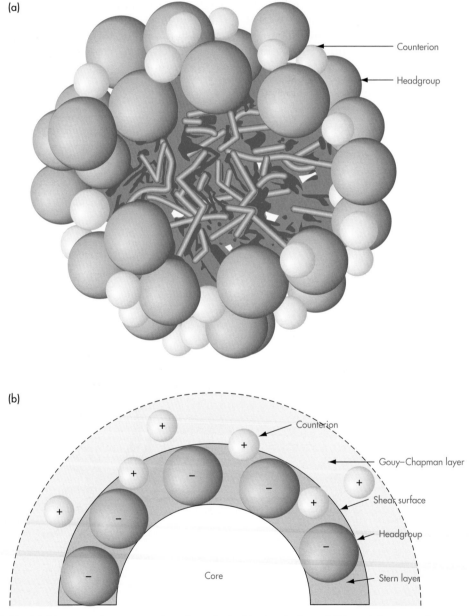

(a)

Counterion

Headgroup

(b)

Counterion

Gouy–Chapman layer

Shear surface

Headgroup

Core

Stern layer

Figure 6.26 (a) Diagrammatic representation of a spherical ionic micelle and (b) partial cross-section of an anionic micelle showing charged layers.

Ionic micelles

As we have seen from consideration of the simple geometrical packing model, charged micelles of low aggregation number have a CPP < 1/3 and consequently adopt a spherical or near-spherical shape at concentrations not too far removed from the cmc. The hydrophobic part of the amphiphile is located in the core of the micelle. Around this core is a concentric shell of hydrophilic head groups with $(1 - \alpha)N$ counterions, where α is the degree of ionisation. This compact region is termed the *Stern layer* (see Fig. 6.26). For most ionic micelles the degree of ionisation α is between 0.2 and 0.3; that is, 70–80% of the counterions may be considered to be bound to the micelles.

The outer surface of the Stern layer is the shear surface of the micelle. The core and the Stern layer together constitute what is termed the *kinetic micelle*. Surrounding the Stern layer is a diffuse layer called the *Gouy–Chapman electrical double layer*, which contains the αN counterions required to neutralise the charge on the kinetic micelle. The thickness of the double layer is dependent on the ionic strength of the solution and is greatly compressed in the presence of electrolyte.

In highly concentrated solution, a gradual change in micellar shape is thought to occur with many ionic systems, the micelles elongating to form cylindrical structures (see Fig. 6.27).

Nonionic micelles

In general, nonionic surfactants form larger micelles than their ionic counterparts. The reason for this is clearly attributable to the removal of electrical work which must be done when a monomer of an ionic surfactant is added to an existing charged micelle. As a consequence of the larger size, the nonionic micelles are frequently asymmetric. The micelles of Cetomacrogol 1000 ($C_{16}H_{33}$ $(OCH_2CH_2)_{21}OH$, abbreviated to $C_{16}E_{21}$), for example, are thought to be ellipsoidal with an axial ratio not exceeding 2 : 1.

Nonionic micelles have a hydrophobic core surrounded by a shell of oxyethylene chains which is often termed the *palisade layer* (Fig. 6.28). This layer is capable of mechanically entrapping a considerable number of water molecules, as well as those that are hydrogen-bonded to the oxyethylene chains. Micelles of nonionic surfactants tend, as a consequence, to be highly hydrated. The outer surface of the palisade layer forms the shear surface; that is, the hydrating molecules form part of the kinetic micelle.

6.3.4 Factors affecting the critical micelle concentration and micellar size

Structure of the hydrophobic group

The hydrophobic group plays an important role in determining the type of association of the amphiphile. Compounds with rigid aromatic or heteroaromatic ring structures (many dyes, purines and pyrimidines, for example) associate by a nonmicellar process involving the face-to-face stacking of molecules one on top of the other, rather than by micellisation. Such systems do not exhibit cmcs. Association

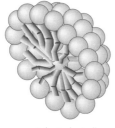

Spherical micelle

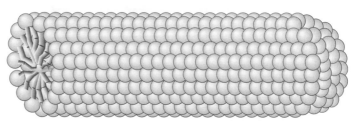

Cylindrical micelle

Figure 6.27   Elongation of a spherical micelle to form a cylindrical micelle at high concentration.

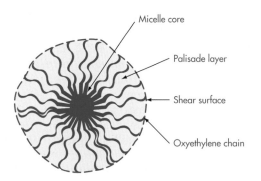

Figure 6.28 Diagrammatic representation of the cross-section of a nonionic micelle.

usually commences at very low concentrations and growth of aggregates may occur by the stepwise addition of monomers. Consequently, the aggregates continuously increase in size rather than attaining an equilibrium size as in micellisation. Some drugs are thought to associate in this manner.[1, 2]

Micellar amphiphiles of the most common type have hydrophobic groups constructed from hydrocarbon chains. Increase in length of this chain results in a decrease in cmc, and for compounds with identical polar head groups this relationship is expressed by the linear equation

$$\log[\text{cmc}] = A - Bm \qquad (6.23)$$

where m is the number of carbon atoms in the chain and A and B are constants for a

homologous series. A corresponding increase in micellar size with increase in hydrocarbon chain length is also noted.

Many drugs are surface active and form small micelles in aqueous solution. For these and other amphiphiles with more complex hydrophobic regions, the effect of substituents on hydrophobicity can be roughly estimated from Table 5.4 (section 5.2.1). In the series of micellar diphenylmethane drugs shown in Table 6.3 there is an increased hydrophobicity (as evidenced by a decrease in cmc and increase in aggregation number) following the introduction of —CH$_3$, —Br and —Cl substituents to the hydrophobic ring systems.

Nature of the hydrophilic group

The most important point to be noted here is the pronounced difference in properties between amphiphiles with ionic hydrophilic groups and those in which this group is uncharged. In general, nonionic surfactants have very much lower cmc values and higher aggregation numbers than their ionic counterparts with similar hydrocarbon chains, mainly because the micellisation process for such compounds does not involve any electrical work.

The properties of the polyoxyethylated nonionic surfactants show a pronounced dependence on the length of the polyoxyethylene chain. An increase in the chain length confers

Table 6.3 Effect of substituents on the micellar properties of some diphenylmethane drugs[a]

Drug	R^1	R^2	R^3	Critical micellar concentration (mol kg^{-1})	Micellar aggregation number
Diphenhydramine	H	H	H	0.132	3
Orphenadrine	H	CH$_3$	H	0.096	7
Bromodiphenhydramine	Br	H	H	0.053	11
Chlorphenoxamine	Cl	H	CH$_3$	0.045	13

[a] Reproduced from D. Attwood, *J. Pharm. Pharmacol.*, 24, 751 (1972); 28, 407 (1976).

a greater hydrophilicity to the molecule and the cmc increases, as shown in Table 6.4.

Nature of the counterion

The counterion associated with the charged group of ionic surfactants has a significant effect on the micellar properties. There is an increase in micellar size for a particular cationic surfactant as the counterion is changed according to the series $Cl^- < Br^- < I^-$, and for a particular anionic surfactant according to $Na^+ < K^+ < Cs^+$. Generally, the more weakly hydrated a counterion, the larger the micelles formed by the surfactant. This is because the weakly hydrated ions can be adsorbed more readily in the micellar surface and so decrease the charge repulsion between the polar groups. A greater depression of cmc and a greater increase in micellar size is noted with organic counterions such as maleates than with inorganic ions.

Addition of electrolytes

Addition of electrolytes to ionic surfactants decreases the cmc and increases the micellar size. The effect is simply explained in terms of a reduction in the magnitude of the forces of repulsion between the charged head groups in the micelle and a consequent decrease in the electrical work of micellisation. At sufficiently high electrolyte concentration the reduction of head group interaction is sufficient to increase CPP to such an extent that spherical micelles can no longer form. Table 6.5 shows the effect of sodium chloride addition on the micellar properties of the cationic surfactant dodecyltrimethylammonium bromide. The micellar properties of nonionic surfactants, in contrast, are little affected by electrolyte addition.

Effect of temperature

If aqueous solutions of many nonionic surfactants are heated, they become turbid at a characteristic temperature called the *cloud point* (see Fig. 6.31 in section 6.4). Other nonionic surfactants have cloud points above 100°C. The process is reversible, that is, cooling the solution restores clarity. The turbidity at the cloud point is due to separation of the solution into two phases. At temperatures up to the cloud point an increase in

Table 6.4 Values of cmc and micellar weights of hexadecyl polyoxyethylene ethers $CH_3(CH_3)_{15}(CH_2CH_2)_nOH$[a]

Property	$n =$					
	6	7	9	12	15	21
10^6 cmc (mol kg^{-1})	1.7	1.7	2.1	2.3	3.1	3.9
10^{-5} Micellar weight	12.3	3.27	1.4	1.17	–	0.82
Aggregation number	2430	590	220	150	–	70

[a] Reproduced from P. H. Elworthy and C. B. Macfarlane, *J. Chem. Soc.*, 907 (1963); 537 (1962).

Table 6.5 Effect of electrolyte on the micellar properties of dodecyltrimethylammonium bromide $CH_3(CH_2)_{11}N^+(CH_3)_3Br^-$[a]

NaCl concentration (mol dm^{-3})	Critical micellar concentration (mol dm^{-3})	Aggregation number
0.00	0.014 6	61
0.10	0.004 28	74
0.50	0.001 71	90

[a] Reproduced from E. W. Anacker, in *Cationic Surfactants* (ed. E. Jungermann), Marcel Dekker, New York, 1970.

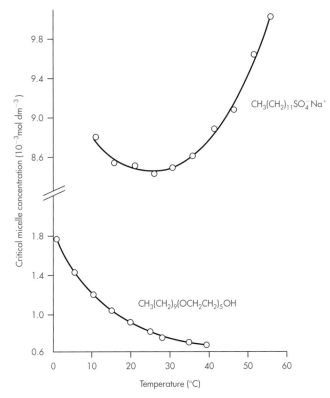

Figure 6.29 Variation of cmc with temperature for: sodium dodecyl sulfate ($CH_3(CH_2)_{11}SO_4^-Na^+$) and pentaoxyethylene glycol monodecyl ether ($CH_3(CH_2)_9(OCH_2CH_2)_5OH$).
Modified from E. D. Goddard and G. C. Benson, *Can. J. Chem.*, 35, 986 (1957) with permission.

micellar size and a corresponding decrease in cmc is noted for many nonionic surfactants (Fig. 6.29). The cloud point is very sensitive to additives in the system, which can increase or decrease the clouding temperature.

Temperature has a comparatively small effect on the micellar properties of ionic surfactants. The temperature dependence of the cmc of sodium lauryl (dodecyl) sulfate shown in Fig. 6.29 is typical of the effect observed.

6.4 Liquid crystals and surfactant vesicles

6.4.1 Liquid crystals

Lyotropic liquid crystals

Surfactant solutions at concentrations close to the cmc are clear and isotropic; that is, the magnitudes of such physical properties as viscosity and refractive index do not depend on the direction in which these properties are measured. As the concentration is increased there is frequently a transition from the typical spherical micellar structure to a more elongated or rod-like micelle. Further increase in concentration may cause the orientation and close packing of the elongated micelles into hexagonal arrays. A new phase containing these ordered arrays separates out from the remainder of the solution, which contains randomly orientated rods, but remains in equilibrium with it. This new phase is a liquid crystalline state termed the *middle phase* or *hexagonal phase*. With some surfactants, further increase of concentration results in the separation of a second liquid crystalline state, the *neat phase* or *lamellar phase*. In some surfactant systems another liquid crystalline state, the *cubic phase*, occurs between the

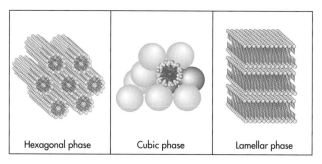

Figure 6.30 Diagrammatic representation of forms of lyotropic liquid crystals.

middle and neat phases. The most common type of cubic phase is the micellar cubic phase formed by the close packing of spherical micelles; a more complex cubic phase, the bicontinuous cubic phase, occurs with some amphiphilic lipids such as glyceryl monooleate (see section 6.4.2). Finally, in all systems, surfactant separates out of solution. The liquid crystalline phases that occur on increasing the concentration of surfactant solutions are referred to as *lyotropic* liquid crystals; their structure is shown diagrammatically in Fig. 6.30. The phase diagram in Fig. 6.31 shows the transition from micellar solution to liquid crystalline phase and finally to pure amphiphile

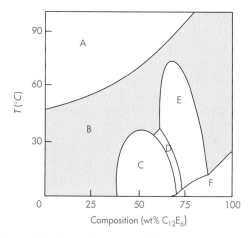

Figure 6.31 Phase diagram of the $CH_3(CH_2)_{11}(OCH_2$ $CH_2)_6OH(C_{12}E_6)/H_2O$ system: A, two isotropic liquid phases; B, micellar solution; C, middle or hexagonal phase; D, cubic phase; E, neat or lamellar phase; F, solid phase. The boundary between phases A and B is the cloud point.
Modified from J. S. Clunie, J. F. Goodman and P. C. Symons, *Trans. Farad. Soc.*, 65, 287 (1969).

for the polyoxyethylated nonionic surfactant $C_{12}E_6$ $(CH_3(CH_2)_{11}(OCH_2CH_2)_6OH)$.

Liquid crystals are anisotropic; that is, their physical properties vary with direction of measurement. The middle phase, for example, will flow only in a direction parallel to the long axis of the arrays. It is rigid in the other two directions. On the other hand, the neat phase is more fluid and behaves as a solid only in the direction perpendicular to that of the layers. Similarly, plane-polarised light is rotated when travelling along any axis except the long axis in the middle phase and a direction perpendicular to the layers in the neat phase. Because of this ability to rotate polarised light, the liquid crystals are visible when placed between crossed polarisers, and this provides a useful means of detecting the liquid crystalline state.

Thermotropic liquid crystals

A second category of liquid crystals is the type produced when certain substances, notably the esters of cholesterol, are heated. These systems are referred to as *thermotropic* liquid crystals and, although not formed by surfactants, their properties will be described here for purposes of comparison. The formation of a cloudy liquid when cholesteryl benzoate is heated to temperatures between 145 and 179°C was first noted in 1888 by the Austrian botanist Reinitzer. The name 'liquid crystal' was applied to this cloudy intermediate phase because of the presence of areas with crystal-like molecular structure within this solution.

Although the compounds that form thermotropic liquid crystalline phases are of a variety of chemical types such as azo compounds, azoxy compounds or esters, the molecular geometries of the molecule have some characteristic features in that they are generally elongated, flat and rigid along their axes. The presence of easily polarisable groups often enhances liquid crystal formation.

The arrangement of the elongated molecules in thermotropic liquid crystals is generally recognisable as one of three principal types:

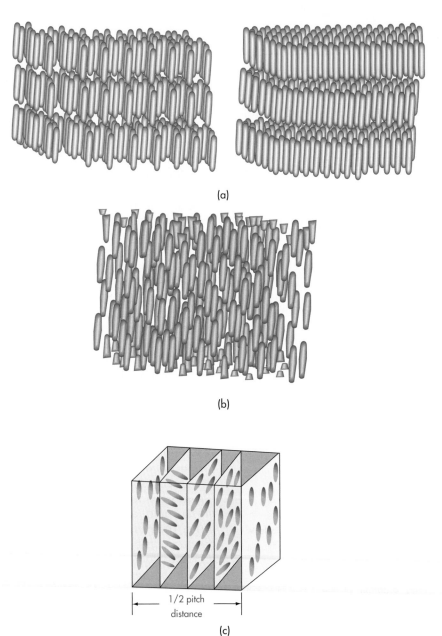

Figure 6.32 Diagrammatic representation of forms of thermotropic liquid crystals: (a) smectic, (b) nematic, and (c) cholesteric liquid crystals.

namely, *smectic* (soap-like), *nematic* (thread-like) and *cholesteric*. The molecular arrays are illustrated diagrammatically in Fig. 6.32.

In the nematic liquid crystalline state, groups of molecules orientate spontaneously with their long axes parallel, but they are not ordered into layers. Because the molecules have freedom of rotation about their long axis, the nematic liquid crystals are quite mobile and are readily orientated by electric or magnetic fields. Nematic liquid crystals are formed, for example, when *p*-azoxyanisole is heated.

The molecules in smectic liquid crystals are more ordered than the nematic since, not only are they arranged with their long axes parallel, but they are also arranged into distinct layers. As a result of this two-dimensional order the smectic liquid crystals are viscous and are not orientated by magnetic fields. Examples of compounds forming smectic liquid crystals are octyl *p*-azoxycinnamate and ethyl *p*-azoxy-benzoate.

If a nematic liquid crystal is made of chiral molecules, i.e. the molecules differ from their mirror image, a cholesteric (or chiral nematic)

Box 6.4   Some vesicle-forming amphiphiles

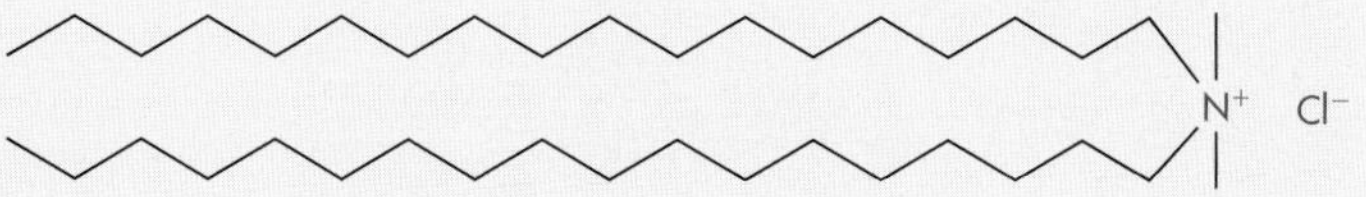

Dioctadecyldimethylammonium chloride

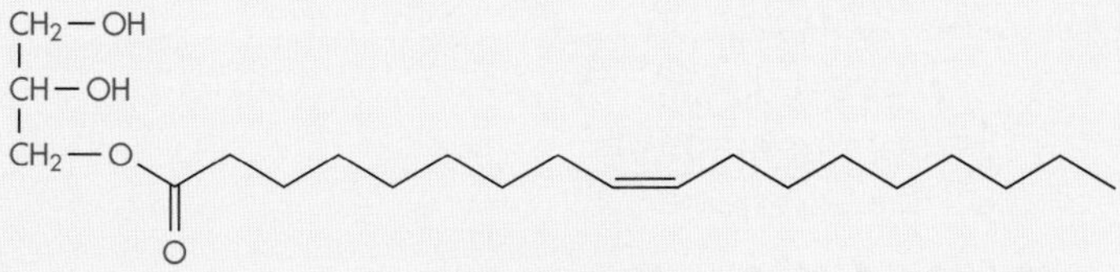

Glyceryl monooleate

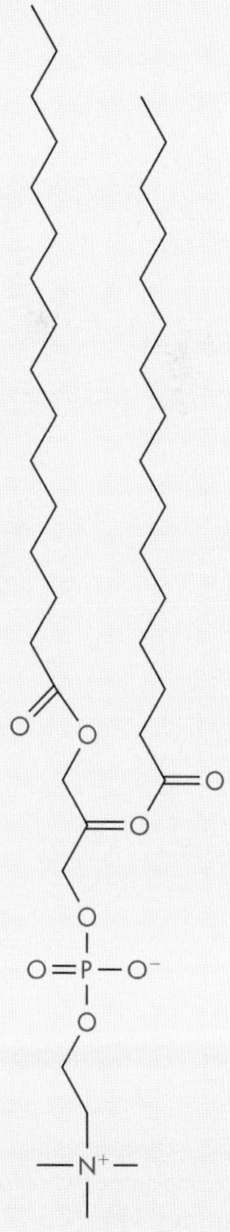

Lecithin

liquid crystal is obtained. The cholesteric phase is formed by several cholesteryl esters and can be visualised as a stack of very thin two-dimensional nematic-like layers in which the elongated molecules lie parallel to each other in the plane of the layer. The orientation of the long axes in each layer is displaced from that in the adjacent layer and this displacement is cumulative through successive layers, so that the overall displacement traces out a helical path through the layers. The helical path causes very pronounced rotation of polarised light, which can be as much as 50 rotations per millimetre. The pitch of the helix (the distance required for one complete rotation) is very sensitive to small changes in temperature and pressure and dramatic colour changes can result from variations in these properties. When nonpolarised light is passed through the cholesteric material, the light is separated into two components, one with the electric vector rotating clockwise and the other with the electric vector rotating anticlockwise. One of these components is transmitted and the other reflected, depending on the material involved. This process is called *circular dichroism* and it gives the cholesteric phase a characteristic iridescent appearance when illuminated by white light.

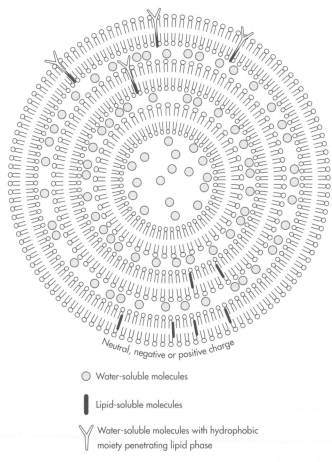

Neutral, negative or positive charge

○ Water-soluble molecules

❙ Lipid-soluble molecules

Y Water-soluble molecules with hydrophobic moiety penetrating lipid phase

Figure 6.33 Diagrammatic representation of a liposome in which three bilayers of polar phospholipids alternate with aqueous compartments. Water-soluble and lipid-soluble substances may be accommodated in the aqueous and lipid phases, respectively. Certain macromolecules can insert their hydrophobic regions into the lipid bilayers with the hydrophilic portions extending into water.

Reproduced from G. Gregoriadis, *N. Engl. J. Med.*, 295, 704 (1976) with permission.

6.4.2 Liposomes, niosomes and surfactant vesicles

Phospholipids and other surfactants having two hydrophobic chains have CPP values of approximately 1 (see section 6.3.3) and tend to form lamellar phases. When equilibrated with excess water, these lamellar phases may form vesicles that can entrap drug and these have potential use as drug carriers. In this section we will consider several types of vesicular structures; Box 6.4 (p. 213) shows some of the amphiphiles that form such structures.

Liposomes

Liposomes are formed by naturally occurring phospholipids such as lecithin (phosphatidylcholine). When first formed in solution they are usually composed of several bimolecular lipid lamellae separated by aqueous layers (*multilamellar liposomes*). Figure 6.33 shows a diagrammatic representation of a multilamellar liposome with three phospholipid bilayers. Sonication of these units can give rise to *unilamellar liposomes*. The net charge of the liposome can be varied by incorporation of, for example, a long-chain amine such as stearyl amine (to give positively charged vesicles) or dicetyl phosphate (to give negatively charged species). Positively charged vesicles are being used experimentally as carriers for DNA: the anionic DNA condenses around the cationic vesicles to provide compact units for cell delivery. Water-soluble drugs can be entrapped in liposomes by intercalation in the aqueous layers, while lipid-soluble drugs can be solubilised within the hydrocarbon interiors of the lipid bilayers (see Fig. 6.33). The use of liposomes as drug carriers has been reviewed.[12] Since liposomes can encapsulate drugs, proteins and enzymes, the systems can be administered intravenously, orally or intramuscularly in order to decrease toxicity, to increase specificity of uptake of drug and in some cases to control release. Liposomes have several disadvantages as carriers to deliver drugs, however; for example, phospholipids are liable to oxidative degradation and must be stored and handled in a nitrogen atmosphere.

Surfactant vesicles and niosomes

Surfactants having two alkyl chains can pack in a similar manner to the phospholipids (see Box 6.4 for examples). Vesicle formation by the dialkyldimethylammonium cationic surfactants has been studied extensively. As with liposomes, sonication of the turbid solution formed when the surfactant is dispersed in water leads ultimately to the formation of optically transparent solutions which may contain single-compartment vesicles. For example, sonication of dioctadecyldimethylammonium chloride for 30 s gives a turbid solution containing bilayer vesicles of 250–450 nm diameter, while sonication for 15 min produces a clear solution containing monolayer vesicles of diameter 100–150 nm. The main use of such systems has been as membrane models rather than as drug delivery vehicles because of the toxicity of ionic surfactants.

Some dialkyl polyoxyethylene ether nonionic surfactants also form vesicles, as do mixtures of cholesterol and a single-alkyl-chain nonionic surfactant with a glyceryl head group. The resultant vesicles have been termed *niosomes*. These vesicles behave *in vivo* like liposomes, prolonging the circulation of entrapped drug and altering its organ distribution and metabolic stability. As with liposomes, the properties of niosomes depend both on the composition of the bilayer and on the method of production; Fig. 6.34 shows a freeze-fracture electron micrograph of a multilamellar niosome. Being nonionic, niosomes are likely to be less toxic than vesicles produced from ionic surfactants and represent promising vehicles for drug delivery.[13, 14]

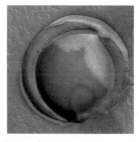

Figure 6.34 Freeze-fracture electron micrograph of a multilamellar niosome.

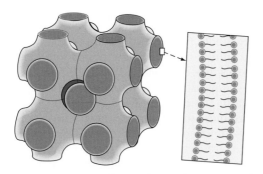

Figure 6.35 Structure of glyceryl monooleate–water cubic phase with inset showing the lipid bilayer.
Redrawn from J. C. Shah, Y. Sadhale and D. M. Chilukuri, *Adv. Drug Delivery Rev.*, **47**, 229 (2001).

Monoolein vesicles

Polar amphiphilic lipids such as glyceryl monooleate (monoolein) also form bilayers, the nature of which depends on the temperature and concentration. An interesting phase formed at monoolein concentrations of 60–80% w/w is the bicontinuous cubic phase. The structure of this phase is unique and consists of a curved bicontinuous lipid bilayer extending in three dimensions, separating two networks of water channels with pores of about 5 nm diameter (see Fig. 6.35). On dilution, these structures coexist with excess water and there is the formation of dispersed cubic phase vesicles or *cubosomes*. Cubic phases have been shown to incorporate and deliver small molecule drugs and large proteins by oral and parenteral routes, in addition to local delivery in vaginal and periodontal cavities.[15]

6.5 Properties of some commonly used surfactants

6.5.1 Anionic surfactants

Sodium Lauryl Sulfate BP is a mixture of sodium alkyl sulfates, the chief of which is sodium dodecyl sulfate, $C_{12}H_{25}SO_4^-Na^+$. It is very soluble in water and is used pharmaceutically as a preoperative skin cleaner, having bacteriostatic action against Gram-positive bacteria, and also in medicated shampoos. It is a component of Emulsifying Wax BP.

Sodium dodecyl sulfate has been studied in depth. The cmc at 25°C is 8.2×10^{-3} mol dm^{-3} (0.23% w/v). The effect of temperature on the cmc is shown in Fig. 6.29.

6.5.2 Cationic surfactants

The quaternary ammonium and pyridinium cationic surfactants are important pharmaceutically because of their bactericidal activity against a wide range of Gram-positive and some Gram-negative organisms. They may be used on the skin, especially in the cleaning of wounds. Aqueous solutions are used for cleaning contaminated utensils.

Cetrimide BP consists mainly of tetradecyltrimethylammonium bromide together with smaller amounts of dodecyl- and hexadecyltrimethylammonium bromides. The properties of the individual components have been studied in detail and are summarised in Table 6.6. Solutions containing 0.1–1% of cetrimide are used for cleaning the skin, wounds and burns, for cleaning contaminated vessels, polythene tubing and catheters, and for storage of sterilised surgical instruments. Solutions of cetrimide are also used in shampoos to remove scales in seborrhoea. In the form of Cetrimide Emulsifying Wax BP, it is used as an emulsifying agent for producing oil-in-water creams suitable for the incorporation of cationic and nonionic medicaments (anionic medicaments would, of course, be incompatible with this cationic surfactant).

Benzalkonium chloride is a mixture of alkylbenzyldimethylammonium chlorides of the general formula $[C_6H_5CH_2N(CH_3)_2R]Cl$, where R represents a mixture of the alkyls from C_8H_{17} to $C_{18}H_{37}$. In dilute solution (1 in 1000 to 1 in 2000) it may be used for the preoperative disinfection of skin and mucous membranes, for application to burns and wounds, and for cleaning polythene and nylon tubing and catheters. Benzalkonium chloride is also used as a preservative for eye-drops and as a permitted vehicle for the preparation of certain eye-drops.

Table 6.6 Micellar properties of a commercial sample of Cetrimide and its main constituents at 25°C[a]

Constituent	Percentage (calculated on dry weight basis)	Critical micellar concentration (mmol dm^{-3})	Micellar molecular weight ($\times 10^{-4}$)
Tetradecyltrimethylammonium bromide	68	3.3	2.7
Dodecyltrimethylammonium bromide	22	5.3	2.1
Hexadecyltrimethylammonium bromide	7	0.82	3.3
Cetrimide	–	2.9	2.5

[a] Data from B. W. Barry et al., J. Colloid Interface Sci., 33, 554 (1970); 40, 174 (1972).

6.5.3 Nonionic surfactants

The amphiphilic nature of nonionic surfactants is often expressed in terms of the balance between the hydrophobic and hydrophilic portions of the molecule. An empirical scale of HLB (hydrophile–lipophile balance) numbers has been devised (see Chapter 7, section 7.3.2). The lower the HLB number, the more lipophilic is the compound and vice versa. HLB values for a series of commercial nonionic surfactants are quoted in Tables 6.7 and 6.8. The choice of surfactant for medicinal use involves a consideration of the toxicity of the substance, which may be ingested in large amounts. The following surfactants are widely used in pharmaceutical formulations.

Sorbitan esters

Commercial products are mixtures of partial esters of sorbitol and its mono- and dianhydrides with oleic acid. They are generally insoluble in water and are used as water-in-oil emulsifiers and as wetting agents. The main sorbitan esters are listed in Table 6.7 together with a space-filling model of a representative component of sorbitan palmitate.

Polysorbates

Commercial products are complex mixtures of partial fatty acid esters of sorbitol and its mono- and dianhydrides copolymerised with approximately 20 moles (usually) of ethylene oxide for each mole of sorbitol and

Table 6.7 HLB values of sorbitan esters

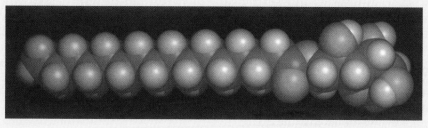

Chemical name	Commercial name	HLB
Sorbitan laurate	Span 20	8.6
Sorbitan palmitate	Span 40	6.7
Sorbitan stearate	Span 60	4.7
Sorbitan tristearate	Span 65	2.1
Sorbitan oleate	Span 80	4.3
Sorbitan trioleate	Span 85	1.8

Table 6.8 HLB and cmc values of polysorbates

Chemical name	Commercial name	HLB	cmc[a] (g dm^{-3})
Polyoxyethylene (20) sorbitan laurate	Polysorbate (Tween) 20	16.7	0.060
Polyoxyethylene (20) sorbitan palmitate	Polysorbate (Tween) 40	15.6	0.031
Polyoxyethylene (20) sorbitan stearate	Polysorbate (Tween) 60	14.9	0.028
Polyoxyethylene (20) sorbitan tristearate	Polysorbate (Tween) 65	10.5	0.050
Polyoxyethylene (20) sorbitan oleate	Polysorbate (Tween) 80	15.0	0.014
Polyoxyethylene (20) sorbitan trioleate	Polysorbate (Tween) 85	11.0	0.023

[a] Data from L. S. Wan and P. F. S. Lee., *J. Pharm. Sci.*, 63, 136 (1974).

its anhydrides. The space-filling model of a representative component of polysorbate 20 is shown in Table 6.8. The polysorbates are miscible with water, as reflected in their higher HLB values (see Table 6.8), and are used as emulsifying agents for oil-in-water emulsions.

Cetomacrogol 1000 BP and other macrogol ethers

Cetomacrogol is a water-soluble substance with the general structure $CH_3(CH_2)_m(OCH_2CH_2)_nOH$, where m may be 15 or 17 and the number of oxyethylene groups, n, is between 20 and 24. It is used in the form of Cetomacrogol Emulsifying Wax BP in the preparation of oil-in-water emulsions and also as a solubilising agent for volatile oils. The cmc and micellar molecular weight in aqueous solution are 6×10^{-2} g dm^{-3} and 1.01×10^5, respectively. Other macrogol ethers are com-

mercially available as the Brij series – for example, Brij 30 [polyoxyethylene (4) lauryl ether, $C_{12}H_{35}(OCH_2CH_2)_4OH$], Brij 72 [polyoxyethylene (2) stearyl ether, $C_{18}H_{37}(OCH_2CH_2)_2OH$] and Brij 97 [polyoxyethylene (10) oleyl ether, $C_{18}H_{35}(OCH_2CH_2)_{10}OH$].

Cremophor EL is a polyoxyethylated castor oil containing approximately 40 oxyethylene groups to each triglyceride unit. It is used as a solubilising agent in the preparation of intravenous anaesthetics and other products.

Poloxamers

Poloxamers are synthetic block copolymers of hydrophilic poly(oxyethylene) and hydrophobic poly(oxypropylene) with the general formula $E_mP_nE_m$, where E = oxyethylene (OCH_2CH_2) and P = oxypropylene (OCH_2CHCH_3) and the subscripts *m* and *n* denote chain lengths. Properties such as viscosity, HLB and physical state (liquid, paste or solid) are dependent on the relative chain lengths of the hydrophilic and hydrophobic blocks. The convention for naming these compounds is to use a number of which the first two digits, when multiplied by 100, correspond to the approximate average molecular weight of the poly(oxypropylene) block and the third digit, when multiplied by 10, corresponds to the percentage by weight of the poly(oxyethylene) block. For example, the poly(oxypropylene) block of poloxamer 188 has a molecular weight of approximately 1800 and about 80% by weight of the molecule is poly(oxypropylene). These copolymers were

introduced to the market in 1951 by the Wyandotte Chemical Corp. (now BASF-Wyandotte) under the trade name Pluronic. The nomenclature adopted by this company indicates the physical state by a letter (F, P or L, denoting solid, paste or liquid, respectively) followed by a two- or three-digit number. The last digit of this number is the same as that for the equivalent poloxamer and is approximately one-tenth of the weight percentage of poly(oxyethylene), the first digit (or two digits in a three-digit number) multiplied by 300 gives a rough estimate of the molecular weight of the hydrophobe. So, for example, Pluronic F68 is a solid, the molecular weight of the hydrophobe is approximately 1800 and the poly(oxyethylene)

Table 6.9 Nomenclature of $E_mP_nE_m$ and $P_nE_mP_n$(*) block copolymers[a]

Poloxamer	Pluronic	Mol. wt. of P block	Chain length, n	Weight % of E block	Chain length, m	Mol. wt. of copolymer
188	F68	1 750	30	80	80	8 750
217	F77	2 050	35	70	54	6 835
237	F87	2 250	39	70	60	7 500
238	F88	2 250	39	80	102	11 250
288	F98	2 750	47	80	125	13 750
338	F108	3 250	56	80	148	16 250
407	F127	4 000	69	70	106	13 335
105	L35	5 950	103	50	68	11 900
123	L43	1 200	21	30	6	1 715
124	L44	1 200	21	40	9	2 000
181	L61	1 750	30	10	2	1 945
182	L62	1 750	30	20	5	2 190
183	L63	1 750	30	30	9	2 500
184	L64	1 750	30	40	13	2 915
212	L72	2 050	35	20	6	2 565
231	L81	2 250	39	10	3	2 500
282	L92	2 750	47	20	8	3 440
331	L101	3 250	56	10	4	3 610
401	L121	4 000	69	10	5	4 445
402	L122	4 000	69	20	11	5 000
185	P65	1 750	30	50	20	3 500
333	P103	3 250	56	30	16	4 645
334	P104	3 250	56	40	25	5 415
335	P105	3 250	56	50	37	6 500
403	P123	4 000	69	30	19	5 715
171*	17R1	1 410	–	10	–	1 565
252*	25R2	2 100	–	20	–	2 625
258*	25R8	2 100	–	80	–	10 500
311*	31R1	2 450	–	10	–	2 720

[a] Modified from M. W. Edens, in *Nonionic Surfactants. Polyoxyalkylene Block Copolymers* (ed. V. M. Nace), Surfactant Science Series 60, Marcel Dekker, New York, 1996, pp. 185–210.

content is approximately 80% of the molecule by weight. A grid was developed by BASF to interrelate the properties of the Pluronics (Fig. 6.36a). The BASF nomenclature has been adopted by the other major supplier of poloxamers, Uniqema, who market the copolymers as the Synperonic series. The relationship between the Pluronic (and Synperonic) and poloxamer nomenclatures is shown in Table 6.9, which also gives the composition of each copolymer.

Included in Table 6.9 are examples of block copolymers of poly(oxyethylene) and poly(oxypropylene) with the general formula $P_nE_mP_n$ (meroxapols). The nomenclature for these 'reverse' block copolymers uses three digits, the first two (approximately one-hundredth of the molecular weight of the poly(oxypropylene) block) separated from the third (approximately one-tenth of the weight percentage of poly(oxyethylene) in the molecule) by the letter R. For example, 25R4 contains 40% by weight of poly(oxyethylene), and the total molecular weight of the poly(oxypropylene) blocks is approximately 2500. The properties of the Pluronic R series are interrelated using the grid shown in Fig. 6.36b.

The poloxamers are water soluble and, as might be expected from their amphiphilic structure, are also surface active. Many of the series form micelles, the properties of which have been reviewed by several authors.[16, 17]

Poloxamers are used as emulsifying agents for intravenous fat emulsions, as solubilising agents to maintain clarity in elixirs and syrups, and as wetting agents for antibacterials. They may also be used in ointment or suppository bases and as tablet binders or coaters.

6.6 Solubilisation

As we have seen in section 6.3, the micellar core is essentially a paraffin-like region and as such is capable of dissolving oil-soluble molecules. This process, whereby water-insoluble substances are brought into solution by incorporation into micelles, is termed *solubilisation* and the incorporated substance is referred to as the *solubilisate*. The subject of solubilisation has been reviewed extensively[1, 18] and it is only possible in this book to give an outline of this phenomenon.

6.6.1 Determination of maximum additive concentration

The maximum amount of solubilisate that can be incorporated into a given system at a fixed

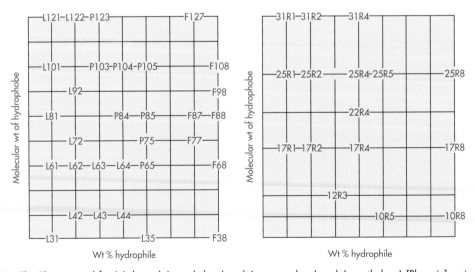

Figure 6.36 The Pluronic grid for (a) the poly(oxyethylene)–poly(oxypropylene)–poly(oxyethylene) [Pluronic] series and (b) the poly(oxypropylene)–poly(oxyethylene)–poly(oxypropylene) [Pluronic R] series of block copolymers.

concentration is termed the *maximum additive concentration* (MAC). The simplest method of determining the MAC is to prepare a series of vials containing surfactant solution of known concentration. Increasing amounts of solubilisate are added and the vials are then sealed and agitated until equilibrium conditions are established. The maximum concentration of solubilisate forming a clear solution can be determined by visual inspection or from extinction or turbidity measurement on the solutions.

Solubility data are expressed as a solubility–concentration curve or as phase diagrams. The latter are preferable since a three-component phase diagram completely describes the effect of varying all three components of the system – namely, the solubilisate, the solubiliser and the solvent. The axes of the phase diagram form an equilateral triangle (see Fig. 6.37), each side of which is divided into 100 parts to correspond to percentage composition.

A typical phase diagram of a solubilised system is shown in Fig. 6.38. In solutions of high water content the oil is solubilised in the micelles of the nonionic surfactant Brij 97 $(C_{18}H_{35}(OCH_2CH_2)_{10}OH)$, forming an isotropic micellar solution (often referred to as the L_1 region). When the concentration of the oil is increased, stable oil-in-water emulsions may be formed, while an increase in the surfactant concentration results in the formation of the liquid crystalline regions, labelled middle and neat phases (see section 6.4). It is important in formulation to avoid boundary regions, as otherwise there is a danger of unwanted phase transitions.

6.6.2 Location of the solubilisate

The site of solubilisation within the micelle is closely related to the chemical nature of the solubilisate (see Fig. 6.39). It is generally accepted that nonpolar solubilisates (aliphatic hydrocarbons, for example) are dissolved in the hydrocarbon core of ionic and nonionic micelles. Water-insoluble compounds containing polar groups are orientated with the polar group at the core/surface interface of the

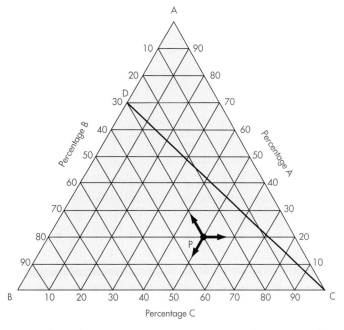

Figure 6.37 Three-component phase diagram. Point P represents a system of composition 20% A, 30% B and 50% C. Line CD represents the dilution of a mixture, originally containing 70% A and 30% B, with component C.

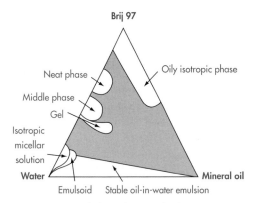

Figure 6.38   Partial phase diagram for the Brij 97 ($C_{18}H_{35}$ $(OCH_2CH_2)_{10}OH$)–water–mineral oil solubilised system.
Redrawn from R. Lachampt and R. M. Vila, Am. Perfum. Cosmet., 82, 29 (1967).

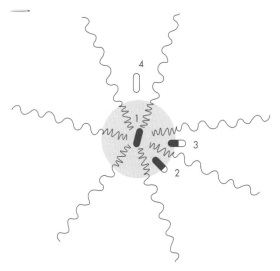

Figure 6.39   Schematic representation of sites of solubilisation depending on the hydrophobicity of the solubilisate. Completely water-insoluble hydrophobic molecules are incorporated in the micelle core (case 1); water-soluble molecules may be solubilised in the polyoxyethylene shell of a nonionic micelle (case 4); solubilisates with intermediate hydrophobicities (cases 2 and 3) are incorporated in the micelle with the hydrophobic region (black) in the core and the hydrophilic region (white) at the micelle/water interface.
Redrawn from V. Torchilin, J. Control. Release, 73, 137 (2001).

micelle and the hydrophobic group buried inside the hydrocarbon core of the micelle. In addition, solubilisation in nonionic polyoxyethylated surfactants can occur in the polyoxyethylene shell (palisade layer) which surrounds the core. p-Hydroxybenzoic acid, for example, is solubilised entirely within this

region of the cetomacrogol micelle, whilst esters of p-hydroxybenzoic acid are located at the palisade–core junction, with the ester group just within the core.

Solubilisates that are located within the micellar core increase the size of the micelles in two ways. Micelles become larger not only because their core is enlarged by the solubilisate but also because the number of surfactant molecules per micelle (the aggregation number) increases in an attempt to cover the swollen core. Solubilisation within the palisade layer, on the other hand, tends not to alter the aggregation number, the increase in micellar size resulting solely from the incorporation of solubilisate molecules.

6.6.3   Factors affecting solubilisation

Nature of the surfactant

Chain length of hydrophobe
It is difficult to generalise about the way in which the structural characteristics of a surfactant affect its solubilising capacity because this is influenced by the solubilisation site within the micelle. In cases where the solubilisate is located within the core or deep within the micelle structure, the solubilisation capacity increases with increase in alkyl chain length as might be expected. Table 6.10 clearly shows an increase of solubilising capacity of a series of polysorbates for selected barbiturates as the alkyl chain length is increased from C_{12} (Polysorbate 20) to C_{18} (Polysorbate 80). Similar effects have been noted for the solubilisation of barbiturates in polyoxyethylene surfactants with the general structure $CH_3(CH_2)_m(OCH_2CH_2)_nOH$ with increasing alkyl chain length, m. There is a limit, however, to the improvement of solubilising capacity caused by increase of alkyl chain length in this way: an increase of m from 16 to 22, although producing larger micelles, does not result in a corresponding increase of solubilisation.[19]

Ethylene oxide chain length
The effect of an increase in the ethylene oxide chain length of a polyoxyethylated nonionic

Table 6.10   Solubilising capacity of polysorbates for the barbiturates at 30°C[a]

Drug	Surfactant	Solubility (mg drug per g surfactant)
Phenobarbital	Polysorbate 20	55
	Polysorbate 40	61
	Polysorbate 60	63
	Polysorbate 80	66
Amobarbital	Polysorbate 20	32
	Polysorbate 40	38
	Polysorbate 80	40
Secobarbital	Polysorbate 20	111
	Polysorbate 80	144

[a] Reproduced from A. A. Ismail, M. W. Gouda and M. M. Motawi, *J. Pharm. Sci.*, 59, 220 (1970).

surfactant on its solubilising capacity is again dependent on the location of the solubilisate within the micelle and is complicated by corresponding changes in the micellar size. Table 6.11 shows the solubilisation capacity of a series of polyoxyethylated nonionic surfactants with a hydrocarbon chain length of 16 (C_{16}) and an increasing number of ethylene oxide units (E) in the polyoxyethylene chain. As seen from this table, the aggregation number decreases with increase in the hydrophilic chain length so, although the number of steroid molecules solubilised per micelle also decreases, the total amount solubilised per mole of surfactant (number of steroid molecules per micelle × number of micelles per mole) actually increases because of the increasing number of micelles.

Similar results were observed in a study of the solubilisation of the poorly water-soluble mydriatic drug tropicamide by a series of poloxamers.[20] Fig. 6.40 shows an increase of solubilisation (expressed as moles of tropicamide per mole of poloxamer) with increase of the oxyethylene content of the poloxamer. When the data were expressed as the number of moles of drug solubilised per ethylene oxide unit of the poloxamer, however, the solubilisation capacity decreased with increasing ethylene oxide chain length. Again, the reason for this decrease is that the micellar size per ethylene oxide equivalent decreases with increasing length of the ethylene oxide chain.

Nature of the solubilisate

Although many possible relationships between the amount solubilised and various physical properties of the solubilisate molecule (for example, molar volume, polarity,

Table 6.11   Micellar solubilisation parameters for steroids in *n*-alkyl polyoxyethylene surfactants C_nE_m (where n = alkyl (C) chain length and m = polyoxyethylene (E) chain length) at 25°C[a]

Surfactant	Aggregation number	Micelles per mole ($\times 10^{-21}$)	Steroid molecules per micelle			
			Hydrocortisone	Dexamethasone	Testosterone	Progesterone
$C_{16}E_{17}$	99	6.1	9.1	6.7	6.0	5.6
$C_{16}E_{32}$	56	10.8	7.6	5.3	4.6	4.3
$C_{16}E_{44}$	39	15.4	5.8	4.2	3.6	3.3
$C_{16}E_{63}$	25	24.1	4.0	3.3	2.4	2.3

[a] Reproduced from B. W. Barry and D. I. D. El Eini, *J. Pharm. Pharmacol.*, 28, 210 (1976).

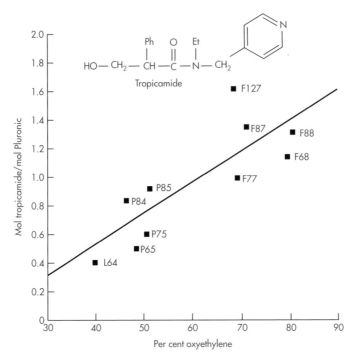

Figure 6.40 Moles of tropicamide solubilised per mole of Pluronic plotted against the oxyethylene content of the poloxamer (see Table 6.9 for details of the Pluronics).

Reproduced from M. F. Saettone, B. Giannaccini, G. Delmonte, et al., Int. J. Pharm., 43, 67 (1988) with permission.

polarisability and chain length) have been explored, it has not been possible to establish simple correlations between them. In general, a decrease in solubility in a surfactant solution occurs when the alkyl chain length of a homologous series is increased. Unsaturated compounds are generally more soluble than their saturated counterparts. Branching of the hydrocarbon chain of the solubilisate has little effect, but increased solubilisation is often noted following cyclisation. Unfortunately, these generalisations apply only to very simple solubilisates.

More specific rules can be formulated for particular series of solubilisates. For example, it is clear from studies of the effect of steroid structure on solubilisation by a series of surfactants that the more hydrophilic is the substituent in position 17 of the ring structure the lower is the quantity of surfactant required to effect solubilisation of the hormone. Thus the extent of solubilisation of hormones in sodium lauryl sulfate follows the series proges-

terone < testosterone < deoxycorticosterone, the C17 substituents being $-COCH_3$, $-OH$ and $-COCH_2OH$, respectively (Box 6.5).

A relationship between the lipophilicity of the solubilisate, expressed by the partition coefficient between octanol and water, $P_{octanol}$ (see Chapter 5), and its extent of solubilisation has been noted for the solubilisation of substituted barbituric acids by polyoxyethylene stearates, of substituted benzoic acids by polysorbate 20, and of several steroids by polyoxyethylene nonionic surfactants. An exhaustive survey of data for the solubilisation of some 64 drugs by bile salt micelles revealed linear relationships between $\log P_m$ (partition coefficient between micelles and water) and $\log P_{octanol}$ for each of seven bile salts examined.[21]

Effect of temperature

In most systems the amount solubilised increases as temperature increases. The effect

---

Box 6.5 Structures of some steroid solubilisates

Progesterone	$R = -COCH_3$
Testosterone	$R = -OH$
Deoxycorticosterone	$R = -COCH_2OH$

---

is particularly pronounced with some non-ionic surfactants, where it is a consequence of an increase in the micellar size with increase in temperature. Table 6.12 shows an increased solubilisation of two drugs by aqueous micellar solutions of bile salts as temperature is increased over the range 27 to 45°C.

A complicating factor when considering the effect of temperature on the amount solubilised is the change in the aqueous solubility of the solubilisate with temperature increase. In some cases, although the amount of drug that can be taken up by a surfactant solution increases with temperature increase, this may simply reflect an increase in the amount of drug dissolved in the aqueous phase rather than an increased solubilisation by the micelles. This point is illustrated by a study of the solubilisation of benzoic acid by a series of polyoxyethylated nonionic surfactants, details of which are given in Table 6.13. Although the extent of solubilisation of benzoic acid increases with temperature, the micelle/water distribution coefficient, P_m, shows a minimum at about 27°C. The decrease in P_m (and therefore the amount of drug solubilised in the micelles) with temperature increase up to this temperature is possibly due to the increase in aqueous solubility of benzoic acid; the subsequent increase of P_m at higher temperatures is due to a rapid increase of micellar size as the cloud point is approached and a consequent ability of the micelles to incorporate more solubilisate.

6.6.4 Pharmaceutical applications of solubilisation

A wide range of insoluble drugs has been formulated using the principle of solubilisation. Only a few representative examples will be discussed in this section.

Phenolic compounds such as cresol, chlorocresol, chloroxylenol and thymol are frequently solubilised with soap to form clear solutions which are widely used for disinfection. Solution of Chloroxylenol BP, for example, contains 5% w/v chloroxylenol with terpineol in an alcoholic soap solution.

Table 6.12 The effect of temperature on the maximum additive concentrations (MAC) of griseofulvin and hexestrol in bile salts[a]

Solubilisate	Bile salt	10^3 MAC (moles solubilisate/mole surfactant)		
		27°C	37°C	45°C
Griseofulvin	Sodium cholate	5.36	6.18	6.80
	Sodium deoxycholate	4.68	6.18	7.54
	Sodium taurocholate	3.77	4.90	6.15
	Sodium glycocholate	3.85	5.13	5.29
Hexestrol	Sodium cholate	187	195	197
	Sodium deoxycholate	164	167	179
	Sodium taurocholate	220	225	223
	Sodium glycocholate	221	231	251

[a] Reproduced from T. S. Wiedmann and L. Kamel, *J. Pharm. Sci.*, **91**, 1743 (2002).

Table 6.13 Micelle/water distribution coefficients, P_m, for the solubilisation of benzoic acid by n-alkyl poly-oxyethylene surfactants C_nE_m (where n = alkyl (C) chain length and m = polyoxyethylene (E) chain length) as a function of temperature[a]

Surfactant formula	18°C	25°C	31°C	37°C	45°C
$C_{16}E_{16}$	59.51	50.07	43.75	44.11	–[b]
$C_{16}E_{30}$	47.80	45.55	35.42	38.23	38.66
$C_{16}E_{40}$	37.07	32.72	28.76	29.90	37.06
$C_{16}E_{96}$	31.22	27.43	25.43	27.46	32.35

[a] Reproduced from K. J. Humphries and C. T. Rhodes, *J. Pharm. Sci.*, 57, 79 (1968).
[b] No P_m value determined at this temperature for $C_{16}E_{16}$ because the cloud point temperature was exceeded.

Nonionic surfactants are efficient solubilisers of iodine, and will incorporate up to 30% by weight, of which three-quarters is released as available iodine on dilution. Such iodine–surfactant systems (referred to as *iodophors*) are more stable than iodine–iodide systems. They are preferable in instrument sterilisation since corrosion problems are reduced. Loss of iodine by sublimation from iodophor solutions is significantly less than from simple iodine solutions such as Iodine Solution NF. There is also evidence of an ability of the iodophor solution to penetrate hair follicles of the skin, so enhancing the activity.

The low solubility of steroids in water presents a problem in their formulation for ophthalmic use. The requirements of optical clarity preclude the use of oily solutions or suspension and there are many examples of the use of nonionic surfactants as a means of producing clear solutions which are stable to sterilisation. In most formulations, solubilisation has been achieved using polysorbates or polyoxyethylene sorbitan esters of fatty acids.

Essential oils are extensively solubilised by surfactants, polysorbates 60 and 80 being particularly well suited to this purpose.

The polysorbate nonionics have also been employed in the preparation of aqueous injections of the water-insoluble vitamins A, D, E and K. Table 6.14 shows the solubility of these vitamins in 10% polysorbate solutions, polysorbate 20 and 80 being the best two solubilisers.

One of the problems encountered with the use of nonionic surfactants as solubilisers is that they are prone to clouding on heating (see section 6.3.4), and the presence of solubilisate can reduce the cloud point. For this reason, sucrose esters may be more suitable as alternative solubilisers for the vitamins, although they do have the disadvantage of a slightly higher haemolytic activity.

It has been possible to give only a brief description of the types of drugs that have been formulated using solubilisation. Many

Table 6.14 Solubilisation of vitamins by 10% polysorbate solutions[a]

Polysorbate	Vitamin D_2 (IU cm^{-3})	Vitamin E (mg cm^{-3})	Vitamin K_3 (mg cm^{-3})	Vitamin A alcohol (IU cm^{-3})
20	20 000	5.7	4.7	80 000
40	16 000	3.8	4.0	60 000
60	15 000	3.2	3.7	60 000
80	20 000	4.5	4.5	80 000

[a] Reproduced from F. Gstirner and P. S. Tata, *Mitt. dt. Pharm. Ges.*, 28, 191 (1958).

other drugs have been formulated in this way, including the analgesics, sedatives, sulfonamides and antibiotics. The reader is referred to reference 1 for a more complete survey of this topic and for a discussion of the effects of solubilisation on drug activity and absorption characteristics.

Summary

- Surface and interfacial tensions arise because of an imbalance of attractive forces on the molecules of a liquid at these interfaces such that the surface or interface has a tendency to contract.
- Surfactant molecules have hydrophilic and hydrophobic regions and adsorb at interfaces in such a way that their hydrophobic regions are removed from the aqueous environment. The forces of attraction between surfactant and water molecules in the interface are less than those between two water molecules and hence the surface tension is reduced as a result of adsorption.
- The extent of adsorption at the interface can be calculated using the Gibbs equation. The lowering of surface tension increases with increase of surfactant concentration until the critical micelle concentration is reached, i.e. until the surfactant forms micelles; at higher concentrations the surface tension remains effectively constant.
- Insoluble amphiphilic compounds will also form films on water surfaces and these may be tightly packed, as in condensed films, or more loosely packed, as in expanded and gaseous films. We have seen that polymers and proteins may also form insoluble monolayers.
- Adsorption of solutes onto solid surfaces from solution can occur by physical adsorption, involving weak van der Waals forces, or by a chemical process. Adsorption data can be analysed using the Langmuir equation or, if multilayer adsorption occurs, by the Freundlich equation.
- The extent of adsorption increases as the ionisation of the solute decreases and is at a maximum for an unionised compound. The greater the solubility of a solute in a particular solvent, the lower is the extent of its adsorption. The adsorption processes can be used advantageously, as in the removal of toxic drugs in the case of overdosing, or can cause problems, as in the unintentional adsorption of drugs by antacids from the gastrointestinal tract, or the adsorption of drugs on to the walls of the container.
- Micelles form at the critical micelle concentration, which has a characteristic value for a particular surfactant under a given set of conditions. The main driving force for the formation of micelles is the increase of entropy that occurs when the hydrophobic regions of the surfactant are removed from water and the ordered structure of the water molecules around this region of the molecule is lost.
- We have examined the structure of both ionic and nonionic micelles and some of the factors that affect their size and critical micelle concentration. An increase in hydrophobic chain length causes a decrease in the cmc and increase of size of ionic and nonionic micelles; an increase of polyoxyethylene chain length has the opposite effect on these properties in nonionic micelles. About 70–80% of the counterions of an ionic surfactant are bound to the micelle and the nature of the counterion can influence the properties of these micelles. Electrolyte addition to micellar solutions of ionic surfactants reduces the cmc and increases the micellar size, sometimes causing a change of shape from spherical to ellipsoidal. Solutions of some nonionic surfactants become cloudy on heating and separate reversibly into two phases at the cloud point.
- An important property of surfactant micelles is their ability to solubilise water-insoluble compounds. The location of solubilisates in the micelles is closely related to the chemical nature of the solubilisate; in

general, nonpolar solubilisates are dissolved in the micelle core and water-insoluble compounds having polar groups are orientated with the polar group at the surface and the hydrophobic group in the core. Some pharmaceutical applications of solubilisation have been discussed.

References

1. D. Attwood and A. T. Florence. *Surfactant Systems*, Chapman and Hall, London, 1983

2. D. Attwood. The mode of association of amphiphilic drugs in aqueous solution. *Adv. Coll. Interface Sci.*, 55, 271–303 (1995)

3. J. L. Zatz, N. D. Weinder and M. Gibaldi. Monomolecular film properties of protective and enteric film formers. II. Evaporation resistance and interactions with plasticizers of poly (methyl vinyl ether-maleic anhydride). *J. Pharm. Sci.*, 58, 1493–6 (1969)

4. A. A. Hidalgo, W. Caetano, M. Tabak and O. N. Oliveira. Interaction of two phenothiazine derivatives with phospholipid monolayers. *Biophys. Chem.*, 109, 85–104, (2004)

5. S. El-Masry and S. A. H. Khalil. Adsorption of atropine and hyoscine on magnesium trisilicate. *J. Pharm. Pharmacol.*, 26, 243–8 (1974)

6. L. Chin, A. L. Picchioni, W. M. Bourn and H. E. Laird. Optimal antidotal dose of activated charcoal. *Toxicol. Appl. Pharmacol.*, 26, 103–8 (1973)

7. W. J. Decker. H. J. Combs and D. G. Corby. Absorption of drugs and poisons by activated charcoal. *Toxicol. Appl. Pharmacol.*, 13, 454–60 (1968)

8. W. J. Decker, R. A. Shpall, D. G. Corby, *et al.* Inhibition of aspirin absorption by activated charcoal and apomorphine. *Clin. Pharm. Ther.*, 10, 710–13 (1969)

9. J. Kolthammer. *In vitro* adsorption of drugs from horse serum onto carbon coated with an acrylic hydrogel. *J. Pharm. Pharmacol.*, 27, 801–5 (1975)

10. J. A. Vale. A. J. Rees. B. Widdop and R. Goulding. Use of charcoal haemoperfusion in the management of severely poisoned patients. *Br. Med. J.*, 1, 5–9 (1975)

11. C. Rouchotas, O. E. Cassidy and G. Rowley. Comparison of surface modification and solid dispersion techniques for drug dissolution. *Int. J. Pharm.*, 195, 1–6 (2000)

12. D. J. A. Crommelin and H. Schreier. In *Colloidal Drug Delivery Systems* (ed. J. Kreuter), Marcel Dekker, New York, 1994, chapter 3

13. J. A. Bouwstra and H. E. J. Hofland. In *Colloidal Drug Delivery Systems* (ed. J. Kreuter), Marcel Dekker, New York, 1994, chapter 4.

14. I. F. Uchegbu and A. T. Florence. Nonionic surfactant vesicles (niosomes): physical and pharmaceutical chemistry. *Adv. Colloid Interface Sci.*, 58, 1–55 (1995)

15. J. C. Shah, Y. Sadhale and D. M. Chilukuri. Cubic phase gels as drug delivery systems. *Adv. Drug Deliv. Rev.*, 47, 229–50 (2001)

16. C. Booth and D. Attwood. Effect of block copolymer architecture and composition on the association properties of poly(oxyalkylene) copolymers in aqueous solution. *Macromol. Rapid Commun.*, 21, 501–27 (2000)

17. V. M. Nace. *Nonionic Surfactants. Polyoxyalkylene Block Copolymers*, Surfactant Science Series 60, Marcel Dekker, New York, 1996, pp. 185–210

18. P. N. Hurter, P. Alexandridis and T. A. Hatton. Solubilisation in amphiphilic copolymer solutions. In *Solubilisation in Surfactant Aggregates* (ed. S. D. Christian and J. F. Scamehorn), Surfactant Science Series 55, Marcel Dekker, New York, 1995, pp. 191–235

19. T. Arnarson and P. H. Elworthy. Effects of structural variations of nonionic surfactants on micellar properties and solubilization: surfactants based on erucyl and behenyl (C_{22}) alcohols. *J. Pharm. Pharmacol.*, 32, 381–5 (1980)

20. M. F. Saettone, B. Giannaccini, G. Delmonte, *et al.* Solubilization of tropicamide by poloxamers: physicochemical data and activity data in rabbits and humans. *Int. J. Pharm.*, 43, 67–76 (1988)

21. T. S. Wiedmann and L. Kamel. Examination of the solubilisation of drugs by bile salt micelles. *J. Pharm. Sci.*, 91, 1743–64 (2002)

7

Emulsions, suspensions and other disperse systems

Emulsions and suspensions are 'disperse' systems; that is, a liquid or solid phase is dispersed in an external liquid phase. While emulsions are sometimes formulated from oily drugs or nutrient oils their main function is to provide vehicles for drug delivery in which the drug is dissolved in the oil or water phase. Suspensions, on the other hand, are usually prepared from water-insoluble drugs for delivery orally or by injection, usually intramuscular injection. An increasing number of modern delivery systems are suspensions – of liposomes or of polymer or protein microspheres, nanospheres or dendrimers, hence the need to understand the formulation and stabilization of these systems. Pharmaceutical emulsions and suspensions are in the colloidal state, that is where the particles range from the nanometre size to visible (or coarse) dispersions of several micrometres.

After a general introduction to colloidal systems (these being disperse systems with particles below about 1 μm in diameter) this chapter introduces the main types of emulsions namely,

- Oil-in-water (o/w)
- Water-in-oil (w/o)
- Multiple emulsions (w/o/w; o/w/o)
- Microemulsions.

The chapter should allow an appreciation of the factors leading to emulsion stability and physical instability, including flocculation and coalescence. Approaches to the formulation of emulsions to provide vehicles for drug delivery and parenteral nutrition (the main uses in pharmacy) should be understood.

The chapter then deals with aqueous and nonaqueous pharmaceutical suspensions and their formulation and forms of instability, which are principally sedimentation, flocculation and caking. Finally, some newer colloidal systems used pharmaceutically will be discussed.

The word 'colloid' derives from the Greek *kolla* (glue) and was coined from the impression that colloidal substances were amorphous or glue-like rather than crystalline forms of matter. The colloidal state was recognised by Thomas Graham in 1861 and described poetically by Wolfgang Ostwald some fifty years later as the 'world of neglected dimensions', a reference both to the fact that colloid science had somehow remained a Cinderella topic, and to the special world of systems in which the particles are extremely small. Colloid chemistry has re-emerged as important in pharmacy because of the growing interest in nanoparticles and other colloidal systems for drug delivery and targeting.

7.1 Classification of colloids

Colloids can be broadly classified as those that are *lyophobic* (solvent-hating) and those that are *lyophilic* and *hydrophilic*. Surfactant molecules, because of their dual affinity for water and oil and their consequent tendency to associate into micelles, form hydrophilic colloidal dispersions in water. Proteins and gums also form lyophilic colloidal systems. Hydrophilic systems are dealt with in Chapters 8 and 11. Water-insoluble drugs in fine dispersion or clays and oily phases will form lyophobic dispersions, the principal subject of this chapter. While lyophilic dispersions (such as phospholipid vesicles and micelles) are inherently stable, lyophobic colloidal dispersions have a tendency to coalesce because they are thermodynamically unstable as a result of their high surface energy.

Pharmaceutical colloids such as emulsions and suspensions (Fig. 7.1) and aerosols are readily identified (Table 7.1). The *disperse phase* is the phase that is subdivided. The *continuous phase* is the phase in which the disperse phase is distributed. Many natural systems such as suspensions of microorganisms, blood, and isolated cells in culture, are also colloidal dispersions. Colloid science is interdisciplinary, for although dealing with complex systems it is nevertheless a unifying discipline as it bridges the physical and biological sciences. The concepts of the stability of colloidal systems derived for suspensions can be applied with little modification to our understanding of interactions between living cells, for example (see section 7.5).

It is because of the subdivision of matter in colloidal systems that they have special properties. The large surface-to-volume ratio of the particles dispersed in a liquid medium results in a tendency for particles to associate to reduce their surface area, so reducing their contact with the medium. Emulsions and aerosols are thermodynamically unstable two-phase systems which only reach equilibrium when the globules have coalesced to form one macro-phase, for which the surface area is at a minimum. Many pharmaceutical problems revolve around the stabilisation of colloidal systems.

Some biological phenomena can be understood in terms of the association of cells with other cells or with inanimate or other substrates. These, too, are kinds of colloidal

Table 7.1 Main types of colloidal systems

Type	Disperse phase	Continuous phase
o/w emulsion	Oil	Water
w/o emulsion	Water	Oil
Suspension	Solid	Water or oil
Aerosol	Solid or liquid	Air

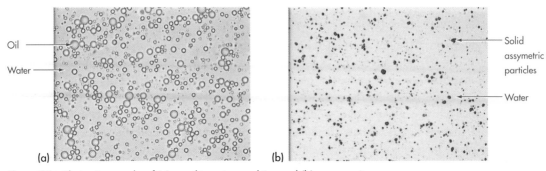

Figure 7.1 Photomicrographs of (a) an oil-in-water emulsion and (b) a suspension.

instability. This chapter describes various colloidal systems, deals in outline with the theories of colloid stability, and discusses the pharmaceutical problems encountered with colloidal dosage forms. At the close of the chapter some of the biological implications of the subject are indicated, which include the increasing use of particles in the nanometre size range (*nanoparticles*) and particles in the micrometre size range (*microparticles*) as carriers for drugs for targeting and for modifying the disposition of drug molecules contained within them.

Obviously the dividing line between the colloidal and noncolloidal systems in terms of the nature of the dispersing medium and the dispersed material is not one that can be defined exactly.

7.2 Colloid stability

In dispersions of fine particles in a liquid (or of particles in a gas) frequent encounters between the particles occur owing to

- Brownian movement
- Creaming
- Sedimentation
- Convection

The rate of creaming depends on the difference in density between the dispersed particles and the dispersion medium, the particle radius, a, and the viscosity of the dispersion medium η. According to Stokes' law the rate of sedimentation (or creaming) of a spherical particle, v, in a fluid medium is given by

$$v = \frac{2ga^2(\rho_1 - \rho_2)}{9\eta} \tag{7.1}$$

where ρ_1 is the density of the particles, ρ_2 is the density of the medium and g is the gravitational constant.

Creaming of an emulsion or sedimentation of a given suspension can be reduced in several ways:

- By forming smaller particles ($a\downarrow$)
- By increasing the viscosity of the continuous phase ($\eta\uparrow$)

- By decreasing the density difference between the two phases (ideally $\rho_1 \approx \rho_2$)

Particles will still collide, but the frequency or the impact of the collisions can be minimised. What happens when the particles do come into close contact? The encounters may lead to permanent contact of solid particles or to coalescence of liquid droplets. If they are allowed to continue unchecked, the colloidal system destroys itself through growth of the disperse phase and excessive creaming or sedimentation of the large particles. Whether these collisions result in permanent contact or whether the particles rebound and remain free depends on the forces of interaction, both attractive and repulsive, between the particles, and on the nature of the surface of the particles.

7.2.1 Forces of interaction between colloidal particles

There are five possible types of force between colloidal particles:

- Electrostatic forces of repulsion
- van der Waals' forces or electromagnetic forces of attraction
- Born forces – essentially short-range and repulsive
- Steric forces, which are dependent on the geometry and conformation of molecules (particularly macromolecules) at the particle interface
- Solvation forces due to changes in quantities of adsorbed solvent on the very close approach of neighbouring particles

Consideration of the electrostatic repulsion and van der Waals' forces of attraction by the Russians Deryagin and Landau and the Dutch scientists Verwey and Overbeek produced a satisfactory quantitative approach to the stability of hydrophobic suspensions. Their theory is known as the DLVO theory of colloid stability, the briefest outline of which is given here.

Van der Waals' forces between particles of the same kind are always attractive. The multiplicity of interactions between pairs of atoms or molecules on neighbouring particles must be taken into account in the calculation of attractive forces. Hamaker first determined equations for these forces on the basis of the additivity of van der Waals energies between neighbouring molecules, assuming that the energies of attraction varied with the inverse 6th power of the distance between them. At greater separations of the particles, the power law changes to the inverse 7th power. The model considers two spherical particles of radius a at a distance H, R being $2a + H$ (Fig. 7.2).

Hamaker calculated the energy of attraction, V_A, to be

$$V_A = -\frac{A}{6}\left(\frac{2a^2}{R^2 - 4a^2} + \frac{2a^2}{R^2} + \frac{R^2 - 4a^2}{R^2}\right) \quad (7.2)$$

The Hamaker constant, A, depends on the properties of the particles and of the medium in which they are dispersed. When H/a is small, that is when the particles are large relative to the distance of separation, equation (7.2) reduces to

$$V_A = -\frac{Aa}{12H}$$

The electrical charge on particles is due either to ionisation of surface groups or to adsorption of ions which confer their charge to the surface. A particle surface with a negative charge is shown in Fig. 7.3 along with the layer of positive ions that are attracted to the surface in the Stern layer, and the diffuse or

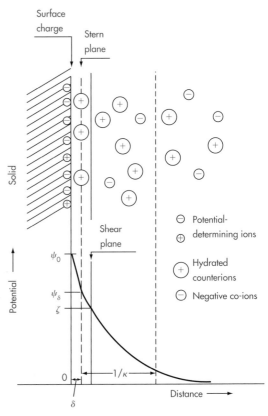

Figure 7.3 Representation of the conditions at a negative surface, with a layer of adsorbed positive ions in the Stern plane. The number of negative ions increases and the number of positive ions decreases (see upper diagram) as one moves away from the surface, the electrical potential becoming zero when the concentrations are equal. The surface potential, ψ_0, and the potential at the Stern plane, ψ_δ, are shown. As the particle moves, the effective surface is defined as the surface of shear, which is a little further out from the Stern plane, and would be dependent on surface roughness, adsorbed macromolecules, etc. It is at the surface of shear that the zeta potential, ζ, is located. The thickness of double layer is given by $1/\kappa$.

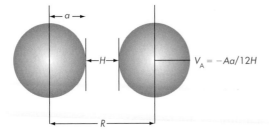

Figure 7.2 Diagram of the interaction between two spheres of radius a at a distance of separation H with a centre to centre distance of $(R = H + 2a)$ used in calculating energies of interaction.

electrical double layer which accumulates and contains both positive and negative ions.

Electrostatic forces arise from the interaction of the electrical double layers surrounding particles in suspension (see Fig. 7.3). This interaction leads to repulsion if the particles have surface charges and surface potentials of the same sign and magnitude. When the surface charge is produced by the adsorption of potential-determining ions the surface potential, ψ_0, is determined by the activity of these ions and remains constant during interaction with other particles, if the extent of adsorption does not change. The interaction therefore takes place at *constant surface potential*. In emulsion systems where the adsorbed layers can desorb, or in conditions of low availability of potential-determining ions, the interaction takes place not at constant surface potential but at *constant surface charge* (or at some intermediate state). The electrostatic repulsive force decays as an exponential function of the distance and has a range of the order of the thickness of the electrical double layer, equal to the Debye–Hückel length, $1/\kappa$:

$$1/\kappa = \left(\frac{\varepsilon\varepsilon_0 RT}{F^2 \sum c_i z_i^2} \right)^{1/2} \tag{7.3}$$

where ε_0 is the permittivity of the vacuum, ε is the dielectric constant (or relative permittivity) of the dispersion medium, R is the gas constant, T is temperature, F is the Faraday constant, and c_i and z_i are the concentration and the charge number of the ions of type i in the dispersion medium. For monovalent ions in water, $c = 10^{-15}\kappa^2$ (with c in mol dm^{-3} and κ in cm^{-1}). No simple equations can be given for the repulsive interactions. However, for small surface potentials and low values of κ (that is, when the double layer extends beyond the particle radius) and at constant ψ_0, the repulsive energy is

$$V_R = 2\pi\varepsilon\varepsilon_0 a\psi_\delta^2 \frac{\exp(-\kappa H)}{1 + H/2a} \tag{7.4}$$

For small values of ψ_δ and $\exp(-\kappa H)$ this simplifies to

$$V_R = 2\pi\varepsilon\varepsilon_0 a\psi_\delta^2 \exp(-\kappa H) \tag{7.5}$$

The equations do not take into account the finite size of the ions; the potential to be used is ψ_δ, the potential at the Stern plane (the plane of closest approach of ions to the surface), which is difficult to measure. The nearest experimental approximation to ψ_δ is often the zeta potential (ζ) measured by electrophoresis.

In the DLVO theory the combination of the electrostatic repulsive energy V_R with the attractive potential energy V_A gives the total potential energy of interaction

$$V_{total} = V_A + V_R \tag{7.6}$$

V_{total} plotted against the distance of separation H gives a potential energy curve showing certain characteristic features, illustrated in Fig. 7.4. The maximum and minimum energy states are shown. At small and at large distances the van der Waals energy (proportional to H^{-x}, where x varies from 1 to 7) is greater than the repulsion, which is proportional to $\exp(-\kappa H)$. If the maximum is too small, two interacting particles may reach the primary

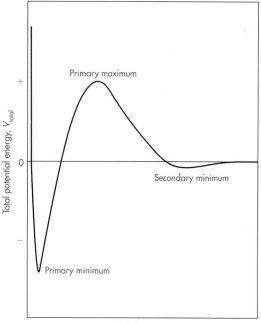

Figure 7.4 Schematic form of the curve of total potential energy (V_{total}) against distance of surface separation (H) for interaction between two particles, with $V_{total} = V_A + V_R$.

minimum and in this state of close approach the depth of the energy minimum can mean that escape is improbable. Subsequent irreversible changes in the system may then occur, such as sintering and recrystallisation in suspensions or coalescence in emulsions forming irreversible structures. When the maximum in V_{total} is sufficiently high, the two particles do not reach the stage of being in close contact. The depth of the secondary minimum is important in determining events in a hydrophobic dispersion. If the secondary minimum is smaller than the thermal energy, kT (where k is the Boltzmann constant), the particles will always repel each other, but when the particles are large enough the secondary minimum can trap particles for some time as there is no energy barrier to overcome. At intermediate distances the energy of repulsion may be the larger of the two.

Effect of electrolytes on stability

Pharmaceutical colloids are rarely simple systems. The influence of additives including simple and complex electrolytes has to be considered. Electrolyte concentration and valence (z) are accounted for in the term $(\Sigma c_i z_i^2)$ in equation (7.3) and thus in equations (7.4) and (7.5). Figure 7.5 gives an example of the influence of electrolyte concentration on the electrostatic repulsive force. In this example, $a = 10^{-5}$ cm, $A = 10^{-19}$ J, and $\psi_0 = RT/F \approx 26.5$ mV. As the electrolyte concentration is increased, κ increases due to compression of the double layer with consequent decrease in $1/\kappa$.

At low electrolyte concentrations (low κ) the range of the double layer is high and V_R extends to large distances around the particles. Summation of V_R and V_A gives a total energy curve having a high primary maximum but no secondary minimum. The decrease of the double layer when more electrolyte is added produces a more rapid decay in V_R and the resultant total energy curve now has a small primary maximum but, more importantly, a secondary minimum. This concentration of electrolyte would produce a stable suspension, since flocculation could occur in the

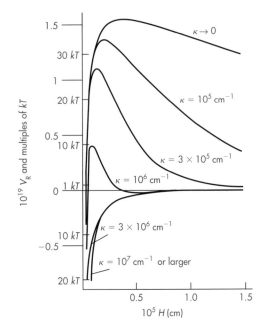

Figure 7.5 The energy of interaction of two spherical particles as a function of the distance, H, between the surfaces. For monovalent ions c (mol dm^{-3}) = $10^{-15}\kappa^2$ (cm^{-1}). In this example, $a = 10^{-5}$ cm, $A = 10^{-19}$ J and $\psi_0 = RT/F = 26.5$ mV.

Reproduced from J. Th. Overbeek, *J. Colloid Interface Sci.*, **58**, 408 (1977).

secondary minimum and the small primary maximum would be sufficient to prevent coagulation in the primary minimum. At high concentrations of added electrolyte, the range of V_R would be so small that the van der Waals attractive forces would dictate the shape of the total energy curve. As a consequence, this curve has no primary maximum and the dispersion would consequently be unstable since there would be no energy barrier to prevent coagulation of the particles in the primary minimum. The practical importance of this can be seen when nanoparticles are dispersed in cell culture media with high levels of electrolyte and flocculate as a result.

We can see from equation (7.3) that the magnitude of the effect of an electrolyte of a given concentration on V_R also depends on the valence of the ion of opposite charge to that of the particles (the counterion): the greater the valence of the added counterion, the greater its effect on V_R. These generalisations are known as the *Schulze–Hardy rule*.

Notice that it does not matter which particular counterion of a given valence is added.

Effect of surface potential on stability

A second parameter which influences the shape of the total energy curve is the surface potential of the particles. We can see from equation (7.4) that V_R will increase with an increase in ψ_0; the changes which occur in the total curve are seen in Fig. 7.6. There is a decrease in the primary maximum as the surface potential decreases and you should note the appearance of a secondary minimum at the intermediate value of ψ_0 (see C).

7.2.2 Repulsion between hydrated surfaces

The increasing use of nonionic macromolecules as stabilisers, which has occurred since the development of the DLVO theory, has led to the awareness of other stabilising forces. The approach of particles with hydrated macromolecules adsorbed to their surfaces leads, on the interaction of these layers, to repulsion (Fig. 7.7), because of the consequent positive enthalpy change ($+\Delta H$) which ensues. In more general terms, the approach of two particles with adsorbed stabilising chains leads

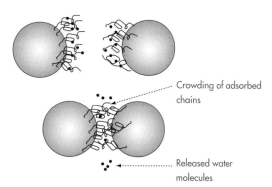

Figure 7.7 Enthalpic stabilisation: representation of enthalpic stabilisation of particles with adsorbed hydrophilic chains. The hydrated chains of the polyoxyethylene molecules $-(OCH_2CH_2)_nOH$ protrude into the aqueous dispersing medium. On close approach of the particles to within 2δ (twice the length of the stabilising chains), hydrating water is released, resulting in a positive enthalpy change which is energetically unfavourable.

to a steric interaction when the chains interact. The repulsive forces may not always be enthalpic in origin. Loss of conformational freedom leads to a negative entropy change ($-\Delta S$). Each chain loses some of its conformational freedom and its contribution to the free energy of the system is increased, leading to repulsion. This volume restriction is compounded by an 'osmotic effect' which arises as the macromolecular chains on neighbouring particles crowd into each other's space, increasing the concentration of chains in the overlap region. The repulsion which arises is due to the osmotic pressure of the solvent attempting to dilute out the concentrated region: this can only be achieved by the particles moving apart.

Quantitative assessments of the steric effect depends on three parameters:

- The hydrophilic polymer chain length, δ
- The interaction of the solvent with the chains
- The number of chains per unit area of interacting surface

The steric effect does not come into play until $H = 2\delta$, so the interaction increases suddenly with decreasing distance. There are many problems in applying such equations in practice, the main ones being the lack of an

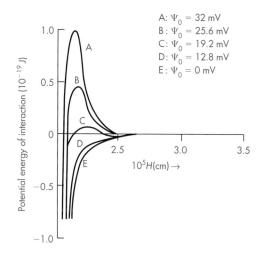

A : $\Psi_0 = 32\,mV$
B : $\Psi_0 = 25.6\,mV$
C : $\Psi_0 = 19.2\,mV$
D : $\Psi_0 = 12.8\,mV$
E : $\Psi_0 = 0\,mV$

Figure 7.6 The influence of the surface potential (ψ_0) on the total potential energy of interaction of two spherical particles.

accurate knowledge of δ, and the difficulty in taking account of desorption and changes in chain conformation or solvation during interaction. When the steric contribution is combined with the electrostatic and van der Waals interactions, a minimum in the energy at large separations still obtains, but repulsion is generally evident at all shorter distances, provided that the adsorbed macromolecules or surfactants do not desorb into the continuous phase or otherwise move away from the points of interaction (Fig. 7.8).

For particles with a hydrated stabilising layer of thickness δ, the volume of the overlapping region (V_{ov}) is as derived in Fig. 7.9:

$$V_{ov} = \frac{2\pi}{3}\left(\delta - \frac{H}{2}\right)^2\left(3a + 2\delta + \frac{H}{2}\right) \quad (7.7)$$

The difference between chemical potential in the overlap volume (μ_H) and the potential when the particles are at an infinite distance apart (μ_∞) is a measure of the repulsive force, an osmotic force, caused by the increased concentration of the polymer chains in the region of overlap:

$$\mu_H - \mu_\infty = -\pi_E \overline{V}_1 \quad (7.8)$$

where $\overline{V}_1$ is the partial molal volume of solvent and by analogy with osmotic pressure

relationships,

$$\pi_E = RTBc^2 \quad (7.9)$$

where B is the second virial coefficient. Now the free energy of mixing is

$$\Delta G_m = 2\int_0^{V_{ov}} \pi_E dV = 2\pi_E V_{ov}$$

and therefore

$$\Delta G_m = 2\pi_E \frac{2\pi}{3}\left(\delta - \frac{H}{2}\right)^2\left(3a + 2\delta + \frac{H}{2}\right) \quad (7.10)$$

Substituting for π_E and using $R = kN_A$, where k is the Boltzmann constant, we obtain

$$\frac{\Delta G_m}{kT} = \frac{4\pi}{3}BN_A c^2\left(\delta - \frac{H}{2}\right)^2\left(3a + 2\delta + \frac{H}{2}\right)$$

$$(7.11)$$

where c is the concentration of surfactant in the interfacial layer and N_A is the Avogadro constant.

This equation probably appears more complex than it is. Apart from telling us the effect of increasing or decreasing δ, for example by using different polymers of different length (δ), we can find out the effect of temperature and additives, as B is proportional to $(1 - \theta/T)$, where θ is the temperature (the

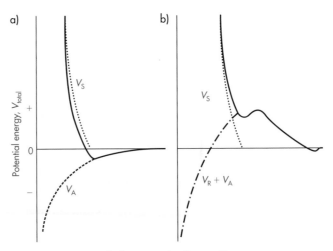

Figure 7.8 Entropic (steric) stabilisation: the potential energy–distance plots for (a) particles with no electrostatic repulsion, $V_{total} = V_S + V_A$; (b) with electrostatic repulsion, $V_{total} = V_S + V_A + V_R$.

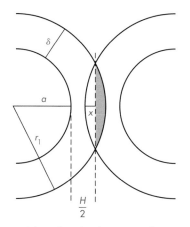

Volume of hatched section $(r_{ov}) = \dfrac{\pi x^2}{3} (3r_1 - x)$

$$= \frac{\pi}{3} (\delta - \frac{H}{2})^2 (3a + 3\delta - \delta + \frac{H}{2})$$

$$= \frac{\pi}{3} (\delta - \frac{H}{2})^2 (3a + 2\delta + \frac{H}{2})$$

V_{ov} = Total volume of overlap = $2r_{ov}$

Figure 7.9 The model used in the derivation of equation (7.7): particles of radius a with adsorbed layer of thickness δ approach to a distance H between the particle surfaces; $r_1 = (a + \delta)$ and x is the distance between the surface and the line bisecting the volume of overlap.
Reproduced from R. H. Ottewill, in *Nonionic Surfactants* (ed. M. J. Schick), Marcel Dekker, New York, 1967.

theta temperature) at which the polymer and solvent have no affinity for each other. Thus when $T = \theta$, B tends to zero, and the stabilising influence of the hydrated layer disappears, as hydration is lost. Heating thus reduces ΔG_m in this case. Additives which salt out the macromolecules from solution will have the same effect.

The requirement for the strict applicability of equations (7.1), (7.2) and (7.4) and subsequent equations is that the particles are monosized, which is rarely the case with conventional pharmaceutical emulsions and suspensions. Where particles of two radii, a_1 and a_2, interact, equation (7.2) is modified to

$$V_A = -\frac{A a_1 a_2}{6(a_1 + a_2)H} \tag{7.12}$$

Similarly, V_R is expressed by an analogue of equation (7.4), namely

$$V_R = \frac{\varepsilon}{4} \frac{a_1 a_2}{(a_1 + a_2)} (\psi_1 + \psi_2)^2 \ln[1 + \exp(-kH)]$$
$$+ (\psi_1 - \psi_2)^2 \ln[1 - \exp(-kH)] \tag{7.13}$$

where ψ_1 and ψ_2 are the surface potentials of particles 1 and 2.

These equations have been applied not only to the study of suspensions but to the reversible interaction of microbial cells with a solid substrate such as glass before permanent adhesion occurs due to the formation of polymeric bridges between cell and glass.

7.3 Emulsions

Emulsions – liquid dispersions usually of an oil phase and an aqueous phase – are a traditional pharmaceutical dosage form. Oil-in-water systems have enjoyed a renaissance as vehicles for the delivery of lipid-soluble drugs (e.g. propofol). Their use as a dosage form necessitates an understanding of the factors governing the formulation and stability of oil-in-water (o/w) and water-in-oil (w/o) emulsions, multiple emulsions (w/o/w or o/w/o) and microemulsions, which occupy a position between swollen micelles and emulsions with very small globule sizes. Photomicrographs of o/w, w/o systems and multiple emulsions are shown in Fig. 7.10. It is also possible to formulate nonaqueous or anhydrous emulsions, that is oil-in-oil systems and even multiple oil-in-oil-in-oil systems.

7.3.1 Stability of o/w and w/o emulsions

Adsorption of a surfactant at the oil/water interface, by lowering interfacial tension

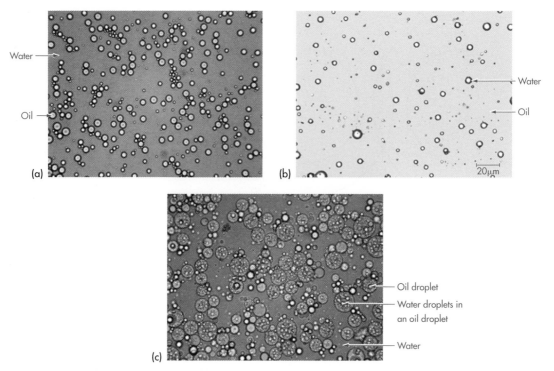

Figure 7.10 Photomicrograph of emulsions: (a) an oil-in-water (o/w) emulsion, (b) a water-in-oil (w/o) system, (c) a water-in-oil-in-water emulsion in which the internal water droplets can be seen in the larger oil droplets.

during manufacture, aids the dispersal of the oil into droplets of a small size and helps to maintain the particles in a dispersed state (Fig. 7.11) Unless the interfacial tension is zero, there is a natural tendency for the oil droplets to coalesce to reduce the area of oil–water contact, but the presence of the surfactant monolayer at the surface of the droplet reduces the possibility of collisions leading to coalescence. Charged surfactants will lead to an increase in negative or positive zeta potential and will thus help to maintain stability by increasing V_R. Nonionic surfactants such as the alkyl or aryl polyoxyethylene ethers, sorbitan polyoxyethylene derivatives and sorbitan esters and polyoxyethylene–polyoxypropylene–polyoxyethylene block copolymers are widely used in pharmaceutical emulsions because of their lack of toxicity and their low sensitivity to additives. These nonionic stabilisers adsorb onto the emulsion droplets and, although they generally reduce zeta potentials, they maintain stability by creating a hydrated layer on the

hydrophobic particle in o/w emulsions. They effectively convert a hydrophobic colloidal dispersion into a hydrophilic dispersion.

In w/o emulsions the hydrocarbon chains of the adsorbed molecules protrude into the oily continuous phase. Stabilisation arises from steric repulsive forces as described in section 7.2.2. Emulsions are more complex than suspensions, because of the possibility (a) of movement of the surfactant into either the continuous or disperse phase, (b) micelle formation in both phases, and (c) the formation under suitable conditions of liquid crystalline phases between the disperse droplets.

It is usually observed that mixtures of surfactants form more stable emulsions than do single surfactants. This may be because complex formation at the interface results in a more 'rigid' stabilising film. Certainly where complex films can be formed, such as between sodium lauryl sulfate and cetyl alcohol, the stability of emulsions prepared with such mixtures is high. Theory has not developed to

(a)

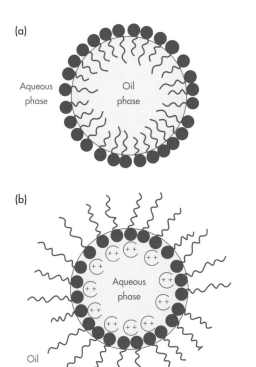

Aqueous phase

Oil phase

(b)

Aqueous phase

Oil phase

Figure 7.11 Surfactant films at the water/oil interface in o/w and w/o emulsions: (a) formation of a monomolecular film at the oil/water interface for the stabilisation of o/w emulsions; (b) stabilisation of w/o emulsions by the oriented adsorption of divalent soap salts (not to scale).

an extent that it can readily cope with mixtures of stabiliser molecules. Complex formation between surfactant and cosurfactants in the bulk phase of emulsion systems is dealt with in section 7.3.5, as this frequently leads to semisolid systems of high intrinsic stability.

7.3.2 HLB system

In spite of many advances in the theory of stability of lyophobic colloids, resort has still to be made to an empirical approach to the choice of emulsifier, devised in 1949 by Griffin. In this system we calculate the hydrophile–lipophile balance (HLB) of surfactants, which is a measure of the relative contributions of the hydrophilic and lipophilic regions of the

molecule. Values of the effective HLB of surfactant mixtures can be calculated.

The HLB number of a surfactant is calculated according to an empirical formula. For nonionic surfactants the values range from 0 to 20 on an arbitrary scale (see Fig. 7.12). At the higher end of the scale the surfactants are hydrophilic and act as solubilising agents, detergents and o/w emulsifiers. To maintain stability, an excess of surfactant is required in the continuous phase; hence, in general, water-soluble surfactants stabilise o/w emulsions and water-insoluble surfactants stabilise w/o emulsions. Oil-soluble surfactants with a low HLB act as w/o emulsifiers. In the stabilisation of oil globules it is essential that there is a degree of surfactant hydrophilicity to confer an enthalpic stabilising force and a degree of hydrophobicity to secure adsorption at the o/w interface. The balance between the two will depend on the nature of the oil and the mixture of surfactants; hence the need to apply the HLB system. The HLB of polyhydric alcohol fatty acid esters such as glyceryl monostearate may be obtained from equation (7.14)

$$HLB = 20\left(1 - \frac{S}{A}\right) \qquad (7.14)$$

where S is the saponification number of the ester and A is the acid number of the fatty acid. The HLB of polysorbate 20 (Tween 20) calculated using this formula is 16.7, with $S = 45.5$ and $A = 276$.

Typically, the polysorbate (Tween) surfactants have HLB values in the range 9.6–16.7; the sorbitan ester (Span) surfactants have HLBs in the lower range of 1.8–8.6.

For those materials for which it is not possible to obtain saponification numbers, for example beeswax and lanolin derivatives, the HLB is calculated from

$$HLB = (E + P)/5 \qquad (7.15)$$

where E is the percentage by weight of oxyethylene chains, and P is the percentage by weight of polyhydric alcohol groups (glycerol or sorbitol) in the molecule.

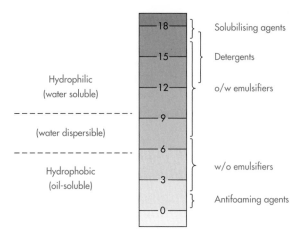

Figure 7.12 The HLB scale and the approximate ranges into which solubilising agents, detergents, emulsifiers and antifoaming agents fall.

Calculation of HLB of a polysorbate

Polysorbate 20 has a molecular weight of approximately 1300 and contains 20 oxy-ethylene groups and two sorbitan rings. Thus,

$$E = \frac{20 \times 44 \times 100}{1300} = 68$$

$$P = \frac{182 \times 100}{1300} = 14$$

Hence,

$$HLB = 82/5 = 16.4$$

If the hydrophile consists only of oxyethylene groups (CH_2CH_2O, mol. wt. = 44), a simpler version of the equation is

$$HLB = E/5 \qquad (7.16)$$

giving the upper end of the scale (20) for polyoxyethelene glycol itself.

Some HLB values of typical surfactants used in pharmacy are given in Table 7.2. A more detailed list is given in Tables 6.7 and 6.8.

Group contribution

The HLB system has been put on a more quantitative basis by Davies, who calculated group contributions (group numbers) to the HLB number such that the HLB was obtained from

$$HLB = \Sigma \text{ (hydrophobic group numbers)}$$
$$- \Sigma \text{ (lyophilic group numbers)} + 7 \quad (7.17)$$

Table 7.2 Typical HLB numbers of some surfactants

Compound	HLB
Glyceryl monostearate	3.8
Sorbitan monooleate (Span 80)	4.3
Sorbitan monolaurate (Span 20)	8.6
Triethanolamine oleate	12.0
Polyoxyethylene sorbitan monooleate (Tween 80)	15.0
Polyoxyethylene sorbitan monolaurate (Tween 20)	16.7
Sodium oleate	18.0
Sodium lauryl sulfate[a]	40.0

[a] Although applied mainly to nonionic surfactants it is possible to obtain numbers for ionic surfactants.

Some group numbers are given in Table 7.3.

Choice of emulsifier or emulsifier mixture

The appropriate choice of emulsifier or emulsifier mixture can be made by preparing a series of emulsions with a range of surfactants of varying HLB. It is assumed that the HLB of a mixture of two surfactants containing fraction f of A and $(1 - f)$ of B is the algebraic mean of the two HLB numbers:

$$HLB_{mixture} = fHLB_A + (1 - f)HLB_B \qquad (7.18)$$

For reasons not explained by the HLB system, but from other approaches, mixtures

Table 7.3 Group contributions to HLB numbers

Group	Group number
Hydrophilic groups	
COO⁻Na⁺	19.1
Ester	2.4
Hydroxyl	1.9
Hydroxyl (sorbitan)	0.5
Lipophilic groups	
—CH—	0.475
—CH$_2$—	0.475
—CH$_3$	0.475
=CH—	0.475

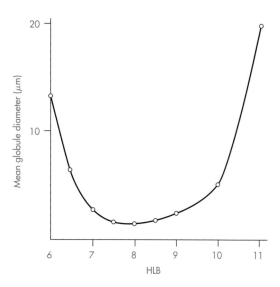

Figure 7.13 Variation of mean globule size in a mineral oil-in-water emulsion as a function of the HLB of the surfactant mixtures present at a level of 2.5%. Surfactants: Brij 92–Brij 96 mixtures.
Source: P. Depraetre, M. Seiller, A. T. Florence and F. Puisieux (unpublished).

of high HLB and low HLB give more stable emulsions than do single surfactants. Apart from the possibility of complex formation at the interface, the solubility of surfactant components in both the disperse and the continuous phase maintains the stability of the surfactant film at the interface from the reservoirs created in each phase. In the experimental determination of optimum HLB, creaming of the emulsion is observed and is taken as an index of stability. The system with the minimum creaming or separation of phases is deemed to have an optimal HLB. It is therefore possible to determine optimum HLB numbers required to produce stable emulsions of a variety of oils. Table 7.4 shows the required HLB of surfactants to achieve stability of five oils. A more sensitive method would be to determine the mean globule size in emulsions using modern techniques such as laser diffraction methods to produce data such as those in Fig. 7.13. For the mineral oil-in-water emulsion stabilized by a mixture of two nonionic surfactants, an optimal HLB of between 7.5 and 8 is identified.

At the optimum HLB the mean particle size of the emulsion is at a minimum (Fig. 7.13) and this factor would explain to a large extent the stability of the system (see equations 7.1 and 7.2, for example).

Although the optimum HLB values for forming o/w emulsions are obtained in this way, it is possible to formulate stable systems with mixtures of surfactants well below the optimum. This is sometimes because of the formation of a viscous network of surfactant in the continuous phase. The high viscosity of the medium surrounding the droplets prevents their collision and this overrides the influence of the interfacial layer and barrier forces due to the presence of the adsorbed layer.

The HLB system has several drawbacks. The calculated HLB, of course, cannot take account of the effect of temperature or that of additives. The presence in emulsions of agents which salt-in or salt-out surfactants will

Table 7.4 Required HLB for different oils for o/w emulsion formation

Oil	HLB
Cottonseed oil	7.5
Vaseline oil	8.5
Dodecane	9–9.5
Mineral oil	10–12
Cyclohexane	12

respectively increase and decrease the effective (as opposed to the calculated) HLB values. Salting-out the surfactant (for example, with NaCl) will make the molecules less hydrophilic and one can thus expect a higher optimal calculated HLB value for the stabilising surfactant for o/w emulsions containing sodium chloride. Examples are shown in Fig. 7.14 in which the effects of NaCl and NaI are compared.

7.3.3 Multiple emulsions

Multiple emulsions are emulsions whose disperse phase contains droplets of another phase[1,2] (Fig. 7.10). Water-in-oil-in-water (w/o/w) or o/w/o emulsions may be prepared, both forms being of interest as drug delivery systems. Water-in-oil emulsions in which a water-soluble drug is dissolved in the aqueous phase may be injected by the subcutaneous or intramuscular routes to produce a delayed-action preparation, as to escape the drug has to diffuse through the oil to reach the tissue fluids. The main disadvantage of a w/o emulsion is generally its high viscosity, brought about through the influence of the oil on the bulk viscosity. Emulsifying a w/o emulsion using surfactants which stabilise an oily disperse phase can produce w/o/w emulsions with an external aqueous phase and lower viscosity than the primary emulsion. On injection, into muscle for example, the external aqueous phase dissipates rapidly, leaving behind the w/o emulsion. Nevertheless, biopharmaceutical differences have been observed between w/o and multiple emulsion systems. (Fig. 7.15)

Physical degradation of w/o/w emulsions can arise by several routes: (Fig. 7.16a):

- Coalescence of the internal water droplets
- Coalescence of the oil droplets surrounding them
- Rupture of the oil film separating the internal and external aqueous phases

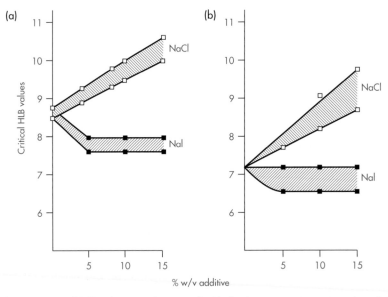

Figure 7.14 The change in critical HLB values as a function of added salt concentration, where the salt is either NaCl or NaI. Results were obtained from measurements of particle size, stability, viscosity and emulsion type as a function of HLB for liquid paraffin-in-water emulsions stabilised by Brij 92–Brij 96 mixtures. Data from different experiments showed different critical values; hence, on each diagram hatching represents the critical regions while data points actually recorded are shown. Results in (a) show particle size and stability data; those in (b) show the HLB at transition from pseudoplastic to Newtonian flow properties (see section 7.3.10) and emulsion type (o/w → w/o) transitions.
Reproduced from A. T. Florence, F. Madsen and F. Puisieux, J. Pharm. Pharmacol., 27, 385 (1975).

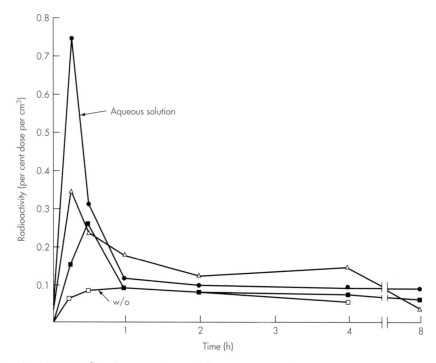

Figure 7.15 Blood levels of (^{3}H)5-fluorouracil (5-FU) following intramuscular injection of (●) an aqueous solution, (□) a w/o emulsion prepared with hexadecane, and a w/o/w emulsion prepared with (△) isopropyl myristate or (■) hexadecane as the oil phase.

- Osmotic flux of water to and from the internal droplets, possibly associated with inverse micellar species in the oil phase

The external oil particles may coalesce with others (which may or may not contain internal aqueous droplets), as in route (a); the internal aqueous droplets may be expelled individually (routes b, c, d, e) or more than one may be expelled (route f), or less frequently they may be expelled in one step (route g); the internal droplets may coalesce before being expelled (routes h, i, j, k); or water may pass by diffusion through the oil phase, gradually resulting in shrinkage of the internal droplets (routes l, m, n). Figure 7.16 is oversimplified; in practice the number of possible combinations is large. Several factors will determine the breakdown mechanisms in a particular system, but one of the main driving forces behind each step will be the reduction in the free energy of the system brought about by the reduction in the interfacial area.

Mechanisms of drug release from multiple emulsion systems include diffusion of the drug molecules from the internal droplets (1), from the medium of the external droplets (2), or by mass transfer due to the coalescence of the internal droplets (3), as shown in Fig. 7.16(b)

Nonaqueous emulsions

Few studies have been carried out on non-aqueous emulsions, but these can be useful as topical vehicles or reservoirs for the delivery of hydrolytically unstable drugs. Systems such as castor oil or propylene glycol in silicone oil can be formulated using silicone surfactants; the HLB number clearly does not help in the formulation, especially if the continuous phase has low polarity. The key to stabilisation lies in the sufficient solubility of the emulsifier in the continuous phase.

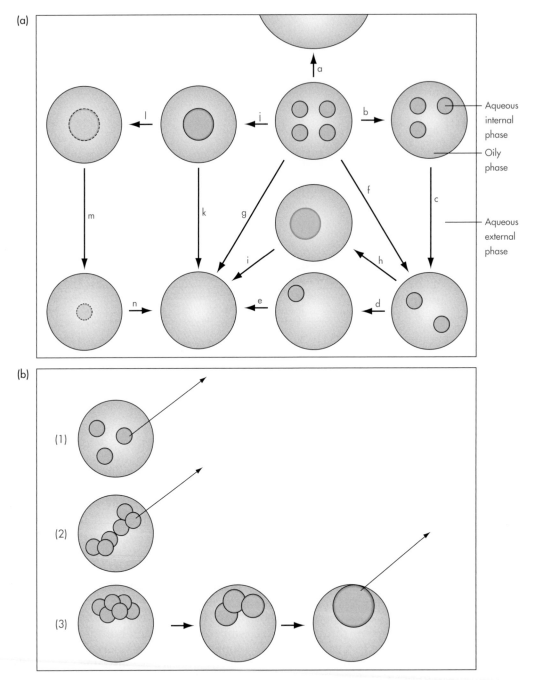

Figure 7.16 (a) Possible breakdown pathways (see text) in w/o/w multiple emulsions (Whitehill and Florence). (From reference 1.) (b) Diagrammatic representation of mechanisms of drug release (see text). (From S. S. Davis, *J. Clin. Pharm.*, 1, 11 (1976).) See text for explanation.

7.3.4   Microemulsions

Microemulsions consist of apparently homogeneous transparent systems of low viscosity which contain a high percentage of both oil and water and high concentrations (15–25%) of emulsifier mixture. They were first described by Schulman as disperse systems with spherical or cylindrical droplets in the size range 8–80 nm. They are essentially swollen micellar systems, but obviously the distinction between a swollen micelle and small emulsion droplet is difficult to assess.

Microemulsions form spontaneously when the components are mixed in the appropriate ratios and are thermodynamically stable. In their simplest form, microemulsions are small droplets (diameter 5–140 nm) of one liquid dispersed throughout another by virtue of the presence of a fairly large concentration of a suitable combination of surfactants. They can be dispersions of oil droplets in water (o/w) or water droplets in oil (w/o). An essential requirement for their formation and stability is the attainment of a very low interfacial tension γ. Since microemulsions have a very large interface between oil and water (because of the small droplet size), they can only be thermodynamically stable if the interfacial tension is so low that the positive interfacial energy (given by γA, where A is the interfacial area) can be compensated by the negative free energy of mixing ΔG_m. We can calculate a rough measure of the limiting γ value required as follows: ΔG_m is given by $-T \Delta S_m$ (where T is the temperature), and the entropy of mixing (ΔS_m) is of the order of the Boltzmann constant. Hence $k_B T = 4\pi r^2 \gamma$. Hence for a droplet radius r of about 10 nm, an interfacial tension of 0.03 mN m^{-1} would be required. The role of the surfactants in the system is thus to reduce the interfacial tension between oil and water (typically about 50 mN m^{-1}) to this low level.

Use of cosurfactants

With the possible exception of double alkyl chain surfactants and a few nonionic surfactants, it is generally not possible to achieve the required interfacial area with the use of a single surfactant. If, however, a second amphiphile is added to the system, the effects of the two surfactants can be additive provided that the adsorption of one does not adversely affect that of the other and that mixed micelle formation does not reduce the available concentration of surfactant molecules. The second amphiphile is referred to as the *cosurfactant*.

The importance of the cosurfactant is illustrated in the following example. The interfacial tension between cyclohexane and water is approximately 42 mN m^{-1} in the absence of any added surfactant. The addition of the ionic surfactant sodium dodecyl sulfate (SDS) in increasing amounts causes a gradual reduction of γ to a value of about 2 mN m^{-1} at an SDS concentration of 10^{-4} g cm^{-3}. Further reduction of interfacial tension does not occur, since the cyclohexane/water interface is now saturated with SDS and any SDS added in excess of this limiting concentration forms micelles in the aqueous solution. Addition of 20% pentanol to the cyclohexane–water system in the absence of SDS reduces the interfacial tension to 10 mN m^{-1}. It is then theoretically possible by the addition of SDS to achieve a negative interfacial tension at SDS concentrations below the level at which it forms micelles (the critical micelle concentration, cmc). The changes in interfacial tension occurring in this system are illustrated in Fig. 7.17. Although pentanol is not generally regarded as a surfactant, it has the ability to reduce interfacial tension by virtue of its amphiphilic nature (a short hydrophobic chain and a terminal hydrophilic hydroxyl group) and functions as the cosurfactant in this system. Its presence means that the SDS is now required to produce a much smaller lowering of the interfacial tension (10 mN m^{-1} rather than 42 mN m^{-1} in its absence) in order to produce a microemulsion.

The simplest representation of the structure of microemulsions is the droplet model in which microemulsion droplets are surrounded by an interfacial film consisting of both surfactant and cosurfactant molecules, as illustrated in Fig. 7.18. The orientation of the amphiphiles at the interface will, of course, differ in o/w and w/o microemulsions. As

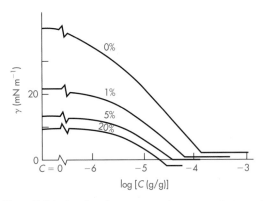

Figure 7.17 Interfacial tension, γ, between solutions of sodium dodecyl sulfate (SDS) of concentration C in aqueous 0.30 mol dm^{-3} NaCl and solutions of 1-pentanol in cyclohexane with the percentage concentrations indicated.
Reproduced from J. Th. G. Overbeek, *Proc. R. Dutch. Acad. Sci. Ser. B*, 89(1), 61 (1986) with permission.

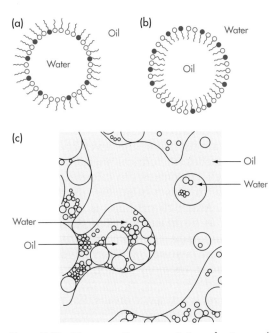

Figure 7.18 Diagrammatic representation of microemulsion structures: (a) a water-in-oil microemulsion droplet; (b) an oil-in-water microemulsion droplet; and (c) an irregular bicontinuous structure.

shown in Fig. 7.18, the hydrophobic portions of these molecules will reside in the dispersed oil droplets of o/w systems, with the hydrophilic groups protruding in the continuous phase, while the opposite situation will be true

of w/o microemulsions. For systems of known composition, an estimation may be made of the droplet radius r using $r = 3\phi C_s a_0$, where ϕ is the volume fraction of the disperse phase, C_s is the number of surfactant molecules per unit volume, and a_0 is the surface area of a surfactant molecule at the interface. In practice not all of the surfactant can be assumed to be associated with the interface, and C_s is consequently seldom known with any certainty, although it is often assumed that the amount of surfactant in the continuous phase approximates to the surfactant cmc.

Whether the systems form o/w or w/o microemulsions is determined to a large extent by the nature of the surfactant. The geometry of the surfactant molecule is important. If the volume of the surfactant molecule is v, the cross-sectional area of its head group a, and its length l, then when the critical packing parameter v/al (see section 6.3.3) has values of between 0 and 1, o/w systems are likely to form, but when v/al is greater than 1, w/o microemulsions are favoured. Values of the critical packing parameter close to unity can result in the formation of a bicontinuous structure in which areas of water can be imagined to be separated by a connected amphiphile-rich interfacial layer as depicted in Fig. 7.18(c). Values of the parameters v, a and l can be readily estimated, but it should be noted that the critical packing parameter is based purely on geometric considerations. Penetration of oil and cosurfactant into the surfactant interface and hydration of the surfactant head groups will also influence the packing of the molecules in the interfacial film around the droplets. In many systems, inversion from w/o to o/w microemulsions can occur as a result of changing the composition or the temperature. In general, o/w microemulsions are favoured when small amounts of oil are present and w/o systems form in the presence of small amounts of water. Under such conditions the droplet model is a reasonable representation of the system. The structure of microemulsions containing almost equal amounts of oil and water is best represented by a bicontinuous structure.

A microemulsion formulation

A formulation of ciclosporin (Sandimmun Neoral, Novartis) incorporates the drug in a preconcentrate which forms a microemulsion on dilution in aqueous fluids.[3,4] This formulation offers an alternative to the oil formulation of ciclosporin (Sandimmun) which *in vivo* would be emulsified by bile salts and pancreatic enzymes. The residence time of ciclosporin in the gastrointestinal tract is shorter and the rate of absorption is faster with the microemulsion formulation[5] (Fig. 7.19).

W/o microemulsions incorporating medium-chain glycerides have been used to deliver calcein intraduodenally and produce significantly higher plasma levels of the drug compared to an aqueous formulation.[6]

7.3.5 Structured (semisolid) emulsions

In sections 7.3.1–7.3.4 we have considered only relatively simple dilute emulsions. Many pharmaceutical preparations, lotions or creams are, in fact, complex semisolid or structured systems which contain excess emulsifier over that required to form a stabilising monolayer at the oil/water interface. The excess surfactant can interact with other components either at the droplet interface or in the bulk (continuous) phase to produce complex semisolid multiphase systems. Theories derived to explain the stability of dilute colloidal systems cannot be applied directly. In many cases the formation of stable interfacial films at the oil/water interface cannot be considered to play the dominant role in maintaining

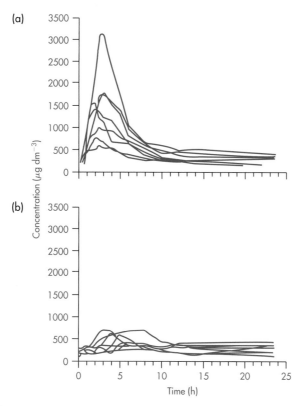

Figure 7.19 Blood ciclosporin concentration–time curves obtained following single oral doses (10 mg kg^{-1}) of (a) microemulsion and (b) conventional formulations in eight liver transplant recipients with external biliary diversion.
Reproduced from A. K. Trull *et al.*, *Br. J. Clin. Pharmacol.*, 39, 627 (1995) with permission.

stability. Rather it is the structure of the bulk phase which maintains the disperse phase at a distance. Even very complex emulsions are often mobile at some point in their lifetime, e.g. during manufacture at elevated temperatures, or may become so during application of high shear rates in use. Under these conditions globules previously unable to interact become free to do so.

Stable o/w creams prepared with ionic or nonionic emulsifying waxes are composed of (at least) four phases (Fig. 7.20): (1) dispersed oil phase, (2) crystalline gel phase, (3) crystalline hydrate phase, and (4) bulk aqueous phase containing a dilute solution of surfactant. The interaction of the surfactant and fatty alcohol components of emulsifying mixtures to form these structures (body) is critical. It is also time-dependent, giving the name 'self-bodying' to these emulsions. The overall stability of a cream is dependent on the stability of the crystalline gel phase.

Emulsion stability is increased by the presence of liquid crystalline phases, as they form multilayers at the oil/water interface. These multilayers thus protect against coalescence by reducing the van der Waals forces of attraction and by retarding film thinning between approaching droplets, the viscosity of the liquid crystalline phases being at least 100 times that of the continuous phase in the absence of these structures.

It is apparent from the nature of these self-bodied systems that, at equilibrium, contacts between droplets are prevented, although in the long term processes equivalent to syneresis may occur due to rearrangement of the matrix structure and the 'squeezing out' of the oil phase.

Certain guidelines have been devised for the formulation of self-bodied emulsions:[7]

- The *lipophilic component* should be an amphiphile that promotes the formation of w/o emulsions and is capable of complexing with the hydrophilic surfactant at the o/w interface. Its concentration should be at least sufficient to form a close-packed

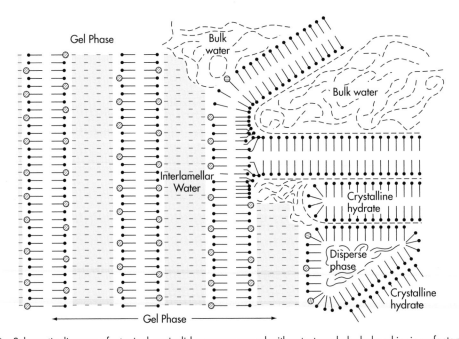

Figure 7.20 Schematic diagram of a typical semisolid cream prepared with cetostearyl alcohol and ionic surfactant. Note the four phases: (1) the dispersed oil phase; (2) the crystalline gel phase containing interlamellar-fixed water; (3) phase composed of crystalline hydrates of cetostearyl alcohol; (4) bulk water phase.
Reproduced from G. M. Eccleston, *Pharm. Int.*, 7, 63 (1986).

mixed monolayer with the hydrophilic component. To promote the formation of semisolid emulsions at room temperature, it should be near or above its saturation concentration in the oil. Excess material should diffuse readily from the warm oil phase into the warm micellar phase and there be solubilised. The melting point should be sufficiently high to precipitate solubilised material at room temperature.

- The *hydrophilic component* should be a surfactant that promotes the formation of o/w systems and is capable of complexing with the lipophilic component at the o/w interface. Its concentration should be at least sufficient to form a close-packed monolayer with the lipophilic component and it should be in excess of its cmc in the aqueous phase. It should be capable of solubilising the lipophilic component when warm.

The rigidity and strength of networks prepared with cetostearyl alcohol and alkyltrimethyl-ammonium bromides (C_{12}–C_{18}) increase as the alkyl chain length increases. The rheological stability of ternary systems is markedly dependent on the alcohol chain length; networks prepared with ionic or nonionic surfactants and pure cetyl or pure stearyl alcohol are weaker than those prepared with cetostearyl alcohol. In particular, emulsions prepared with stearyl alcohol are mobile and eventually separate.

7.3.6 Biopharmaceutical aspects of emulsions

Traditionally, emulsions have been used to deliver oils (castor oil, liquid paraffin) in a palatable form. This is now a minor use, but there is a growing interest in the possibility of improving delivery by the use of lipid o/w emulsions as vehicles for lipophilic drugs (e.g. diazepam, propofol) for intravenous use. Griseofulvin, presented as an emulsion, exhibits enhanced oral absorption; an emulsion of indoxole has superior bioavailability over other oral forms. Medium-chain triglycerides and mono- and diglycerides promote the absorption of ceftriaxone and cefoxitin as well as ciclosporin.

In the case of griseofulvin, administration in a fatty medium enhances absorption. Fat is emulsified by the bile salts, and the administration of an already emulsified form increases the opportunity for solubilisation and hence transport across the microvilli by fat absorption pathways. The influence of the emulsifier on membrane permeability is one factor that must be considered. Knowledge that particles may be absorbed from the gut by the gut-associated lymphoid tissue suggests that we may have to revise our views on the nature of absorption of many drugs from the gastrointestinal tract.

Drug release from emulsions is related to the partition coefficient of the drug and the volume of the disperse phase, as well as to the concentration of surfactant which might solubilise the drug in the aqueous phase.

7.3.7 Preservative availability in emulsified systems

Microbial spoilage of emulsified products is avoided by the inclusion of appropriate amounts of a preservative in the formulation. Infected topical emulsions have been the cause of outbreaks of pseudomonal and other bacterial skin infections. The incorporation of preservatives into pharmaceutical emulsions is not without problems as most agents partition to the oily or micellar phases of complex systems; some are inactivated by surfactants.

The amount of preservative remaining in the aqueous phase (C_w) is related to the total amount (C) of preservative with a partition coefficient P in an emulsion with an oil/water phase ratio of Φ by equation (7.19):

$$C_W = \frac{C(\Phi + 1)}{R(P\Phi + 1)} \tag{7.19}$$

where R is the preservative/emulsifier ratio or interaction ratio.[8] If the volume of oil is V_o and the total volume of the emulsion is V_t, then the volume of the aqueous phase is $V_t - V_o$, and therefore

$$\Phi = \frac{V_o}{V_t - V_o} \tag{7.20}$$

0.4–3.0 μm. These natural emulsion globules are called *chylomicrons*. There are pronounced physical similarities between chylomicrons and the fat particles of the Intralipid emulsion.

The addition of electrolyte or drugs to intravenous fat emulsions is generally contraindicated because of the risk of destabilising the emulsion. Addition of cationic local anaesthetics reduces the electrophoretic mobility of the dispersed fat globules, and this contributes to instability.[9] Minimum stability (and minimum zeta potential) is caused by addition to Intralipid of 3×10^{-3} mol dm^{-3} CaCl$_2$ and 2.5×10^{-1} mol dm^{-3} NaCl, which are thus

recommended as the maximum additive levels (see Fig. 7.23).

Prostaglandin E$_1$ (PGE$_1$) formulations

Lipid emulsion formulations of prostaglandin E$_1$ have been used in the treatment of vascular disorders. They exhibit a reduced incidence of side-effects at the site of injection, as does the diazepam lipid emulsion. A soybean emulsion stabilized by egg-yolk lecithin[10] releases the PGE$_1$ over a period of 4–16 hours depending on pH (Fig. 7.24). The partition coefficients of PGE$_1$ between soybean emulsion and aqueous buffers at 20°C are shown in Fig. 7.25, explaining why

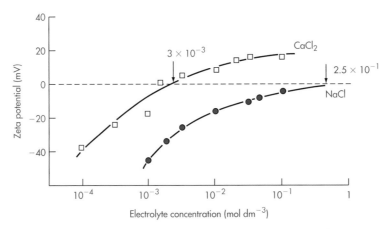

Figure 7.23   Zeta potential of Intralipid 20% diluted into varying concentrations (mol dm^{-3}) of (●) NaCl, (□) CaCl$_2$. Reproduced from reference 9 with permission.

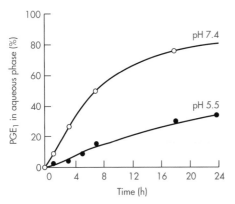

Figure 7.24   Release profiles of PGE$_1$ from particles in Lipo-PGE$_1$ diluted tenfold with buffer solutions at 5°C: (●), pH5.5; (○), pH7.4.
Reproduced from reference 10.

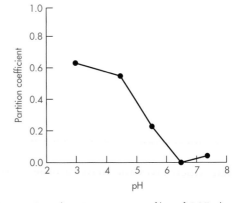

Figure 7.25   The pH–partition profiles of PGE$_1$ between soybean oil and water at 20°C, explaining why the release profiles have the pH dependency shown in Fig. 7.24.
Reproduced from reference 10.

the release profiles have the pH dependency shown in Fig. 7.24. The release profile follows the expected pH trend, but a more detailed analysis shows that the majority of the drug is associated with the phospholipid.

7.3.10 The rheology of emulsions

Most emulsions, unless very dilute, display both plastic and pseudoplastic flow behaviour rather than simple Newtonian flow. The flow properties of fluid emulsions should have little influence on their biological behaviour, although the rheological characteristics of semisolid emulsions may affect their performance. The 'pourability', 'spreadability' and 'syringeability' of an emulsion will, however, be directly determined by its rheological properties. The high viscosity of w/o emulsions leads to problems with intramuscular administration of injectable formulations. Conversion to a multiple emulsion (w/o/w), in which the external oil phase is replaced by an aqueous phase, leads to a dramatic decrease in viscosity and consequent improved ease of injection.

The influence of phase volume on the flow properties of an emulsion is shown in Fig. 7.26. In this diagram the relative viscosity (η_{rel}) of the system increases with increasing ϕ, and at any given phase volume increases with decreasing mean particle size, D_m. These and other factors which affect emulsion viscosity are listed in Table 7.6.

Table 7.6 Factors that influence emulsion viscosity

Internal (disperse) phase
Volume fraction (ϕ)
Viscosity
Particle size and size distribution
Chemical nature

Continuous phase
Viscosity
Chemical constitution and polarity

Emulsifier
Chemical constitution and concentration
Solubility in the continuous and internal (disperse) phase
Physical properties of the interfacial film
Electroviscous effects

Presence of additional stabilisers, pigments, hydrocolloids, etc.

As most emulsions are polydisperse, the influence of particle size and, in particular, of particle size distribution on viscosity is important. Figure 7.26 shows the viscosity of w/o emulsions varying in mean particle size (D_m) stabilised with sorbitan trioleate.

Several equations for the viscosity of emulsion systems take the form

$$\eta_{rel} - 1 = \eta_{sp} = \frac{\alpha\phi}{1 - h\phi} \tag{7.24}$$

where $\alpha = 2.5$, and h is a measure of the fluid immobilised between the particles in concentrated emulsions and dispersions, which

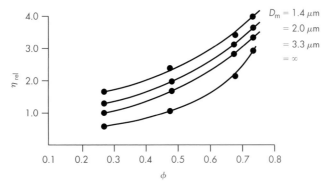

Figure 7.26 The relative viscosities of w/o emulsions stabilised with sorbitan trioleate; four emulsions have been studied with different mean particle diameters, D_m.
Reproduced from P. Sherman, *J. Pharm. Pharmacol.*, 16, 1 (1964).

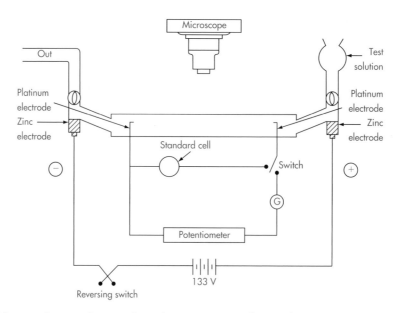

Figure 7.29 Schematic drawing of a microelectrophoresis apparatus showing the positioning of the anode and cathode and the capillary in which the velocity of particulates is monitored to allow calculation of zeta potential.

fashion. Flocculation, unlike coalescence, can be a reversible process and partial or controlled flocculation is attempted in formulation, as discussed above.

Caking of the suspension, which arises on close packing of the sedimented particles, cannot be eliminated by reduction of particle size or by increasing the viscosity of the continuous phase. Fine particles in a viscous medium settle more slowly than coarse particles but, after settling, they form a more closely packed sediment which may be difficult to redisperse. Particles in a close-packed condition brought about by settling and by the pressure of particles above thus experience greater forces of attraction. Flocculating agents can prevent caking; deflocculating agents increase the tendency to cake. The addition of flocculating and deflocculating agents is often monitored by measurement of the zeta potential of the particles in a suspension.

Zeta potential and its relationship to stability

Most suspension particles dispersed in water have a charge acquired by specific adsorption of ions or by ionisation of ionisable surface groups, if present. If the charge arises from ionisation, the charge on the particle will depend on the pH of the environment. As with other colloidal particles, repulsive forces arise because of the interaction of the electrical double layers on adjacent particles. The magnitude of the charge can be determined by measurement of the electrophoretic mobility of the particles in an applied electrical field. A microelectrophoresis apparatus in which this mobility may be measured is shown schematically in Fig. 7.29.

The velocity of migration of the particles (μ_E) under unit applied potential can be determined microscopically with a timing device and an eyepiece graticule. For nonconducting particles, the Henry equation is used to obtain ζ from μ_E. This equation can be written in the form

$$\mu_E = \frac{\zeta\varepsilon}{4\pi\eta} f(\kappa a) \qquad (7.28)$$

where $f(\kappa a)$ varies between 1 for small κa and 1.5 for large κa; ε is the dielectric constant of the continuous phase and η is its viscosity. In systems with low values of κa, the equation can be written in the form

$$\mu_E = \frac{\zeta\varepsilon}{4\pi\eta}$$

The zeta potential (ζ) is not the surface potential (ψ_0) discussed earlier but is related to it. Therefore ζ can be used as a reliable guide to the magnitude of electric repulsive forces between particles. Changes in ζ on the addition of flocculating agents, surfactants and other additives can then be used to predict the stability of the system.

The changes in a bismuth subnitrate suspension system on addition of dibasic potassium phosphate as flocculating agent are shown in Fig. 7.30. Bismuth subnitrate has a positive zeta potential; addition of phosphate reduces the charge and the zeta potential falls to a point where maximum flocculation is observed. In this zone there is no caking. Further addition of phosphate leads to a negative zeta potential and a propensity towards caking. Flocculation can therefore be controlled by the use of ionic species with a charge opposite to the charge of the particles dispersed in the medium.

The rapid clearance of the supernatant in a flocculated system is undesirable in a pharmaceutical suspension. The use of thickeners such as sodium carboxymethylcellulose or bentonite hinders the movement of the particles by production of a viscous medium, so that sedimentation is delayed. The incompatibility of these anionic agents with cationic flocculating agents has to be considered. A technique to overcome the problem is the conversion of the particle surfaces into positive surfaces so that they require anions and not cations to flocculate them. Negatively charged or neutral particles can be converted into positively charged particles by addition of a surface-active amine. Such a suspension can then be treated with phosphate ions to induce flocculation.

It is perhaps not surprising that with some complex systems the interpretation of behaviour is open to debate. Consider the system shown in Fig. 7.31. One starts with a clumped suspension of sulfamerazine, a flocculated system which produces non-caking sediments. Addition of the surfactant sodium dioctyl sulfosuccinate (docusate sodium) confers a greater negative charge on the suspension particles and deflocculation results. Addition of aluminium chloride as a flocculating agent reduces the negative charge in a controlled way to produce the loose clusters illustrated in

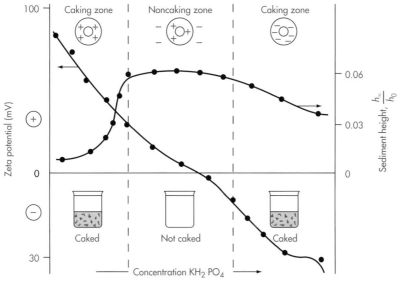

Figure 7.30 Caking diagram showing controlled flocculation of a bismuth subnitrate suspension employing dibasic potassium phosphate as the flocculating agent.

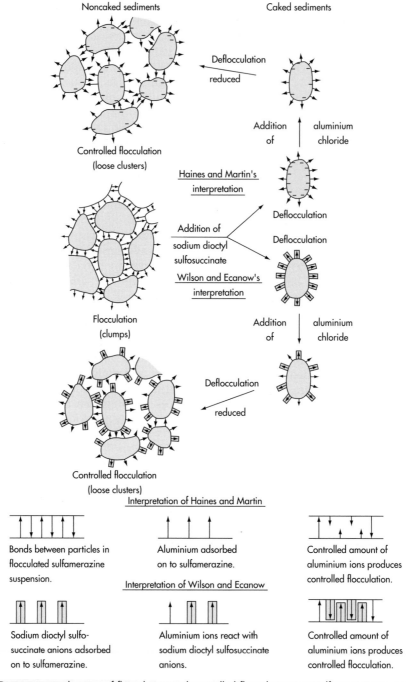

Noncaked sediments

Caked sediments

Controlled flocculation
(loose clusters)

Haines and Martin's
interpretation

Addition of
sodium dioctyl
sulfosuccinate

Wilson and Ecanow's
interpretation

Flocculation
(clumps)

Deflocculation
reduced

Addition   aluminium
of   chloride

Deflocculation

Deflocculation

Addition   aluminium
of   chloride

Deflocculation
reduced

Controlled flocculation
(loose clusters)

Interpretation of Haines and Martin

Bonds between particles in
flocculated sulfamerazine
suspension.

Aluminium adsorbed
on to sulfamerazine.

Controlled amount of
aluminium ions produces
controlled flocculation.

Interpretation of Wilson and Ecanow

Sodium dioctyl sulfo-
succinate anions adsorbed
on to sulfamerazine.

Aluminium ions react with
sodium dioctyl sulfosuccinate
anions.

Controlled amount of
aluminium ions produces
controlled flocculation.

Figure 7.31 Diagrammatic drawing of flocculation and controlled flocculation in a sulfamerazine suspension: the effect of the addition of sodium dioctyl sulfosuccinate (docusate sodium) and aluminium chloride is shown and two interpretations of the results are outlined.
Reproduced from R. Woodford, *Pharmacy Digest*, 29, 17 (1966).

the diagram. These are the observable results of these procedures. The different interpretations of the effects are diagrammatically realised, the difference lying in the manner in which the aluminium ions adsorb onto the sulfamerazine particles; in one view they adsorb directly, and in the other view they interact with the surfactant ions on the surface.

Barium sulfate as an X-ray contrast medium

The formulation of barium sulfate ($BaSO_4$) suspensions as a radio-opaque material has to be carefully controlled for use. Flocculation of the suspended particles, which can be caused by the mucin in the gastrointestinal tract, causes artefacts to be seen in radiography. Such factors as particle size, zeta potential, pH-dependence of the properties of adjuvants and the whole suspension, and the film-forming characteristics of the formulation must be taken into account. The preparation must flow readily over the mucosal surface, penetrate into folds and coat the surface evenly with a thin radio-opaque layer. A film 2 μm thick will absorb twice as much radiation as a layer 1 μm thick if the average $BaSO_4$ particle size and concentration are the same in both cases. The adhesion of wet films of barium sulfate suspensions to surfaces and their thickness have been assessed *in vitro* by a simple method in which a clean microscope slide is dipped into the suspension and allowed to drain for 30 s. The gross appearance displays evidence of irregular coating caused by foaming, bubble formation, or coagulation of particles. Commercially available suspensions preferred by radiologists are strongly negative at low pH, presumably resisting flocculation because of strong interparticle repulsion.

Polymers as flocculating agents

In many applications, such as water purification, suspended particles have to be removed by filtration. Flocculated particles are more readily removed than deflocculated particles. Polymers have been widely used as flocculating agents. Polymers used as flocculating or destabilising agents frequently act by adsorption and interparticle bridging. To be effective, the polymer must contain chemical groups that can interact with the surface of the colloidal particles. A particle–polymer complex is then formed, with polymer emerging into the aqueous phase. This free end will attach itself to another particle ('bridging') and thus promote flocculation. If there are no particles with which to interact, the polymer can coat the particle, leading to restabilisation. As can be seen in Fig. 7.32, however, the action of polymeric agents which can anchor at the particle surface is very concentration-dependent.

Polyacrylamide (30% hydrolysed) is an anionic polymer which can induce flocculation in kaolinite at very low concentrations. Restabilisation occurs by 'overdosing', probably by the mechanism outlined in Fig. 7.32. Dosages of polymer which are sufficiently large to saturate the colloidal surfaces produce a stable colloidal system, since no sites are available for the formation of interparticle bridges. Under certain conditions, physical agitation of the system can lead to breaking of polymer–suspension bonds and to a change in the state of the system.

7.4.3 Extemporaneous suspensions

Extemporaneous preparation of suspensions of drugs available commercially only in other dose forms is widely practised in hospital pharmacy, particularly for paediatric use. Drugs such as acetazolamide, amiodarone and mercaptopurine are examples. In such formulations, alternatives to traditional suspending agents such as tragacanth should be examined. The ideal suspending agent should:

- Be readily and uniformly incorporated in the formulation
- Be readily dissolved or dispersed in water without resort to special techniques
- Ensure the formation of a loosely packed system which does not cake
- Not influence the dissolution rate or absorption rate of the drug

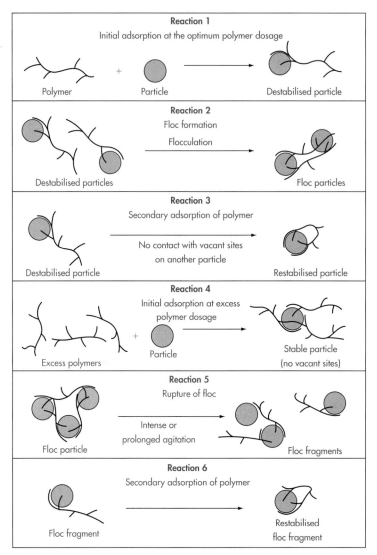

Figure 7.32 Schematic representation of the bridging model for the destabilisation of colloids by polymers: the concentration dependence of the process is illustrated.
Reproduced from W. J. Weber, *Physicochemical Processes for Water Quality Control*, Wiley, New York, 1972.

- Be inert, nontoxic and free from incompatibilities

Among the alternatives are sodium carboxymethylcellulose, microcrystalline cellulose, aluminium magnesium silicate (Veegum), sodium alginate (Manucol) and sodium starch (Primojel). Pregelatinised starches, Primojel and Veegum, are promising alternatives to compound tragacanth powder.

7.4.4 Suspension rheology

In deriving an equation for the viscosity of a suspension of spherical particles, Einstein considered particles which were far enough apart to be treated independently. The particle volume fraction ϕ is defined by

$$\phi = \frac{\text{volume occupied by the particles}}{\text{total volume of the suspension}} \quad (7.29)$$

The suspension could be assigned an effective viscosity, η_*, given by

$$\eta_* = \eta_0(1 + 2.5\phi) \qquad (7.30)$$

where η_0 is the viscosity of the suspending fluid. As we have seen, the assumptions involved in the derivation of the Einstein equation do not hold for colloidal systems subject to Brownian forces, electrical interactions and van der Waals forces. Brownian forces result from 'the random jostling of particles by the molecules of the suspending fluid due to thermal agitation and fluctuation on a very short time scale'.

A charged particle in suspension with its inner immobile Stern layer and outer diffuse Gouy (or Debye–Hückel) layer presents a different problem from that arising with a smooth and small nonpolar sphere. In movement such particles experience electroviscous effects which have two sources: (a) the resistance of the ion cloud to deformation, and (b) the repulsion between particles in close contact. When particles interact, for example to form pairs in the system, the new particle will have a different shape from the original and will have different flow properties. The coefficient 2.5 in Einstein's equation (7.30)

applies only to spheres; asymmetric particles will produce coefficients greater than 2.5.

Other problems in deriving *a priori* equations result from the polydisperse nature of pharmaceutical suspensions. The particle size distribution will determine η. A polydisperse suspension of spheres has a lower viscosity than a similar monodisperse suspension.

Structure formation during flow is an additional complication. Structure breakdown occurs also and is evident particularly in clay suspensions, which are generally flocculated at rest. Under flow there is a loss of the structure and the suspension exhibits thixotropy and a yield point. The viscosity decreases with increasing shear stress (Fig. 7.33).

Addition of electrolytes to a suspension decreases the thickness of the double layer and reduces electroviscous effects, an effect reflected in the reduced viscosity of the suspension.

7.4.5 Nonaqueous suspensions

Many pharmaceutical aerosols consist of solids dispersed in a nonaqueous propellant. Few studies have been published on the behaviour

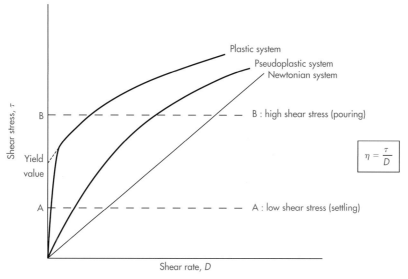

Figure 7.33 A plot of shear stress τ against shear rate D for plastic and pseudoplastic suspensions. As $\eta = \tau/D$, the slope of the line represents the viscosity at each rate of shear; in both the plastic and pseudoplastic systems the viscosity at level A is greater than that at level B.
Modified from J. C. Samyn, *J. Pharm. Sci.*, 50, 517 (1961).

of such systems, although their sensitivity to water is well established. Low amounts of water adsorb at the particle surface and can lead to aggregation of the particles with each other or to deposition on the walls of the container, which adversely affects the product.

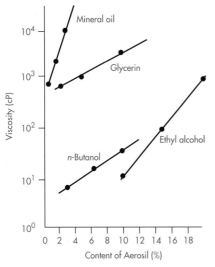

Figure 7.34 Influence of the polarity of the medium on the increase in viscosity attainable with Aerosil 200, a coagulated silica sol.
Reproduced from *Degussa's Technical Bulletin* No. 4 on Aerosil.

Oleogels

Lipophilic ointment bases and nonaqueous suspensions may be thickened with materials such as Aerosil, a coagulated silica sol. Incorporation of the silica into an oil leads to an increase in viscosity, which is brought about by hydrogen bonding between the silica particles. Silica (Aerosil 200) at 8–10% imparts a paste-like consistency to a range of oils such as isopropyl myristate, peanut oil and silicone oil. The degree to which viscosity is increased is a function of the polarity of the oil, the silica being more effective in nonpolar media (see Fig. 7.34). Suspensions of silica in oils are thixotropic; on storage for several days the viscosity increases owing to the slow aggregation of the silica particles, shown schematically in Fig. 7.35.

7.4.6   Adhesion of suspension particles to containers: immersional, spreading and adhesional wetting

When the walls of a container are wetted repeatedly, an adhering layer of suspension particles may build up, and this subsequently

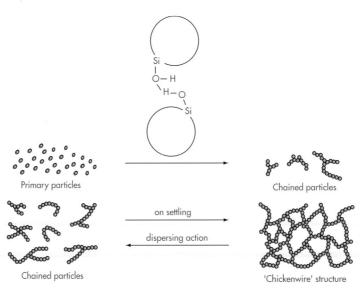

Figure 7.35 Schematic representation of the interaction between two Aerosil particles (top), the formation of a chain structure (centre), and the development of a 'chickenwire' structure as well as thixotropy (bottom). The mean particle diameter of Aerosil is 10 nm.
Reproduced from *Degussa's Technical Bulletin* No. 4 on Aerosil.

dries to a hard and thick layer. In Fig. 7.36 three types of wetting are shown. Where the suspension is in constant contact with the container wall, immersional wetting occurs, in which particles are pressed up to the wall and may or may not adhere. Above the liquid line, spreading of the suspension during shaking or pouring may also lead to adhesion of the particles contained in the spreading liquid. Adhesional wetting occurs when a liquid drop remains suspended, like a drop of water on a clothes line. Evidently the surface tension of the suspension plays a part in the spreading and wetting processes.

Adhesion increases with increase in suspension concentration, and with the number of contacts the suspension makes with the surfaces in question.

Additives, especially surfactants, will modify the adhesion of suspension particles. They will act in two ways: (a) by decreasing the surface tension; and (b) by adsorption modifying the forces of interaction between particle and container. The example illustrated in Figs. 7.37 and 7.38 refers to the addition of benzethonium chloride to chloramphenicol suspensions. Benzethonium chloride converts both the glass surface and the particles into positively charged entities (see Fig. 7.37). Adhesion in the presence of this cationic surfactant is concentration-dependent, the process being akin to flocculation. At low concentrations the surfactant adsorbs by its cationic head to the negative glass and to the suspension particle. The glass is thus made hydrophobic. At higher concentrations hydrophobic interactions occur between coated particle and surface (Fig. 7.38). Further increase in concentration results in multilayer formation of surfactant, rendering the surfaces hydrophilic. In this condition the particles repel, reducing adhesion.

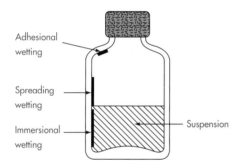

Figure 7.36 Adhesion. (a) Three types of wetting giving rise to adhesion of suspension particles. (Modified from H. Uno and S. Tanaka, *Kolloid Z. Z. Polym.*, 250, 238 (1972).) Suspended particles adhering to the surface of a glass vial can be seen in Figure 7.27 on page 255.

Miscellaneous colloidal systems

Several colloidal systems have not been mentioned in this chapter because they are dealt with elsewhere. These include nanoparticle suspensions used in drug delivery and targeting, and vesicular dispersions (liposomes,

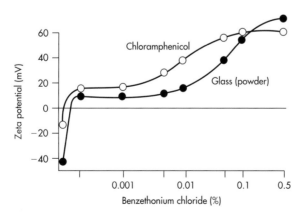

Figure 7.37 Zeta potential of glass (powder) and chloramphenicol in aqueous benzethonium chloride solutions.
Reproduced from H. Uno and S. Tanaka, *Kolloid Z. Z. Polym.*, 250, 238 (1972).

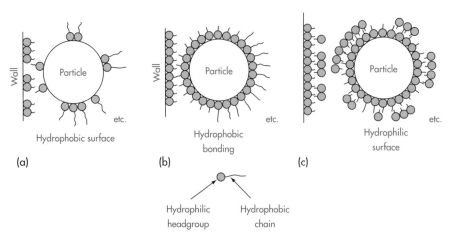

Figure 7.38 Adsorption of benzethonium chloride on particle and wall surfaces creating in (a) hydrophobic surfaces and in (b) hydrophobic bonding between the adsorbed molecules. In (c) further additions of the benzethonium chloride results in the conversion to hydrophilic surfaces.
Modified from H. Uno and S. Tanaka, *Kolloid Z. Z. Polym.*, 250, 238 (1972).

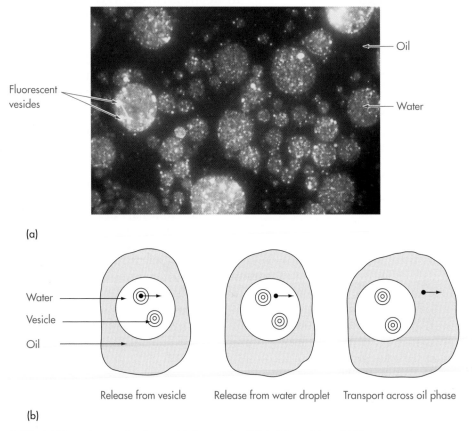

Figure 7.39 (a) Photomicrograph of a vesicle-in-water-in-oil (v/w/o) emulsion. (b) Diagrammatic representation of the modes of release of solutes from the formulation (● = drug).

niosomes, etc). Variations on the emulsion theme include microsphere-in-water-in-oil systems (s/w/o) and vesicle-in-water-in-oil (v/w/o) formulations. (Fig. 7.39).

7.5 Applications of colloid stability theory to other systems

There are several colloidal systems other than synthetically produced emulsions and suspensions which are of interest – blood and other cell suspensions, for example – whose behaviour can now be better understood by application of colloid stability theory. The adhesion of cells to surfaces, the aggregation of platelets, the spontaneous sorting out of mixed cell aggregates and other such phenomena, depend to a large extent on interaction between the surfaces of the objects in question, although the surfaces are frequently more labile and less homogeneous than those encountered in model colloids. The extended circulation in the blood of 'long life' or 'stealth' liposomes whose surfaces are modified by protruding long surface bonded hydrophilic chains (usually polyoxyethylene glycols) may also be ascribed to their modified interactions *in vivo* with opsonins and with scavenging cells of the reticuloendothelial system.

7.5.1 Cell–cell interactions

A simple way of considering interactions between free-floating cells is to treat the cells as spheres. Adhesion between cells in contact is, however, best considered as interaction between planar surfaces (Fig. 7.40).

Cell adhesion and separation occur during the interaction of sperm and egg, in cell fusion and in parasitism; phagocytosis may also have an adhesive component. Cell adhesion can occur with a variety of nonliving materials such as implanted prosthetic devices.

Adhesion is primarily a surface phenomenon. The main factors which act to produce adhesion are:

- Bridging mechanisms (sensitisation)
- Electrostatic interactions
- Interactions involving long-range forces

As in suspension flocculation, the bridging agent will be a molecule which combines in some way with both surfaces and thus links them together. Macromolecules may adsorb onto the surface of the particle and, if the length of the molecule is greater than twice the range of the electrostatic forces of repulsion, the other end of the molecule may adsorb on to a second surface. Flexible molecules may adsorb on to the same cell or particle. Alternatively, polyvalent ions may bind to charged groups on the two adjacent surfaces. Brownian motion may provide the means for close approach of the particles or the polyvalent ion and may so reduce the electrostatic repulsion that the cells can approach each other.

Electrostatic forces of attraction will come into play when the surfaces have opposite sign or charge or when the surfaces possess mosaics of charges such that interaction can occur. The long-range forces are those discussed earlier in the chapter. In studying echinoderm egg attachment to glass, an inverse relationship was found between zeta potential and adhesiveness, when zeta potential was controlled by the addition of monovalent cations. Low pH, high ionic strength and the presence of covalent cations all favour cell–cell adhesion.

Artificial bridging adhesion between cells is known. Immunological procedures which involve the agglutination of cells by an antibody (or antigen when the cells are coated with antibody) appear to be bridging reactions.

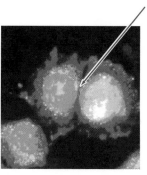

Flattened surface between two adhering cells

Figure 7.40 Interacting cells with a planar interface formed between them.
Photograph: J Ivaska, Centre for Biotech, Finland.

Polycations may be used to flocculate cells; erythrocytes have been flocculated with poly-lysine, and polyvinylamine hydrochloride and protamine sulfate clump cells. Lectins (phyto-haemagglutinins) stimulate cell adhesion by combining with certain sugar groupings on the plasmalemma glycolipids or glycoproteins. Instances of such specific interactions can be vital in targeting drugs to cells, but this is outside the scope of this chapter.

It is not possible to discuss all cell–cell reactions rigorously. Often adhesion results in the secretion of complex chemicals which further induce interaction which cannot be treated by any physicochemical model.

7.5.2 Adsorption of microbial cells to surfaces

The contamination of pharmaceutical suspensions for oral use is a cause of concern. The behaviour of organisms in such suspensions therefore needs to be examined before interpretation of experimental results can be undertaken. Under some conditions, bacteria may be strongly adsorbed and therefore more resistant to the effects of preservatives; in other cases, the bacteria may be free in suspension.

Two distinct phases of bacterial adsorption onto glass have been observed;[12] the first, reversible, phase may be interpreted in terms of DLVO theory. Reversible sorption of a non-mobile strain (*Achromobacter*) decreased to zero as the electrolyte concentration of the medium was increased, as would be expected. The second, irreversible, phase is probably the result of polymeric bridging between bacterial cell and the surface in contact with it. It is obviously not easy to apply colloid theory directly, but the influence of factors such as surface potential, pH and additives can usually be predicted and experimentally confirmed.

In the agglutination of erythrocytes and the adsorption of erythrocytes to virus-infected cells, projections of small radius of curvature have been observed and could well account for the local penetration of the energy barrier and strong adhesion at the primary minimum. The various modes of cell sorption are shown diagrammatically in Fig. 7.41.

Sorption of microbial cells is selective but there is no obvious relation between Gram-staining characteristics and attachment. In Fig. 7.41, bacterial cells are shown adsorbing onto larger solid particles (a) or free in suspension (b); (c) illustrates the opposite effect – small particles are shown adsorbed onto bacterial cells. The bacterial cells are adsorbed onto flocculated particles in (d), onto solid surfaces in (e); (f)–(i) show the more complicated behaviour of bacterial forms with coats, cilia and flagella. The adsorption affects growth partly by masking the cell surface and

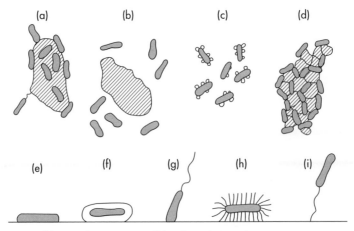

Figure 7.41 Various types of bacterial sorption on solid surfaces (see text).

Reproduced from D. Zvyagintsev, *Interaction between Microorganisms and Solid Surfaces*, Moscow University Press, Moscow, 1973.

partly by altering the release of metabolites from the cell.

Addition of HCl and NaOH to drug suspensions alters the adhesion of *E. coli* to kaolinite (Fig. 7.42). The negative charge of the cell surfaces will decrease with decrease in pH; the isoelectric point of many bacteria lies between pH 2 and 3. At pH values lower than the isoelectric point the cell surface carries a positive charge. The flat surface of the clay also carries a negative charge, which also diminishes with decrease of pH; the positive charge localised on the edge of the clay platelet will be observed only in acidic solution.

In addition to the van der Waals and electrical forces, steric forces resulting from protruding polysaccharide and protein molecules affect interactions; specific interactions between charged groups on the cell surface and on the solid surface, hydrogen bonding or the formation of cellular bridges may all occur to complicate the picture. The ten possible forces of interaction between cells and surfaces have been listed as:

- Chemical bonds between opposed surfaces
- Ion-pair formation
- Forces due to charge fluctuation
- Charge mosaics on surfaces of like or opposite overall charge
- Electrostatic attraction between surfaces of opposite charge
- Electrostatic repulsion between surfaces of like charge
- Van der Waals' forces
- Surface energy
- Charge repulsion
- Steric barriers

7.5.3 Blood as a colloidal system

Blood is a non-Newtonian suspension showing a shear-dependent viscosity. At low rates of shear, erythrocytes form cylindrical aggregates (rouleaux), which break up when the rate of shear is increased. Calculations show that the shear rate (D) associated with blood flow in large vessels such as the aorta is about 100 s^{-1}, but for flow in capillaries it rises to about 1000 s^{-1}. The flow characteristics of blood are similar to those of emulsions except that, while shear deformation of oil globules can occur with a consequent change in surface tension, no change in membrane tension

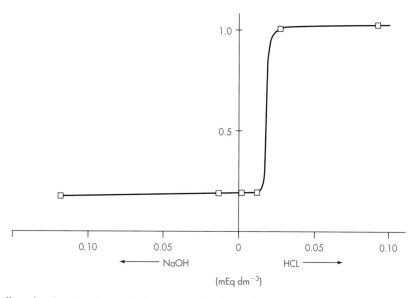

Figure 7.42   Effect of HCl and NaOH on the formation and stability of *E. coli*–kaolinite complexes. The ordinate signifies the number of cells adhering to one clay particle. Addition of sodium hydroxide decreases adhesion.
Reproduced from T. Hattori, *J. Gen. Appl. Microbiol.*, 16, 351 (1970).

occurs on cell deformation. Figure 7.43 shows the viscosity of blood at low shear rates, measured in a Brookfield LVT micro cone-plate viscometer.

Figure 7.43 also shows the influence of a surfactant on blood flow: low concentrations of sodium oleate decrease the viscosity but concentrations higher than 60 mg per 100 cm^3 increase it. One would anticipate changes in viscosity on addition of an anionic surfactant, but strict interpretation is complicated by the fact that a reversible morphological effect takes place in the erythrocyte. Surfactants such as sodium oleate are able to disaggregate

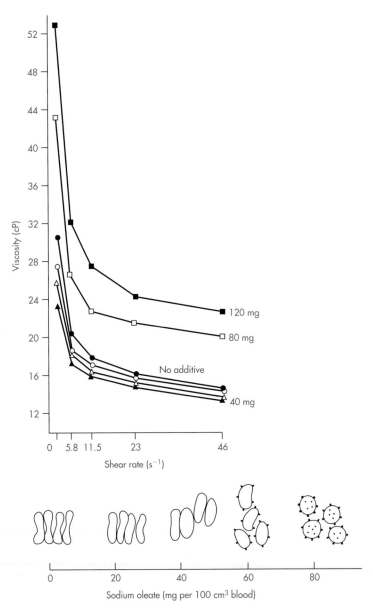

Figure 7.43 The influence of varying concentrations of sodium oleate on the viscosity of blood at different rates of shear; each value represents an average of 8 subjects.
Reproduced from A. M. Ehrly, *Biorheology*, 5, 209 (1968).

clumped cells and consequently would be expected to reduce the viscosity. At higher concentrations the increase in viscosity may be due to an electroviscous effect or the altered shape of the erythrocytes.

Velocity gradients in blood vessels are reduced in cases of retarded peripheral circulation, especially in shock. Under these conditions erythrocytes may aggregate and the discovery of agents that are capable of reducing this structural viscosity is thus of great clinical value. Dextrans and polyvinylpyrrolidones diminish attraction between individual cells in blood and improve flow properties.

Aggregation of platelets involves a contact phase and an adhesive phase, shown diagrammatically in Fig. 7.44. There is good evidence that most thrombi forming within the arterial tree after endothelial injury consist initially of a mass of associated particles on the surface of the vessel. The shearing effects of blood may dislodge platelets.

Interest in platelet interaction with simpler surfaces has been stimulated by the increasing use of plastic prosthetic devices which come into contact with blood. While we do not have a clear idea of the physical and chemical properties of surfaces that are responsible for the attraction of platelets, a relationship between adhesion and the critical surface tension of uncharged hydrophobic surfaces has been demonstrated. The number of platelets adsorbed increases as the critical surface tension increases. There is other evidence that platelets adhere readily to a high-energy hydrophilic surface and less readily to low-energy hydrophobic surfaces. Thus platelet adhesion to glass is reduced following coating the latter with dimethylsiloxane.

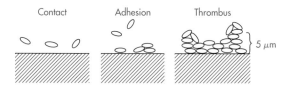

Figure 7.44 Sequence in the formation of a thrombus at a surface involving three stages: contact, adhesion and thrombus growth.

7.6 Foams and defoamers

Aqueous foams are formed from a three-dimensional network of surfactant films in air. Foams can be used as formulations for the delivery of enemas and topical products. Foams which develop in production of liquids or in ampoules are troublesome; hence there is an interest in breaking foams and preventing foam formation. The breaking and prevention of liquid foams is less well understood than the stabilisation of foams. It is recognised, however, that small quantities of specific agents can reduce foam stability markedly. There are two types of such agent:

- *Foam breakers*, which are thought to act as small droplets forming in the foam lamellae (see Fig. 7.45)
- *Foam preventatives*, which are thought to adsorb at the air/water interface in preference to the surfactants which stabilise the thin films

The latter, however, do not have the capacity, once adsorbed, to stabilise the foam. It is well established that pure liquids do not foam. Transient foams are obtained with solutes such as short-chain aliphatic alcohols or acids which lower the surface tension moderately; really persistent foams arise only with solutes that lower the surface tension strongly in dilute solution – the highly surface-active materials such as detergents and proteins. The physical chemistry of the surface layers of the solutions is what determines the stability of the system.

Foam is a disperse system with a high surface area, and consequently foams tend to collapse spontaneously. Ordinarily, three-dimensional foams of surfactant solutes persist for a matter of hours in closed vessels. Gas slowly diffuses from the small bubbles to the large ones (since the pressure and hence thermodynamic activity of the gas within the bubbles is inversely proportional to bubble radius). Diffusion of gas leads to a rearrangement of the foam structures and this is often sufficient to rupture the thin lamellae in a well-drained film.

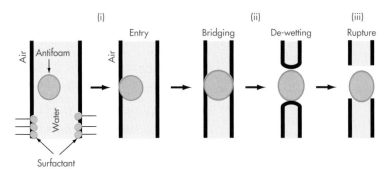

Figure 7.45 A schematic drawing of the antifoaming mechanism of antifoam droplets (i) entering a foam lamella, (ii) bridging–de-wetting and (iii) rupturing the foam wall.
Reproduced from D. Perry, J. Zeng and V. O'Neil, *Foam Control in Aqueous Coatings*, Dow Corning Corporation, 2001.

The most important action of an antifoam agent is to eliminate surface elasticity – the property that is responsible for the durability of foams. To do this it must displace foam stabiliser. It must therefore have a low interfacial tension in the pure state to allow it to spread when applied to the foam, and it must be present in sufficient quantity to maintain a high surface concentration. Many foams can be made to collapse by applying drops of liquids such as ether, or long chain alcohols such as octanol. Addition of ether, which has a low surface tension, to an aqueous foam will locally produce regions with a low surface tension. These regions are rapidly pulled out by surrounding regions of higher tension. The foam breaks because the ethereal region cannot stretch. Long-chain alcohols also break foams because the surface is swamped by rapidly diffusing molecules so that changes in surface tension are rapidly reversed (that is, elasticity disappears).

Generally more effective and more versatile than any soluble antifoams are the silicone fluids, which have surface tensions as low as 20 mN m^{-1}. Quantities of the order of 1–60 ppm prevent foaming in fermentation vats, sewage tanks and dyebaths. Polyfluorinated hydrocarbons will lower surface tensions to the order of 10 mN m^{-1}.

Antifoam droplets are seen in Fig. 7.45 entering the foam lamella, bridging between the surfaces, dewetting and then rupturing the foam wall.

Table 7.7 *In vivo* effects of polydimethylsiloxane (PDMS)[a]

Treatment by mouth	Volume (cm^3)	Dose (mg/rat)		Mean percentage reduction[b] in foam height (± SEM).
		PDMS	Silica	
PDMS	0.25	250		19 ± 4
	0.50	500		29 ± 6
	1.00	1000		56 ± 6
	2.00	2000		84 ± 3
PDMS containing 65 w/v silica	0.005	4.7	0.2	45 ± 6
	0.01	9.4	0.6	58 ± 5
	0.02	18.9	1.1	61 ± 5
	0.04	37.7	2.0	87 ± 2

[a] Reproduced from R. D. N. Birtley, J. S. Burton *et al.*, *J. Pharm. Pharmacol.*, 25, 859 (1973).
[b] 10 rats in each group; foam induced by saponin.

Table 7.8 *In vitro* froth test: time taken for antifoam agent to remove experimental foam[a]

Frothing system	Antacid preparation[b]	Froth reduction	
		Time(s)	Extent (%)
Cetomacrogol–0.1 mol dm^{-3} HCl	Asilone tablet	17	100
	Asilone	60	80
Cetomacrogol–saturated NaHCO$_3$	Asilone tablet	20	100
	Asilone (ether-extracted)	–	0–10

[a] Reproduced from reference 14.
[b] Ether extraction removes dimethicone.

7.6.1 Clinical considerations

X-ray studies have clearly shown the presence of foam in the upper gastrointestinal tract in humans. Silicone antifoaming agents derive their value from their ability to change the surface tension of the mucus-covered gas bubbles in the gut and thus to cause the bubbles to coalesce. A range of polydimethyl-siloxanes is available commercially, including Dimethicones 20, 200, 350, 500 and 1000 (the numbers refer to the viscosity of the oil in centistokes). In simple *in vitro* tests polydi-methylsiloxane, of molecular weight used in pharmaceutical formulations (Dimethicone 1000), has poor antifoaming properties. The addition of a small percentage (2–8%) of hydrophobic silica, which on its own is a weak defoamer, increases the antifoaming effect, the finely divided silica particles being suspended in the silicone fluid. The product is a simple physical mixture of silica and poly-dimethylsiloxane. Some *in vivo* results are listed in Table 7.7. The incorporation of these materials into antacid tablets is widespread; certain antacids have been found, however, to adsorb the polydimethylsiloxane and reduce its antifoaming potential.[13] Unbound extract-able silicone is primarily responsible for the antifoaming properties of the tablets[14] (Table 7.8). The ability of silica to defoam has been attributed to the fine particles, which cause the small bubbles to coalesce.

Summary

This chapter has covered the topic of pharma-ceutical colloids, with a special emphasis on emulsions and suspensions. These have been rather traditional pharmaceutical forms, but they are attracting increasing interest because of increased knowledge of the biodistribution and fate of colloidal particles in the body, and the need to deliver highly lipophilic and often very potent drugs in carriers. Emulsions, microemulsions and solid suspensions are all, therefore, important in modern drug delivery.

The chapter has dealt with the stability and stabilisation of colloidal systems and covered topics such as their formation and aggrega-tion. If the particle size of a colloidal particle determines its properties (such as viscosity or fate in the body), then maintenance of that particle size throughout the lifetime of the product is important. The emphasis in the section on stability is understandable. Various forms of emulsions, microemulsions and multiple emulsions have also been discussed, while other chapters deal with other impor-tant colloidal systems, such as protein and polymer micro- and nanospheres and phos-pholipid and surfactant vesicles.

Towards the end of the chapter we point out the biological importance of an understanding of colloid chemistry and several examples of biological importance are covered. Pharma-ceutical and biological colloids are often very complex systems, but even so the fundamental principles can be applied to obtain an appreciation of the behaviour of systems such as blood, platelets and microorganisms when they come in contact with inert or biological surfaces. In simplifying the concepts here, we do not pretend that there are no other forces at work. It is nonetheless useful to think of complex systems in a straightforward physico-chemical manner, as pointed out in the introduction to the book.

References

1. A. T. Florence and D. Whitehill. Some features of breakdown in water-in-oil-in-water multiple emulsions. *J. Colloid Interface Sci.*, 79, 243–56 (1981)

2. A. T. Florence and D. Whitehill. Stability and stabilization of water-in-oil-in-water multiple emulsions. In *Macro- and Micro-Emulsions* (ed. D. O. Shah), ACS Symposium Series No. 272, American Chemical Society, Washington DC, 1983, pp. 359–80

3. J. M. Kovarik, L. Vevnillet, E. A. Mueller, *et al.* Cyclosporine disposition and metabolite profiles in renal transplant patients receiving a micro-emulsion formulation. *Ther. Drug. Monit.* 16, 519–25, (1994)

4. J. M. Kovarik, E. A. Mueller, J. B. van Bree, *et al.* Cyclosporine pharmacokinetics and variability from a microemulsion formulation – a multicenter investigation in kidney transplant patients. *Transplantation*, 58, 658–63 (1994)

5. E. A. Mueller, J. M. Kovarik, J. B. van Bree, *et al.* Improved dose linearity of cyclosporine pharmacokinetics from a microemulsion formulation. *Pharm Res.*, 11, 301–4 (1994)

6. P. P. Constantinides, G. Welzel, H. Ellens, *et al.* Water-in-oil microemulsions containing medium-chain fatty acids/salts: formulation and intestinal absorption enhancement evaluation. *Pharm Res.*, 13, 210–15 (1996)

7. B. W. Barry. Structure and rheology of emulsions stabilized by mixed emulsifiers. *Rheol. Acta*, 10, 96–105 (1971)

8. G. H. Konning. Effects of formulation on preservative availability in fixed oil emulsified systems. *Can. J. Pharm. Sci.*, 9, 103–7 (1974)

9. T. L. Whateley, G. Steele, J. Urwin and G. A. Smail. Particle size stability of Intralipid and mixed total parenteral nutrition mixtures. *J. Clin. Hosp. Pharm.*, 9, 113–26 (1984)

10. T. Yamaguchi, N. Tanabe, Y. Fukushima, *et al.* Distribution of prostaglandin E_1 in lipid emulsion in relation to release rate from lipid particles. *Chem. Pharm. Bull.*, 42, 646–50 (1994)

11. N. L. Henderson, P. M. Meer and H. B. Kostenbauder. Approximate rates of shear encountered in some pharmaceutical processes. *J. Pharm. Sci.*, 50, 788–91 (1961)

12. K. C. Marshall, R. Stout and R. Mitchell. Mechanism of the initial events in the sorption of marine bacteria to surfaces. *J. Gen. Microbiol.*, 68, 337–48 (1971)

13. M. J. Rezak. *In vitro* determination of deforming inactivation of silicone antacid tablets. *J. Pharm. Sci.*, 55, 538–9 (1966)

14. J. E. Carless, J. B. Stenlake and W. D. Williams. Effect of particulate dispersing agents on the antifoaming properties of dimethicone 1000 in antiflatulent products. *J. Pharm. Pharmacol.*, 25, 849–53 (1973)

8

Polymers and macromolecules

This survey of the pharmaceutical aspects of polymers and macromolecules emphasises their use in formulation. It stresses the key features of polymers – their molecular weight distribution and their versatility in terms of their morphology, crystallinity, solubility and performance.

It is convenient to think of polymeric systems as either water-soluble or water-insoluble. This division, while not rigid as some polymers are water-dispersible, is useful in that it separates the two main areas of use which form the basis of this chapter. Water-soluble materials are used to modify the viscosity of aqueous solutions and to maintain the stability of suspensions, to form the basis of film coatings and as the basis of water-soluble matrices (for example, the higher molecular weight polyoxyethylene glycols as suppository bases). Adhesives for use in the buccal mucosa (bioadhesives) are usually water soluble, while pressure sensitive adhesives for use in transdermal particles tend to be polyacrylates and polysiloxanes. Water-insoluble materials form membranes and matrices. The factors affecting the transport of drugs in the systems should be understood: the thickness of the membrane, the solubility of the drug in the membrane and the relationship of this to its lipophilicity generally, copolymer ratios, porosity and heterogeneity of the mix caused by fillers or plasticisers.

Water-soluble polymers can be crosslinked electrostatically or covalently to give hydrogels. Crosslinked hydrogels absorb water but do not dissolve. The differences in release of drugs from water-insoluble matrices and from swelling hydrogels should be appreciated.

Homopolymer architectures

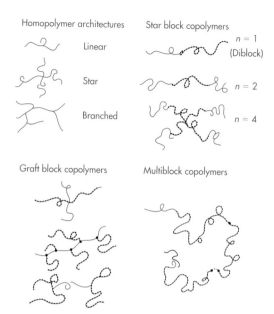

Figure 8.2 The range of structures of homopolymers and star block, graft block and multiblock copolymers.

reactions (generations); such chemical architecture has virtually no bounds. Dendrons are partial dendrimers.

8.1.2 Polydispersity

Nearly all synthetic polymers and naturally occurring macromolecular substances exist with a range of molecular weights; exceptions to this are proteins and natural polypeptides, each of which occurs as a substance with a single well-defined molecular weight. The molecular weight of a polymer or macromolecular subtance is thus an average molecular weight, which may be determined by chemical analysis or by osmotic pressure or light-scattering measurements. When determined by chemical analysis or osmotic pressure measurement a *number average* molecular weight, M_n, is found, which in a mixture containing n_1, n_2, n_3, ... moles of polymer with molecular weights M_1, M_2, M_3, ..., respectively, is defined by

$$M_n = \frac{n_1 M_1 + n_2 M_2 + n_3 M_3 + \cdots}{n_1 + n_2 + n_3 + \cdots} = \frac{\Sigma n_i M_i}{\Sigma n_i}$$

(8.1)

The individual molecular weights M_1, M_2, ... cannot be determined separately – the equation merely explains the meaning of the value M_n. In light-scattering techniques, larger molecules produce greater scattering; thus the weight (or more strictly the mass) rather than the number of the molecules is important, giving a *weight average* molecular weight, M_w:

$$M_w = \frac{m_1 M_1 + m_2 M_2 + m_3 M_3 + \cdots}{m_1 + m_2 + m_3 + \cdots} = \frac{\Sigma n_i M_i^2}{\Sigma n_i M_i}$$

(8.2)

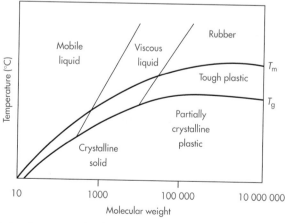

Figure 8.3 Approximate relation between molecular weight, T_g (glass transition temperature), T_m (melting point), and polymer properties.
Reproduced from F. W. Billmeyer, *Textbook of Polymer Science*, 2nd edn, Wiley, New York, 1971.

Table 8.1 Structural formulae of some macromolecular compounds

Name	Chain structure	Monomer
Polymers with a carbon chain backbone:		
Polyethylene	$-CH_2-CH_2-CH_2-CH_2-CH_2-$	$CH_2{=}CH_2$
Polypropylene	$-CH_2-CH-CH_2-CH-CH_2-CH-CH_2-$ with CH_3 groups	$CH_2{=}CH$, CH_3
Polystyrene	$-CH_2-CH-CH_2-CH-CH_2-CH-CH_2-$ with phenyl groups	$CH{=}CH_2$ with phenyl
Poly(vinyl chloride)	$-CH_2-CH-CH_2-CH-CH_2-CH-CH_2-$ with Cl groups	$CH_2{=}CH$, Cl
Polytetrafluoroethylene	$-C-C-C-C-C-C-$ with F groups	$F_2C{=}CF_2$
Polyacrylonitrile	$-CH_2-CH-CH_2-CH-CH_2-CH-CH_2-$ with CN groups	$CH_2{=}CH$, CN
Poly(vinyl alcohol)	$-CH_2-CH-CH_2-CH-CH_2-CH-CH_2-$ with HO groups	$CH_2{=}CH$, OH
Poly(vinyl acetate)	$-CH_2-CH-CH_2-CH-CH_2-CH-CH_2-$ with $O-C{=}O-CH_3$ groups	$CH_2{=}CH$, $O-C{=}O-CH_3$
Polyacrylamide	$-CH_2-CH-CH_2-CH-CH_2-CH-CH_2-$ with $CONH_2$ groups	$CH_2{=}CH$, $O{=}C-NH_2$
Poly(methyl methacrylate)	$-CH_2-C-CH_2-C-CH_2-C-CH_2-$ with CH_3 and $COOCH_3$ groups	$CH_2{=}C$ with CH_3 and $COOCH_3$
Polyvinylpyrrolidone	$-CH_2-CH-CH_2-CH-CH_2-CH-CH_2-$ with N-pyrrolidone groups	$CH_2{=}CH$ with N-pyrrolidone
Polymers with a heterochain backbone:		
Poly(ethylene oxide)	$-O-CH_2-CH_2-O-CH_2-CH_2-O-CH_2-CH_2-O-$	CH_2-CH_2 (epoxide)
Poly(propylene oxide)	$-O-CH_2-CH-O-CH_2-CH-O-CH_2-CH-O-$ with CH_3 groups	$CH_2-CH-CH_3$ (epoxide)
Cellulose (polyglucoside, $\beta \rightarrow 14$)		Glucose

The bulk viscosity of polymer solution is an important parameter also when polymers are being used as suspending agents to maintain solid particles in suspension by prevention of settling (see Chapter 7) and when they are used to modify the properties of liquid medicines for oral and topical use.

8.3 General properties of polymer solutions

8.3.1 Viscosity of polymer solutions

The presence in solution of large macromolecular solutes may have an appreciable effect on the viscosity of the solution. From a study of the concentration dependence of the viscosity it is possible to gain information on the shape or hydration of these polymers in solution and also their average molecular weight. The assumption is made in this section that the solution exhibits Newtonian flow characteristics.

The viscosity of solutions of macromolecules is conveniently expressed by the *relative viscosity*, defined as the ratio of the viscosity of the solution, η, to the viscosity of the pure solvent η_0:

$$\eta_{rel} = \frac{\eta}{\eta_0} \qquad (8.4)$$

Another useful expression is the *specific viscosity*, η_{sp}, of the solution, defined by

$$\eta_{sp} = \eta_{rel} - 1 \qquad (8.5)$$

For ideal solutions the ratio η_{sp}/c (called the *reduced viscosity*) is independent of solution concentration. In real solutions the reduced viscosity varies with concentration owing to molecular interactions and it is usual to extrapolate plots of η_{sp}/c versus c to zero concentration. The extrapolated value is called the *intrinsic viscosity* $[\eta]$.

Einstein showed from hydrodynamic theory that for a dilute system of rigid, spherical particles

$$\eta_{rel} = 1 + 2.5\phi \qquad (8.6)$$

i.e.

$$\lim_{\phi \to 0}(\eta_{sp}/\phi) = 2.5 \qquad (8.7)$$

where ϕ is the volume fraction of the particles, defined as the volume of the particles divided by the total volume of the solution.

Departure of the limiting value of η_{sp}/ϕ from the theoretical value of 2.5 may result from either hydration of the particles, or from particle asymmetry, or from both as discussed in Box 8.1.

Box 8.1   Effect of shape and hydration on viscosity

Effect of particle shape

A more general form of equation (8.6) allowing for particle asymmetry is

$$\eta_{rel} = 1 + \nu\phi \qquad (8.8)$$

where ν is a shape factor related to the axial ratio of an ellipsoid. In the case of nonhydration spheres ν reduces to 2.5. The volume is usually replaced by the weight concentration, c. For a macromolecule of hydrodynamic volume v_h and molecular weight M

$$\phi = \frac{N_A c v_h}{M} \qquad (8.9)$$

and equation (8.8) becomes

$$\eta_{rel} - 1 = \nu\phi = \frac{\nu N_A v_h c}{M} \qquad (8.10)$$

Hydration effects

Consider a hydrated macromolecule containing δ_1 grams of solvent per gram of dry macromolecular material. The specific volume v_0 (volume per gram) of the entrapped water may be considerably different from that of pure solvent, $v_1^{\ominus}$. If v_2 is the average specific volume of the macromolecular material, then the total hydrodynamic volume of the particle, v_h, is

$$v_h = \frac{M}{N_A}(v_2 + \delta_1 v_1) \qquad (8.11)$$

The total volume V of a solution containing g_1 grams of solvent and g_2 grams of dry macromolecular solute is

$$
\begin{aligned}
V &= \text{volume of solute} \\
&\quad + \text{volume of water of hydration} \\
&\quad + \text{volume of free solvent} \\
&= g_2 v_2 + g_2 \delta_1 v_1 + (g_1 - g_2 \delta_1) v_1^{\ominus} \qquad (8.12)
\end{aligned}
$$

Therefore,

$$\overline{v}_2 = \left(\frac{\partial V}{\partial g_2}\right)_{P,T,g_1} = v_2 + \delta_1 v_1 - \delta_2 v_2^{\ominus} \tag{8.13}$$

Substituting for v_2 in equation (8.11) gives

$$v_h = \frac{M}{N}(\overline{v}_2 + \delta_1 v_1^{\ominus}) \tag{8.14}$$

Substituting for v_h in equation (8.10),

$$[\eta] = \lim_{c \to 0}\left(\frac{\eta_{rel} - 1}{c}\right) = \nu(\overline{v}_2 + \delta_1 v_1^{\ominus}) \tag{8.15}$$

If the particle can be assumed to be unhydrated, or if the degree of hydration can be estimated with certainty from other experimental techniques, equation (8.15) may be used to determine the asymmetry of the particle. Alternatively, if the macromolecule may be assumed to be symmetrical or its asymmetry is known from other techniques, then this equation may be used to estimate the extent of hydration of the macromolecule.

Shape and solvent

As the shape of molecules is to a large extent the determinant of flow properties, change in shape due to changes in polymer–solvent interactions and the binding of small molecules with the polymer may lead to significant changes in solution viscosity. The nature of the solvent is thus of prime importance in this regard. In so-called 'good' solvents linear macromolecules will be expanded as the polar groups will be solvated. In a 'poor' solvent the intramolecular attraction between the segments is greater than the segment–solvent affinity and the molecule will tend to coil up (see Fig. 8.6). The viscosity of ionised macromolecules is complicated by charge interactions which vary with polymer concentration and additive concentration. Flexible charged macromolecules will vary in shape with the degree of ionisation. At maximum ionisation they are stretched out owing to mutual charge repulsion and the viscosity increases. On addition of small counterions the effective charge is reduced and the molecules contract; the viscosity falls as a result. Some of the effects are illustrated later in this

chapter in discussion of individual macromolecules, for example, gum Arabic (acacia).

The viscosity of solutions of globular proteins (which are more or less rigid) is only slightly affected by change in ionic strength. The intrinsic viscosity of serum albumin varies only between 3.6 and 4.1 $cm^3 g^{-1}$ when the pH is varied between 4.3 and 10.5 and the ionic strength between zero and 0.50.

Viscosity in pharmacopoeial specifications

In cases where control of molecular weight is important, for example in the use of dextran fractions as plasma expanders, a viscosity method is specified, for example, in the BP monograph. Staudinger proposed that the reduced viscosity of solutions of linear high polymers is proportional to the molecular weight of the polymer or its degree of polymerisation, p:

$$\frac{\eta_{sp}}{c} = K_m p \tag{8.16}$$

This empirical law has been modified to

$$\lim_{c \to 0} \frac{\eta_{sp}}{c} = [\eta] = KM^a \tag{8.17}$$

where a is a constant in the range 0–2, which for most high polymers has a value between 0.6 and 0.8, $[\eta]$ is the intrinsic viscosity as defined previously, and M is the molecular weight of the polymer. For a given polymer–solvent system, K and a are constant. Values of these constants may be determined from measurements on a series of fractions of known molecular weight and hence the molecular weight of an unknown fraction can be determined by measurement of the intrinsic viscosity. The *viscosity average* molecular weight is essentially a weight average since the larger macromolecules influence viscosity more than the smaller ones. The intrinsic viscosity of Dextran 40 BP is stated to be not less than 16 $cm^3 g^{-1}$ and not more than 20 $cm^3 g^{-1}$ at 37°C, while that of Dextran 110 is not less than 27 $cm^3 g^{-1}$ and not more than 32 $cm^3 g^{-1}$.

Ethylhydroxyethylcellulose is an ether of cellulose with both ethyl and hydroxyethyl substituents attached via ether linkages to the anhydroglucose rings. It swells in water to form a clear viscous colloidal solution. Preparation of solutions of cellulose derivatives requires hydration of the macromolecules, the rate of which is a function of both temperature and pH, as shown in the example in Fig. 8.18.

Ethylmethylcellulose contains ethyl and methyl groups, a 4% solution having approximately the same viscosity as acacia mucilage. *Hydroxyethylcellulose* is soluble in hot and cold water but does not gel. It has been used in ophthalmic solutions. More widely used for the latter, however, is *hydroxypropylmethylcellulose* (hypromellose) which is a mixed ether of cellulose containing 27–30% of $-OCH_3$ groups and 4–7.5% of $-OC_3H_6OH$ groups. It forms a viscous colloidal solution. There are various pharmaceutical grades. For example, hypromellose 20 is a 2% solution which has a viscosity between 15 and 25 cS (centistokes) at 20°C; the viscosity of a 2% hypromellose 15 000 solution lies between 12 000 and 18 000 cS. Hypromellose prolongs the action of medicated eyedrops and is employed as an artificial tear fluid.

Sodium carboxymethylcellulose is soluble in water at all temperatures. Because of the carboxylate group its mucilages are more sensitive to change in pH than are those of methylcellulose. The viscosity of a sodium carboxymethylcellulose mucilage is decreased markedly below pH 5 or above pH 10. Addition of heavy metal ions (Al^{3+}, Zn^{2+}, Fe^{2+}) causes changes in solution properties.

8.4.3 Natural gums and mucilages

Gum arabic (acacia) has been used in pharmacy as an emulsifier. It is a polyelectrolyte whose solutions are highly viscous owing to the branched structure of the macromolecular chains; its adhesive properties are also believed to be due to, or in some way related to, this branched structure. Molecular weights of between 200 000 and 250 000 (M_n) have been determined by osmotic pressure, values between 250 000 and 3×10^6 by sedimentation and diffusion, and values of 10^6 by light scattering, which also points to the shape of the molecules as short stiff spirals with numerous side-chains. Arabic acid prepared from commercial gum arabic by precipitation is a moderately strong acid whose aqueous solutions have a pH of 2.2–2.7. It has a higher viscosity than its salts, but emulsions prepared with arabic acid cream are not as stable as those made with its salts.

Whereas most gums are very viscous in aqueous solution, gum arabic is unusual in that, being extremely soluble, it can form solutions over a wide range of concentrations up to about 37% at 25°C. The marked variation in viscosity means that the gum arabic molecules must be flexible, with the ionic acid carboxyl groups distributed along the chain. At low pH the carboxyl groups are unionised. On increase of pH the carboxyl groups become progressively ionised and the folded chains expand owing to repulsion between the charged groups, causing an increase in viscosity. On addition of NaOH to the system the viscosity falls again as the concentration of counterion (Na^+) increases and effectively shields the acidic groups. The molecule then folds on itself. Similar falls in viscosity are exhibited on addition of sodium chloride.

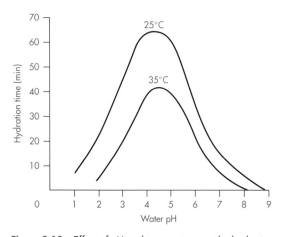

Figure 8.18 Effect of pH and temperature on the hydration time of fast-dissolving grades of hydroxyethylcellulose.
Reproduced from R. L. Whistler (ed.), *Industrial Gums*, 2nd edn, Academic Press, New York, 1973.

The effect of salt addition to the gum at fixed pH reflects the decrease in effective charge on the molecules of gum with resultant contraction and reduction in viscosity.

The gum arabic molecule is, in addition, surface-active, a 4% solution at 30°C has a surface tension of 63.2 mN m^{-1}. Addition of electrolytes makes the molecule more surface-active either by causing a change in conformation of the molecule at the interface, allowing closer packing, or by increasing the hydrophobicity of the molecule. It is an effective emulsifier, the stabilisation of the emulsion being dependent mainly on the coherence and elasticity of the interfacial film, which is by no means monomolecular.

Gum arabic is incompatible with several phenolic compounds (phenol, thymol, cresols, eugenol) and under suitable conditions forms coacervates (see section 8.6.3) with gelatin and positively charged polyelectrolytes.

Gum tragacanth partially dissolves in water; the soluble portion is called tragacanthin and this can be purified by precipitation from water by acetone or alcohol. Tragacanthin is a highly viscous polyelectrolyte with a molecular weight of 800 000 (as determined by sedimentation). It is one of the most widely used natural emulsifiers and thickeners. As its molecules have an elongated shape, its solutions have a high viscosity which, as with gum arabic, is dependent on pH. The maximum viscosity occurs at pH 8 initially, but because of ageing effects the maximum stable viscosity is near pH 5.

It is an effective suspending agent for pharmaceuticals and is used in conjunction with acacia as an emulsifier, the tragacanth imparting a high structural viscosity while the gum arabic adsorbs at the oil/water interface. It is also used in spermicidal jellies, acting by immobilising spermatozoa and as a viscous barrier.

Alginates: although the solutions of alginate are very viscous and set on addition of acid or calcium salts, they are less readily gelled than pectin and are used chiefly as stabilisers and thickening agents. Propylene glycol alginate does not precipitate in acid and as it is non-toxic is widely used as a stabiliser for foodstuffs. The molecules are highly asymmetric, with molecular weights in the range 47 000–370 000. Sodium alginate has the structure given in **X**.

Pectin is a purified carbohydrate product from extracts of the rind of citrus fruits and consists of partially methoxylated polygalacturonic acid (**XI**). It has remarkable gelling qualities but is also used therapeutically, often with kaolin, in the treatment of diarrhoea. It has been established that the longer the pectin chains, the greater its capacity for gel formation. The presence of inorganic cations and the degree of esterification of the carboxyl groups are important factors; in the case of calcium pectate gel it can be assumed that the calcium or indeed other polyvalent cations can interlink the chains by binding through $COO^- \cdots Ca^{2+} \cdots {}^-OOC$ interactions. Thus a high degree of esterification will disfavour

Structure **X** Sodium alginate

Structure 8.11 **XI** Partially methylated chain of poly(galacturonic acid) of pectin gelation in this case. In the absence of inorganic cations, however, a high degree of esterification aids gelation, suggesting that hydrophobic interactions cause the chains to associate. The properties of the formed gels also depend on the degree of esterification; the rigidity of the 40–60% ester pectin gels is higher than that of 70–80% ester jellies. This suggests that rigidity is due to hydrogen bonding between the hydroxyl groups and the free carboxyls.

8.4.4 Chitosan

Chitosan is a polymer obtained by the deacetylation of chitin, one of the most abundant polysaccharides. Chitosan, or poly[α-(1, 4)-2-amino-2-deoxy-D-glucopyranose] has the structure (**XII**). As might be expected the degree of deacetylation has a significant effect on the solubility and rheological properties of the polymer. At low pH, the polymer is soluble, with the sol–gel transition occurring at approximate pH 7. Chitosan also has filmforming abilities and its gel- and matrix-forming abilities make it useful for solid dosage forms, such as granules or microparticles.[5] The molecular weight, crystallinity and degree of deacetylation are all factors that can be varied to control the release rates from chitosan-based granules. When the positively charged chitosan is mixed in solution with polyanions such as gelatin, alginic acid and hyaluronic acid, interesting new matrix materials are formed.[6]

Structure XII The chemical structure of chitosan. The amine groups on the polymer have a pK_a in the range 5.5–6.5, depending on the source of the polymer

8.4.5 Dextran

Certain fractions of partially hydrolysed dextran are used as plasma substitutes or 'expanders'. Certain strains of *Leuconostoc meserentoides* are cultivated to synthesise dextran (**XIII**), which is a polymer of anhydroglucose, linked through α–1,6 glucosidic linkages. The chains are branched; on the average, one branch occurs for every 10–12 glucose residues. The intrinsic viscosity [η] is related to M by the relationship

$$[\eta] = 10^{-3}M^{1/2} \tag{8.23}$$

in the molecular weight range 20 000–200 000. The dextrans produced by fermentation are hydrolysed and fractionated to give a range of products suitable for injection. Dextran, being a hydrophilic colloid, exerts an osmotic pressure comparable to that of plasma and it is thus used to restore or maintain blood volume. Other substances that have been used in a similar way include hydroxyethyl starch, polyvinylpyrrolidone and gelatin.

Dextran injections are sterile solutions of dextran with weight average molecular weights of about 40 000–110 000. Dextrans with a molecular weight of about 50 000 or less are excreted in the urine within 48 hours of injection. Dextran molecules with higher molecular weights disappear more slowly from the bloodstream and are temporarily stored in the reticuloendothelial system.

Dextran 70 (mol. wt. ~70 000) and Dextran 110 (mol. wt. ~110 000) are used to maintain blood volume, and Dextran 40 is used primarily to prevent intravascular aggregation of blood cells and for assisting capillary blood flow. This latter effect is the result of dextran adsorption and stabilisation of the erythrocyte suspensions. If the higher molecular weight fractions exceed about 1% concentration in the blood, rouleaux tend to form. The sensitivity of blood to the concentration and molecular weight of dextran is clearly seen in Fig. 8.19, where aggregation and relative viscosity of red-cell suspensions are shown in the presence of varying amounts of five different dextrans. Molecular weight control is thus important and may be exercised by measurement of intrinsic viscosity, [η].

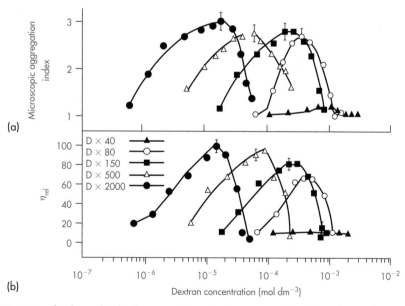

Structure XIII Dextran

Figure 8.19 Variation of indices of red-cell aggregation with the concentration of five dextran fractions of different molecular weight: (a) microscopic aggregation index; (b) relative viscosity at a shear rate of $0.1 \ s^{-1}$. Note that the maximum of each curve (that is, maximum aggregation of the red cells) corresponds to a well-defined concentration of a particular dextran fraction. Maxima in both indices of aggregation of red cells occur at about the same concentration of dextran fraction.

Reproduced from S. Chien, *Bibl. Anat. Basel*, 11, 244 (1973).

Iron–dextran complexes are soluble, non-ionic and suitable for injection for the treatment of anaemia; the complex is stable on storage in the pH range 4–11. More recently aminoethyldextran–methotrexate complexes have been prepared, the object being to influence uptake of the drug selectively into tumour cells. Attachment of the drug to the macromolecule allows selective uptake into malignant cells, as such cells are more active than normal cells in pinocytosis, the mechanism by which macromolecules are taken into many cells.

8.4.6 Polyvinylpyrrolidone

Polyvinylpyrrolidone (PVP) is used as a suspending and dispersing agent, as a tablet binding and granulating agent, and as a vehicle for drugs such as penicillin, cortisone, procaine and insulin to delay their absorption and prolong their action. It forms hard films which are utilised in film-coating processes. Chemically it is a homopolymer of *N*-vinyl-pyrrolidone (**XIV**). It is available in a number of grades designated by numbers ranging from K15 to K90. The *K* values represent a function of the mean molecular weight, since

$$\frac{\log \eta_{rel}}{c} = \frac{75K_0^2}{1 + 1.5K_c} + K_0 \qquad (8.24)$$

where c = concentration in g per 100 cm^3 and η_{rel} is the viscosity relative to the solvent. $K = 1000K_0$. Viscosity is essentially independent of pH over the range 0–10 and aqueous solutions exhibit a high tolerance for many inorganic salts. Its wide solubility in organic solvents is unusual. The viscosity of a range of aqueous solutions of PVP is shown in Fig. 8.20.

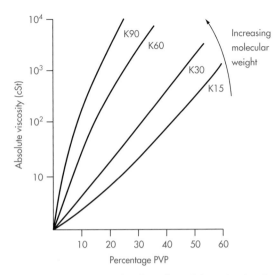

Figure 8.20 Viscosity of polyvinylpyrrolidone (PVP) solutions as a function of molecular weight (PVP K15 (mol. wt. 40 000) to PVP K90 (mol. wt. 700 000)) and concentration of the polymer in water.
Reproduced from J. L. Azorlosa and A. J. Martinelli, in *Water Soluble Resins* (ed. R. L. Davidson and M. Sittig), Reinhold, New York. 1962.

PVP forms molecular adducts with many substances. Insoluble complexes are formed when aqueous solutions of PVP are added to tannic acid, poly(acrylic acid) and methyl vinyl ether–maleic anhydride copolymer. Soluble complexes, called *iodophors*, are formed with iodine: the solubility of iodine is increased from 0.034% in water at 25°C to 0.58% by 1% PVP. The resulting iodophor retains the germicidal properties of iodine. It is thought that the iodine is held in a PVP helix in solution. The influence of two samples of PVP on the solubility of testosterone is shown in Fig. 8.21. The PVP correspondingly increases the rate of solution of the steroid from solid dispersions.

8.4.7 Polyoxyethylene glycols (Macrogols)

Macrogols (polyoxyethylene glycols. PEGs, **XV**) are liquid over the molecular weight range 200–700; the liquid members and semisolid members of the series are hygroscopic. Macrogol 200 has a hygroscopicity 70% of that of glycerol, but this decreases with

Structure XIV Polyvinylpyrrolidine

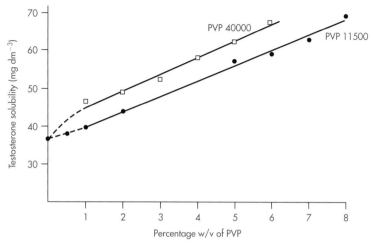

Figure 8.21 The influence of PVP 11 500 and PVP 40 000 on the aqueous solubility of testosterone at 37°C.
Reproduced from A. Hoelgaard and N. Muller, *Arch. Pharm. Chem.*, 3, 34 (1975).

molecular weight: the comparable value for Macrogol 1540 is only 30%. They are used as solvents for drugs such as hydrocortisone. The macrogols are incompatible with phenols and can reduce the antimicrobial activity of other preservatives. Higher molecular weight PEGs are more effective on a molecular basis as complexing agents. Up to four phenol molecules bind to each PEG molecule; the complex formed is of the donor–acceptor type. The semisolid and waxy members of the series may be used as suppository bases; in such cases their potential to interact with medicaments must be borne in mind.

Use of polyoxyethylene glycols, and other hydrophilic polymers, in high concentrations

$$HO(CH_2CH_2O)_nH$$

Structure XV Polyoxyethylene glycol

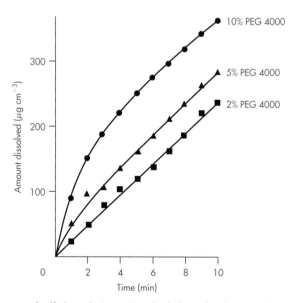

Figure 8.22 Dissolution rates of sulfathiazole (Form I)–polyethylene glycol 4000 physical mixtures.
Reproduced from S. Niazi, *J. Pharm. Sci.*, 65, 302 (1976).

in formulations can influence the behaviour of drugs even when the drug is present as a physical mixture with the polymer. For example, combination of polyoxyethylene glycol 4000 with sulfathiazole increases the solution rate of sulfonamides (Fig. 8.22). Probable mechanisms include an increase in drug solubility or increased wetting of the drug surrounded by the hydrophilic polymer.

8.4.8 Bioadhesivity of water-soluble polymers

Adhesion between a surface of a hydrophilic polymer, or a surface to which a hydrophilic polymer has been grafted or adsorbed, and a biological surface arises from interactions between the polymer chains and the macromolecules on the mucosal surface. From Fig. 8.23(a) it is clear that to achieve maximum adhesion there should be maximum interaction between the polymer chains of the bioadhesive (A) and the mucus (B). The charge on the molecules will be important, and for two anionic polymers maximum interaction will occur when they are not charged. Penetration and association must be balanced. Table 8.5 shows the adhesive performance of a

range of polymers, many of which have been discussed in this chapter. Of these, two classes have been approved by the FDA: anionic poly(acrylic acid) (carbophil) derivatives and the cationic chitosans. Polycarbophil and carbomer (Carbopol 934P) have pK_a values of about 4.5 and display maximum mucoadhesivity at pH values where they are mostly undissociated[6] (see Fig. 8.23b).

8.4.9 Polymers as wound dressings

Several polymers are now used in the preparation of synthetic wound dressings. Synthaderm is a 'synthetic skin' of a modified polyurethane foam, hydrophilic on one side and hydrophobic on the other. The hydrophilic side is placed in contact with the wound. The system has been described as an 'environmental dressing'[7] as it (a) maintains a high humidity at the dressing interface, (b) removes excess exudate, (c) allows gaseous exchange and (d) provides insulation; moreover, it is impermeable to bacteria, the outer surface remaining dry unlike many saturable dressings. Lyofoam is a similar product.[8] Laminates of polypeptides and elastomers have

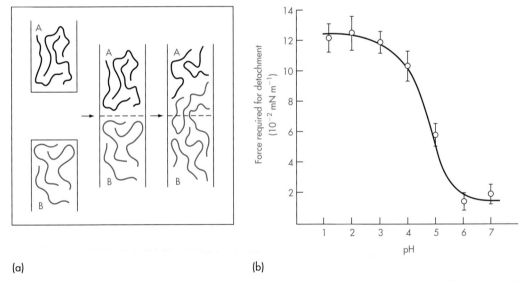

(a)   (b)

Figure 8.23 (a) Schematic representation of two phases, adhesive (A) and mucus (B), which adhere due to chain adsorption and consecutive chain entanglement during mucoadhesion. (Reproduced from N. A. Peppas and A. G. Mikos, in *Bioadhesion* (ed. R. Gurney and H. Junginger), Wiss. Verlagsgesellschaft, Stuttgart, 1990.) (b) Effect of pH on *in vitro* bioadhesion of polycarbophil to rabbit gastric tissue. (From reference 6.)

Table 8.5 Some representative mucoadhesives and their relative mucoadhesivities

Substance	Adhesive performance
Carboxymethylcellulose	Excellent
Carbopol	Excellent
Carbopol and hydroxypropylmethylcellulose	Good
Carbopol base with white petrolatum/hydrophilic petrolatum	Fair
Carbopol 934 and EX 55	Good
Poly(methyl methacrylate)	Excellent
Polyacrylamide	Good
Poly(acrylic acid)	Excellent
Polycarbophil	Excellent
Homopolymers and copolymers of acrylic acid and butyl acrylate	Good
Gelatin	Fair
Sodium alginate	Excellent
Dextran	Good
Pectin	Poor
Acacia	Poor
Povidone	Poor
Poly(acrylic acid) crosslinked with sucrose	Fair

been proposed as burn wound coverings to provide a film with the appropriate strength and physical properties.[9]

Crosslinked dextran gels are insoluble hydrophilic gels that can be partially depolymerised to the required molecular weight. The gel is produced in a bead shape; the degree of crosslinking determines the water uptake and pore size. Dextranomer (Debrisan) is a crosslinked dextran with pores large enough to allow substances with a molecular weight of less than 1000 to enter the beads. Each gram of beads abstracts approximately 4 cm^3 of fluid. Applied to the surface of secreting wounds, dextranomer removes by suction various exudates that tend to impede tissue repair, while leaving behind high molecular weight materials such as plasma proteins and fibrinogen.

8.4.10 Polymer crystallinity

Polymers form perfect crystals with difficulty simply because of the low probability of arranging the chains in regular fashion, especially at high molecular weights. Advantage can be taken of defects in crystals in the preparation of microcrystals. Microcrystalline cellulose (Avicel) is prepared by disruption of larger crystals. It is used as a tablet excipient and as a binder-disintegrant. Dispersed in water it forms colloidal gels, and it can be used to form heat-stable o/w emulsions. Spheroidised forms of microcrystalline cellulose with accurately controlled diameters can be prepared and drugs can be incorporated during preparation. The concept of crystallinity is potentially important when considering polymer membranes, as discussed below.

8.5 Water-insoluble polymers and polymer membranes

In defining the properties of polymers for drug formulation, certain characteristics are important. Obviously molecular weight and molecular weight distribution must be known, as these affect solvent penetration and crystallinity. The functionality of the polymer is best described by a series of parameters such as

- Glass transition temperature, T_g
- Tensile strength
- Diffusion coefficient
- Hardness (crystallinity)
- Solubility

Crystallinity defines several features of polymers: rigidity, fluidity, the resistance to diffusion of small molecules in the polymer, and degradation.

In hydrogels T_g can be measured and is a measure of polymer structure, crosslinking density, solvent content and polymer–solvent interactions, as can be seen from Table 8.6.

8.5.1 Permeability of polymers

Hydrophobic polymers also play an important role in pharmacy. When these materials are used as membranes, containers or tubing material, their surfaces may come into contact

Table 8.6 Effect of hydrogel structure and characteristics on T_g

Feature	Effect on T_g
Presence of flexible groups in main chain	↓
Bulky, inflexible side-chains	↑
Flexible side-chains	↓
Increase in main chain polarity	↑
Increase in crosslinking	↑
Plasticiser content	↓

with solutions. The surfaces of insoluble polymers are not as inert as might be thought. The interaction of drugs and preservatives with plastics depends on the structure of the polymer and on the affinity of the compound for the plastic. The latter is determined by the degree of crystallinity of the polymer, as permeability is a function of the degree of amorphous content of the polymer. The crystalline regions of the solid polymer present an impenetrable barrier to the movement of most molecules. Diffusing molecules thus have to circumnavigate the crystalline islands, which act as obstructions. The greater the volume fraction of crystalline material (ϕ_c) the slower the movement of molecules.

Diffusion

Diffusion in nonporous solid polymer is of course a more difficult process than in a fluid because of the necessity for the movement of polymer chains to allow passage of the drug molecule, and it is therefore slower. The equation which governs the process is Fick's first law (see Section 3.6, equation (3.90)):

$$J = -D \frac{dc}{dx} \tag{8.25}$$

where J is the flux, D is the diffusion coefficient of the drug in the membrane, and dc/dx is the concentration gradient across the membrane. If the membrane is of thickness l, and Δc represents the difference in solution concentration of drug at the two faces of membrane,

$$J = \frac{DK \, \Delta c}{l} \tag{8.26}$$

where K is the distribution coefficient of the permeant towards the polymer. Therefore alteration of polymer/membrane thickness, coupled with appropriate choice of polymer, can give rise to the desired flux. Within a given polymer, permeability is a function of the degree of crystallinity, itself a function of polymer molecular weight. If P is the permeability of drug in a partially crystalline polymer (see Fig. 8.24), the volume fraction of the crystalline regions being ϕ_c, and P_a is the permeability in an amorphous sample, then

$$\frac{P}{P_a} = (1 - \phi_c)^2 \tag{8.27}$$

Permeation of drug molecules through the solid polymer, which may be acting as a drug depot, is a function of the solubility of the drug in the polymer as

$$P = DK \tag{8.28}$$

Addition of inorganic fillers in which the

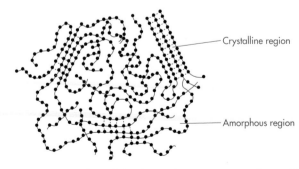

Figure 8.24 Diagrammatic representation of a solid polymer showing regions of crystallinity and regions which are amorphous; the total volume fraction of crystalline regions, ϕ_c, can be calculated from measurements of density.

drug is insoluble alters the overall solubility of the drug in the polymer and hence alters the permeation characteristics. The equation for overall solubility (S) is given by

$$S = S_f \phi_f + S_p \phi_p \qquad (8.29)$$

where f refers to filler and p to polymer. Thus, when $S_f \to 0$, as happens when inorganic fillers such as zinc oxide are employed, an obstruction-type equation may be written:

$$\frac{S}{S_p} = 1 - \phi_f \qquad (8.30)$$

The natural permeabilities of polymers vary over a wide range and this widens the choice, provided one can select a polymer which is compatible with the tissues with which it comes into contact. Once a polymer has been chosen that gives a flux of drug sufficient to provide adequate circulating levels, use of fillers and plasticisers can give fine control of permeability (Table 8.7).

The method of preparation also influences the properties of the film. Cast films of varying properties can be prepared by variation *inter alia* of the solvent power of the casting solution containing the polymer, although the complex processes involved in film formation are not yet fully understood. It is clear, however, that the conformation of the polymer chains in concentrated solution just prior to solvent evaporation will determine the density of the film, and the number and size of pores and voids. Drug flux through dense (nonporous) polymer membranes is by diffusion; flux through porous membranes will be by diffusion and by transport in solvent through pores in the film. With porous films, control can be exercised on porosity, and hence overall permeability, by the use of swelling agents. Dense membranes can be subjected to certain post-formation treatments such as thermal annealing which modify their structural and performance characteristics.

The solubility of sterilising gases in polymers is important in determining the retention of residues which may, as in the case of ethylene oxide residues, be toxic. The quality control problems of polymers and plastics are considerable. Both the chemical and physical nature of the material has to be taken into account, as well as purity.

Permeability of polymers to gases

The permeability of polymers to the gaseous phase is of importance when the use of polymers as packaging materials is considered. Figure 8.25 shows oxygen penetration through a wide range of plastic materials ranging from Teflon to dimethylsilicone rubber, which has the highest permeability. Ether, nitrous oxide, halothane and cyclopropane diffuse through silicone rubbers, and general anaesthesia in dogs has been achieved by passing the vapours of these substances through a coil of silicone rubber tubing, each end of which is placed in an artery or vein. Aspects of the permeability of polymeric films of interest pharmaceutically include the process of gas diffusion, water sorption and permeation and dialysis processes. With few exceptions, there is an inverse relationship between water-vapour transmission and oxygen permeability. Water-vapour permeability has been shown to be dependent on the polarity of the polymer. More polar films tend to be more ordered and less porous, hence less oxygen-permeable. The less polar films are more porous, permitting the permeation of oxygen but not necessarily of the larger water molecules. Being more lipophilic, the less polar films have less affinity for water. Because of the importance of water as a solvent and permeant species, much work has been directed towards the synthesis of polymeric membranes with controlled hydrophilic/hydrophobic balance. The

---

Table 8.7 Factors that influence diffusivity in polymers

Factor	Net effect on D
Increased polymer molecular weight	↓
Increased degree of crosslinking	↓
Diluents and plasticisers	↑
Fillers	↓
Increased crystallinity of polymers	↓
Increased drug molecular size	↓

types, such as polacrilin potassium (Amberlite IRP 88, sulfonated polystyrene resin) are used as tablet disintegrants because of the high degree of swelling the dry resins undergo on interaction with water.

8.5.3   Silicone oligomers and polymers

The *silicones* are examples of hydrophobic liquid polymers, although in high molecular weight they exist as waxes and resins. Silicones are polymers with a structure containing alternate atoms of Si and O; the dimethicones are fluid polymers with the general formula **XIX** in which each unit has two methyl groups and an oxygen atom attached to the silicon atom in the chain. The viscosity range extends from 0.65 cS to 3×10^6 cS. The dimethicones 20, 200, 350 and 1000 (the number representing the average viscosity in centistokes at 25°C) have rheological properties which allow them to be used in ophthalmology and in rheumatoid arthritis. Dimethicone 200 has been used as a lubricant for artificial eyes and to replace

the degenerative vitreous fluid in cases of retinal detachment. It can also act as a simple lubricant in joints. More common uses are as barrier substances, silicone lotions and creams acting as water-repellent applications protecting the skin against water-soluble irritants. Methylphenylsilicone is used as a lubricant for hypodermic syringes. Glassware which has been treated with a thin film of silicone is rendered hydrophobic; solutions and aqueous suspensions thus drain completely from such vessels.

Activated dimethicone (activated polymethylsiloxane) is a mixture of liquid dimethicones containing finely divided silica to enhance the defoaming properties of the silicone. The mechanism by which dispersion of colloidal silica antifoams improves their action is not well understood.

By varying the amounts of polymer in resin a variety of products, catheters, tubing materials for reconstructive surgery and membranes for drug reservoirs can be formed.

The release of lipophilic steroids from silicone elastomer matrices is dependent on the cross linking density of the polymer and the content of filler, but also on the lipophilicity of the drug. A relationship between the solubility parameters of a number of drugs and their release rate is shown in Fig. 8.27.

An interesting application of the silicone fluids is their coformulation with adhesives to

Structure XIX Dimethicone

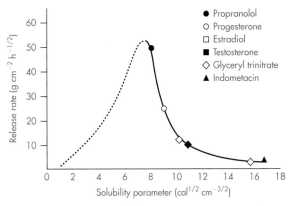

Figure 8.27   Comparative release rates of different drugs from a pressure-sensitive silicone matrix as a function of their solubility parameter.

Reproduced from L. C. Clauss, in *Proceedings of the International Conference on Pharmaceutical, Ingredients and Intermediates (1990)*, Expoconsult, Maarssen, 1991, p. 116.

Table 8.11 Pressure-sensitive adhesives in trans-dermal patches[a]

Adhesive class	Adhesive polymer
	Polyisoprene Polybutene Polyisobutylene
	Ethyl acrylate 2-Ethylhexyl acrylate Isooctyl acrylate
	Polydimethylsiloxane Polysilicate resin Siloxane blends

[a] Reproduced from W. R. Pfister *et al.*, *Pharm. Tech.*, 16(1), 42 (1992).

increase 'tack' and in elastomers to soften the product.

Pressure-sensitive silicone adhesives are formed from the most highly crosslinked systems based on the structure **XIX**.

Other pressure-sensitive adhesives used in transdermal delivery device include those shown in Table 8.11.

8.6 Some applications of polymeric systems in drug delivery

Control of the rate of release of a drug when administered by oral or parenteral routes is aided by the use of polymers that function as a barrier to drug movement.

8.6.1 Film coating

Polymer solutions allowed to evaporate produce polymeric films which can act as protective layers for tablets or granules containing sensitive drug substances or as a rate-controlling barrier to drug release. Film coats have been divided into two types; those that dissolve rapidly and those that behave as dialysis

membranes, allowing slow diffusion of solute or some delayed diffusion by acting as gel layers. Materials that have been used as film formers include shellac, zein, glyceryl stearates, paraffins and a range of anionic and cationic polymers such as the Eudragit polymers (**XX** to **XXIII**). Newer materials used for the same purpose include cellulose acetate phthalate.

Different film coats applied to tablet surfaces can lead to quite different rates of solution.

Structure XX Poly(methacrylic acid, methyl methacrylate) 1 : 1 copolymer (Eudragit L12.5, L100)

Structure XXI Poly(ethylacrylate, methacrylic acid) 1 : 1 (Eudragit L 30 D, L 100–55)

XX and XXI: Chemical structure of various preparations of Eudragit L range (anionic)

In Fig. 8.28, hydroxypropylmethylcellulose, an acrylic derivative and zein are compared for their effect on sodium chloride dissolution from discs. Two plasticisers have been used: glycerin and diethyl phthalate. Times for 50% dissolution range from a few minutes to 450 minutes, indicating the scope of the technique for retard formulations, and the possibility of unwittingly extending dissolution times by the injudicious choice of coating material.

8.6.2 Matrices

The use of a barrier film coating is only one of several procedures that can be adopted to

DMEMA   MMA/BMA

Structure XXII Poly(butylmethacrylate, 2-dimethylamino-ethyl methacrylate, methyl methacrylate) 1 : 2 : 1 (Eudragit E 100, E 12.5)

EA   MMA

Structure XXIII Poly(ethylacrylate, methyl methacrylate) 2 : 1 (Eudragit E 30 D)

XXII and XXIII: Chemical structure of various preparations of Eudragit E range (cationic)

control release of drugs (Fig. 8.29a). Various methods are shown schematically in Table 8.12. If hydrophobic water-soluble polymers are used, the mechanism of release is the passage of drug through pores in the plastic, or by leaching or slow diffusion of drug through the polymer wall (Fig. 8.29b), as discussed earlier in this chapter. Release may also be effected by erosion of the polymer (Fig. 8.29c). When water-soluble polymers are employed, for example as hydrophilic matrices, the entry of water into the polymer is followed by swelling and gelation and the drug must diffuse through the viscous gel, a process obviously slower than diffusion through plain solvent.

Release of drugs from matrices

Equations describing the rate of drug release from hydrophobic and hydrophilic matrices

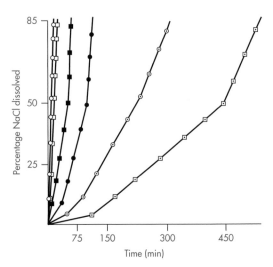

Figure 8.28 Dissolution of sodium chloride from tablets coated with hydroxypropylmethylcellulose (O), a vinyl polymer (●) and zein (⊙) with glycerin as an additive, and the same polymers with diethyl phthalate as additive (□, ■, and ⊡ respectively).
Reproduced from O. Laguna et al., Ann. Pharm. Franc., 33, 235 (1975).

are useful in determining which factors may be altered to change the measured release rate of drug. Higuchi[11] proposed the following equation for the amount of drug, Q, released per unit area of tablet surface in time t, from an insoluble matrix:

$$Q=\left[\frac{D\varepsilon}{\tau}(2A-\varepsilon C_s)C_s t\right]^{1/2} \quad (8.33)$$

D is the diffusion coefficient of the drug in the release medium, C_s is the solubility of drug in the medium, ε is the porosity of the matrix, τ is the tortuosity of the matrix, and A is the total amount of drug in the matrix per unit volume.

If the same matrix is saturated with a solution of the drug (as in medicated soft contact lenses, see Chapter 9) the appropriate equation becomes, if C_0 is the concentration of drug solution:

$$Q=2C_0\varepsilon\left(\frac{Dt}{\tau\pi}\right)^{1/2} \quad (8.34)$$

That is, for a given drug in a given matrix, $Q \propto t^{1/2}$. The more porous the matrix the more

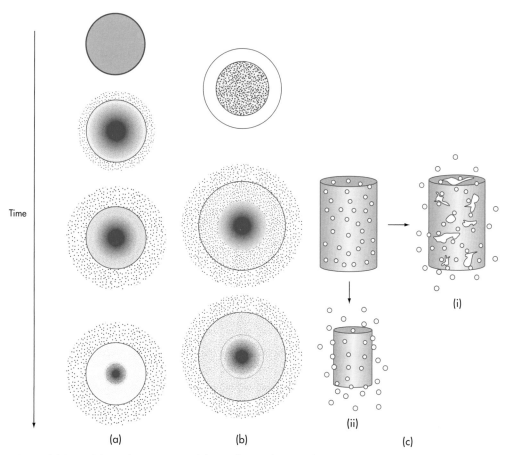

Time

(a)   (b)   (c)

(i)

(ii)

Figure 8.29 (a) Drug delivery from a matrix delivery device showing diagrammatically the depletion of drug from the system and the release of the drug. (b) Release from a typical reservoir system with a membrane controlling release from the internal store of drug. (c) Illustrating release from (i) a bulk-eroding system and (ii) a surface-eroding system.
After Lisa Brannon-Peppas, Polymers in Controlled Drug Delivery, *Medical Plastics and Biomaterials*, 1997(Nov.), p. 34.

rapid the release. The more tortuous the pores the longer the path for diffusing molecules, thus the lower is Q. More-soluble drugs diffuse more quickly form the matrix.

The extension of these equation to hydrophilic matrices is difficult because the conditions in a hydrophilic matrix change with time as water penetrates into it. If the polymer does not dissolve but simply swells and if the drug has not completely dissolved in the incoming solvent, diffusion of drug commences from a saturated solution through the gel layer, and

$$Q = \frac{D\varepsilon}{\tau}\left[\left(\frac{2W_0}{V} - \varepsilon C_s\right)tC_s\right]^{1/2} \qquad (8.35)$$

Equation 8.35 is similar to equation (8.33) except that the effective volume V of the hydrated matrix is used as this is not a fixed quantity. W_0 is the dose of the drug in the matrix. If the drug completely dissolves on hydration of the matrix, an analogue of equation (8.34) is used:

$$Q = \frac{2W_0}{V}\left(\frac{Dt}{\tau\pi}\right)^{1/2} \qquad (8.36)$$

In the initial stages of the process the rate of movement of water into the matrix may be important in determining release characteristics. When a homogeneous barrier wall is present diffusion through the walls has to take place and equations in section 8.5 apply.

Table 8.12 Depot forms employing polymeric films and matrices[a]

Type	Materials[b]	Diagrammatic representation	Mechanisms
1 Barrier coating	Beeswax, glyceryl monostearate, ethylcellulose, nylon (Ultramid IC), acrylic resins (Eudragit retard)	drug, coating	Diffusion
2 Fat embedment	Glycerol palmitostearate (Precirol), beeswax, glycowax, castorwax, aluminium monostearate, carnauba wax, glyceryl monostearate, stearyl alcohol	drug, fat	Erosion, hydrolysis of fat, dissolution
3 Plastic matrix	Polyethylene Poly(vinyl acetate) Polymethacrylate Poly(vinyl chloride) Ethylcellulose	drug, polymer	Leaching, diffusion
4 Repeat action	Cellulose acetylphthalate	enteric coat	Dissolution of enteric coat
5 Ion exchange	Amberlite Dowex		Dissociation of drug–resin complex
6 Hydrophilic matrix	Carboxymethylcellulose Sodium carboxymethylcellulose Hydroxypropylmethylcellulose	hydrophilic polymer, drug	Gelation, diffusion
7 Epoxy resin beads	Epoxy resins	epoxy resin bead or microcapsule	Dissolution of resin or swelling, diffusion
8 Microcapsules	Polyamides, gelatin		
9 Soft gelatin depot capsules	Shellac–PEG Poly(vinyl acetate)–PEG		Diffusion

[a] Modified from W. A. Ritschel, in *Drug Design*, vol. IV (ed. A. J. Ariens), Academic Press, New York, 1974.
[b] Materials are not all polymeric. The waxes are included for completeness; these depend on conferring a hydrophobic layer on the drug, tablet or granule to prevent access of solvent.

8.6.3 Microcapsules and microspheres

Microencapsulation is a technique which, as its name suggests, involves the encapsulation of small particles of drug, or solution of drug, in a polymer film or coat. Microspheres, on the other hand, are solid but not necessarily homogenous particles which can entrap drug. Although the terms tend to be used interchangeably, we retain the distinction here. Microspheres can be prepared also by a variety of techniques which are briefly discussed in the section on nanoencapsulation below.

Typical photomicrographs of poly(ε-caprolactone) microphores are shown in Fig. 8.30.

Microcapsules can be prepared by three main processes:

- *Coacervation* of macromolecules around the core material, this being induced by temperature change, solvent change or addition of a second macromolecule of appropriate physical properties.
- *Interfacial polymerisation of a monomer* around the core material by polymerisation at the interface of a liquid dispersion.

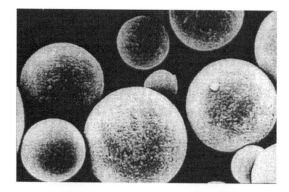

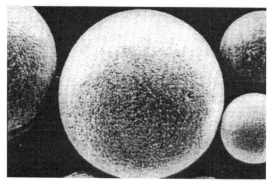

Figure 8.30 Scanning electron micrographs of bovine serum albumin-loaded microspheres prepared from a ternary blend of poly(ε-caprolactone). Protein entrapment efficiency and mean particle size were 28.6% and 2.9 μm respectively.
Reproduced from H. Huatan, J. H. Collett and D. Attwood, J. Microencaps., 12, 557 (1995).

- *Spray coating and other methods* in which larger particles may be coated in suspension.

Any method which will cause a coherent barrier to deposit itself on the surface of a liquid droplet or a solid particle of drug may be applied to the formation of microcapsules. Many so-called microencapsulation procedures result in the formation of macroscopic 'beads' which are simply coated granules.

Coacervation

Coacervation is the term used to describe the separation of macromolecular solutions into colloid-poor and colloid-rich (coacervate) phases when the macromolecules are desolvated. The liquid or solid to be encapsulated is dispersed in a solution of a macromolecule (such as gelatin, gum arabic, carboxymethylcellulose or poly(vinyl alcohol)) in which it is immiscible. A nonsolvent, miscible with the continuous phase but a poor solvent for the polymer, under certain conditions will induce the polymer to form a coacervate (polymer-rich) layer around the disperse phase. This coating layer may then be treated to give a rigid coat of capsule wall. This is the process of *simple coacervation*. Successful application of the technique relies on the determination of the appropriate conditions for coacervate deposition, which can be achieved not only by the addition of nonsolvents such as ethanol and isopropanol and salts (sodium and ammonium sulfates) but also by the choice of macromolecules incompatible under selected conditions with the first species. The latter process is termed *complex coacervation*. In both simple and complex coacervation utilising hydrophilic macromolecules it is the decrease in solubility which results in deposition of the macromolecule layer at the particle–solution interface.

Desolvation of water-insoluble macromolecules in nonaqueous solvents leads to the deposition of a coacervate layer around aqueous or solid disperse droplets. Table 8.13 lists both water-soluble and water-soluble macromolecules which have been used in coacervation processes. Desolvation, and thus coacervation, can be induced thermally and

Table 8.13 Materials used in coacervation microencapsulation

Water-soluble macromolecules	Water-insoluble macromolecules
Arabinogalactan	Cellulose acetate phthalate
Carboxymethylcellulose	Cellulose nitrate
Gelatin	Ethylcellulose
Gum arabic (acacia)	Poly(ethylene vinyl acetate)
Hydroxyethylcellulose	Poly(methyl methacrylate)
Poly(acrylic acid)	
Polyethyleneimine	
Poly(vinyl alcohol)	
Polyvinylpyrrolidone	
Methylcellulose	
Starch	

this is the basis of some preparative techniques. Conditions for phase separation are best obtained using phase diagrams.

For example, in the region pH 6–8, gelatin will be positively and gum arabic negatively charged. In admixture, complex coacervates will form under the conditions described in Fig. 8.31, which shows the partial phase diagram of the ternary system gum arabic–gelatin–water. The hatched area at the top of the phase diagram is the restricted region in which coacervation occurs. At higher concentrations of the macromolecules, macroscopic precipitates of the complex will occur.

Interfacial reaction

Reactions between oil-soluble monomers and water-soluble monomers at the oil/water interface of w/o or o/w dispersions can lead to

interfacial polymerisation resulting in the formation of polymeric microcapsules, the size of which is determined by the size of the emulsion droplets. Alternatively, reactive monomer can be dispersed in one of the phases and induced to polymerise at the interface, or to polymerise in the bulk disperse phase and to *precipitate* at the interface due to its insolubility in the continuous phase. There are many variations on this theme. Probably the most widely studied reaction has been the interfacial condensation of water-soluble alkyl diamines with oil-soluble acid dichlorides to form polyamides. Representative examples of other wall materials are polyurethanes, polysulfonamides, polyphthalamides and poly(phenyl esters). The selection of polymer is restricted to those that can be formed from monomers with the requisite preferential solubilities in one phase so that polymerisation

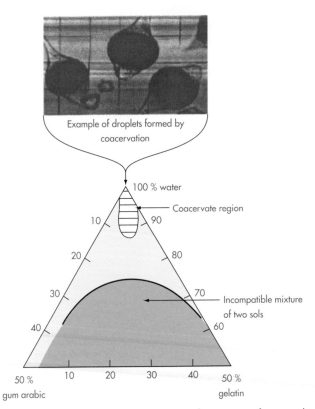

Figure 8.31 Ternary diagram showing complex coacervation region for mixtures of gum arabic and gelatin at pH 4.5; below the curved line the mixture separates into two sols (US Patent 2800457). Insert: Typical droplets formed by coacervation (Ronald T. Dodge).

takes place only at the interface. The process for the preparation of nylon 6.10 micro-capsules is represented diagrammatically in Fig. 8.32.

Physical methods of encapsulation

Various physical methods of preparing micro-capsules such as spray drying and pan coating are available.

Pan coating application of films to particles can only be used for particles greater than 600 μm in diameter. The process has been applied in the formation of sustained-release beads by application of waxes such as glyceryl monostearate in organic solution to granules of drug.

The *spray drying* process involves dispersion of the core material in a solution of coating sub-stance and spraying the mixture into an envi-ronment which causes the solvent to evaporate. In an analogous *spray congealing* process the coating material is congealed thermally or by introducing the core coat mixture into a non-solvent mixture. Both processes can produce microcapsules in the size range 5000–6000 μm.

Spray polycondensation is a variant based on the polycondensation of surface-active mono-mers on a melamine–formaldehyde base on the surface of suspended particles during spray drying. A dispersion of the core material is prepared in a continuous phase containing aminoplast monomers or precondensates of relatively low molecular weight, in addition to other film-forming agents and catalyst. The reactive monomers derived from hexamethylol melamine derivatives are selectively adsorbed at the surface of the disperse phase. Spray drying at 150–200°C results in vaporisation of the water and causes simultaneous poly-condensation of the monomers and precon-densates by acid catalysis.

Pharmaceutical nanotechnology

Nanotechnology – the science of small objects in the size range around 2 nm to 250 nm – has attracted much attention in recent years. In drug delivery the interest in nanoparticles and other nanosized container systems (Fig. 8.33) lies in the fact that they can be injected readily and can gain access to tissues beyond the capillary blood supply. Once there, they can diffuse in tissues more easily than larger par-ticles. Scheme 8.2 is an attempt to summarise the range of the subject, the nature of the nanosystems used in pharmacy, their charac-terisation and their biological uses. Biodegrad-able nanoparticles from poly(lactic acid)–poly(glycolic acid) (PLGA), polycaprolactone and polyalkylcyanoacrylates have been widely studied experimentally.

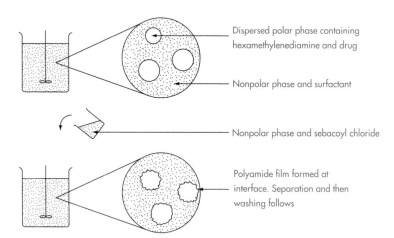

Figure 8.32 Process for the preparation of nylon 6.10 microcapsules by interfacial polymerisation: the hexamethylene-diamine in the aqueous phase reacts with the sebacoyl chloride in the nonpolar phase to form an interfacial polyamide film.

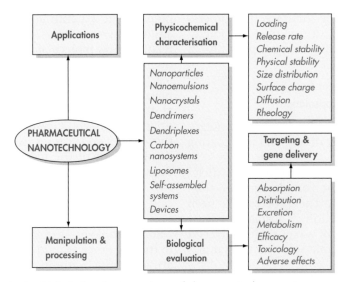

Scheme 8.2 Characterisation, biological evaluation and uses of pharmaceutical nanosystems

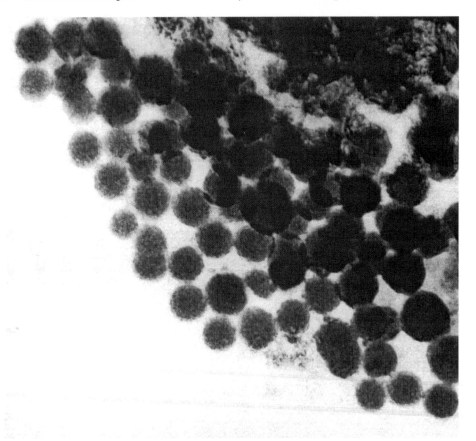

Figure 8.33   Nanosystems formed by association of dendrimers in aqueous solution. These structures are around 50 nm in diameter.

Reproduced from K. T. Al-Jamal, C. Ramaswamy, B. Singh and A. T. Florence, *J. Drug Sci. Technol.*, 15, 11–18 (2005).

Nanoencapsulation

Polymer nanoparticles with diameters of 50–500 nm are now widely used. As with microspheres and microcapsules, one can differentiate between solid polymeric spheres (nanoparticles) and those spheres with thin polymeric walls (nanocapsules). The locus of polymerisation is not an emulsion droplet as in microencapsulation, but a micelle. The process involves the solubilisation of a water-soluble monomer such as acrylamide along with the drug or other agent such as antigen to be encapsulated. An organic liquid such as n-hexane serves as the outer phase. Polymerisation is induced by irradiation (γ-rays, X-rays, UV light), exposure to visible light or heating with an initiator.

Appropriate modification or control of the coacervation process has been shown to produce nanoparticles of gelatin. Gelatin nanoparticles have been prepared by desolvation (for example, with sodium sulfate) of a gelatin solution containing drug bound to the gelatin, in a process which terminates the desolvation just before coacervation begins. In this manner, colloidal particles rather than the larger coacervate droplets are obtained. The general method has been applied to yield nanoparticles of human and bovine serum albumin, ethylcellulose and casein.

Hardening of the gelatin nanoparticles is achieved by glutaraldehyde, which crosslinks with gelatin and is more efficient than formaldehyde. To achieve a high percentage incorporation of drug in the nanoparticles, the drug substance must have an affinity for the macromolecule used; thus water-soluble drugs are unlikely to be trapped in the embryo particles. Highly water-soluble drugs would be better incorporated in a nonaqueous system.

General considerations

In all techniques discussed there are several factors which are of importance in relation to the use of the product as a drug delivery vehicle or carrier.

- The efficiency of encapsulation of the active ingredient
- The effect of the encapsulation process on the properties of the encapsulated agent
- The presence of potentially toxic residue (e.g. monomer, salts) in the final product
- The reproducibility of the process and ease of separation
- The biocompatibility of the encapsulating agent
- The biodegradability of the material (in some cases)
- The properties of the microcapsule in relation to use, size distribution, porosity and permeability of the wall

The different processes and materials produce microcapsules in which optimum properties are not always obtained. Polyamide microcapsules are not biodegradable, hence the search for alternatives for forming microcapsules based on natural materials such as albumin. Biodegradable polymers cannot always be induced to form microcapsules and a polymer found to be degradable in solid or film form may not be degradable when formed into microcapsules if crosslinking of the polymer chains occurs during formation. In their application in medicine, the permeability of the capsule wall is probably the most important feature of the product. The effects of the various parameters relating to wall material, capsule and environment on permeability are outlined in Table 8.14.

Protein microspheres

Aqueous solutions of proteins such as albumin can be emulsified in an oil and induced to form microspheres, either by crosslinking the protein molecules with glutaraldehyde or other agents or by coagulating the protein by heating. Incorporation of a drug within the initial protein solution results in drug-laden microspheres which are biodegradable. The particle size of the microspheres (generally 0.2–300 μm diameter) is determined by the size distribution of the initial emulsion.

Protein microspheres have been used for physical drug targeting, i.e. the entrapment of carrier and therefore drug in, for example, the capillaries of the lung. Microspheres greater

Table 8.14 General parameters affecting capsule wall permeability[a]

Parameter	For lower permeability
Properties of wall polymer	
Density	Increase
Crystallinity	Increase
Crosslinking	Increase
Plasticiser content	Decrease
Fillers	Increase
Solvents used in film formation	Use good solvents versus poor
Properties of capsule	
Size	Increase
Wall thickness	Increase
Treatment	Utilise (e.g. crosslinking, sintering)
Multiple coatings	Utilise
Environmental properties	
Temperature	Decrease

[a] Reproduced from J. E. Vandegaer (ed.), *Microencapsulation, Processes and Applications*, Plenum Press, New York, 1974.

than about 7 μm in diameter will be physically trapped in capillary beds. On intra-arterial injection of large microspheres, the blood supply to an organ is reduced; the process of chemo-embolisation involves both blockage and delivery of drugs to the organ. External control over intravenously administered protein microspheres has been achieved by incorporation of magnetite (Fe_3O_4) particles into the microspheres, which then respond to an externally applied magnetic field.

8.6.4 Rate-limiting membranes and devices

The use of rate-limiting membranes to control the movement of drugs from a reservoir has been referred to above. Implants of silicone rubber or other appropriate polymeric material in which drug is embedded can be designed by choice of polymer, membrane thickness and porosity, to release drug at preselected rates. The Progestasert device (Fig. 8.34c) is designed to be implanted into the uterine

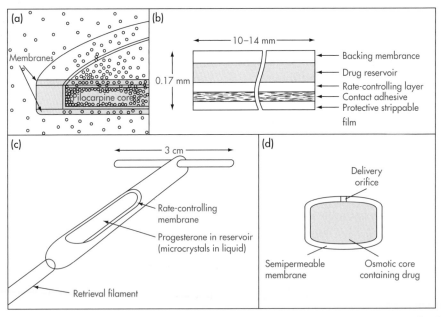

Figure 8.34 Examples of drug-delivery systems employing polymeric membranes. (a) Ocusert system for the eye with two rate-controlling membranes. (b) Transiderm system for transdermal medication with one rate-controlling layer. (c) The Progestasert device for intrauterine insertion in which the body of the device serves as the rate-controlling barrier. (d) The oral Oros device in which the membrane is a semipermeable membrane which forbids drug transport, allowing water ingress only.

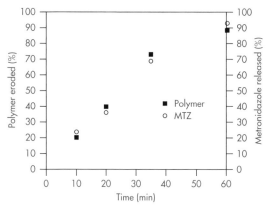

Figure 8.35 Characteristics of *in vivo* polymer erosion and metronidazole (MTZ) release from 50/50 CAP/Pluronic L101 films (with 10% metronidazole loading) in a dorsal rat model. Reproduced from K. A. Gates *et al.*, *Pharm. Res.*, 11, 1605 (1994).

cavity and to release there 65 μg progesterone per day to provide contraceptive cover for one year. The Ocusert device and the Transiderm therapeutic system (also shown in Fig. 8.34) which are discussed in Chapter 9, are products of the Alza Corporation (USA) and rely on rate-limiting polymeric membranes to control drug release. The opportunities for prolonged release of drugs given by the oral route are fewer. The aim in oral dose forms is for controlled rather than prolonged release, so that dosage frequency can be reduced or so that side-effects resulting from fast dissolution of drug can be minimised. Ion-exchange resin–drug complexes have also been used, and drugs may also be embedded in hydrophilic or hydrophobic matrices.

$t \times \lambda_a = 0.042$

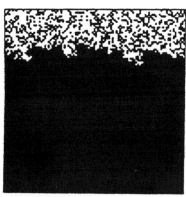

$t \times \lambda_a = 0.104$

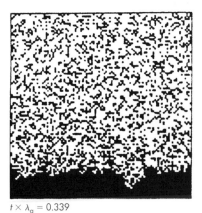

$t \times \lambda_a = 0.339$

Figure 8.36 Theoretical representation of a polymer matrix: changes during erosion (dark pixels = nondegraded areas, white pixels = degraded areas), where λ_a (a rate constant) = 2.7×10^{-7} s^{-1} for a sample containing 50% polyanhydride CPP.

Reproduced from A. Göpferich *et al.*, in *Formulation and Delivery of Proteins and Peptides* (ed. J. L. Cleland and R. Langer), ACS Symposium Series no. 567, ACS, Washington, 1994.

9

Drug absorption and routes of administration

This chapter provides basic information on the physicochemical mechanisms of drug absorption and how the processes of absorption are affected by the physicochemical properties of the drug and its formulation, by the interaction of the drug with the aqueous phase and by the nature of the membrane. Oral absorption is discussed in some detail and the influence of the following in determining bioavailability should become clear:

- The extent and rate of dissolution of the drug
- The rate of gastric emptying
- The site of absorption

The pH of the contents of the gastrointestinal tract (GI tract, gut) and the effect of pH on the ionisation of the drug (discussed also in section 5.2.4) are crucial.

The application of the so-called pH–partition hypothesis and its limitations should be understood, so that the effects of the nature of the drug and the medium on absorption can be assessed. In the case of the oral route, the effect of concomitant medication (cimetidine, ranitidine, antacids, etc.), which might alter the pH of the gut contents, can be approximated by calculating the change in the drug ionisation.

Many routes of entry into the body are used for both systemic and local action of drugs. We deal here with the essentials of formulations used by the following routes:

- Oral
- Buccal and sublingual
- Subcutaneous and intramuscular
- Topical or transdermal
- Ocular
- Aural
- Vaginal
- Rectal
- Respiratory or inhalational
- Nasal
- Intrathecal

Factors affecting drug absorption after delivery of the drug by these routes, often in special formulations designed for the given route, are important, particularly with regard to the comparative advantages and disadvantages of the different routes.

Absorption, whether it be from the gastrointestinal tract, from the buccal mucosa, or from the rectal cavity, generally requires the passage of the drug in a molecular form across one or more barrier membranes and tissues. Most drugs are presented to the body as solid or semisolid dosage forms and obviously these must first release the drug contained within them. Tablets or capsules will disintegrate, and the drug will then dissolve either completely or partially. Many tablets contain granules or drug particles which should preferably deaggregate to facilitate the solution process. If the drug has the appropriate physicochemical properties, its molecules will pass by passive diffusion from a region of high concentration to a region of low concentration across the membrane separating the site of absorption from tissues containing the blood supply. Soluble drugs can, of course also be administered as solutions, e.g. intravenously.

The special features of the different routes of administration are dealt with in separate sections of this chapter, after a brief summary of the general properties of biological membranes and drug transport, a knowledge of which is important in understanding all absorption processes. It is impossible to be comprehensive in this one chapter, but we will concentrate on factors unique to the routes discussed, such as the properties of the vehicle in topical therapy, and the aerodynamic properties of aerosols in inhalation therapy, to give a flavour of the different problems that face formulators. Where attempts have been made to quantify absorption, equations are presented, but the derivations of most equations have been omitted.

9.1 Biological membranes and drug transport

The main function of biological membranes is to contain the aqueous contents of cells and separate them from an aqueous exterior phase. To achieve this, membranes are lipoidal in nature and, to allow nutrients to pass into the cell and waste products to move out, biological membranes are selectively permeable. Membranes have specialised transport systems to assist the passage of water-soluble materials and ions through their lipid interior. Lipid-soluble agents can pass by passive diffusion through the membrane from a region of high concentration to one of low concentration. Biological membranes differ from polymer membranes in that they are composed not of polymers but of small amphipathic molecules,

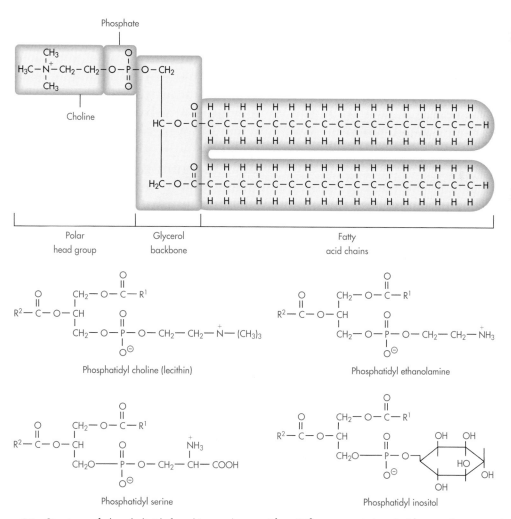

Scheme 9.1 Structures of phospholipids found in membranes. R^1 and R^2 may vary in length. R^1 is usually saturated and R^2 is usually unsaturated.

phospholipids (see Scheme 9.1) with two hydrophobic chains and cholesterol or other related structures, which associate into lipoidal bilayers in aqueous media. Embodied in the matrix of lipid molecules are proteins, which are generally hydrophobic in nature, embedded in the matrix of lipid molecules. Thus the membrane has a hydrophilic exterior and a hydrophobic interior.

Cholesterol is a major component of most mammalian biological membranes; its removal causes the membrane to lose its structural integrity and to become highly permeable. Cholesterol complexes with phospholipids and its presence reduces the permeability of phospholipid membranes to water, cations, glycerol and glucose. The shape of the cholesterol molecule allows it to fit closely in bilayers with the hydrocarbon chains of unsaturated fatty acids (Fig. 9.1). The present consensus of opinion is that cholesterol condenses and rigidifies membranes without solidifying them. The flexibility of biological membranes is an important feature, giving them their ability to re-form and to adapt to changed environments, a vital part of their function. The dynamic characteristics of biological membranes are due to their unique construction from small amphipathic molecules. On stretching (as with a soap film), the molecules at the surfaces become less concentrated in the bilayer but are replenished from the bulk phase to maintain the original tension.

Figure 9.2 shows a diagram of the 'fluid mosaic' model of a biological membrane.

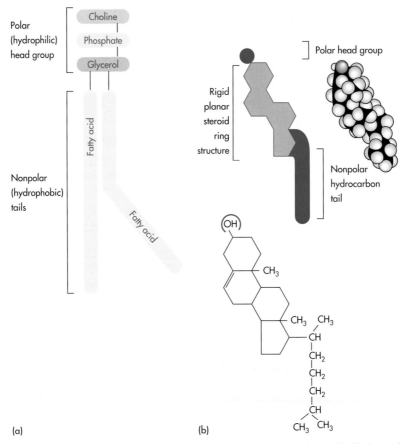

Figure 9.1 (a) Cell membranes are composed primarily of phospholipid amphiphiles. (b) Cholesterol molecules act as rigidifiers which make the membrane stiffer. Three representations of cholesterol are shown: a space-filling molecule (top right), a structural diagram (bottom) and a simplified block diagram (top left).
Source: http://physioweb.med.uum.edu.

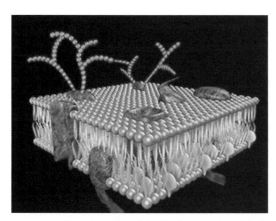

Figure 9.2 Representation of the 'fluid mosaic' model of a biological membrane, showing embedded protein and protruding glycoproteins. From Funhouse Films.

Although most of the data on permeation of nonelectrolytes across biological membranes can be explained on the basis of the membrane behaving as a continuous hydrophobic phase, a fraction of the membrane may be composed of aqueous channels which are continuous across the membrane. That is, there are pores which offer a pathway parallel to the diffusion pathway through the lipid. In the absence of bulk flow (that is flow of water in one direction or the other (see below)) these pores play a minor part in the transfer of drugs, although in the case of ions and charged drugs such as the quaternary ammonium compounds the pore pathway must be important. The low electrical resistance of membranes compared with synthetic lipid membranes suggests that the ions move in the pores. These pores may be provided by the conjunction of hydrophilic faces of proteins or the polar heads of fatty acids and phospholipids orientated in the appropriate direction. The fluid mosaic model, in particular, allows the protein–lipid complexes to form either hydrophilic or hydrophobic 'gates' to allow transport of materials with different characteristics.

It has been suggested that the permeability of the lipid bilayer is regulated by the density of hydrogen bonding in the outer polar layers of the membranes which contain the phosphate, ammonium and carboxyl head groups of phospholipids and the hydroxyl groups of cholesterol. Overall, membrane permeability is controlled by the nature of the membrane, its degree of internal bonding and rigidity, its surface charge and the nature of the solute being transported.

There are some similarities between solute transport in biological membranes and in synthetic membranes. As we have discussed in Chapter 8, the permeation of drugs and other molecules through hydrophobic membranes made of polydimethylsiloxane, for example, depends primarily on the solubility of the drug in the membrane. Drugs with little affinity for the membrane are unlikely to permeate, although in porous membranes, such as those of cellophane or collagen, even drugs with little affinity for the polymer may be transported through the pores.

Most biological membranes bear a surface negative charge, so one would imagine that this might influence permeation. Membranes with unionized surfaces (such as cellophane) or positively charged surfaces such as collagen have different permeability characteristics for ionic drugs. Indeed, molecular forms of solutes permeate faster than ionic forms through membranes composed of collagen, which have been used as potential haemodialysis membranes or release-controlling membranes for medication of the eye. Crucially, anionic solutes permeate faster than cationic solutes. With amphoteric drugs such as sulfasomidine and sulfamethizole, a similar order of permeation may be observed depending on the pH of the medium, namely: unionised > anionic > cationic form. The most likely explanation is that the basic groups in collagen, which are mainly the basic amino acids lysine, arginine and histidine, are positively charged, as the pK_a of lysine and of arginine is about 10. In acidic media the membrane is positively charged and cationic drugs will therefore be repelled from the surface.

pH has little effect on the passage of drugs through cellophane membranes, a fact that can be rationalised by the lack of charge on the cellophane surface. In biological membranes, one might expect some preference for cationic drugs, other things being equal, but we have to remember that biological membranes are more complex and more dynamic than synthetic membranes and there are many confounding factors. One of these, which is outside the scope of this book, is the existence of efflux mechanisms centred on P-glycoproteins (P-gp). Some drugs are ejected from cells by the efflux pump, so that these drugs have a lower apparent absorption than predicted on physicochemical grounds.

In Chapter 5 we examined some relationships between the lipophilicity of drugs and their activity, which was usually controlled by their ability to pass across lipid membranes and barriers. Although of the same basic con-struction, biological membranes in different sites in the body serve different functions and thus one might expect them to have different compositions and physicochemical properties, as indeed they do. Tissues derived from the ectoderm (the epidermis, the epithelium of nose and mouth and the anus, and the tissues of the nervous system) have protective and sensory functions. Tissues evolved from the endoderm, such as the epithelium of the gastrointestinal tract, have evolved mainly to allow absorption.

9.1.1 Lipophilicity and absorption

If one measures the absorption of a suffi-ciently wide range of substances in a homo-logous series, one generally finds that there is an optimal point in the series for absorption. In other words, a plot of percentage absorp-tion versus log P would be parabolic with the optimum value designated as log P_o (Fig. 9.3). By noting the values of optimal partition coefficient for different absorbing membranes and surfaces, one can deduce something about their nature. Some values are given in Table 9.1.

The parabolic nature of activity–log P plots is due to a combination of factors: with drugs with high log P values, protein binding, low solubility and binding to extraneous sites cause a lower measured activity than if it were

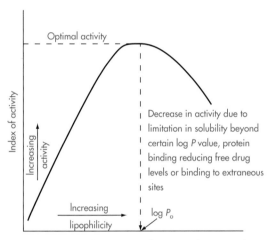

Figure 9.3 Parabolic nature of a typical activity–log P plot: the decrease in biological activity beyond the optimal log P_o probably is due to the factors listed.

Table 9.1	Ideal lipophilic character of drugs (log P_o) in different regions of the body	
System	Solute or drug	Log P_o (octanol/water) for maximal transport
Buccal cavity (human)	Bases	5.52 (undissociated)
		3.52 (dissociated)
	Acids	4.19 (undissociated)
Epidermis (human)	Steroids	3.34
Whole skin (rabbit)	Non-electrolytes	2.55
Small intestine (rat)	Sulfonamides	2.56–3.33
Stomach (rat)	Barbiturates	2.01
	Acids	1.97
Cornea (rabbit)	Steroids	2.8
Biliary excretion	Sulfathiazoles	0.60
Milk/plasma	Sulfonamides	0.53
Prostatic/plasma ratio	Sulfonamides	0.23

possible to take the drug and place it at the receptor without it having to traverse the various lipid and aqueous hurdles that it finds on its way to the site of action.

Molecular weight and drug absorption

The larger drug molecules are, the poorer will be their ability to traverse biological membranes. The change of permeability with increasing molecular size is shown in Fig. 9.4.

In a survey of over 2000 drugs only 11% had molecular weights above 500, and only 8% had molecular weights above 600. Lipinski[1] devised the so-called 'Rule of 5' which refers to drug-like properties of molecules. It states that poor oral absorption is more likely when the drug molecule:

- Has more than five hydrogen-bond donors (—OH groups or —NH groups)
- Has a molecular weight >800
- Has a log $P > 5$
- Has more than 10 H-bond acceptors

and that compounds that are substrates for transporters are exceptions to the rule.

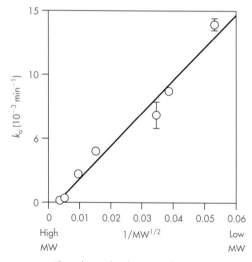

Figure 9.4 The relationship between the molecular weight of compounds and absorption rate constant. The membrane studied is the rat kidney surface, but similar plots hold for other sites.
Reproduced from K. Nishida et al., Eur. J. Pharm. Biopharm., 58, 705–711 (2004).

9.1.2 Permeability and the pH–partition hypothesis

If, in the first instance, the plasma membrane is considered to be a strip of lipoidal material, homogeneous in nature and with a defined thickness, one must assume that only lipid-soluble agents will pass across this barrier. As most drugs are weak electrolytes it is to be expected that the unionised form (U) of either acids or bases, the lipid-soluble species, will diffuse across the membrane, while the ionised forms (I) will be rejected. This is the basis of the *pH–partition hypothesis* in which the pH dependence of drug absorption and solute transport across membranes is considered. The equations of Chapters 3 and 5 are relevant here.

For weakly acidic drugs such as acetylsalicylic acid (aspirin) and indometacin, the ratio of ionised to unionised species is given by the equations

$$pH - pK_a = \log \frac{[\text{ionised form}]}{[\text{unionised form}]} = \log \frac{[I]}{[U]}$$

(9.1)

For weak bases the equation takes the form

$$pK_a - pH = \log \frac{[\text{ionised form}]}{[\text{unionised form}]} = \log \frac{[I]}{[U]}$$

(9.2)

One can calculate from these equations (and equations 3.70–3.73) the relative amounts of absorbable and nonabsorbable forms of a drug substance ([U] and [I], respectively), given the prevailing pH conditions in the lumen of the gut or the site of absorption. The profiles for unionised drug (%) versus pH for several drugs are given in Fig. 9.5. In very broad terms, one would expect acids to be absorbed from the stomach and bases from the intestine.

A comparison of the intestinal absorption of several acids and bases at several pH values (Table 9.2) indicates the expected trend. Surprisingly, however, it will be seen that salicylic acid is absorbed from the rat intestine at pH 8, although with a pK_a of 3.0 it is virtually completely ionised at this pH. There are two explanations: one is that absorption and

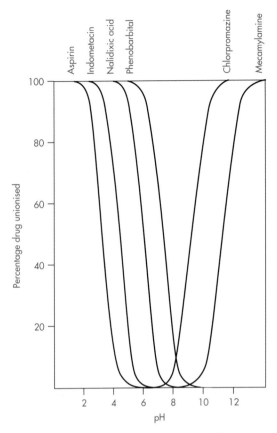

Figure 9.5 Plot of percentage drug unionised (that is, in its lipid-soluble form) as a function of solution pH, for the *acidic* drugs aspirin, indometacin, nalidixic acid and phenobarbital, and for the *basic* drugs chlorpromazine and mecamylamine.

Table 9.2 Intestinal absorption of acids and bases in the rat at several pH values[a]

Acid/base	pK_a	Perentage absorption			
		pH 4	pH 5	pH 7	pH 8
Acids					
Salicylic acid	3.0	64	35	30	10
Acetylsalicylic acid (aspirin)	3.5	41	27	–	–
Benzoic acid	4.2	62	36	35	5
Bases					
Amidopyrine	5.0	21	35	48	52
Quinine	8.4	9	11	41	54

[a] Reproduced from B. B. Brodie, in *Absorption and Distribution of Drugs* (ed. T. Binns), Livingstone, Edinburgh, 1964.

Box 9.1   Calculation of percentage ionisation

Absorption values for acetylsalicylic acid at pH 4, 5, 7 and 8 are quoted in Table 9.2. The amount of drug in the unionised form at these pH values is obtained from equation (9.1). For example, at pH 4,

$$4 - 3.5 = \log \frac{[I]}{[U]}$$

$$\therefore \frac{[I]}{[U]} = 3.162$$

Percentage unionised

$$= \frac{[U] \times 100}{[U] + [I]} = \frac{100}{1 + \dfrac{[I]}{[U]}}$$

$$= \frac{100}{1 + 3.162} = \frac{100}{4.162} = 24.03\%$$

In the same way, we find 3.07% unionised at pH 5; 0.032% at pH 7; and less than 0.009% unionised at pH 9. Absorption is much greater than one would expect, being 41% at pH 4 and 27% at pH 5, although the trend is as predicted.

---

ionisation are both dynamic processes and that the small amount of unionised drug absorbed is replenished; the second is that the bulk pH is not the actual pH at the membrane. Nevertheless, instilling solutions of different pH directly into the lumen of the rat stomach indicates the correct qualitative trends of absorption (62% absorption at pH 1 for salicylic acid and 13% at pH 8).

In attempts to explain away such discrepancies between theoretical prediction and observed results we have already hinted that a local pH exists at the membrane surface which differs from the bulk pH (see below). This local pH is due to the attraction of hydrogen ions by the negative groups of membrane components so that, in the intestine, while the bulk

pH is around 7 the surface pH is nearer 6. One can calculate a 'virtual' surface pH which will allow results such as those in Table 9.2 to be explained. If we take as another example salicylic acid, again calculating the percentage of unionised species by equation (9.1), we obtain the following figures (taken from Table 9.2):

pH	4	5	7	8
Percentage unionised	9.09	0.99	0.009 999	0.001
Percentage absorbed	64	35	30	10

To have 30% of this compound in its unionised form when the bulk pH is 7, would require a surface pH of about 3.4, which is lower than anticipated. Again, however, we must remember that absorption and ionisation processes are dynamic processes. As the unionised species is absorbed, so the level of [U] in the bulk falls and, because of a shift in equilibrium, more of the unionised species appears in the bulk. In fact, if a pH of 5.3 is taken as the pH of the absorbing surface, the results in Table 9.2 become more explicable, as we discuss in the next section.

9.1.3   Problems in the quantitative application of the pH–partition hypothesis

There are several reasons why the pH–partition hypothesis cannot be applied quantitatively in practical situations. Some are discussed here.

Variability in pH conditions

The variation in the stomach pH in human subjects is remarkable, bearing in mind that each pH unit represents a ten-fold difference in hydrogen ion concentration. While the normally quoted range of stomach pH is 1–3, studies using pH-sensitive radiotelemetric capsules have shown a greater spread of values, ranging up to pH 7 as seen in Fig. 10.2 in Chapter 10. This means that the dissolution rate of many drugs will vary markedly in individuals – this is indeed one of the reasons for individual-to-individual variation in drug availability.

The scope for variation in the small intestine is less, although in some pathological states the pH of the duodenum may be quite low owing to hypersecretion of acid in the stomach. Table 9.3 lists the normal pH of

Table 9.3   pH of blood and contents of the human alimentary tract[a]

Sample	pH
Blood	7.35–7.45
Buccal cavity	6.2–7.2
Stomach	1.0–3.0
Duodenum	4.8–8.2
Jejunum and ileum	7.5–8.0
Colon	7.0–7.5

[a] Reproduced from W. C. Bowman, M. J. Rand and G. B. West, *Textbook of Pharmacology*, Blackwell, London, 1967.

the blood and of different regions of the alimentary tract.

pH at membrane surfaces

Data on the relationship between absorption and pH of the intestinal contents on the one hand, and the percentage of drug in the unionised state on the other, can generally be rationalised if the apparent pH is reduced below the pH of the intestine. As described above, this pH 'shift' is thought to be due to the existence of a pH at the membrane surface that is lower than that of the bulk pH. One might expect that the hydrogen ion concentration at the surface would be greater (and hence pH lower) at the membrane surface as hydrogen ions would accumulate near anionic groups, leading to an effect which can be quantified by the equation

$$[H^+]_{surface} = [H^+]_{bulk} \exp \frac{-F\zeta}{RT} \qquad (9.3)$$

where F is the Faraday constant, R is the gas constant, T is absolute temperature and ζ is the zeta potential of the surface (see Chapter 7). Thus, in terms of pH,

$$pH_{surface} = pH_{bulk} + \frac{\zeta}{60} \qquad (9.4)$$

where ζ is expressed in millivolts.

The secretion of acidic and basic substances in many parts of the gut wall is also a complicating factor in the application of the equations, as the local pH in the region of the microvilli of the small intestine will undoubtedly influence the absorption of weak electrolytes. A drug molecule in the bulk will diffuse towards the membrane surface and so meet different pH conditions from those in the bulk phase. Whether or not this influences the extent of absorption will depend on the pH changes and the pK_a of the drug in question. The negative charge on the membrane will attract small cations towards the surface and small anions will be repelled; one might thus expect some selectivity in the absorption process. The existence of this 'microclimate' has been questioned, but experimental evidence for its existence has been forthcoming from the use of microelectrodes, which revealed the existence of a layer on the (rat) jejunum with a pH of 5.5 when the pH of the bathing buffer was 7.2. The existence of this more acid layer has also been demonstrated on the surface of the human intestine.

Other complications include convective water flow and unstirred layers, discussed here.

Convective water flow

The movement of water molecules into and out of the alimentary canal will affect the rate of passage of small molecules across the membrane. The reasons for water flow are the differences in osmotic pressure between blood and the contents of the lumen, and differences in hydrostatic pressure between lumen and perivascular tissue, resulting, for example, from muscular contractions. It can be appreciated that the absorption of water-soluble drugs will be increased if water flows from the lumen to the blood side across the mucosa, provided that drug and water are using the same route. Water movement is greatest within the jejunum.

It has been shown in animals that the absorption of lipid-soluble molecules is affected by solvent flow induced by addition of salts to the lumen.[2] Absorption of benzoic acid, salicylic acid, benzyl alcohol and digitoxin has been shown to be increased by efflux of water from the lumen and decreased by flow into the lumen (see Fig. 9.6). One likely

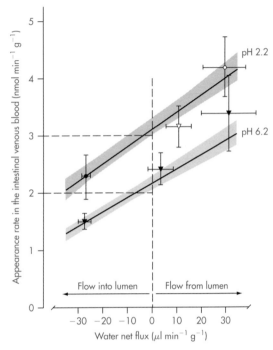

Figure 9.6 The dependence of salicylic acid absorption on the net water flux (positive sign: flow directed from the lumen and towards the blood) in the rat jejunal loop perfused with hypo-, iso- and hypertonic solutions at pH 6.2 and 2.2. The lines, mean values with 95% confidence limits (shaded areas), were calculated by means of the parameters determined by a kinetic model with the following constants: concentration of salicylic acid in the perfusion solution 32.3 μmol dm^{-3}, wet tissue weight 0.453 g, perfusion rate 0.11 cm^3 min^{-1}, intestinal blood flow 0.945 at pH 6.2 and 0.968 cm^3 min^{-1} at pH 2.2.
Reproduced from reference 2.

explanation is that when water flows from the lumen the drug becomes concentrated and drug absorption is increased because of the more advantageous concentration gradient. Suggestions that water flow affects the 'unstirred' layers close to the membrane may also be valid in interpreting these data.

Unstirred water layers

A layer of relatively unstirred water lies adjacent to all biological membranes. The boundary between the bulk water and this unstirred layer is indistinct but, nevertheless, it has a real thickness. During absorption, drug molecules must diffuse across this layer and then on through the lipid layer. The overall rate of transfer is the result of the resistance in both water layer and lipid layer. The flux, J, for a substance across the unstirred layer is given by the expression

$$J = (C_1 - C_2)\frac{D}{\delta} \qquad (9.5)$$

where C_1 and C_2 are the concentrations of the substance in the bulk water phase and in the unstirred water layer respectively, D is the diffusion coefficient and δ is the effective thickness of the unstirred layer. The flux of molecules which pass by passive diffusion through the lipid membrane can be written as

$$J = C_2 P_c \qquad (9.6)$$

where P_c is the permeability coefficient. The rate of absorption must equal the rate of transport across the unstirred layer; that is

$$J = (C_1 - C_2)\frac{D}{\delta} = C_2 P_c \qquad (9.7)$$

The rate of movement across the unstirred layer, as can be seen from the equations, is proportional to D/δ; the rate of absorption is proportional to P_c. Compounds with a large permeability coefficient may be able to penetrate across cell membranes much faster than they can be transported through the unstirred layer. Under these circumstances diffusion through the water layer becomes the rate-limiting step in the absorption process. Neglect of the unstirred layer causes errors in the interpretation of experimental flux data.

Effect of the drug

Drugs, as we have seen, must be in their molecular form before diffusional absorption processes take place. We would expect bases to be more soluble than acids in the stomach, but it is impossible to generalise in this way. Although the basic form of a drug as its hydrochloride salt should be soluble to some extent in this medium, this is not always so. Indeed the free bases of, for example, chlortetracycline, dimethylchlortetracycline and methacycline are more soluble than their corresponding hydrochlorides in the pH range

of the stomach (see Chapter 5). It has been shown that mean plasma levels following administration of the free base and the hydrochloride of these tetracyclines reflect the differences in solubility, the bases giving higher levels. The reason is most likely that discussed in section 5.7.2, namely the influence of high ionic strength on the solubility of the drug substance (the common ion effect). As absorption of the tetracyclines takes place mainly from the duodenum, it is vital that they reach the intestine in a dissolved or readily soluble form, as their solubility is low at the pH conditions prevailing in the duodenum (pH 4–5).

The presence of buffer components in the formulation also creates a pH microenvironment around dissolving particles which may aid drug dissolution. If dissolution is the rate-limiting step in the absorption process, this will be significant in determining absorption. Bulk pH will then give little help in calculating the solution rate on the basis of a knowledge of saturation solubilities in bulk conditions.

Other complicating factors

The very high area of the surface of the small intestine also upsets the calculation of absorption based on considerations of theoretical absorption across identical areas of absorbing surface. The sheer complexity of the situation precludes mathematical precision, yet the pH–partition hypothesis is useful especially in predicting what follows from a change in bulk pH – for example, on ingestion of antacids or drugs such as cimetidine which reduce gastric acid secretion. The extent of the change in pH after administration of cimetidine can be seen from the diagram in Fig. 9.7, which shows a rise in resting pH from below 2 to near neutrality and which in turn depends on the formulation used. The fact that aspirin, an acid with a pK_a of 3.5, is absorbed from the small intestine is due partly to the massive surface area available for absorption (which allows significant absorption to occur even though the percentage of absorbable species is very low) and partly to the dynamics of the process referred to earlier.

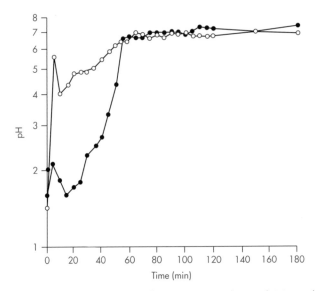

Figure 9.7 Intragastric pH after administration of (O) effervescent cimetidine and (●) standard cimetidine, plotted as median values from 13 patients with gastro-oesophageal flux given 800 mg orally of the preparations.
Reproduced from M. Ström, S. Madsen and B. Norlander, Lancet, 337, 433 (1991).

A warning, however: drugs that are unstable in the gastrointestinal tract (for example, erythromycin), drugs that are metabolised on their passage through the gut wall, drugs that are hydrolysed in the stomach to active forms (prodrugs), and drugs that bind to mucin or form complexes with bile salts may not always be absorbed in the manner expected.

Ion pairing

The interaction of drugs in the charged form with other ions to form absorbable species with a high lipid solubility is a possible explanation for the ability of molecules such as quaternary ammonium compounds, ionised under all pH conditions, to be usefully absorbed. The origin of the ions which pair with drug ions is not clear, but there is evidence that ion-pair formation will aid absorption.

One could assume that small organic ions are absorbed through water-filled pores or channels in the membrane, but the effective diameter of such pores means that large drug ions would be excluded from this route. Although membranes are impermeable to large organic ions, nevertheless ion-pairing

between a drug ion and an organic ion of opposite charge forming an absorbable neutral species is possible.

Two ionic species A^+ and B^- may exist in solution in several states:

$$
\begin{array}{cccc}
A:B & \rightleftharpoons A^+, B^- & \rightleftharpoons A^+B^- & \rightleftharpoons A^+ + B^- \\
\text{undissociated} & \text{'tight'} & \text{'loose'} & \text{free ions} \\
\text{species} & \text{ion pair} & \text{ion pair} &
\end{array}
$$

The formation of tight or loose ion pairs will depend on solvent–ion interactions: hydrophobic ions might be encouraged to form ion pairs by the mechanism of *water-structure enforced ion pairing* in which the water attempts to minimise the disturbance on its structuring, and achieves this end by reducing the polarity of the species in solution by ion-pair formation. Ion pairing in highly structured solvents, then, is due not to an electrostatic interaction but to a solvent-mediated effect. The significance of the phenomenon is that ion pairs have the property of being almost neutral species, so that the ion pair can partition into an oily phase when its parent ionic species cannot, a property that is important in drug absorption and drug extraction procedures, and that is put to use in chromatography.

The two reactions below are examples (i) of a quaternary amine pairing with a weak acid, and (ii) of an alkyl sulfate with a weak base, both under pH conditions in which the solute is charged:

(i) $RCOO^- + N^+(C_4H_9)_4 \rightleftharpoons$
$$RCOON(C_4H_9)_4$$

(ii) $RNH_3^+ + {}^-O_3SO(CH_2)_{11}CH_3 \rightleftharpoons$
$$RNH_3O_3SO(CH_2)_{11}CH_2$$

| hydrophilic | ion-pair agent |
| solute | hydrophobic ion pair |

In extraction procedures using methylene chloride as organic phase, bromothymol blue has been used as an ion-pairing counterion for amfetamine, and picrate ions for atropine. Tetrabutylammonium ion has been used for the extraction of penicillins into chloroform.

Figure 9.8 shows clearly the effect of chloride ion and other anions such as methane sulfonate on the apparent partition coefficient of chlorpromazine. The nature of the anion significantly affects the partitioning of the drug. Ion pairing in the gastrointestinal tract obviously could influence absorption.

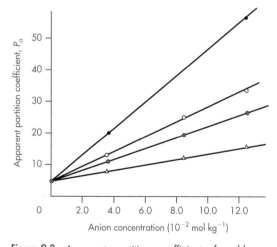

Figure 9.8 Apparent partition coefficients for chlorpromazine between *n*-octanol and aqueous buffers at pH 3.9, in the presence of various anions at 30°C: ○, chloride; ●, propanesulfonate; ⊗, ethanesulfonate; △, methanesulfonate. Reproduced from L. S. Murthy and G. Zografi, *J. Pharm. Sci.*, 59, 1281 (1970).

9.2 The oral route and oral absorption

9.2.1 Drug absorption from the gastrointestinal tract

The oral route is the most popular and convenient route of drug administration for those drugs which can survive the acid of the stomach, which are resistant to enzymatic attack, and which are absorbed across gastrointestinal membranes. The functions of the gastrointestinal tract are the digestion and absorption of foods and other nutrients and it is not easy to separate these two functions from that of drug delivery. Indeed, the natural processes in the gut frequently influence the absorption of drugs. This is not surprising when it is considered that approximately 500 g of solid and up to 2.5 litres of fluid are ingested on average each day. As well as this oral intake, an estimated 30 litres of endogenous fluid are excreted each day into the intestine.

The pH of the gut contents and the presence of enzymes, foodstuffs, bile salts, fat and the microbial flora will all influence drug absorption. The complexity of the absorbing surfaces means that a simple physicochemical approach to drug absorption remains an *approach* to the problem and not the complete picture, as described above. Whatever the limitations of theory – and one should not expect simple theories to hold in the complex and dynamic circumstances which are involved in drug absorption – theory provides a starting point in rationalising the behaviour of drugs in the gastrointestinal tract. While most drugs are absorbed by passive diffusion across the lipid membranes separating the gut contents from the rest of the body, certain molecules that resemble naturally occurring substances are actively transported by special mechanisms.

We first consider the physiological situation which might impinge on passive drug absorption. The delivery of macromolecules, including peptides and proteins, is treated in a separate chapter.

Particulate absorption from the gut

While the general rule is that only drugs in

(a)

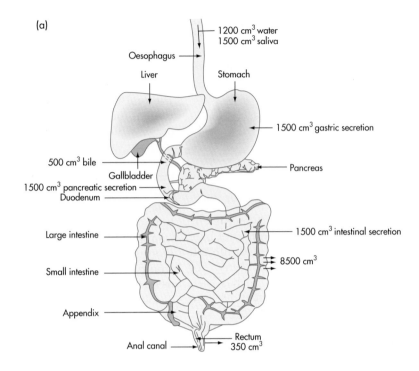

(b)

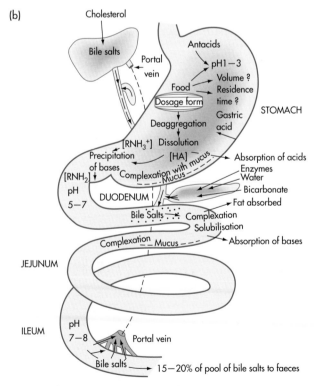

Figure 9.9   Representation of the processes occurring along the gastrointestinal tract, and of the factors that must be taken into account in considering drug absorption.

solution are absorbed from the gastrointestinal tract, colloidal particles, some viruses, bacteria and prion proteins can gain entry to the lymphatic system after absorption by specialised cells (M-cells) in the gut-associated lymphoid tissue (GALT).[3,4]. A discussion of this route of uptake is outside the scope of this book, but it is a route which is likely to be increasingly explored as a means of developing proteins and perhaps genes in carrier nanoparticles and for oral vaccination.

9.2.2 Structure of the gastrointestinal tract

Figure 9.9(a) and (b) diagrammatically represents the gastrointestinal tract and some of the factors involved in the process of drug absorption from this complex milieu. The stomach is not an organ designed for absorption, the main site of absorption being the small intestine. The stomach may be divided into its two main parts: (i) *the body of the stomach* (a receptacle or hopper), which includes the pepsin- and HCl-secreting areas; and (ii) *the pyloris* (a churning chamber), the mucus-secreting area of the gastric mucosa. The stomach varies its luminal volume with the content of food and this is

one reason why food intake can be so important in relation to drug absorption; the stomach may contain a few millilitres or a litre or more of fluid. Hydrochloric acid is liberated from the parietal cells at a concentration of 0.58%, or 160 mmol dm^{-3}. The gastric glands produce some 1000–1500 cm^3 of gastric juice per day. It is in this environment that pharmaceutical dosage forms find themselves. Some of the issues are shown in Fig. 9.9(b).

The small intestine is divided anatomically into three sections: *duodenum*, *jejunum* and *ileum*. Histologically there is no clearly marked transition between these parts. All three are involved in the digestion and absorption of foodstuffs, absorbed material being removed by the blood and the lymph. The absorbing area is enlarged by surface folds in the intestinal lining which are macroscopically apparent: the surface of these folds possess villi and microvilli (Fig. 9.10). It has been calculated that with a maximum of 3000 microvilli per cell in the epithelial brush border (so called because of its physical appearance) the number of microvilli in the small intestine mucosa, even of the rat, is 2×10^8 per mm^2. Although one would expect organic acids to be absorbed only from the stomach where

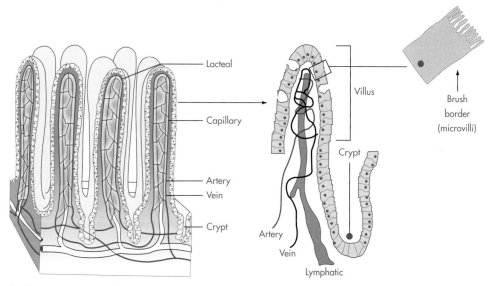

Figure 9.10 Representation of the epithelium of the small intestine at different levels of magnification. From left to right: the intestinal villi and microvilli which comprise the brush border.

they will exist in the unionised lipid-soluble and membrane-diffusible form, the enormous surface area in the intestine allows significant absorption of acidic drugs from the intestine even though (as noted earlier) the fraction of unionised molecules is very small.

Over the entire length of the large and small intestines and the stomach, the brush border has a uniform coating (3 nm thick) of mucopolysaccharides which consist of multi-branched polymeric chains. This coating layer appears to act as a mechanical barrier to bacteria, cells or food particles, or as a filter. Whatever its function, the weakly acidic, sulfated mucopolysaccharides influence the charge on the cell membrane and complicate the explanations of absorption.

The goblet cells of the epithelium form mucus; secretions are stored in granule form in the apical cell region and are liquefied on contact with water to form mucus, which is composed of protein and carbohydrate.

The large intestine is concerned primarily with the absorption of water and the secretion of mucus to aid the intestinal contents to slide down the intestinal 'tube'. Villi are therefore completely absent from the large intestine, but there are deep crypts distributed over its surface.

Differences in the absorptive areas and volumes of gut contents in different animals are important when comparing experimental results on drug absorption in various species.[5] The human small intestine has a calculated active surface area of approximately 100 m^2. No analogous calculations are available for the most commonly used laboratory animals, although the surface area of the small intestine of the rat is estimated to be 700 cm^2.

Passive transport, carrier-mediated transport and specialised transport

In discussing the pH–partition hypothesis, it has been considered that drugs are absorbed by passive diffusion through epithelial cells – the enterocytes of the GI tract for example. In fact there is the possibility of some passage of drugs by way of the tight junctions (the paracellular route) and there are transcellular carrier-mediated uptake mechanisms as well as endocytosis. Figure 9.11 summarises these. The possibility of specialised membranous epithelial cells (M-cells) contributing to the uptake of macromolecules and proteins is referred to later.

9.2.3 Bile salts and fat absorption pathways

Fat is absorbed by special mechanisms in the gut. The bile salts which are secreted into the jejunum are efficient emulsifiers and disperse fat globules, allowing the action of lipase at the much increased globule surface. Medium-chain triglycerides are thought to be directly absorbed. Long-chain triglycerides are hydrolysed, and the monoglycerides and fatty acids produced form mixed micelles with the bile salts and are absorbed either directly in the micelle or, more probably, brought to the microvillus surface by the micelle and transferred directly to the mucosal cells, the bile salts remaining in the lumen. The bile salts are reabsorbed in the ileum and transported via the portal vein back into the bile salt pool.

There have been suggestions that lipid-soluble drugs may be absorbed by fat absorption pathways. Certainly, administration of drugs in an oily vehicle can significantly affect absorption, increasing it in the case of griseofulvin and ciclosporin, but decreasing it in the case of vitamin D.

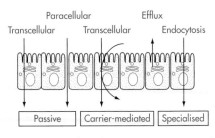

Figure 9.11 GI membrane transport. Transport through the enterocyte barrier can be divided into active, passive and specialized transport; and into the paracellular and transcellular routes. Efflux mechanisms can reduce absorption by these routes.

9.2.4   Gastric emptying, motility and volume of contents

The volume of the gastric contents will determine the concentration of a drug which finds itself in the stomach. The time the drug or dosage form resides in the stomach will determine many aspects of absorption. If the drug is absorbed lower down the gut, the residence time will determine the delay before absorption begins; if the drug is labile in acid conditions, longer residence times in the stomach will lead to greater stability; if the dosage form is nondisintegrating then retention in the stomach can influence the pattern of absorption. Gastroretentive dosage forms are designed to achieve that control.

The stomach empties liquids faster than solids. The rate of transfer of gastric contents to the small intestine is retarded by the activity of receptors sensitive to acid, fat, osmotic pressure and amino acids in the duodenum and the small intestine and stimulated by material that has arrived from the stomach. Gastric emptying is a simple exponential or square-root function of the volume of a test meal – a pattern that holds for meals of variable viscosity. To explain the effect of a large range of substances on emptying, an osmoreceptor has been postulated which, like a red blood cell, shrinks in hypertonic solutions and swells in hypotonic solutions.

Acids in test meals have been found to slow gastric emptying; acids with higher molecular weights (for example, citric acid) are less effective than those, such as HCl, with very low molecular weights. Natural triglycerides inhibit gastric motility, linseed and olive oils being effective. The formulation of a drug may thus influence drug absorption through an indirect physiological effect. The nature of the dose form – whether solid or liquid, whether acid or alkaline, whether aqueous or oily – may thus influence gastric emptying. The question of gastric emptying and transit down the gastrointestinal tract has assumed further importance in relation to the design and performance of sustained-release preparations. The transit of pellets of different densities,[6,7] for example, is shown in Fig. 9.12 and illustrates the influence of both density and food intake.

Food, then, affects not only transit but also pH. The effect of a meal on the hydrogen ion concentration of the stomach contents is shown in Fig. 9.13; the effect of two antacids on gastric volume and pH is shown in Table 9.4. When considering the effect of an antacid, therefore, the effect of volume change and pH change and the effect on gastric emptying must all be considered. In designing delivery systems all these factors have ideally to be taken into account.

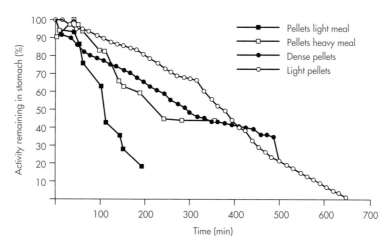

Figure 9.12   Gastric emptying of pellets of different density with various sizes of meal.
Reproduced from C. G. Wilson and N. Washington, *Physiological Pharmaceutics*, Ellis Horwood, Chichester, 1989.

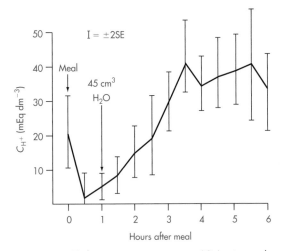

Figure 9.13 Hydrogen ion concentrations (C_{H^+}) at intervals after a test meal (mean results are shown ± 2SEM); the zero samples were taken just before the meal was begun, and the 1 hour sample just before 45 cm^3 of water.
Modified from J. Fordtran, *N. Engl. J. Med.*, 274, 921 (1966).

Table 9.4 Effects of antacids on gastric volume and pH in the rat[a, b]

	Water	Maalox	Amphojel
Volume (cm^3)	0.29 ± 0.03	1.8 ± 0.3	4.0 ± 0.2
pH	2.2 ± 0.2	7.4 ± 0.1	4.7 ± 0.2

[a] Reproduced from M. Hava and A. Hurwitz, *Eur. J. Pharmacol.*, 22, 156 (1973).
[b] Ten rats per group. Measurements on gastric contents made 20 min after the third hourly dose of 1 cm^3 water or antacid by gastric intubation.

9.3 Buccal and sublingual absorption

Mouthwashes, toothpastes and other preparations are introduced into the oral cavity for local prophylactic and therapeutic reasons. It is not known to what extent components of these formulations are absorbed and give rise to systemic effects. The absorption of drugs through the oral mucosa, however, provides a route for systemic administration which avoids exposure to the gastrointestinal system. Drugs absorbed in this way bypass the liver and have direct access to the systemic circulation. The sublingual, buccal and gingival

tissues are shown diagrammatically in Fig. 9.14. There are many drugs that have not been administered sublingually, although some, like glyceryl trinitrate, have been traditionally administered in this way. The oral mucosa functions primarily as a barrier, however, and it is not a highly permeable tissue, resembling skin more closely than gut in this respect. Table 9.5 lists some commercially available sublingual and buccal delivery systems. Mucosal adhesive systems have been studied for administration of buprenorphine through the gingiva (gums).

9.3.1 Mechanisms of absorption

The oral mucosa comprises

- A mucus layer over the epithelium
- A keratinised layer in certain regions of the oral cavity
- An epithelial layer
- A basement membrane
- Connective tissue
- A submucosal region

While cells of the oral epithelium and epidermis are capable of absorbing material by endocytosis, it does not seem likely that drugs or other solutes would be transported by this mechanism across the entire stratified epithelium. It is also unlikely that active transport processes are operative in the oral mucosa. There is considerable evidence that most substances are absorbed by simple diffusion. The linear relationship between percentage absorption through the buccal epithelium and log *P* of a homologous series is seen in Fig. 9.15. For example, the buccal absorption of some basic drugs increases (Fig. 9.16), and that of acidic drugs decreases, with increasing pH of their solutions.

Nicotine in a gum vehicle when chewed is absorbed through the buccal mucosa; nicotine levels obtained are lower than those obtained by smoking cigarettes and the high peak levels are not seen. Buccal glyceryl trinitrate has been found to be an effective drug. The buccal route has the advantages of the sublingual route – the buccal mucosa is similar to sublingual

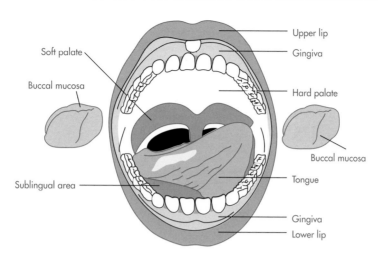

Figure 9.14 The anatomy of the oral cavity including the buccal, sublingual and gingival cavities. (From K. Kunth *et al.*, *Adv. Drug Del. Rev.*, 11, 137 (1993).)

Table 9.5 Commercially available drug-delivery systems for systemic delivery by the oral mucosal route[a]

Mucosal site	Drug	Proprietary name	Dosage form
Sublingual	Glyceryl trinitrate	Nitrostat	Tablets
		Lenitral spray	Spray
		Susadrin	Bioadhesive tablets
	Isosorbide dinitrate	Risordan	Tablets
		Sorbitrate	Chewable tablets
		Isocard spray	Spray
	Erythritol trinitrate	Cardiwell	Tablets
	Nifedipine	Adalat	Tablets
	Buprenorphine	Temgesic	Tablets
	Apomorphine HCl	Apomorphine	Tablets
Buccal	Prochlorperazine	Buccastem	Bioadhesive tablets
		Tementil	Solution
	Phloroglucinol	Spasfon-Lyoc	Lyocs
	Oxazepam	Seresta Expidet	Lyophilised tablets
	Lorazepam	Temesta Expidet	Lyophilised tablets
	Methyltestosterone	Metandren	Tablets
	Nicotine	Nicorette	Chewing-gum

[a] Modified from G. Ponchel, *Adv. Drug Del. Rev.*, 13, 75, (1994).

mucosal tissue – but a sustained-release tablet can be held in the cheek pouch for several hours if necessary. Mucosal adhesive formulations can have obvious advantages.

Experiments with some analgesics showed that the highly lipid-soluble etorphine was absorbed several times more rapidly from the buccal cavity than the less lipid-soluble morphine.[8] Impressive absorption has been obtained with glyceryl trinitrate (which exerts its pharmacological action 1–2 minutes after sublingual administration), methacholine chloride, isoprenaline, some steroids such as desoxycortisone acetate[9] and 17β-estradiol (at one-quarter of its normal oral dose), morphine, captopril and nifedipine.

It has been claimed that an oil/water partition coefficient in the range 40–2000 (log P of

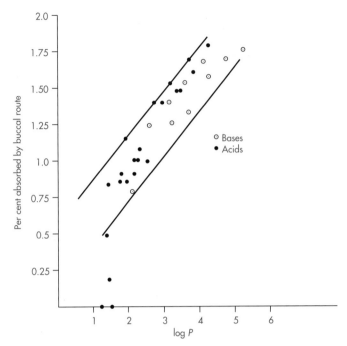

Figure 9.15   Relationship between the log *P* of solute and the percentage absorption through the buccal mucosa of human subjects for bases (O) and acids (●)
Plotted from data from E. Lien *et al.*, *Drug Intell. Clin. Pharm.*, 5, 38 (1971).

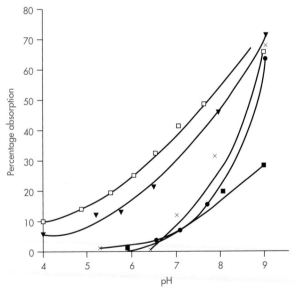

Figure 9.16   Buccal absorption of some basic drugs. The drugs were dissolved in buffered solutions of different pH and placed in the mouth of human subjects; absorption rates were determined from the decrease of drug concentration in expelled solutions: □, chlorphenamine ($pK_a = 8.99$); ▼, methadone ($pK_a = 8.25$); ×, amfetamine ($pK_a = 9.94$); ●, pethidine ($pK_a = 8.72$); ■, nicotine ($pK_a = 8.02$).
Reproduced from A. H. Beckett and E. J. Triggs, *J. Pharm. Pharmacol.*, 19, 31S (1976).

1.6 to 3.3) is optimal for drugs to be used by the sublingual route. Drugs with a $\log P$ greater than 3.3 are so oil-soluble that it is difficult for sufficiently high levels of drug to be soluble in the aqueous salivary fluids. Drugs less lipophilic than those with a $\log P$ of 1 would not be absorbed to any great extent and thus require large doses by this route. A comparison of the sublingual/subcutaneous dose ratio serves as an index of the usefulness of the route.[10] For example, cocaine with a P of 28 requires a sublingual/subcutaneous dosage ratio of 2 to obtain equal effects; atropine with a P of 7 requires 8 times the subcutaneous dose; and for codeine $(P \approx 2)$ over 15 times the subcutaneous dose must be given sublingually.

9.4   Intramuscular and subcutaneous injection

The intramuscular and subcutaneous routes of administration have long been regarded as efficient routes because they bypass the problems encountered in the stomach and intestine, but not all the drug injected will necessarily be bioavailable. Early views that subcutaneous (s.c.) and intramuscular (i.m.) administration of drugs resulted in only local action at the site were dispelled by Benjamin Bell, who wrote in the *Edinburgh Medical Journal* of 1858 that 'absorption from the enfeebled stomach may not be counted on; we possess in subcutaneous injections a more direct, rapid and trustworthy mode of conveying our remedy in the desired quantity to the circulatory blood'. We now know that not all drugs are efficiently or uniformly released from i.m. or s.c. sites. Some of the drugs that are *not* fully absorbed from the i.m. site are listed in Table 9.6.

Where differences in bioavailability between i.m., s.c and oral or i.v. delivery occur, the clinical importance is most marked when the route of administration is changed from one to the other, and, of course, such changes are most important in drugs with a low therapeutic index such as digoxin and phenytoin.

Table 9.6   Widely used drugs that may be incompletely absorbed after intramuscular injection

Ampicillin	Digoxin[a]
Cefaloridine	Insulin[a]
Cefradine	Phenylbutazone
Chlordiazepoxide	Phenytoin[a]
Diazepam	Quinidine
Dicloxacillin	

[a] Clinically important problems have been demonstrated with these.

In order for a drug to have a systemic action following injection, it must be released from the formulation and reach the site of action in sufficient amounts and at a sufficient rate to produce the desired pharmacological effect. The various regions into which injections are given are shown in Fig. 9.17. The subcutaneous region has a good supply of capillaries, although it is generally agreed that there are few, if any, lymph vessels in muscle proper. Drugs with the correct physicochemical characteristics can diffuse through the tissue and pass across the capillary walls and thus enter the circulation via the capillary supply.

If it is assumed that drug absorption proceeds by passive diffusion of the drug, it can be considered to be a first-order process. Thus the rate of absorption is proportional to the concentration, C, of drug remaining at the injection site:

$$\frac{dC}{dt} = -k_a C \tag{9.8}$$

where k_a is the first-order rate constant. The half-life of the absorption process is

$$t_{0.5} = \frac{0.693}{k_a} \tag{9.9}$$

Drug absorption is 90% complete when a time equivalent to three times the half-life has elapsed.

Both dissolution and diffusion are important parameters in defining bioavailability of species by the i.m. or s.c. routes. Soluble neutral compounds disperse from intramuscular sites according to size: Table 9.7 shows that mannitol, a small molecule, rapidly diffuses from the site of injection; insulin

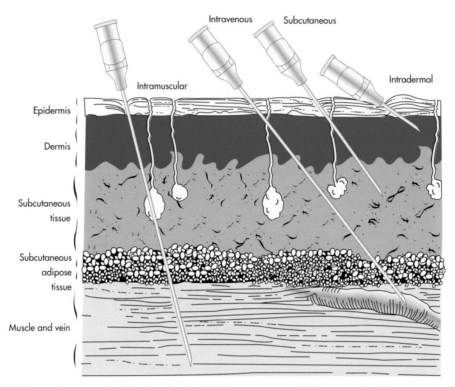

Figure 9.17 Routes of parenteral medication, showing the tissues penetrated by intramuscular, intravenous, subcutaneous and intradermal injections; the needles, with bevel up, penetrate the epidermis (cuticle) consisting of stratified epithelium with an outer horny layer, the corium (dermis or true skin) consisting of tough connective tissue, elastic fibres, lymphatic and blood vessels, and nerves, the subcutaneous tissue (*tela subcutanea*) consisting of loose connective tissue containing blood and lymphatic vessels, nerves, and fat-forming cells, the fascia (a thin sheet of fibrous connective tissue), and the veins, arteries and muscle.
Drawing modified after David S. Quackenbush, in E. W. Martin, *Techniques of Medication*, Lippincott, Philadelphia, 1969.

disperses less rapidly; and dextran (molecular weight 70 000), as might be expected, disperses more slowly.

Molecular size is a minor factor in controlling release of drugs with molecular weights in the range 100–1000, but it assumes greater importance in proteins and other macromolecules. Unless low molecular weight drugs

Table 9.7 Influence of molecular size on clearance from intramuscular sites

Substance	Molecular weight	Fraction cleared (5 min)
Mannitol	182	0.7
Inulin	3 500	0.2
Dextran	70 000	0.07

are attached to a macromolecular backbone, significant retardation cannot be achieved. Hydrophilic molecules such as those listed in Table 9.7 will be transported to the blood after diffusing through muscle fibres and then through the pores in the capillary walls, being incapable of absorption through the lipid walls. The transport through the capillary wall is the rate-limiting step in most cases; the larger the molecule the more slowly it diffuses (as seen from equation (3.91)) and the greater difficulty it has in traversing the aqueous pore in the capillary walls or the cell junction. The 'pores', of whatever character they are, account for only 1% of the available surface of the capillary wall.

Absorption of weak electrolytes across the capillary walls follows the expected patterns, uptake of more lipid-soluble agents being relatively fast. Hydrophobic drugs may bind to muscle protein, leading to a reduction in free drug and perhaps to prolongation of action. Dicloxacillin is 95% bound to protein, ampicillin is bound to the extent of 20%; as a consequence, dicloxacillin is absorbed more slowly from muscle than is ampicillin.

The significance of the diffusion phase through muscle tissue was demonstrated by Duran Reynolds who, in 1928, observed that dye solutions injected together with hyaluronidase spread out more rapidly and over a greater distance in the tissue than in the absence of the enzyme. The enzyme achieves its effect by breaking down the hyaluronic acid in intercellular spaces, thus leading to a decrease in viscosity and so easing the passage of small molecules in the matrix.

Site of injection

The region into which the injection is administered is complex, being composed of both aqueous and lipid components. Muscle tissue is more acidic than normal physiological fluids. Measurement of percutaneous muscle surface pH (pH_m) using microelectrodes gave values of 7.38; patients with peripheral vascular disease demonstrated a mean pH_m of 7.16. pH_m reflects the intramuscular ion concentrations but is stated to be higher than the actual intramuscular pH, which may be as low as 6.4. The pH of the region will determine whether drugs will dissolve in the tissue fluids or precipitate from formulations. In some cases precipitation will occur and may be the cause of the pain experienced on injection (see the discussion on precipitation in section 10.1.2). The rate of solution here, as in many other routes, therefore determines how quickly the drug begins to act or, in some cases, for how long it acts. The deliberate reduction of the solubility of a drug achieves prolonged action by both routes.

9.4.1 Vehicles

Many preparations of drugs for i.m. administration are formulated in water-miscible solvents such as polyethylene glycol (PEG) 300 or 400, or propylene glycol or ethanol mixtures. Dilution by the tissue fluids may cause a drug to precipitate. Drugs formulated as aqueous solutions by adjustment of pH will only momentarily alter the pH of the injection site. Three main types of formulation are used for i.m. and s.c injections: aqueous solutions, aqueous suspensions and oily solutions. Rapid removal of aqueous vehicles is to be expected. If the vehicle is nonaqueous and is an oil such as sesame oil, or other vegetable or mineral oil, the oil phase disperses as droplets in the muscle and surrounding tissue, and is eventually metabolised.

The rate-determining step in the absorption of drug esters such as fluphenazine decanoate (which has an aqueous solubility of about 1 part per million) is the hydrolysis of the drug at the surface of the oil droplet. Hydrolysis of the fluphenazine decanoate to its soluble alcohol therefore depends on the state of dispersion and surface area of the droplets. Dispersing the droplets by rubbing the site of injection or by violent exercise can result in excessive dosage, with toxic effects. Exercise also causes increased blood flow and, as absorption is a dynamic process requiring the sweeping away of the drug from the localised absorption site, this increased flow increases the rate of drug dispersal.

9.4.2 Blood flow

Different rates of blood flow in different muscles mean that the site of i.m. injection can be crucial. Resting blood flow in the deltoid region is significantly greater than in the *gluteus maximus* muscle; flow in the *vastus lateralis* is intermediate. The difference between blood flow in the deltoid and gluteus is of the order of 20% and is likely to be the reason why deltoid injection of lidocaine has been found to give higher blood levels than injection into the lateral thigh. Therapeutic plasma levels for the prevention of arrhythmia with a dose of 4.5 mg kg^{-1} of a 10% solution of lidocaine were achieved only following deltoid injection.

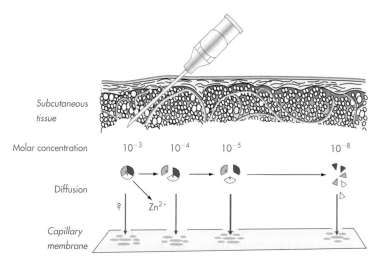

Subcutaneous
tissue

Molar concentration 10^{-3} 10^{-4} 10^{-5} 10^{-8}

Diffusion

? Zn^{2+}

Capillary
membrane

Figure 9.19 Suggested scheme of events after the s.c. administration of soluble human insulin: the concentration of hexameric zinc-insulin, which is the predominant form of insulin in soluble insulin (40 Unit or 100 Unit – i.e. 0.6 mmol dm^{-3}), decreases as diffusion of insulin occurs and as a result the hexamer dissociates into smaller units; to achieve monomeric insulin requires a 1000-fold dilution. The importance of the association state is that the larger species have more difficulty dispersing and passing through the capillary membrane.
Reproduced from J. Brange, D. R. Owens, S. Kang and A. Vølund, *Diabetes Care*, 13, 923 (1990) with permission.

to diffusion and as an active site of degradation.

Figure 9.19 offers a diagrammatic representation of the events following s.c. administration of a soluble human insulin existing initially as a hexameric zinc–insulin complex.

The use of insulins in solution obviates the potential source of error which arises when drawing a suspension into a syringe, but soluble insulins have the drawback that they must be stored at acid pH. Figure 9.20 shows the solubility–pH profiles for soluble insulin and a trilysyl derivative. Injected subcutaneously, the insulin precipitates as amorphous particles.

The hydrogen ion concentration of insulin preparations influences their stability, solubility and immunogenicity. After i.m. administration, short-acting insulin is absorbed about twice as rapidly as after s.c. injection, and therefore the i.m. route is used in the management of ketoacidosis in those cases where continuous i.v. infusion cannot be established. After s.c. injection, absorption of short-acting insulin varies considerably depending in particular on the site of injection. Patient-to-patient variability is as great with these preparations as the variations in the absorption rate of intermediate acting insulins. This can lead to difficulty in control.

Self-regulating systems

A self-regulating delivery system such as the artificial β-cell is of obvious clinical

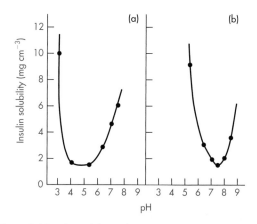

Figure 9.20 The solubility dependence of (a) insulin and (b) trilysyl insulin, a chemically modified insulin with an isoelectric point of 7.4 compared with the isoelectric point of unmodified insulin of 5.3.
Reproduced from F. Fishel-Ghodsian and J. M. Newton, *J. Drug Targeting*, 1, 67 (1993).

relevance.[11] The artificial β-cell consists of an implanted glucose electrode, computer, pump and reservoir. Signals from the glucose electrode cause insulin to be pumped from the reservoir when circulating levels of glucose are high. The reservoir can be topped up through a closure. The advantage of such systems is that the dose administered is in direct response to the levels of glucose in the blood. Insulin delivery in pumps is discussed in Chapter 11.

9.5 Transdermal delivery

A comprehensive account of the pharmaceutics and biopharmaceutics of topical preparations is not possible here. This section has therefore been deliberately restricted in scope to deal with the physicochemical principles involved in the process of treating the skin or in systemic medication by the *transdermal* or *percutaneous* route. Formulation of topical vehicles for the potent drugs applied to the skin is now an exact art. It is readily demonstrated that the

vehicle in which the drug is applied influences the rate and extent of absorption, although it must be remembered that topical formulations can change rather rapidly once they have been spread on the skin, with absorption of some excipients and evaporative loss of water.

Before any drug applied topically can act either locally or systemically it must penetrate the barrier layer of the skin, the *stratum corneum* (Fig. 9.21). This behaves like a passive diffusion barrier with no evidence of metabolic transport processes, drugs being absorbed by transcellular or intercellular pathways.

Penetration of water and low molecular weight nonelectrolytes through the epidermis is proportional to their concentration, and to the partition coefficient of the solute between tissue and vehicle. A form of Fick's law describes steady-state transport through the skin:

$$J = \left(\frac{DP}{\delta}\right)\Delta C_v \qquad (9.10)$$

where J is the solute flux, D is the solute diffusion coefficient in the stratum corneum

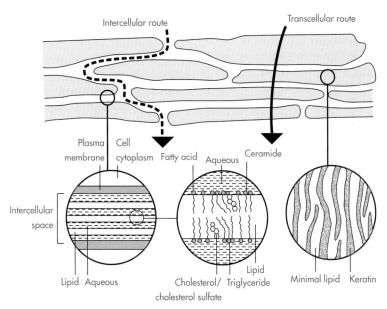

Figure 9.21 'Bricks and mortar' model of the stratum corneum, illustrating possible pathways of drug permeation through intact stratum corneum (transcellular and tortuous intercellular pathways) and the lamellar structure of intercellular lipids. Reproduced from H. R. Moghimi *et al.*, *Int. J. Pharm.*, 131, 117 (1996).

(values range from 1×10^{-12} to 1×10^{-17} m^2 s^{-1} for human stratum corneum), P is the solute partition coefficient between vehicle and skin, and δ is the thickness of the stratum corneum. ΔC_v is the difference in solute concentration between vehicle and tissue. This relation is obtained as shown in Box 9.2.

Box 9.2   Derivation of equation (9.10)

Fick's law of diffusion shows that (for a given vehicle)

$$J \propto \Delta C_v \qquad (9.11)$$

A proportionality constant κ_p may be added. Thus

$$J = \kappa_p \, \Delta C_v \qquad (9.12)$$

where κ_p is the permeability constant, which provides a means of expressing absorption measurements for comparing different vehicles and conditions. The units of a permeability constant are m s^{-1}, the concentration term being mol m^{-3}, so that J has the correct units of mol m^{-2} s^{-1}. It has been shown that

$$\kappa_p = \frac{PD}{\delta} \qquad (9.13)$$

so that equation (9.10) is readily obtained.

Before steady-state penetration is achieved, the rate builds up over a period of time and a lag phase will be apparent (Fig. 9.22). The lag time, τ, does not indicate the point at which steady-state is achieved which, as shown in Fig. 9.22, is obtained by extrapolation. The linear portion of the graph can be described by an equation relating the total amount absorbed at time t, Q_t, to ΔC_v, P, δ, t and D. From equation (9.10), as $Q_t = Jt$,

$$Q_t = \frac{DP \, \Delta C_v}{\delta} t \qquad (9.14)$$

But from Fig. 9.22 it is obvious that the time to be substituted is the time over which steady-state flux has been maintained; namely, $t - \tau$. Thus we write

$$Q_t = \frac{DP \, \Delta C_v}{\delta} (t - \tau) \qquad (9.15)$$

As the lag time, τ, has been shown to be equal to $\delta^2/6D$, the diffusion coefficient D is readily

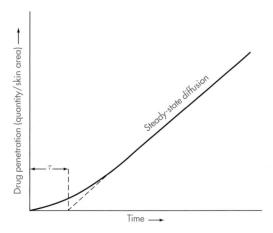

Figure 9.22 Drug penetration–time profile for an idealised drug diffusing through human skin; once steady-state diffusion occurs Q_t can be obtained using equation (9.14) where t = (time elapsed – τ).

obtained from data such as those shown in Fig. 9.22. Values of τ range from a few minutes to several days, so lag times are of obvious clinical relevance.

9.5.1   Routes of skin penetration

Solute molecules may penetrate the skin not only through the stratum corneum but also by way of the hair follicles or through the sweat ducts, but these offer only a comparatively minor route because they represent such a small fraction of the surface area. Only in the case of molecules that move very slowly through the stratum corneum may absorption by these other routes predominate. Passage through damaged skin is increased over normal skin. Skin with a disrupted epidermal layer will allow up to 80% of hydrocortisone to pass into the dermis, but only 1% is absorbed through intact skin.

The physicochemical factors that control drug penetration include the hydration of the stratum corneum, temperature, pH, drug concentration, and the molecular characteristics of the penetrant and the vehicle. The stratum corneum is a heterogeneous structure containing about 40% protein (keratin, a disulfide-crosslinked linear polypeptide), about

40% water and 18–20% lipids (principally triglycerides and free fatty acids, cholesterol and phospholipids). Hydration of the stratum corneum is one determinant of the extent of absorption: increased hydration decreases the resistance of the layer, presumably by causing a swelling of the compact structures in the horny layer. Occlusive dressings increase the hydration of the stratum corneum by preventing water loss by perspiration; certain ointment bases are designed to be self-occluding. The use of occlusive films may increase the penetration of corticosteroids by a factor of 100 and of low molecular weight penetrants 2-fold to 5-fold. As temperature varies little in the clinical use of a topical preparation, this parameter will not be discussed here. A pH in excess of 11 will greatly increase skin permeability.

Occluded skin may absorb up to 5–6 times its dry weight of water. In the idealised model of the stratum corneum shown in Fig. 9.23, L represents the lipid-rich interstitial phase and P the proteinaceous phase. If $\rho = P_L/P_P$ (the ratio of the partition coefficients of the drug between vehicle and the L and P phases), and D_L and D_P are the diffusion coefficients of the drug in these phases, the flux through stratum corneum of average thickness (that is, 40 μm) is found to reduce to

$$J = 0.98\rho \frac{D_L}{D_P} \ (\mu g\ cm^{-2}\ h^{-1})$$

when $\rho(D_L/D_P)$ is very small. When $\rho(D_L/D_P)$ is very large, the flux becomes

$$J = (2.3 \times 10^{-4})\rho \frac{D_L}{D_P} \ (\mu g\ cm^{-2}\ h^{-1})$$

which emphasises the importance of the partition coefficient and diffusion coefficient of the drug in the absorption process.

9.5.2 Influence of drug

The diffusion coefficient of the drug in the skin will be determined by factors such as molecular size, shape and charge; the partition coefficient will be determined not only by the properties of the drug but also by the vehicle as this represents the donor phase, the skin being the receptor phase. The quantity ρ can be approximated by experimentally determined oil/water partition coefficients. Thus, substances that have a very low oil solubility will display low rates of penetration.

The major pathway of transport for water-soluble molecules is transcellular, involving passage through cells and cell walls. The pathway for lipid-soluble molecules is presumably the endogenous lipid within the stratum corneum, the bulk of this being intercellular. Increase in the polar character of the penetrant molecule decreases permeability, as seen from the data on steroids in Table 9.9, in which progesterone and hydroxyprogesterone and desoxycortone and cortexolone should be compared. Each pair differs by a hydroxyl group. The lipid/water partition coefficients of

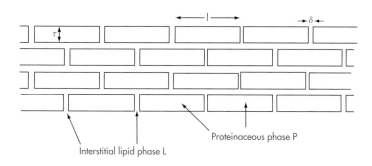

Figure 9.23 Idealised model of the stratum corneum. Lipid (L) and proteinaceous (P) parts of the stratum corneum are represented; this model is used to derive model equations for drug transport across this layer (see text).
Reproduced from A. S. Michaels et al., A. I. Chem. J., 21, 985 (1975).

Table 9.9 Permeability constants of steroids[a]

Steroid	Structure	Permeability constant, κ_P (10^{-6} cm^{-2} h^{-1})
Progesterone		1500
Hydroxyprogesterone		600
Desoxycortone		450
Cortexolone		75

[a] Reproduced from R. Scheuplein, *J. Invest. Dermatol.*, **67**, 672 (1976).

the drugs in Table 9.9 decrease as the number of hydroxyl groups increases, but a simple lipid/water partition coefficient is not an ideal guide, as the stratum corneum is a complex system as described above. If a substance is more soluble in the stratum corneum than in the vehicle in which it is presented, however, the concentration in the first layer of the skin may be higher than that in the vehicle. If depletion of the contact layers of the vehicle occurs, then the nature of the formulation will dictate how readily these are replenished by diffusion and, therefore, will dictate the rate of absorption.

The penetration rates of four steroids through intact abdominal autopsy skin were, in the order of their physiological activity, betamethasone 17-valerate (**I**) > desonide > triamcinolone acetonide (**II**) > hydrocortisone (**III**). Triamcinolone itself is five times more active systemically than hydrocortisone, but has only one-tenth of its topical activity. The acetonide of triamcinolone has a topical activity 1000 times that of the parent steroid because of its favourable lipid solubility. Betamethasone (**IV**) is 30 times as active as hydrocortisone systemically but has only four times the topical potency. Of 23 esters of betamethasone, the 17-valerate ester possesses

Structure I Betamethasone 17-valerate

Structure II Triamcinolone acetonide

Structure III Hydrocortisone

Structure IV Betamethasone

the highest topical activity. The vasoconstrictor potency of betamethasone 17-valerate is 360 (fluocinolone acetonide = 100), that of beta-methasone 0.8, its 17-acetate 114, the 17-propionate 190, and the 17-octanoate 10. The peak activity coincides with an optimal partition coefficient, one which favours neither lipid nor aqueous phase.

9.5.3   Influence of vehicle

Consideration of equation (9.10) shows immediately that the vehicle has an influence on the absorption of the drug; if the vehicle is changed so that the drug becomes less soluble in it, P increases so that permeability increases. The vehicle is more dominant in topical therapy than in most routes of administration because the vehicle remains at the site, although not always in an unchanged form. Evaporation of water from a w/o base would leave drug molecules immersed in the oily phase. Oil-in-water emulsion systems may invert to water-in-oil systems, in such a way that the drug would have to diffuse through an oily layer to reach the skin. Volatile components are driven off, probably altering the state of saturation of the drug and hence its activity. Drug may precipitate owing to lack of remaining solvent. These changes mean that theoretical approaches very much represent the ideal cases.

Formulations

Many modern dermatological formulations are washable oil-in-water systems. Simple aqueous lotions are also used as they have a cooling effect on the skin. Ointments are used for the application of insoluble or oil-soluble medicaments and leave a greasy film on the skin, inhibiting loss of moisture and encouraging the hydration of the keratin layer. Aqueous creams combine the characteristics of the lotions and ointments. A classification of semisolid bases is given in Fig. 9.24.

The descriptions 'ointment' and 'cream' have no universally accepted meaning and generally refer to the completed formulation.

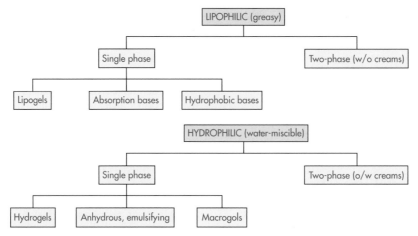

Figure 9.24 Classification of topical semisolid bases into lipophilic and hydrophilic systems in either single-phase or two-phase forms.

Ointments are generally composed of single-phase hydrophobic bases, such as pharmaceutical grades of soft paraffin or microcrystalline paraffin wax.

'Absorption' bases have an alleged capacity to facilitate absorption by the skin, but the term also alludes to their ability to take up considerable amounts of water to form water-in-oil emulsions. Lipogels are gels prepared by dispersion of long-chain fatty acid soaps such as aluminium monostearate in a hydrocarbon base. Hydrogels prepared from Carbopols or cellulose derivatives are discussed in section 8.4.

The complexity of many of the topical bases means that a physicochemical explanation of their influence on the release of medicament is not always possible. It is not difficult, however, to ascertain this influence and to highlight the problem. The interactions between the physical properties of the base and the drug are exemplified by the effect of propylene glycol in simple bases shown in Fig. 9.25, where the percentage of the glycol

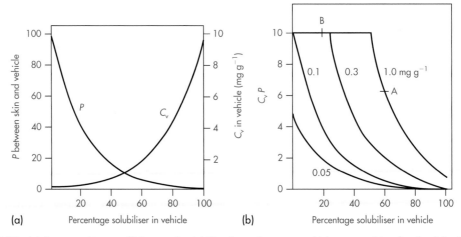

Figure 9.25 (a) Drug partition coefficient and solubility dependence on vehicle composition for the 'ideal' case. (b) Predicted relative steady-state penetration ($C_v P$) as a function of vehicle composition for the 'ideal' case. Point A represents a formulation containing 1.0 mg g^{-1} and 60% solubiliser. On threefold dilution with a base containing no solubiliser, point B is arrived at where $C_v P$ is higher.

Reproduced from B. J. Poulsen, in *Drug Design*, vol. 4 (ed. E. J. Ariens), Academic Press, New York, 1973.

acting as a solvent for the drug significantly affects permeation.

Thermodynamic activity in topical products

The concept of thermodynamic activity is considered in more detail in chapter 3. The thermodynamic activity of the drug is obviously the ultimate determinant of biological activity. If the solubility of the drug in the base is increased by addition of propylene glycol then its partition coefficient, P, towards the skin is reduced. On the other hand, increasing the amount which can be incorporated in the base is an advantage and the concentration (C_v) gradient is increased. It is apparent that there will be an optimum amount of solubiliser. The optimum occurs at the level of additive which just solubilises the medicament. Addition of excess results in desaturation of the system, and therefore a decrease in thermodynamic activity. As the total amount of drug in the vehicle is increased from 0.5 to 1.0 mg g^{-1} (Fig. 9.25b) more propylene glycol has to be added to cause a decrease in $C_v P$. From Fig. 9.25(b) one could postulate that threefold dilution of a formulation containing 1.0 mg g^{-1} and 60% solubiliser with a base with no solubiliser would cause the thermodynamic activity to *increase*. The vehicle affects penetration only when the release of drug is rate-limiting.

In situations where all of the activity gradient is in the applied phase, skin properties play no part. In these cases drug concentration in the vehicle, the diffusion coefficient of the drug in the system and the solubility of the drug are the significant factors. Where these factors are not important, the only significant factor involving the vehicle is the thermodynamic activity of the drug contained in it. Using the simplest model, for a solution of concentration C applied to an area A of the skin, the steady-state rate of penetration, dQ/dt, is given by

$$\frac{dQ}{dt} = \frac{PCDA}{\delta} \qquad (9.16)$$

δ being the thickness of the barrier phase. An equivalent form of this equation expresses release in terms of the thermodynamic activity, a, of the agent in the vehicle:

$$\frac{dQ}{dt} = \frac{a}{\gamma}\frac{DA}{\delta} \qquad (9.17)$$

where γ is the activity coefficient of the agent in the skin barrier phase. Ointments containing finely ground particles of drug where the thermodynamic activity is equal to that of solid drug will have the same rate of penetration, provided that the passage of the drug in the barrier phase is rate-limiting.

Solutes 'held firmly' in the vehicle exhibit low activity coefficients (low escaping tendencies) and thus low rates of penetration. Differences occur in the activity of phenols in mineral oil and polypropylene glycol bases. The latter are bland, the former corrosive. Polyether–phenol complex formation decreases the thermodynamic activity of the phenols, which are therefore less toxic.

Drug release from complex vehicles

In more complex vehicles the activity a is impossible to determine and other approaches must be adopted. For example, in emulsions the relative affinity of drug for the external and internal phases of the emulsion is an important factor. A drug dissolved in an internal aqueous phase of a w/o emulsion must be able to diffuse through the oily layer to reach the skin. Three cases can be considered: solution, suspension and emulsion systems.

Solutions
Release from *solutions* is most readily understood and quantified by equations of the form

$$\frac{dQ}{dt} = C_0\left(\frac{D}{\pi t}\right)^{1/2} \qquad (9.18)$$

$$Q = 2C_0\left(\frac{D}{\pi t}\right)^{1/2} \qquad (9.19)$$

where C_0 is the initial medicament concentration in solution, D is the diffusion coefficient, and t is the time after application of the vehicle. As D is inversely proportional to the viscosity of the vehicle, one would expect that drug release would be slower from a viscous vehicle. There is evidence for this in section 9.11, where the rheological characteristics of rectal formulations are seen to be correlated with bioavailability.

Suspensions

If a drug in *suspension* is to have any action it must have a degree of solubility in the base used. An aged suspension of a drug will therefore have a saturated solution of the drug present in the continuous phase. Release of medicament in these conditions is given by

$$\frac{dQ}{dt} = \kappa_{sp}\left(\frac{C_0 C_s D}{2t}\right)^{1/2} \tag{9.20}$$

where C_s is the total solubility of the drug in the vehicle and C_0 is the concentration in the vehicle. This equation applies only when $C_s \ll C_0$. Only material in solution penetrates the stratum corneum and the depleted layer in the vehicle is replenished only by solution of particles and diffusion of the drug molecules to the depleted layer.

Emulsions

For *emulsion*-type vehicles equations similar to those used to describe germicidal behaviour in two-phase systems can be applied. If D_1 and D_2 are the diffusion coefficients of the medicament in the continuous and disperse phases respectively, ϕ_1 and ϕ_2 are the volume fractions of these two phases, and P is the partition coefficient of the drug between the phases, the effective diffusion coefficient, D_e, is given by

$$D_e = \frac{D_1}{\phi_1 + P\phi_2}\left[1 + 3\phi_2\left(\frac{PD_2 - D_1}{PD_2 + D_1}\right)\right] \tag{9.21}$$

If $\phi_2 \gg \phi_1$ and $D_2 \gg D_1$ (likely if phase 2 is water), then

$$D_e = \frac{D_1}{P\phi_2}(1 + 3\phi_2) \tag{9.22}$$

For a system containing 20% water ($\phi_2 = 0.20$) the equation simplifies even further to

$$D_e = \frac{1.6 D_1}{0.2P} = \frac{8 D_1}{P} \tag{9.23}$$

The importance of P is seen in this equation. The value of D_e obtained here can be used in equations (9.18) and (9.19) above to obtain an approximation of effects.

9.5.4 Dilution of topical steroid preparations

Inappropriate dilution of carefully formulated creams and ointments may result in changes in stability and the effectiveness. The biopharmaceutical considerations will be apparent from the discussion in this chapter. An example would be clobetasol propionate formulated in a base containing the optimum amount of propylene glycol. The solubilities of the steroid as a function of propylene glycol concentration are shown in Fig. 9.26. A 1 in 2

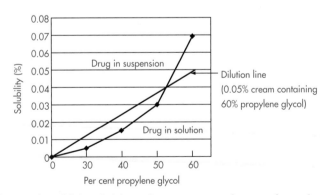

Figure 9.26 A diagram showing the solubility of clobetasol propionate as a function of propylene glycol concentration. The dilution line shows that if a 0.05% cream containing 60% propylene glycol is diluted with a base not containing the glycol, the drug will be precipitated.
Data from M. Busse, *Pharm. J.*, 220, 25 (1978).

dilution of a 0.05% cream, with a vehicle containing water and no propylene glycol will precipitate a large proportion of the steroid. The same principles apply to steroids presented in a fatty acid propylene glycol base.

9.5.5 Transdermal medication: patches and devices

The ease with which some drugs can pass through the skin barrier into the circulating blood means that the transdermal route of medication is a possible alternative to the oral route. Theoretically there are several advantages:[12]

- For drugs that are normally taken orally, administration through the skin can eliminate the vagaries which influence gastrointestinal absorption, such as pH changes and variations in food intake and intestinal transit time.
- A drug may be introduced into the systemic circulation without initially entering the portal circulation and passing through the liver.
- Constant and continuous administration of drugs may be achieved by a simple application to the skin surface.
- Continuous administration of drugs percutaneously at a controlled rate should permit elimination of pulse entry into the systemic circulation, an effect which is often associated with side-effects.
- Absorption of medication can be rapidly terminated whenever therapy must be interrupted.

Not all drugs are suitable for transdermal delivery. The limitations of the route are indicated in Table 9.10, which compares the percutaneous absorption of a range of drugs, from aspirin (22% of which is absorbed even after 120 h) to chloramphenicol, of which only 2% is absorbed. The transdermal route is now routinely used for a range of drugs, oestrogens, clonidine and nicotine included. The range of transdermal patches is growing as discussed in chapter 8. The four basic forms of patch systems are shown in Fig. 9.27.

Maximum flux from a saturated aqueous system of several drugs was estimated to be 300 μg cm^{-2} h^{-1} and from a mineral oil system 250 μg cm^{-2} h^{-1}. Using a 'patch' with a rate-limiting polymeric membrane (see section 8.6.4), delivery is controlled to 40–50 μg cm^{-2} h^{-1}; that is, it is presented to the skin at that rate. A 10 cm^2 device will therefore deliver 0.4–0.5 mg h^{-1}. Control of release can be exercised by altering the membrane's properties and by changing the pH of the reservoir solution for a drug such as hyoscine (Fig. 9.28).

Iontophoresis

Iontophoresis is the process by which the migration of ionic drugs into tissues such as skin is enhanced by the use of an electric current, a technique which has found application favour in facilitating the delivery of peptides and proteins. A typical iontophoretic device is shown in Fig. 9.29.

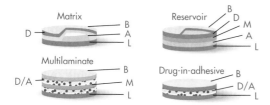

B - Backing   D - Drug   M - Membrane   A - Adhesive   L - Liner

Figure 9.27 The four main types of transdermal patch: matrix, reservoir, multilaminate and drug-in-adhesive designs. The matrix/reservoir systems are cut away to show the drug. Illustration courtesy of 3M.

Table 9.10 Percutaneous absorption of a range of drugs in humans[a]

Drug	Percentage dose absorbed (120 h)
Aspirin	22
Chloramphenicol	2
Hexachlorophene	3
Salicyclic acid	23
Urea	6
Caffeine	48

[a] Reproduced from A. H. Beckett et al., J. Pharm. Pharmacol., 24, 65P (1972).

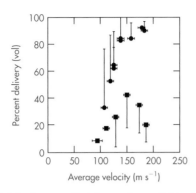

Figure 9.31   Average % delivery of mannitol by jet injection through a 152 μm diameter nozzle into human (●) and porcine (■) skin. The error bars shown are one standard deviation (n = 5–19 for each human skin data point). The magnitude of the delivery into human skin is higher than into porcine skin.

Reproduced from J. Shramm and S. Mitragotri, *Pharm. Res.*, 19, 1673–1679 (2002).

delivery is then possibly due to either or both of skin 'failure' and possibly flow through the skin.[15] The theoretical maximum velocity (v) of the jet is related to the pressure (P) in the nozzle and the density (ρ) of the liquid by

$$v = \left(\frac{2P}{\rho}\right)^{1/2}$$

but the velocity is affected by diameter of the orifice and is reduced by turbulence and friction. Figure 9.31 shows the percentage delivery of mannitol into the skin as a function of the average velocity of the jet.[15]

9.6   Medication of the eye and the eye as a route for systemic delivery

The eye is not, of course, a general route for the administration of drugs to the body, although it has been explored for the systemic delivery of peptides and proteins such as insulin. It is considered here because absorption of drugs does occur from medication applied to the eye, producing sometimes toxic systemic effects, although often the desired local effect is on the eye or its component

parts. We will consider the factors affecting drug absorption from the eye, and those properties of formulations that affect drug performance. A wide range of drug types are placed in the eye, including antimicrobials, antihistamines, decongestants, mydriatics, miotics and cycloplegic agents.

Drugs are usually applied to the eye in the form of drops or ointments for local action. The absorbing surface is the cornea. Drug absorbed by the conjuctiva enters the systemic circulation. It is useful to consider some of the properties of the absorbing surfaces and their environment.

9.6.1   The eye

The eye (Fig. 9.32) has two barrier systems: a blood–aqueous barrier and a blood–vitreous barrier. The former is composed of the ciliary epithelium, the epithelium of the posterior surface of the iris, and blood vessels within the iris. Solutes and drugs enter the aqueous humour at the ciliary epithelium and at blood vessels. Many substances are transported out of the vitreous humour at the retinal surface. Solutes also leave the vitreous humour by diffusing to the aqueous humour of the posterior chamber.

Figure 9.32 is a diagrammatic representation of those parts of the eye involved in drug absorption. The cornea and the conjunctiva are covered with a thin fluid film, the tear film, which protects the cornea from dehydration and infection. Cleansed corneal epithelium is hydrophobic, physiological saline forming a contact angle of about 50° with it, and it has, in this clean condition, a critical surface tension of 28 mN m^{-1}. The aqueous phase of tear fluid is spread by blinking.

Tears

Tears comprise inorganic electrolytes – sodium, potassium and some calcium ions, chloride and hydrogencarbonate counterions – as well as glucose. The macromolecular components include some albumin, globulins and lysozyme. Lipids which form a monolayer over the tear

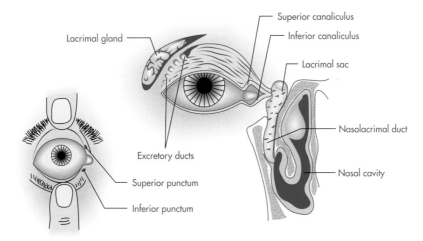

Figure 9.32 Diagrams of parts of the eye of importance in medication: the superior and inferior punctae are the drainage ports for solutions and tear fluids, and medicaments can drain via the canaliculi into the nasolacrimal duct and then to the nasal cavity, from whose surfaces absorption can occur.
Modified from J. R. Robinson (ed.), *Ophthalmic Drug Delivery Systems,* American Pharmaceutical Association, Washington DC, 1980.

fluid surface derive from the Meibomian glands which open on to the edges of the upper and lower lids. This secretion consists mainly of cholesteryl esters with low melting points (35°C) due to the predominance of double bonds and branched-chain structures. This fluid lies on the surface of the cornea (Fig. 9.33) and its importance in formulation lies in the possibility that components of formulations or drugs themselves can so alter the properties of the corneal surface, or interact with components of the tear fluid, that tear coverage of the eye is disrupted. When this occurs the so-called dry-eye syndrome (xerophthalmia) may arise, characterised by the premature break-up of the tear layer resulting in dry spots on the corneal surface.

9.6.2 Absorption of drugs applied to the eye

The cornea, which is the main barrier to absorption, consists of three parts: the epithelium, the stroma and the endothelium. Both the endothelium and the epithelium have a high lipid content and, as with most membranes, they are penetrated by drugs in their unionised lipid-soluble forms. The stroma lying between these two structures has a high water content, however, and thus drugs which

have to negotiate the corneal barrier successfully must be both lipid-soluble and water-soluble to some extent (Fig. 9.33).

Tears have some buffering capacity so, as we noted before, the pH–partition hypothesis has to be applied with some circumspection. The acid neutralising power of the tears when 0.1 cm^3 of a 1% solution of a drug is instilled into the eye is approximately equivalent to $10 \, \mu L$ of a 0.01 mol dm^{-3} strong base. The pH for either maximum solubility (see Chapter 5) or maximum stability (see Chapter 4) of a drug may well be below the optimum in relation to acceptability and activity. Under these conditions it is possible to use a buffer with a low buffering capacity to maintain a low pH adequate to prevent change in pH due to alkalinity of glass or carbon dioxide ingress from the air. When such drops are instilled into the eye the tears will participate in a fairly rapid return to normal pH.

In agreement with the pH–partition hypothesis, raising the pH from 5 to 8 results in a two- to threefold increase in the amount of pilocarpine reaching the anterior chamber. It is also found, however, that glycerol penetration increases to the same extent (Fig. 9.34). The clue to why this should be so lies in the effect of the buffer solutions on lacrimation. Increased tear flow reduces the concentration

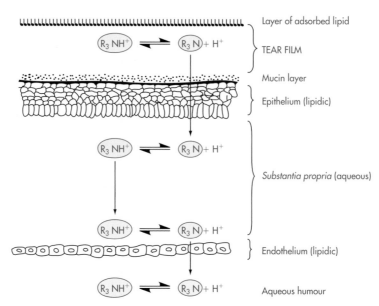

Figure 9.33 Diagrammatic representation of a tear film and the penetration of a base through the cornea; in this example R_3N represents a drug such as homatropine.

Modified from R. A. Moses, *Adler's Physiology of the Eye*, 5th edn, Mosby, St. Louis, 1970.

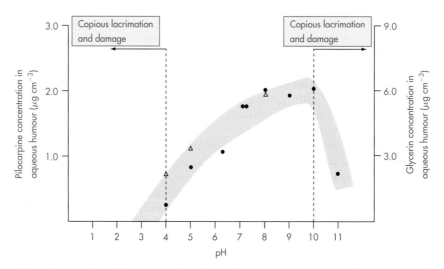

Figure 9.34 The influence of vehicle pH on the aqueous humour concentration of pilocarpine and glycerol. ●, 10^{-2} mol dm^{-3} pilocarpine solutions; △, 0.14 mol dm^{-3} glycerol solutions; all samples obtained at 20 min post-instillation and represent results from a minimum of six eyes.

Reproduced from reference 16.

of drug in the bathing fluid; loss of drug solution through the punctae and nasolacrimal ducts does not affect concentration, as the whole fluid drains away. Solution concentration is reduced only by diffusion of drug across the cornea or conjunctiva or by tear inflow.

The pH 5 solution induced more tear flow than the pH 8 solution; thus the concentration gradient is reduced and transport of both ionised and nonionic drugs is less at pH 5. At pH 11, as will be seen from Fig. 9.34, absorption of pilocarpine is reduced because of the irritant effects of this solution on the eye.[16] Mechanical irritation can produce the same effects and this can override the influence of other formulation factors.

Aqueous humour

As the examples above have shown, both water-soluble and lipid-soluble drugs can enter the aqueous humour. The pH–partition hypothesis thus accounts only imperfectly for different rates of entry into aqueous humour. Sucrose and raffinose pass through the leaky ciliary epithelium and reach steady-state aqueous/plasma concentration ratios of 0.2 and 0.3, respectively. Lipid-soluble drugs, including chloramphenicol and some tetracyclines can achieve higher concentrations as they can enter by both pathways. Penicillins, however, reach only low aqueous/plasma concentration ratios because they are removed from aqueous humour by absorption through the ciliary epithelium. Proteins are excluded, so that protein binding of ophthalmic drugs limits their absorption.

9.6.3 Influence of formulation

Pilocarpine activity has been compared in various formulations. Figure 9.35 shows some of the results on formulations, including results on ointments designed to prolong the contact of the drug with the cornea. One of the most difficult problems is to design vehicles which will retard drainage and prolong contact. Viscous polymer vehicles help to some extent but are not the complete answer. The rate of drainage of drops decreased as their viscosity increased and these factors contribute to an increased concentration of the drug in the precorneal film and aqueous humour.[17] The magnitude of the concentration increase was small considering the 100-fold change in the viscosity, and it was concluded that the viscosity of the solution is not as important a factor in bioavailability as was previously thought.

The results of incorporating pilocarpine (**V**) (a relatively water-soluble drug) and fluorometholone (a lipophilic drug) into a water-in-oil ointment base can be compared in Fig. 9.36. Pilocarpine is thought to be released only when in contact with aqueous tear fluid, whereas the steroid, being soluble in the base, can diffuse through the base to replenish the surface concentrations and thus produce a sustained effect.

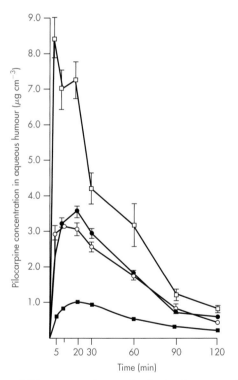

Figure 9.35 Aqueous humour levels of pilocarpine after dosing with 10^{-2} mol dm^{-3} ointment and solution in intact and abraded eyes. ●, 25 mg of ointment, intact eyes; ○, 25 mg of ointment, abraded eyes; ■, 25 mm^3 of solution, intact eyes; □, 25 mm^3 of solution, abraded eyes; all points represent an average of 8–16 eyes.
Reproduced from reference 16.

Structure V Pilocarpine (pK_a = 7.05)

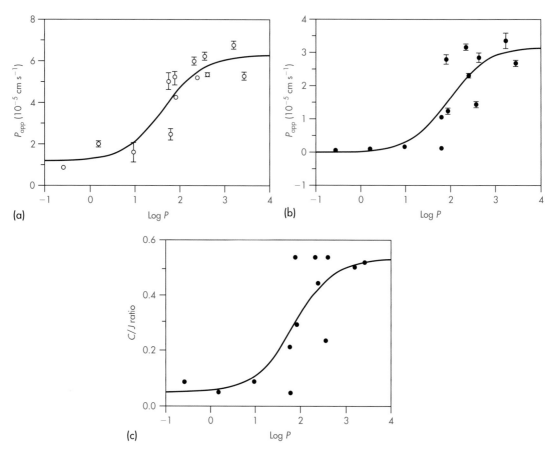

(a)

(b)

(c)

Figure 9.37 Influence of drug lipophilicity (log P) on the permeability coefficients (P_{app}) of beta-blockers across (a) the conjunctiva and (b) the cornea of the pigmented rabbit. Plot (c) shows the influence of log P on the ratio of the corneal (C) and conjunctival (J) permeability coefficients.
Reproduced from W. Wong *et al.*, *Curr. Eye Res.*, 6, 571 (1991).

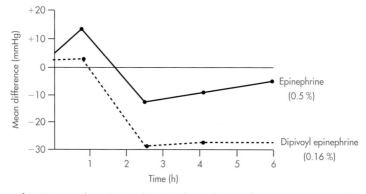

Figure 9.38 The action of 0.5% epinephrine (VI) and 0.16% dipivoyl epinephrine (VII) on intraocular pressure.
Reproduced from D. A. McClure, in *Prodrugs as Novel Drug Delivery Systems* (ed. T. Higuchi and V. Stella), American Chemical Society, Washington DC, 1975.

Structure VI Epinephrine (adrenaline)

Structure VIII Pilocarpine derivatives

R^1 = H, CH_3
R^2 = $(CH_2)_nCH_3$
n = 10–16

Structure VII Dipivoyl epinephrine (dipivefrine; compare with Structure VI)

iris after applications of prednisolone in solution. When the drug was incorporated into the lens, aqueous and corneal levels of the drug were two- to threefold higher 4 hours after insertion.

The Alza Ocusert device (Fig. 9.39) releases controlled amounts of pilocarpine over a period of 7 days and is designed for the treatment of glaucoma. It comprises a drug reservoir in which pilocarpine is embedded in an alginic acid matrix, and this is bounded by

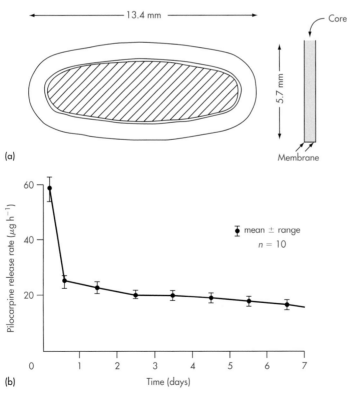

(a)

(b)

Figure 9.39 (a) Dimensions and structure of the Alza Ocusert device. (b) A release rate profile over one week.
Reproduced from J. W. Snell and R. W. Baker, *Ann. Ophthalmol.* **6**, 1037 (1974).

two rate-controlling membranes of polymer (vinyl acetate–ethylene copolymer). The device has a raised rim to aid visibility and handling. It is inserted into the lower conjunctival sac of the eye. The rate-controlling membranes are subject to strict quality control during manufacture and their thicknesses adjusted to give the appropriate flux of drug, either 20 or 40 μg h^{-1}. The difference between the two available systems is effected by altering the amount of di-(2-ethylhexyl)phthalate in the polymer; increasing the concentration of this plasticiser increases the permeability to pilocarpine.

Mucoadhesive systems are discussed in reference 20.

9.6.4 Systemic effects from eye-drops

Most of the dose applied to the eye in the form of drops reaches the systemic circulation and typically less than 5% acts on ocular tissues.

Atropine toxicity resulting from the use of the eye-drops to dilate the pupil has been reported,[21] as has a rise in blood pressure in premature infants following the use of 10% phenylephrine eye-drops in preparation for ophthalmoscopy.[22] The mucosa in the eye, nose and mouth of infants is much thinner and more permeable to a drug than is, say, the skin. Drugs placed in the eye, nose or mouth, moreover, may bypass the metabolic transformations which may inactivate the drug given orally. Reduction in exercise tachycardia in normal volunteers is induced following administration of 0.5% timolol eye-drops, showing the significant effects of beta-blockers.

9.7 The ear

Medications are administered to the ear only for local treatment. Drops and other vehicles administered to the ear will occupy the external auditory meatus, which is separated from the middle ear by the tympanic membrane (Fig. 9.40). Various factors affect drug absorption from the ear or action in it. The sebaceous

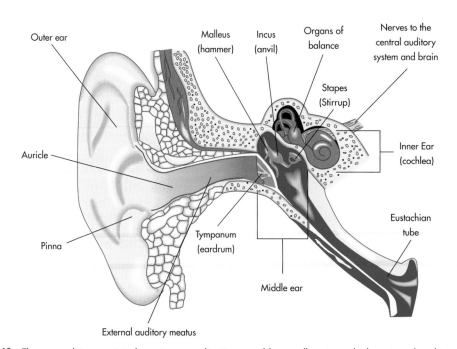

Figure 9.40 The ear and its associated structures; medications would normally enter only the external auditory meatus.

and apocrine glands of the mucosa secrete an oily fluid which, when mixed with exfoliated cells of the stratum corneum forms the cerumon or wax composed of, *inter alia*, fats, fatty acids, protein, pigment, glycoprotein and water.

The acidic environment of the ear skin surface (around pH 6), sometimes referred to as the acid mantle of the ear, is thought to be a defence against invading microorganisms.

Various ceruminolytic agents achieve their action by partially dissolving the wax. Several commercial ear-drops contain poloxamers or sodium dioctyl sulfosuccinate (docusate sodium). In otitis media, infection of the Eustachian tube is involved; antibiotic treatment is indicated along with oral analgesics. There is little evidence that topical analgesics give faster relief, suggesting poor absorption.

9.8 Absorption from the vagina

The vagina cannot be considered to be a route for the systemic administration of drugs, although oestrogens for systemic delivery have been applied intravaginally. Certain medicaments are, however, absorbed when applied to the vaginal epithelium as it is permeable to a wide range of substances including steroids, prostaglandins, iodine and some antibiotics.[23] Econazole and miconazole are also both appreciably absorbed.

The epithelial layer of the vagina (Fig. 9.41a) comprises lamina propria and a surface epithelium of noncornified, stratified squamous cells (Fig. 9.41b). The thickness of the epithelium increases after puberty and then again after menopause. The surface area is increased by folds in the epithelium and by micro-ridges. The pH in the vagina decreases after puberty, varying between pH 4 and 5 depending on the point in the menstrual cycle and also on the location within the vagina, the pH being higher near the cervix. There is little fluid in the vagina. The absorbing surface is under constant change, therefore absorption is variable. While the presence of mucus is likely to retard absorption, there is unlikely to be other

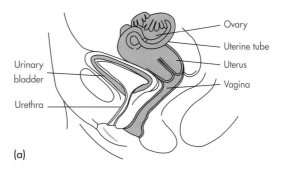

(a)

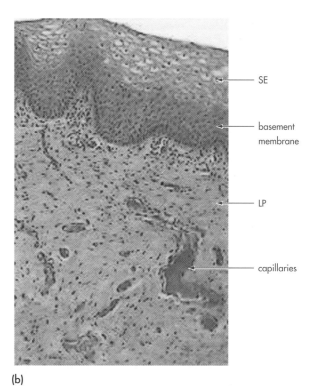

(b)

Figure 9.41 (a) Anatomy of the urethra and vagina; drug-delivery systems for both are available. (b) For other than local vaginal treatment, transport through the absorbing membrane structure (squamous epithelium (SE) lamina propria (LP) and muscularis (M) (not shown)) is important in securing systemic levels of drug; inadvertent absorption after local therapy is, of course, possible.

material in the vagina which will inhibit absorption. The uterine and pudendal arteries are the main sources of blood to the vagina; the venous plexus which surrounds the vagina empties into the internal ileac veins. Lymph vessels drain the vagina, and vaginal capillaries are found in close proximity to the basal epithelial layer.

Proteins and peptides, particularly in the presence of absorption enhancers, can be successfully administered by this route, although surfactant-based enhancers are apparently not effective in the vagina. Vaginal enzymes, especially the proteases, are likely to present problems in the vaginal delivery of proteins and peptides.

9.8.1 Delivery systems

Conventional vaginal delivery systems include vaginal tablets, foams, gels, suspensions and pessaries. Vaginal rings (Fig. 9.42) have been developed to deliver contraceptive steroids. These commonly comprise an inert silicone elastomer ring which is covered with an elastomer layer containing the drug. In some systems a refinement has been to add a third, rate-modifying layer to the external surface of the ring as shown. Some systems contain both an oestrogen and progestogen.

Hydrogel-based vaginal pessaries to deliver prostaglandin E_2 (to assist in ripening of the cervix prior to labour) progesterone and bleomycin have been developed.

Tablets for vaginal use have included hydroxypropylcellulose or sodium carboxymethylcellulose and poly(acrylic acid) (such as Carbopol 934) as excipients. Micropatches in the size range 10–100 μm in diameter prepared from starch, gelatin, albumin, collagen

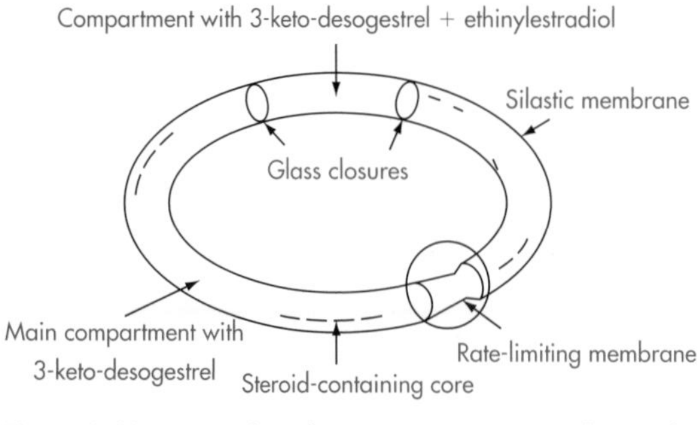

Figure 9.42 A combined contraceptive vaginal ring for the slow release of 3-keto-desogestrel (etonogestrel) and ethinylestradiol.
Reproduced from A. P. Sam., J. Control. Release, 22, 35 (1992).

or dextrose will gel on contact with vaginal mucosal surfaces and adhere, prolonging contact between the delivery system and the absorbing surface.[24]

9.9 Inhalation therapy

The respiratory system provides a route of entry into the body for a variety of airborne substances but is also a route of medication. The large contact area of its surfaces extends to more than 30 m^2. The surfaces have been described[25] as 'gossamer-thin membranes' that separate the lung air from the blood, which courses through some 2000 km of capillaries in the lungs. There is consequently an 'exquisite degree of intimacy between the lung tissue and blood and the atmospheric environment'. The route is thus used for rapid relief of asthmatic conditions, where both local and systemic effects are required, for chronic therapy and for the administration of peptides and proteins.

Orally administered corticosteroids are effective in the treatment of chronic bronchial asthma. The inhalation route has been widely used in attempts to avoid systemic side-effects, such as adrenal suppression, but evidence suggests that inhaled steroids are absorbed systemically to a significant extent. The respiratory tract epithelium has permeability characteristics similar to those of the classical biological membrane, so lipid-soluble compounds are absorbed more rapidly than lipid-insoluble molecules. Cortisone, hydrocortisone and dexamethasone are absorbed rapidly by a nonsaturable diffusion process from the lung, the half-time of absorption being of the order of 1–1.7 min. Quaternary ammonium compounds, hippurates and mannitol have absorption half-times, in contrast, of between 45 and 70 min.

Relative to the gastrointestinal mucosa the pulmonary epithelium possesses a high permeability to water soluble molecules, which is an advantage with drugs such as sodium cromoglicate (**IX**), a bischromone with two carboxylic acid groups and a pK_a of approximately 1.9. The drug is well absorbed from the

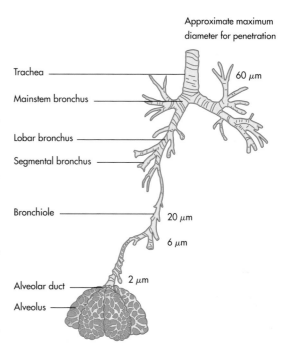

Structure IX Sodium cromoglicate (DSCG; sodium cromoglycate; cromolyn sodium)

lungs with a clearance rate of about 1 hour even though the molecule is completely ionised at physiological pH. The free acid is very insoluble in both polar and non-polar solvents and has virtually no lipid solubility. Because of this, and the insolubility of the unionised form, very little of an oral dose of sodium cromoglicate is absorbed. Powder swallowed after inhalation therefore contributes little to the systemic dose and is subsequently excreted in the urine and bile.

Drugs administered by inhalation are mostly intended to have a direct effect on the lungs. However, the efficiency of inhalation therapy is often not high because of the difficulty in targeting particles to the sites of maximal absorption. Only about 8% of the inhaled dose of sodium cromoglicate administered from a Spinhaler device (see section 9.9.2) reaches the alveoli.[25]

Crude inhalers have been used for medicinal purposes for at least two centuries. Solutions of volatile aromatic substances with a mild irritant action, inhaled as vapour arising from hot aqueous solutions, have been used for many years. Particles from the older nebulisers would settle without reaching the patient's face (a 100 μm particle of unit density settles in still air at a velocity of 8 cm s^{-1}). The duration of existence of a suspension of particles of size around 10 μm is so brief that the upper limit of aerosols of therapeutic interest is well below this size. Special devices are required to generate these.

9.9.1 Physical factors affecting deposition of aerosols

Figure 9.43 shows the order of maximum size of particles that can penetrate to various parts

Figure 9.43 Deposition of particles in various anatomical regions of the respiratory tract from bronchus to alveoli according to particle size.

of the respiratory tract, from trachea to alveoli.

The major processes which influence deposition of drug particles in the respiratory tract are, as illustrated in Fig. 9.44,

- Interception
- Impaction
- Gravitational settling
- Electrostatic attractions
- Brownian diffusion

When a particle contacts the walls of the airways it is removed from the airstream; this process can occur during inspiration or expiration of a single breath, or later if the particle has been transferred to unexhaled lung air. Deposition increases with duration of breath holding and depth of breathing, hence the instructions to patients to breathe deeply when using their inhalers.

As flowing air moves in and out, inertial forces within the nasopharyngeal chamber and at the points of branching of the airways, or wherever the direction of flow changes, result in the collision of particles with

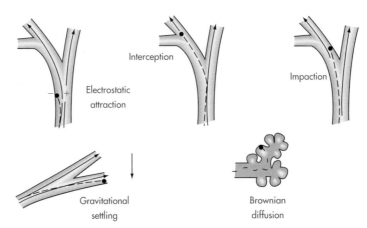

Electrostatic
attraction

Interception

Impaction

Gravitational
settling

Brownian
diffusion

Figure 9.44   Representation of the major processes of particle deposition in the respiratory tract as discussed in the text.

surfaces. Along the narrower airways particles are removed by gravity. Very fine particles ($<0.5\,\mu$m) are deposited on the walls of the smallest airways by diffusion, the result of bombardment of the particles by gas molecules. Particle size, or particle size distribution, is obviously important in several of these processes and will be affected by the nature of the aerosol-producing device and by the formulation. Growth of particles in the hygroscopic environment of the airways may occur, as may agglomeration and deagglomeration of aggregates. Hence appropriate sampling and measuring systems are of great importance. The proportion of the aerosol cloud which actually enters the airways (some will be lost in the delivery device) is also crucial. The use of spacer devices can be critical in optimising efficacy.

The next sections present a more detailed account of deposition in the airways.

Physical diameter and aerodynamic diameter

The aerodynamic diameter of a particle, d_a, is related to the particle diameter (d) and density (ρ) by the equation

$$d_a = \rho^{0.5} d \qquad (9.24)$$

To overcome problems of powder flow and agglomeration, porous particles (i.e. particles with a low density) have been developed. Equation (9.24) shows that a particle of 10 μm

diameter with a density of 0.1 g cm^{-3} has an aerodynamic diameter of ~3 μm.

Gravitational settling

Fine particles falling through the air under the force of gravity do so at a constant velocity such that the resistance of the air balances the mass of the particle. The following equation relates particle diameter, d, and density, ρ, to terminal velocity μ_t

$$\mu_t = \frac{\rho g d^2}{18\eta} \qquad (9.25)$$

where g is the gravitational constant and η is the viscosity of the air. For air, $\eta = 1.9 \times 10^{-7}$ N m^{-2} s and therefore

$$\mu_t = 2.9 \times 10^6 \rho d^2 \;\; (\text{m s}^{-1})$$

Table 9.13 shows the terminal velocities for particles of a range of diameters from 20 to 0.1 μm, reinforcing the importance of small size in preventing removal of particles before entry into the lower reaches of the respiratory tract. In still air, a cloud of powder of about 20 μm diameter takes a few seconds to settle, whereas powder of around 1 μm diameter takes approximately 60 seconds.

Sedimentation

As the particles of drug move with the air in laminar flow in the airways, they fall under the force of gravity a distance equal to $\mu_t t$,

Table 9.13 Terminal velocity (μ_t) of spherical particles of unit density in air[a]

Diameter (μm)	μ_t (cm s^{-1})
20	1.2
10	2.9×10^{-1}
4	5×10^{-2}
1	3.5×10^{-3}
0.6	1.4×10^{-3}
0.1	8.6×10^{-5}

[a] Reproduced from T. F. Hatch and P. Gross, *Pulmonary Deposition and Retention of Inhaled Aerosols*, Academic Press, New York, 1964.

where t is the time of travel. If the tube (or part of the bronchial tree) in which they move is of radius R and is inclined at an angle ψ to the horizontal, the maximum distance of fall will no longer be $2R$ but $2R/\cos \psi$. The ratio, r, of the distance of fall to the maximum distance for deposition to be achieved is thus

$$r = \frac{\mu_t t \cos \psi}{2R} \qquad (9.26)$$

The probability of deposition by sedimentation is proportional to this ratio; the closer $\mu_t t$ is to $2R/\cos \psi$, the greater the likelihood of deposition by this mechanism. If the particles are evenly distributed over the cross-section of an airstream, it is theoretically possible to calculate the probability of deposition in tubular airways and in a spherical alveolus. Individual tubes are of course randomly positioned with reference to the horizontal and therefore an average value of ψ is used. Airflow is also not always laminar, and orderly deposition will not always occur, but in spite of these problems the following calculations of percentage sedimentation (S) may usefully be quoted. If $S = 55\%$ when $d = 2\,\mu$m and the deposition diameter is $1.0\,\mu$m, then for $1\,\mu$m particles $S = 29\%$, and for $0.5\,\mu$m particles $S = 10\%$. Sedimentation, of course, reduces in importance as the drug particle size decreases.

Diffusion

The effectiveness of deposition by diffusion increases as particle size is reduced, which contrasts with the above. There must therefore be a particle diameter for which both processes have a combined minimum value; this occurs with particles approximately 0.5 μm in diameter. Particles of this size have the minimum probability of deposition in the upper respiratory tract.

Inertial impaction

When, during breathing, the airflow suddenly changes direction, a drug particle will continue in its original direction of flow owing to its inertia. In this way the particle may impact on the channel wall. In curved tubes the particle in an airstream which experiences a sudden bend suffers a similar fate, and the effective stopping distance at right-angles to the direction of travel, h_s, is given by

$$h_s = \frac{\mu_t \mu \sin \theta}{g} \qquad (9.27)$$

where μ is the velocity of the airstream with particles approaching a bend of angle θ. The term $\mu \sin \theta$ is therefore a component of initial particle velocity at right-angles to the direction of airflow. The probability of inertial deposition, I, is proportional to the ratio of stopping distance, h_s, to the radius, R, of the airway; that is

$$I \propto \frac{h_s}{R} \propto \frac{\mu_t \mu \sin \theta}{gR} \qquad (9.28)$$

from a calculation similar to that discussed above for sedimentation. Calculated inertial deposition shows a dependence on particle size as follows; 10 μm particles 50%, 7 μm particles 33%, leading to 20% for 5 μm particles, and 1% for 1 μm particles.

9.9.2 Experimental observations

The complexity of the respiratory system prevents a precise mathematical approach to the problem. Many clinical studies, however, clearly demonstrate the importance of particle size.

Particles of hygroscopic materials are removed more effectively than are nonhygroscopic particles, because of the growth of these

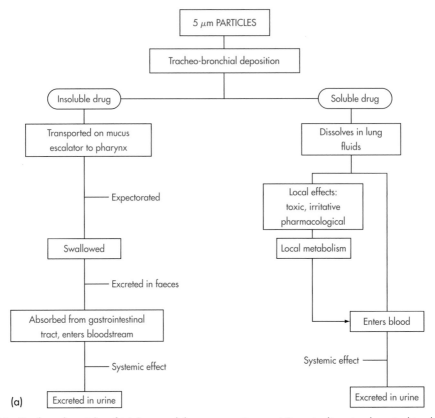

Figure 9.45   The fate of particles of (a) 5 μm and (b, see opposite page) 2 μm in diameter deposited in alveoli.
Reproduced from D. G. Clark, *Proc. Eur. Soc. Study Drug Toxicity*, 15, 252 (1974).

particles by uptake of water from the moist air in the respiratory system. Apart from its importance in determining the efficiency of an aerosol in reaching the alveoli, particle size may be critical in determining response, because of the influence of particle size on rate of solution.

The effect of particle size on the fate of particles inhaled from an aerosol is shown in Fig. 9.45.

When used by patients, the Spinhaler delivers about 25% by weight of sodium cromoglicate, which is normally dispersed as particles below 6 μm in diameter, about 5% being less than 2 μm diameter. The mass medium diameter (and geometric standard deviation) of the sodium cromoglicate particle batches used were, respectively, 2 ± 1.2 and 11.7 ± 1.1 μm. There is no doubt that the biological effect of the small particle material is dramatically greater than that of coarser material, hence the importance of storage conditions of the sodium cromoglicate cartridge capsules to prevent aggregation of the particles of drugs. Although the Spinhaler is designed to break up aggregates, its efficiency will be reduced if moisture uptake is increased by storage in humid conditions, either in the pharmacy or in the home. If aerosols of this drug with large (11 μm diameter) size particles are administered, up to 66% of the dose will end up in the mouth.

An alternative dry powder aerosol device is illustrated in Fig. 9.46 and the mechanism of dispersion of powdered drug in a Ventodisk or Becodisk system is shown in Fig. 9.47

Types of pressurised aerosol

Typical pressurised aerosol systems are discussed in Chapter 7. In two-phase systems the

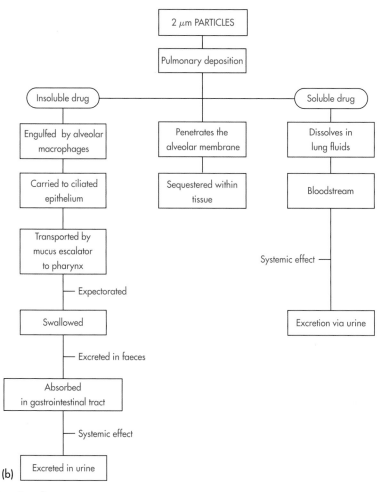

(b)

Figure 9.45 (*continued*).
Reproduced from D. G. Clark, *Proc. Eur. Soc. Study Drug Toxicity*, 15, 252 (1974).

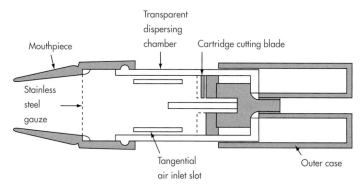

Figure 9.46   Longitudinal view of the Rotahaler.
Reproduced from G. W. Hallworth, *Br. J. Clin. Pharmacol.*, 4, 689 (1977).

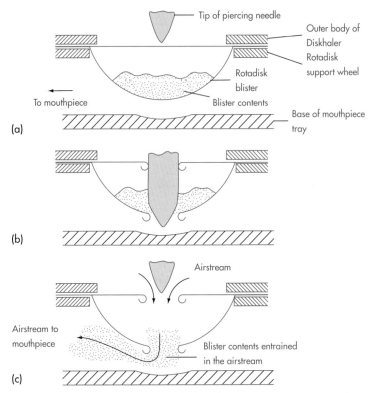

Figure 9.47 Dispersion of Ventodisk or Becodisk contents by breath actuation: a cross-section of a Diskhaler is shown with a disc located on the support wheel. (a) A disc is located beneath an aperture in the body of the Diskhaler through which a piercing needle enters. (b) The needle penetrates the upper and lower surfaces of the blister. (c) The patient inhales through the device and pierced blister, entraining the blister contents into the airstream.
Reproduced from S. J. Farr *et al.*, in *Routes of Drug Administration* (ed. A. T. Florence and E.G. Salole), Wright, London, 1990.

propellant forms a separate liquid phase, whereas in the single-phase form the liquid propellant is the liquid phase containing the drug in solution or in suspension in the liquefied propellant gas. Until recently, materials such as the chlorofluorocarbons were employed, but since the Montreal Treaty replacement non-chlorine-containing materials have been sought which do not affect the ozone layer.

As we have seen in Chapter 2, the formulation of a drug in a chlorofluorocarbon cannot simply be reproduced with another propellant. Optimisation of vapour pressure, drug stability, solubility and spray patterns must take place. Other ingredients of the formulation can include surfactants to act as solubilisers, stabilisers or lubricants to ease the passage the particles when emitted from the valve.

The Autohaler has been devised as a breath-activated pressurised inhaler system because of the difficulty experienced by some patients in coordinating manual operation of an aerosol with inhalation. The Autohaler is activated by the negative pressure created during the inhalation phase of respiration and is specifically designed to respond to shallow inhalation in those with restricted pulmonary capacity.

Nebulisers[26]

Modern nebulisers for domestic and hospital use generate aerosols continuously for chronic therapy of respiratory disorders. A Venturi-type system is shown in Fig. 9.48(a) and an ultrasonic device in Fig. 9.48(b). The particle size distribution and hence efficiency of such

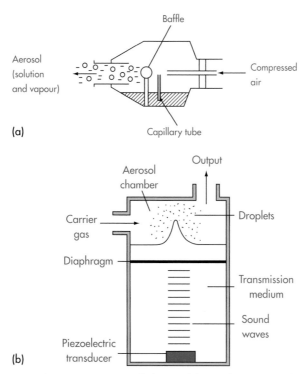

Figure 9.48 Schematic diagrams of (a) a Venturi-type nebuliser and (b) an ultrasonic nebuliser.
Modified from D. F. Egan, *Fundamentals of Respiratory Therapy*, 3rd edn, Mosby, New York, 1977.

systems varies with the design and sometimes with the mode of use. Hence adequate monitoring of particle size is important.

In vitro analysis of the particle size distribution of aerosols and nebulisers is discussed in Chapter 12.

9.10 The nasal route

Two main classes of medicinal agents are applied by the nasal route:

- Drugs for the alleviation of nasal symptoms
- Drugs that are inactivated in the gastro-intestinal tract following oral administration and where the route is an alternative to injection, such as for peptides and proteins

Intranasal beclometasone dipropionate in a dose as low as 200 μg daily is a useful addition to the therapy of perennial rhinitis. Considerable attention is being paid to the delivery by the nasal route of peptides and proteins such as insulin, LHRH analogues such as nafarelin, as well as vasopressin, TRH analogues and ACTH.

A diagram of the structures involved in delivery by the nasal route is given in Fig. 9.49. Formulations have to be efficiently delivered to the epithelial surfaces, so what physical factors affect the utility of this route? Factors such as droplet or particle size which affect deposition in the respiratory tract are involved if administration is by aerosol, but formulations may also be applied directly to the nasal mucosa. The physiological condition of the nose, its vascularity, and mucus flow rate are therefore of importance. So too is the formulation used – the volume, concentration, viscosity, pH and tonicity of the applied medicament can affect activity. As the condition of the nasal passages changes with changes in the environment, temperature and humidity, it is clearly not an ideal route for absorption of drugs or vaccines, but may be the only feasible route for some agents. As

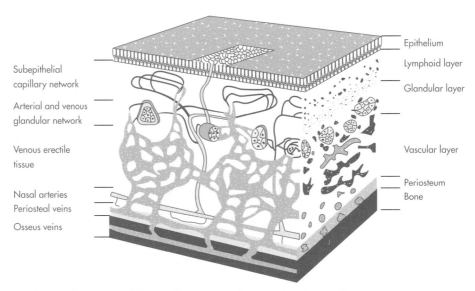

Subepithelial
capillary network

Arterial and venous
glandular network

Venous erectile
tissue

Nasal arteries
Periosteal veins

Osseus veins

Epithelium

Lymphoid layer

Glandular layer

Vascular layer

Periosteum
Bone

Figure 9.49 The vascular network of the nasal mucous membrane in the inferior turbinate.

with all routes, however, absorption decreases with the increasing molecular weight of the active as seen in Fig. 9.50 with a series of model molecules.

The air passages through the nasal cavity begin at the nares (nostrils) and terminate at the choanae (posterior nares). Immediately above the nares are the vestibules, lined by skin which bears relatively coarse hairs and sebaceous glands in its lower portion. The hairs curve radially downward providing an

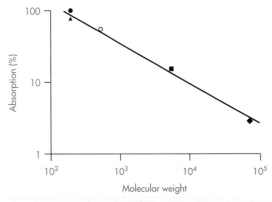

Figure 9.50 Correlation between the percentage dose absorbed after nasal administration and molecular weight: 4-oxo-4H–1-benzopyran-2-carboxylic acid (chromocarb) (●); p-aminohippuric acid (▲); sodium cromoglicate (○); inulin (■); dextran (◆); $r = -0.996$.
Reproduced from A. N. Fisher et al., J. Pharm. Pharmacol., 39, 357 (1987).

effective barrier to the entry of relatively large particles. The division of the nasal cavity exposes the air to maximal surface area. As in the other parts of the respiratory tree, sudden changes in the direction of airflow cause impingement of large particles through inertial forces. The respiratory portion of the nasal passage is covered by a mucous membrane which has a mucous blanket secreted in part by the goblet cells. The ciliary streaming here is directed posteriorly so that the nasal mucus is transported towards the pharynx. Figure 9.51 shows the fractional deposition of inhaled particles in the nasal chamber as a function of their particle size. A diameter of not less than 10 μm minimizes the loss of drug to the lung. In the external nares, removal of particles occurs on nasal hairs; further up inertial deposition takes place, and in the more tortuous upper passages deposition is assumed to be by inertia and sedimentation.

Comparison of the nasal route with other routes has been made in some instances. Desmopressin (1-desamino-8-D-arginine vasopressin) administered as a 20 μg dose elicits a response equivalent to approximately 2 μg administered by i.v. injection. Also, a greater dose of virus is required to obtain an equivalent response to a nasal vaccine than when administered by other routes.

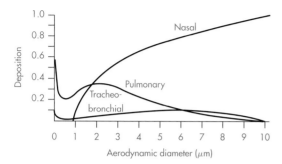

Figure 9.51 Regional deposition of inhaled particulate matter as a function of particle size; nose breathing at 15 respirations per minute and 730 cm³ tidal volume (the 'pulmonary compartment' refers to deposition beyond the terminal bronchiole).
Reproduced from C. D. F. Muir, *Clinical Aspects of Inhaled Particles*, Heinemann, London, 1972.

In the treatment of nasal symptoms the patient adjusts the dose so that, perhaps, the theoretical bases of droplet and particle retention are less vital. Although formulation of the nasal drops, or sprays from plastic squeeze-bottles must obviously influence the efficiency of medication, little work has in the past been carried out relating formulation to the effect of intranasal medicines. Microsphere delivery systems have received some attention, however, with special interest being directed to bioadhesive microspheres.

9.11   Rectal absorption of drugs

Drugs administered by the rectal route in suppositories are placed in intimate contact with the rectal mucosa, which behaves as a normal lipoidal barrier. The pH in the rectal cavity lies between 7.2 and 7.4, but the rectal fluids have little buffering capacity. As with topical medication, the formulation of the suppository can have marked effects on the activity of the drug. Factors such as retention of the suppository for a sufficient duration of time in the rectal cavity also influence the outcome of therapy; the size and shape of the suppository and its melting point may also determine bioavailability.

The once traditional suppository base, cocoa butter (theobroma oil) is a variable natural product which undergoes a polymorphic transition on heating. It is primarily a triglyceride. Four polymorphic forms exist: γ, m.p. 18.9°C; α, m.p. 23°C; β', m.p. 28°C; and the stable β form, m.p. 34.5°C. Heating above 38°C converts the fat to a metastable mixture solidifying at 15–17°C instead of 25°C, and this subsequently melts at 24°C instead of at 31–35°C. Reconversion to the stable β-form takes 1–4 days depending on storage conditions.[27]

Modern bases include polyoxyethylene glycols of molecular weight 1000–6000 and semisynthetic vegetable fats. The appropriate bases must be selected carefully for each substance. The important features of excipient materials are melting point, speed of crystallisation and emulsifying capacity. If the medicament dissolves in the base, it is likely that the melting point of the base will be lowered, so that a base with a melting point higher than 36–37°C has to be chosen. If the drug substance has a high density, it is preferable that the base crystallises rapidly during production of the suppositories to prevent settling of the drug. Preservatives, hardening agents, emulsifiers, colouring agents and materials which modify the viscosity of the base after melting are common formulation additives.

The rectal cavity

The rectum is the terminal 15–19 cm of the large intestine. The mucous membrane of the rectal ampulla, with which suppositories and other rectal medications come into contact, is made up of a layer of cylindrical epithelial cells, without villi.

Figure 9.52 shows the blood supply to the rectal area. The main artery to the rectum is the superior rectal (haemorrhoidal) artery. Veins of the inferior part of the submucous plexus become the rectal veins, which drain to the internal pudendal veins. Drug absorption takes place through this venous network. Superior haemorrhoidal veins connect with the portal vein and thus transport drugs absorbed in the upper part of the rectal cavity

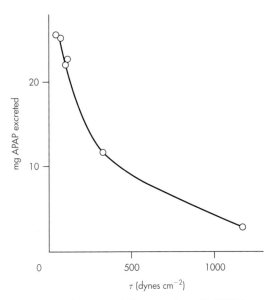

Figure 9.55 Variation of the excretion of APAP (paracetamol) in the urine 2 h after rectal administration of a formulation as a function of the limiting shear stress, τ, of the excipient drug-mixture at 37°C.
Modified from A. Moës, *J. Pharm. Belg.*, 29, 319 (1974).

the rectal cavity and, if the base is not emulsified, on the contact area between molten excipient and rectal mucosa. Addition of surfactants may increase the ability of the molten mass to spread and tends to increase the extent of absorption. Significant increases in absorption can be obtained with polyoxyethylene sorbitan monostearate (polysorbate 60), sodium lauryl sulfate and cetyltrimethylammonium (cetrimonium) bromide. Surfactants increase wetting and spreading and may increase the permeability of the rectal mucosal membrane.

A study of the effect of polyoxyethylene glycols on the rectal absorption of unionised sulfafurazole demonstrated the importance of the affinity of the drug substance for base and for rectal mucosa. As the amount of Macrogol 4000 (polyoxyethylene glycol 4000) was increased, the partition coefficient (lipid/ vehicle) fell and absorption decreased correspondingly, because the affinity of the drug for the suppository base increased and its tendency to partition to the rectal lipids decreased. In a similar way, incorporation of

water-soluble drug into a water-in-oil emulsified suppository base tends to decrease bioavailability as the drug is transferred in dispersed aqueous droplets in the molten base.

Hygroscopicity of some hydrophilic bases such as the polyoxyethylene glycols results in the abstraction of water from the rectal mucosa. This causes a stinging sensation and discomfort and probably affects the passage of drugs across the rectal mucosa.

The hygroscopicity of the glycols decreases as the molecular weight increases. The problem, however, may be overcome by the incorporation of water into the base, although the presence of water may affect drug stability. Glycerogelatin bases are also hygroscopic.

Deliberate incorporation of water into a formulation gives rise to the possibility that, on storage, water will be lost by evaporation and drug may crystallise as a result. Reactions between components of the formulation are more likely to occur in the presence of moisture than in its absence.

Incompatibility between base and drug

Various incompatibilities have been noted with polyoxyethylene glycol bases. Phenolic substances complex with glycol, probably by hydrogen bonding between the phenolic hydroxyl group and the glycol ether oxygens. Polyoxyethylene glycol bases are incompatible with tannic acid, ichthammol, aspirin, benzocaine, clioquinol and sulfonamides.[27] High concentrations of salicylic acid alter the consistency of the bases to a more fluid state.

Glycerogelatin bases are prepared by heating together glycerin, gelatin and water. Although primarily used *per se* as an intestinal evacuant, the glycerogelatin base may be used to deliver drugs to the body. For this purpose the USP XVIII specified two types of gelatin to avoid incompatibilities. Type A is acidic and cationic with an isoelectric point between pH 7 and 9; type B is less acidic and anionic with an isoelectric point between pH 4.7 and 5. Use of untreated gelatin renders the base incompatible with acidic and basic drugs.

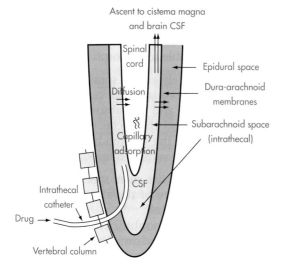

Figure 9.56 Anatomical structures and pathways of drug movement important in intrathecal drug administration; the lower part (sacral, lumbar) of the spinal cord is shown in this diagram.
Reproduced from J. S. Kroin, *Clin. Pharmacokinet.*, 22, 319 (1992).

9.12 Intrathecal drug administration

Administration of drugs in solution by intra-thecal catheter provides an opportunity to delivery drugs to the brain and spinal cord.

Relatively hydrophilic drugs such as metho-trexate ($\log P = -0.5$) which do not cross the blood–brain barrier in significant amounts, have been infused intrathecally to treat meningeal leukaemia, and baclofen ($\log P = -1.0$) to treat spinal cord spasticity. High lumbar CSF concentrates are achieved as a result. Figure 9.56 shows the anatomy of the epidural space and routes of drug transport. The spinal CSF has a small volume (70 cm^3) and a relatively slow clearance (20–40 cm^3 h^{-1}) for hydrophilic drugs.

The intrathecal route is more invasive than i.v, i.m. or s.c routes. Both percutaneously implanted catheters and subcutaneously implantable pumps have been used to reduce the risk of infection on repeated puncture.

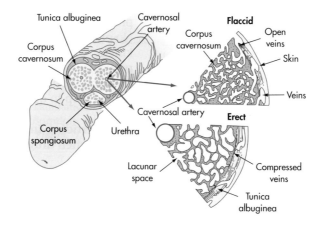

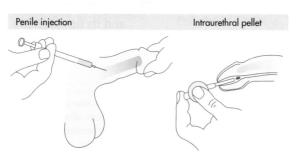

Figure 9.57 Cross-section of the penis, showing differences in the corpora cavernosa between erection and flaccidity. Diffusion path lengths following direct injection are short.

10

Physicochemical drug interactions and incompatibilities

This chapter deals with some practical consequences of the physical chemistry of drugs – particularly their interactions with each other, with solvents and with excipients in formulations. Sometimes the interaction is beneficial and sometimes not. In reading this chapter you should appreciate that there are several causes of interactions and incompatibilities which include:

- pH effects – changes in pH which may lead to precipitation of the drug
- Change of solvent characteristics on dilution, which may also cause precipitation
- Cation–anion interactions in which complexes are formed
- Salting-out and salting-in – the influence of salts in decreasing or increasing solubility, respectively
- Chelation – in which a chelator molecule binds with a metal ion to form a complex
- Ion-exchange interactions – in which ionised drugs interact with opposites charged resins
- Adsorption to excipients and containers – causing loss of drug
- Interactions with plastics – another source of loss of material
- Protein binding – through which the free concentration of drugs *in vivo* is reduced by binding to plasma proteins

Equations can be written to describe most of these interactions, but these formulae can be applied *in vivo* only to provide an indication of behaviour because of the complexity of the body. Nevertheless, the equations are important to allow some prediction of the magnitude of effects.

The chapter discusses the topic of drug interactions from a physicochemical rather than a pharmacological or pharmacodynamic viewpoint. Many drug interactions *in vitro* are, not surprisingly, readily explained by resorting to the physical chemistry discussed in earlier chapters of this book. There is no reason why the same forces and phenomena that operate *in vitro* cannot explain many of the observed interactions that occur *in vivo*, although of course the interplay of physicochemical forces and physiological conditions makes simple interpretations a little hazardous. Interactions such as protein binding, whether as a result of hydrophobic or electrostatic interactions, adsorption of drugs onto solids, or chelation and complexation, all occur in physiological conditions and are predictable to a large degree, provided that certain assumptions are made. We can also observe interactions between drugs themselves (drug–drug interactions) or interactions between drugs and excipients (drug–excipient interactions).

Drug–drug or drug–excipient interactions can take place before administration of a drug. These may result in precipitation of the drug from solution, loss of potency, or instability. They can occur even in the solid state under some circumstances. With the decline in traditional forms of extemporaneous dispensing, this aspect of pharmaceutical incompatibility may seem to have decreased somewhat in importance, but other forms of extemporaneous preparation occur today. One example is the addition of drugs to intravenous fluids, a practice which should be carried out with pharmaceutical oversight to avoid incompatibilities and instabilities, particularly with new drugs and formulations and during clinical trials.

An *incompatibility* occurs when one drug is mixed with other drugs or agents producing a product unsuitable for administration either because of some modification of the effect of the active drug, such as increase in toxicity, or because of some physical change, such as decrease in solubility or stability. Some drugs designed to be administered by the intravenous route cannot safely be mixed with all available intravenous fluids. If, as discussed in Chapter 5, the solubility of a drug in a particular infusion fluid is low, crystallisation may occur (sometimes very slowly) when the drug and fluid are mixed. Microcrystals may be formed which are not immediately visible. When infused, these have potentially serious effects. The mechanism of crystallisation from solution will often involve a change in pH; the problem is a real one because the pH of commercially available infusion fluids can vary within a pH range of perhaps 1–2 units. Therefore, a drug may be compatible with one batch of fluid and not another. The proper application of the equations relating pH and pK_a to solubility discussed in section 5.2.4 should allow additions of drugs to be safely made or to be avoided.

We now discuss, in turn, pH effects *in vitro* and *in vivo*, cation–anion interactions, electrolyte effects, formation of complexes, ion-exchange interactions, adsorption and protein binding.

10.1 pH effects *in vitro* and *in vivo*

The pH of a medium, whether in a formulation or in the body, can be a primary determinant of drug behaviour. For convenience we discuss here pH effects *in vitro* and *in vivo* separately.

10.1.1 *In vitro* pH effects

Chemical, as well as physical, instability may result from changes in pH, buffering capacity, salt formation or complexation. Chemical instability may give rise to the formation of inactive or toxic products. Although infusion times are generally not greater than 2 h, chemical changes following a change in pH may occur rapidly. pH changes often follow from the addition of a drug substance or solution to an infusion fluid, as shown in Table 10.1. This increase or decrease in pH may then produce physical or chemical changes in the system.

The titratable acidity or alkalinity of a system may be more important than pH itself in determining compatibility and stability.[1] For example, an autoclaved solution of dextrose may have a pH as low as 4.0, but the titratable acidity in such an unbuffered solution is low,

Table 10.1 Changes in pH of 5% dextrose (1000 cm³) following addition of three drugs[a]

Drug	Quantity	ΔpH	Final pH
Aminophylline	250 mg	+4.2	8.5
	500 mg	+4.2	8.5
Cefalothin sodium	1 g	+0.1	4.2
	2 g	+0.2	4.3
Oxytetracycline	500 mg	−1.25	2.9
hydrochloride	1 g	−1.45	2.7

[a] Reproduced from M. Edwards. *Am. J. Hosp. Pharm.*, **24**, 440 (1967).

and thus the addition of a drug such as benzylpenicillin sodium, or the soluble form of an acidic drug whose solubility will be reduced at low pH, may not be contraindicated. As seen from Table 10.1, the additive may itself change the pH of the solution or solvent to which it is added. As little as 500 mg of ampicillin sodium can raise the pH of 500 cm³ of some fluids to over 8, and carbenicillin or benzylpenicillin may raise the pH of 5% dextrose or dextrose saline to 5.6 or even higher. Both drugs are, however, stable in these conditions.[2]

The solubility of calcium and phosphate in total parenteral nutrition (TPN) solutions is dependent on the pH of the solution. TPN solutions are, of course, clinically acceptable only when precipitation can be guaranteed not to occur. Dibasic calcium phosphate, for example, is soluble only to the extent of 0.3 g dm⁻³ whereas monobasic calcium phosphate has a solubility of 18 g dm⁻³. At low pH the monobasic form predominates, while at higher pH values the dibasic form becomes available to bind with calcium and precipitates tend to form.[3]

Calcium solubility curves for TPN solutions containing 1.5% (w/v) amino acid and 10% (w/v) dextrose at pH 5.5 are shown in Fig. 10.1. The broken straight lines show the calcium and phosphate concentrations at 3 : 1 and 2 : 1 ratios. The dotted curve for Aminosyn solutions shows the concentrations at which precipitation occurs after 18 h at 25°C followed by 30 min in a water bath at 37°C. The full curve is for TrophAmine solutions, and represents calcium or phosphate concentrations at which visual or microscopic precipitation or crystallisation occurs. Compositions to the left of the curves represent physically compatible solutions.

10.1.2 *In vivo* pH effects

The sensitivity of the properties of most drugs to changes in the pH of their environment

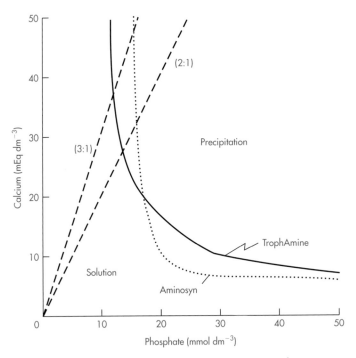

Figure 10.1 Solubility curves for TPN solutions containing amino acid (15 g dm^{-3}) and 10% dextrose at pH 5.5. Dotted line: Aminosyn. Solid line: TrophAmine. Dashed lines: relative calcium to phosphate ratios.
Modified from reference 3 with permission.

means that the hydrogen-ion concentration will be an important determinant of solubility, crystallisation and partitioning. Gastric pH is 1–3 in normal subjects, but the measured range of pH values in the human stomach is wide. Figure 10.2 shows the changes in pH that occur. Remembering that pH is a logarithmic scale, the order of the change in the gut and its effect on aqueous and lipid solubility in particular can be appreciated. Changes in the acid–base balance therefore have a marked influence on the absorption and thus on the activity of drugs.

Ingestion of antacids, food, and weak electrolytes will all change the pH of the stomach. Weakly acidic drugs, being unionised in the stomach, will be absorbed from the stomach by passive diffusion. One might expect, therefore, that concomitant antacid therapy would delay or partially prevent absorption of certain acidic drugs. The main mechanism would be an increase in pH of the stomach, increasing ionisation of the drug and reducing absorp-

tion. A problem in generalisations of this kind is that the acid-neutralising capacity of

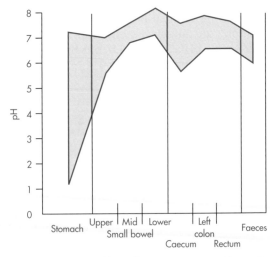

Figure 10.2 pH profile in the gut as measured by radio-telemetric capsule; the shaded area represents extremes of values observed in 9 subjects.
Reproduced from S. J. Meldrum et al., Br. Med. J., 2, 104 (1972).

antacids is very variable, as the results quoted in Table 10.2 show. Some acidic drugs, listed in Table 10.3 are also known to be absorbed in the intestine, in which case the co-administration of an antacid is not necessarily prohibited, as its effects may be transitory.

Effects are not always clear-cut, as pointed out at the beginning of this chapter. There are contradictory reports of the effect of antacids on the absorption of levodopa, as one example. Levodopa is metabolised within the gastro-intestinal tract and more rapidly degraded in the stomach than in the intestine, so the rate at which the drug is emptied from the stomach can affect its availability. It has been suggested that when an antacid is administered prior to the drug, serum levodopa concentration is increased.

The use of cimetidine, ranitidine, nizatidine, famotidine and other H_2-antagonists has given rise to the possibility of a drug interaction involving the increase in gastric pH, as these drugs inhibit gastric acid secretion (see Fig. 9.7 in section 9.1.3). A few subjects have transient achlorhydria after oral cimetidine, so increased absorption of acid-labile drugs is a predictable side-effect, as breakdown is reduced.

Sodium bicarbonate (sodium hydrogen carbonate) is one of the most effective antacids in terms of neutralising capacity. It can greatly

Table 10.2   Amounts of various antacids required to neutralise 50 mEq HCl[a]

Antacid	Neutralising capacity of 1 g or 1 cm³		Dose required to neutralise 50 mEq	Weight of tablet (g)	No. of tablets
	cm³ 0.1 mol dm⁻³ HCl	mEq HCl			
Powders					
$NaHCO_3$	115	11.5	4.4 g		
MgO	85	8.5	5.9 g		
$CaCO_3$	110	11.0	4.5 g		
Magnesium trisilicate	10	1.0	50 g		
$MgCO_3$	8	0.8	63 g		
Suspensions					
$Al(OH)_3$ gel	0.7	0.07	715 cm³		
Milk of Magnesia	27.7	2.8	17.8 cm³		
Titralac	24	2.4	20.6 cm³		
Aludrox	1.7	0.17	294 cm³		
Oxaine	2.4	0.24	208 cm³		
Mucaine	1.7	0.17	294 cm³		
Kolantyl gel	3.4	0.34	147 cm³		
Tablets					
Gastrogel	5.0	0.5	100 g	1.08	93
Gastrobrom	15.0	1.5	33.3 g	1.48	23
Glyzinal	2.5	0.25	200 g	0.72	278
Actal	7.7	0.77	65 g	0.60	109
Amphotab	2.5	0.25	200 g	1.04	192
Gelusil	2.5	0.25	200 g	1.36	147
Nulacin	10.0	1.0	50 g	3.12	17
Kolantyl wafer	5.0	0.5	100 g	1.64	61
Titralac	42.5	4.25	11.8 g	0.65	18
Almacarb	3.0	0.3	167 g	1.28	130
Dijex	4.6	0.46	109 g	1.65	66

[a] Reproduced from D. W. Piper and B. H. Fenton, *Gut*, 5, 585 (1964).

Note that proprietary preparations available in different countries may not have the same formulation.

Table 10.3 Drugs whose absorption may be affected by antacid administration

Drug whose activity would be reduced	Drug whose activity would be potentiated
Tetracyclines	Theophylline
Nalidixic acid	Chloroquine
Nitrofurantoin	Mecamylamine
Benzylpenicillin	Amfetamine
Sulfonamides	Levodopa

depress the absorption of tetracycline – the mean amount of drug appearing in the urine of patients receiving only drug was 114 mg at 48 h and was 53 mg for those also given sodium bicarbonate. Chelation (see section 10.5) is not possible with the monovalent Na$^+$ ion as it is with the multivalent components of other antacids, nor does adsorption occur. If the drug is dissolved prior to administration, the antacid does not affect the excretion of the antibiotic, suggesting that in normal dosage forms it is the rate of dissolution of the drug that is affected by the antacid, as explained below in the case of tetracycline.

The aqueous solubility of tetracycline at pH 1–3 is a hundred-fold greater than at pH 5–6. Consequently, its rate of solution, dc/dt, at this pH is greatly reduced as, according to equation (10.1) (see also section 1.5),

$$\frac{dc}{dt} = kc_s \tag{10.1}$$

where c_s is the solubility. A 2 g dose of $NaHCO_3$ will increase the intragastric pH above 4 for a period of 20–30 min, sufficient time for 20–50% of the undissolved tetracycline particles to be emptied into the duodenum where the pH (at 5–6) is even less favourable for solution to occur. The fraction of drug absorbed is decreased.

Effects of antacids other than directly on pH

The effect of antacids on gastric emptying rate is a factor which makes difficult a direct physicochemical analysis of the problem. The difficulty in predicting the effect of antacids is clearly shown by studies with naproxen, a weakly acidic nonsteroidal anti-inflammatory with a pK_a of 4.2. Several textbooks of drug interactions state that antacids decrease the absorption of acidic drugs such as nalidixic acid, nitrofurantoin and benzylpenicillin (as indicated in Table 10.3), but antacids both increase and decrease the absorption of naproxen. Magnesium carbonate, magnesium oxide and aluminium hydroxide decrease absorption and, as these are insoluble agents, adsorption effects which reduce the quantity of free drug in solution are suspected (see Fig. 10.3). On the other hand intake of Maalox, which contains magnesium and aluminium hydroxides, slightly increased the area under the curve. The extent to which Al^{3+} and Mg^{2+} ions chelate with nalidixic acid is not clear, but the structure of the drug suggests it has chelating potential (see section 10.5).

Even though gastric emptying tends to become more rapid as the gastric pH is raised, antacid preparations containing aluminium or calcium are prone to retard emptying, and magnesium preparations to promote it. The caution about the co-administration of antacids containing divalent or trivalent metals and tetracyclines should be extended to antacids containing sodium bicarbonate or any substance capable of increasing intragastric pH.

Similar principles, of course, can be applied to intestinal absorption, but here the pH gradients between the contents of the intestinal lumen and capillary blood are smaller. Sudden changes in the acid–base balance will, none the less, change the concentration of drugs able to enter cells, providing that the pH change does not alter binding of the drug to protein, or drug excretion, which of course it invariably does. Phenobarbital owes its biological effect to the concentration of drug available inside cells. Breathing CO_2 decreases the concentration of phenobarbital in the plasma and causes an increased affinity for the cell phase and therefore increases its potency. Conversely, the hypotensive activity of the ganglion blocker mecamylamine is increased by inhalation of CO_2, as its activity is dependent on plasma levels. Thus, accurate prediction of the effect of a change in the acid–base balance on the activity of any drug requires a

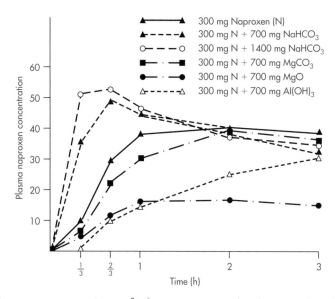

Figure 10.3 Mean plasma concentrations (μg cm^{-3}) of naproxen in 14 male volunteers with and without intake of sodium bicarbonate, magnesium oxide or aluminium hydroxide.
Modified from E. J. Segre, H. Sevelius and J. Varaday, *N. Engl. J. Med.*, 291, 582 (1974).

knowledge of its site of action and the potential effect of pH changes on its excretion and biotransformation, and requires knowledge of the extent of pH changes throughout the body.

Ingestion of some antacids over a period of 24 h will increase urinary pH and hence affect renal resorption and handling of the drug. For example, administration of sodium bicarbonate with aspirin reduces blood salicylate levels by about 50%, probably owing to its increased excretion in the urine. Although high doses of alkalising agents which raise the pH of the urine will increase the renal excretion of free salicylate and result in lowering of plasma salicylate levels, in commercial buffered aspirin tablets (such as Bufferin) there is insufficient antacid to cause a change in the pH of the gastric fluids. The small amount of antacid is sufficient, however, to aid the dissolution of the acetylsalicylic acid (aspirin) (see Chapter 5) and this leads to more favourable absorption rates.[4]

The importance of urinary pH

Change in the pH of urine will change the rate of urinary excretion (as represented in Fig.

10.4). When a drug is in its unionised form it will more readily diffuse from the urine to the blood. In an acidic urine, acidic drugs will diffuse back into the blood from the urine. Acidic compounds such as nitrofurantoin are excreted faster when the urinary pH is alkaline. Amfetamine, imipramine and amitriptyline are excreted more rapidly in acidic urine. The control of urinary pH in studies of pharmacokinetics is thus vital. It is difficult, however, to find compounds to use by the oral route for deliberate adjustment of urinary pH. Sodium bicarbonate and ammonium chloride may be used but are unpalatable. Intravenous administration of acidifying salt solutions presents one approach, especially for the forced diuresis of basic drugs in cases of poisoning.

Urinary pH can be important in determining drug toxicity more directly. A preparation containing methenamine mandelate and sulfamethizole caused turbidity in the urine of 9 out of 32 patients. The turbidity was higher in acidic urine, and was caused by precipitation of an amorphous sulfonamide derivative containing 63% of sulfamethizole. *In vitro*, methenamine causes the precipitation of the sulfonamide at pH values from 5 to 6. The

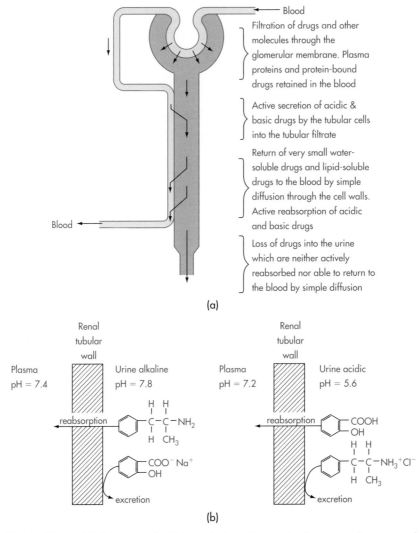

(a)

(b)

Figure 10.4 (a) A highly simplified diagram of a kidney tubule to illustrate the filtration and secretion of drugs from the blood into the tubular filtrate, and their subsequent reabsorption or loss in the urine. (b) Schematic representation of the influence of urinary pH on the passive reabsorption of a weak acid and a weak base from the urine in the renal tubules; at a high pH the passive reabsorption of the weak base and the excretion of the weak acid are enhanced, while at a low pH values the reabsorption of the weak acid and the excretion of the weak base are enhanced.

efficacy of both agents is reduced by precipitation and the danger of renal blockade is, of course, increased.[5]

Precipitation of drugs *in vivo*

Pain on injection may be the result of precipitation of a drug at the site of injection brought about either by solvent dilution or by alteration in pH. Precipitation of drugs from formulations used intravenously can, of course, lead to thromboembolism. The kinetics of precipitation under realistic conditions must be appreciated, since a sufficiently slow rate of infusion may obviate problems from this source as the drug precipitates and then redissolves. A simple equation[6] yields the flow rate (*Q*) of blood or normal saline required to maintain a drug in solution during its addition to an i.v. fluid:

$$Q = \frac{R}{S_m} \qquad (10.2)$$

where R is the rate of injection of drug in mg min^{-1} and S_m is the drug's apparent maximum solubility in the system (mg cm^{-3}). Using diazepam and normal saline as an example, if R is 5 mg min^{-1}, S_m is approximately 0.3 mg cm^{-3}, so Q would have to exceed 17 cm^3 min^{-1} to prevent *observable* precipitation. As this is a high rate of infusion, it is evident that the administration of diazepam through the tubing of an i.v. drip is likely to result in precipitate formation. Too rapid injection of the preparation directly into the venous supply might result in precipitation; slow venous blood flow would contribute to the effect. This would perhaps explain a finding that thrombophlebitis occurs less frequently when smaller veins are avoided and when injection of diazepam is followed by rigorous flushing of the infusion system with normal saline.[7]

10.2 Dilution of mixed solvent systems

In several cases the special nature of a formulation will preclude dilution by an aqueous infusion fluid. Injectable products containing phenytoin, digoxin and diazepam may come into this category if they are formulated in a nonaqueous but water-miscible solvent (such as an alcohol–water mixture) or as a solubilised (e.g. micellar) preparation. Addition of the formulation to water may result in precipitation of the drug, depending on the final concentration of the drug and solvent. It has been suggested that precipitation of the relatively insoluble diazepam may account for the high (3.5%) incidence of thrombophlebitis which occurs when diazepam is given intravenously.

Other additives in formulations may give rise to subtle problems which are not immediately obvious. Valium injection contains 40% propylene glycol and 10% ethanol; it is

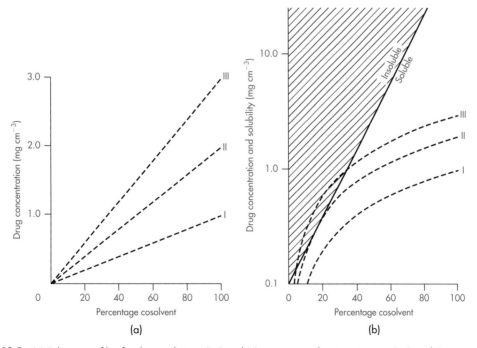

Figure 10.5 (a) Dilution profiles for three solutions (I, II and III) in pure cosolvent containing 1, 2 and 3 mg cm^{-3} drug, respectively. (b) Curves from (a) plotted on semilog scale along with typical solubility line.
Reproduced from S. H. Yalkowsky and S. Valvani, *Drug Intell. Clin. Pharm.*, 11, 417 (1997).

buffered with sodium benzoate and benzoic acid and preserved with benzyl alcohol. Addition of this formulation to normal saline results in the formation of a precipitate. The maximum dilution that produces an observable precipitate after mixing is about 15-fold; a precipitate also forms on addition of the diazepam solution to human plasma.

A graphical technique has been described to predict whether a solubilised drug system will become supersaturated and thus have the potential to precipitate. When a drug dissolved in a cosolvent system is diluted with water, both drug and cosolvent are diluted. The logarithm of the solubility of a drug in a cosolvent system generally increases linearly with the percentage of cosolvent present (Fig. 10.5a). On dilution, the drug concentration falls linearly with a fall in the percentage of cosolvent. The aim of the graphical method

is to plot dilution curves and solubility curves on the same graph. This is achieved in Fig. 10.5(b), where the dilution curves have been plotted semilogarithmically for three systems containing initially 1, 2 and 3 mg cm^{-3} of drug substance (plots I, II and III, respectively). With solution III, dilution below about 30% cosolvent causes the system to be supersaturated; with solution II, below 20% cosolvent the solubility line and the dilution line touch. Only with solutions containing 1 mg cm^{-3} can there be dilution without precipitation.

10.3 Cation–anion interactions

The interaction between a large organic anion and an organic cation may result in the formation of a relatively insoluble precipitate.

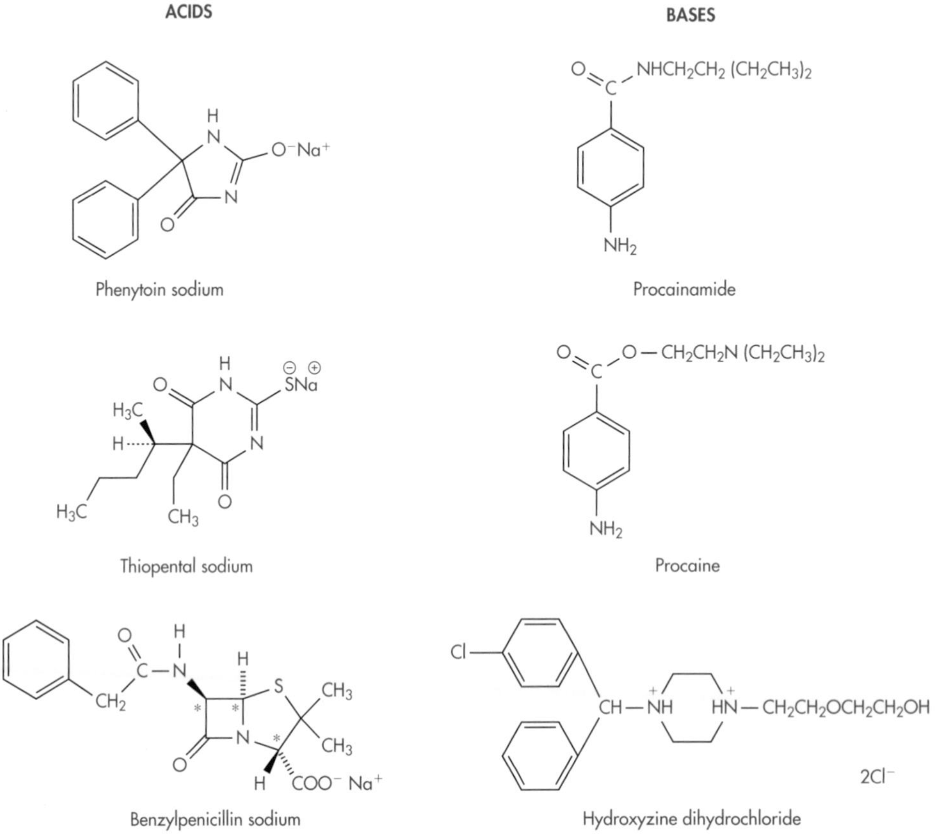

ACIDS

Phenytoin sodium

Thiopental sodium

Benzylpenicillin sodium

BASES

Procainamide

Procaine

Hydroxyzine dihydrochloride

Scheme 10.1

Complexation, precipitation or phase separation can occur in these circumstances, the product being affected by changes in ionic strength, temperature and pH. Examples of cation–anion interactions include those between procainamide and phenytoin sodium, procaine and thiopental sodium, and hydroxyzine hydrochloride and benxylpenicillin (Scheme 10.1). The nature of many of these interactions has not been studied in detail. In the absence of such work it is necessary to predict possible incompatibilities from a knowledge of the physical properties of the drug and other components in the formulation. Sometimes, however, as when chlorpromazine and morphine injections are mixed, the incompatibility is not due to an interaction between the two drugs but to drug–bactericide interaction, the chlorocresol contained in the morphine injection (prepared by heating with a bactericide) precipitated with the chlorpromazine, possibly by an anion–cation interaction. Nitrofurantoin sodium must be diluted prior to use with 5% dextrose or with sterile water for injection;

alkyl *p*-hydroxybenzoates (parabens), phenol or cresol, all of which tend to precipitate the nitrofurantoin, must be absent.

Phase diagrams such as that shown in Fig. 10.6 are useful in determining regions of incompatibility and compatibility in cation–anion mixtures because admixture is not always contraindicated. The example shown here is for mixtures of disodium cromoglicate (DSCG, sodium cromoglicate) – a di-anionic drug – with a cationic surfactant, tetradecyldimethylammonium bromide (C_{14}BDAC). As can be seen, the interaction is strongly concentration dependent. In some regions, below the line AB, the two ions coexist. Ion pairs (see below) form in the shaded region below AB. Above this solubility product line, turbidity occurs in the hatched region. On increasing the concentration of surfactant, the complex is solubilised so that the interaction is masked.[8]

In a study of the incompatibility of organic iodide contrast media and antihistaminic drugs (added to reduce anaphylactic reactions) it was found that the acidity of the antihistamine solutions used caused the precipitation

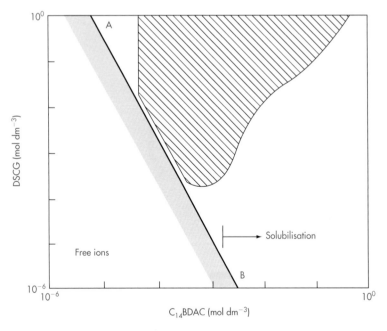

Figure 10.6 Phase diagram for mixtures of disodium cromoglicate (DSCG, sodium cromoglicate) and tetradecyldimethylammonium bromide (C_{14}BDAC).
Reproduced from reference 8.

of the organic iodide.[9] One of the antihistamines, promethazine, reacted strongly with all the contrast media, probably because its solution had the lowest pH of the drugs studied. It is not only with intravenous fluids that such interactions may occur. Examples have been quoted of the inadvisable mixture of syrups; for example, immediate precipitation in a prescribed mixture of a syrup containing cloxacillin sodium (Orbenin) and a syrup (Phensedyl) containing the bases codeine and promethazine. Precipitation was followed by a 20% loss in antibiotic activity in 5 h and 99% loss in 5 days. The double-decomposition reactions involved are likely to be those shown in Fig. 10.7.

Complexes which form are not always fully active. A well-known example is the complex between neomycin sulfate and sodium lauryl sulfate that will form when Aqueous Cream BP is used as a vehicle for neomycin sulfate. Aqueous cream comprises 30% emulsifying ointment, which itself is a mixture of emulsifying wax which contains 10% of sodium lauryl sulfate or a similar anionic surfactant.

Interactions are not always visible. The formation of visible precipitates depends to a large extent on the insolubility of the two combining species in the particular mixture and the size to which the precipitated particles grow. One might assume that in an atropine and phenobarbital mixture, a barbiturate–atropine complex may precipitate. Atropine base is soluble to the extent of 1 part in 460 parts of water. There is only 0.6 mg atropine in a 5 cm^3 dose and it is therefore well within its solubility limit. The solubility of phenobarbital is 1 mg cm^{-3}. The 15 mg of phenobarbital sodium (13.5 mg of phenobarbital) which would result if all the sodium salt were to be precipitated would be in excess of its solubility. Only 0.4 mg of phenobarbital is precipitated by 0.6 mg of atropine sulfate, however, and the phenobarbital therefore remains in solution also. There is thus no precipitation.

Interactions between drugs and ionic macromolecules are another potential source of problems. Heparin sodium and erythromycin lactobionate are contraindicated in admixture, as are heparin sodium and chlorpromazine

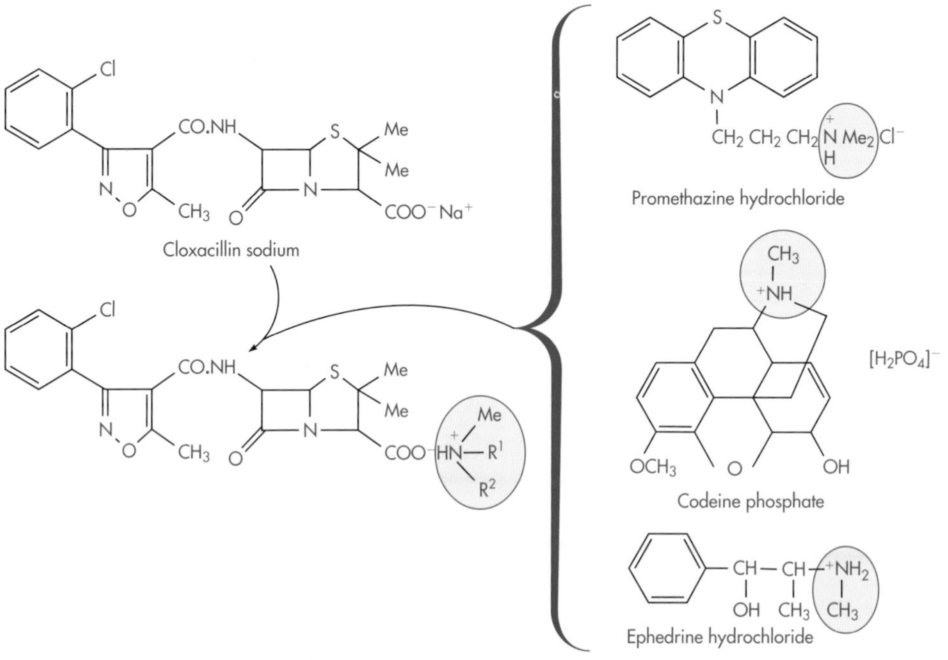

Figure 10.7 The interaction of cloxacillin sodium with promethazine hydrochloride, codeine phosphate and ephedrine hydrochloride.

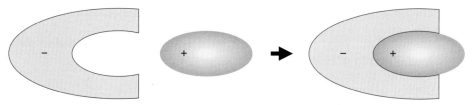

Figure 10.8 Representation of an organic ion-pair – the anion is shown here interacting with a cationic molecule of complementary shape (purely schematic) thus masking the exposure of the charge to the aqueous environment.

hydrochloride or gentamicin sulfate. Tables of incompatibilities abound with such examples. Interference with the sulfate groups reduces the anticoagulant activity of heparin. The activity of phenoxymethylpenicillin against *Staphylococcus aureus* is reduced in the presence of various macromolecules such as acacia, gelatin, sodium alginate and tragacanth.[10] The interaction will not, in each case, be electrostatic in origin but may involve binding through hydrophobic interactions.

Ion-pair formation

Ion-pair formation may be responsible for the absorption of highly charged drugs such as the quaternary ammonium salts and sulfonic acid derivatives, the absorption of which is not explained by the pH–partition hypothesis.[11] Ion pairs may be defined as neutral species formed by electrostatic attraction between oppositely charged ions in solution, which are often sufficiently lipophilic to dissolve in non-aqueous solvents. The formation of an ion pair (Fig. 10.8) results in the 'burying' of charges and alteration to the physical properties of the drug. This is discussed more fully at the end of section 9.1.2. Interactions between charged drug species and appropriate lipophilic ions of opposite charge may constitute a drug interaction and may occur *in vitro* or *in vivo*.

both weak electrolytes and nonelectrolytes can occur through salting out, a phenomenon discussed in section 5.2.3.

Sodium sulfadiazine and sulfafurazole diolamine in therapeutic doses (1 mg) added to 5% dextrose and 5% dextrose and saline solution have been found to be compatible, yet when added to commercial polyionic solutions (such as Abbott Ionosol B, Baxter electrolyte No.2) both rapidly form heavy precipitates. pH and temperature are two vital parameters, but the pH effect is not simply a solubility-related phenomenon. Polyionic solutions of a lower initial pH (4.4–4.6) cause crystallisation of sulfafurazole at room temperature within 2.5 h, the pH values of the admixtures being 5.65 and 5.75 respectively. Other solutions with slightly higher initial pH levels (6.1–6.6) formed crystals only after preliminary cooling to 20°C at pH values from 4.25 to 4.90. If the temperature remains constant, the intensity of precipitation varies with the composition and initial pH of the solution used as a vehicle.[12]

Most physicochemically based drug interactions can take place in the body, or outside it, or during concomitant drug administration, so it is probably not profitable to consider them separately. Some interactions, such as complexation, which are probably more important *in vivo* than *in vitro* are discussed in detail below.

10.4 Polyions and drug solutions

The extensive clinical use of polyionic solutions for intravenous therapy means that drugs are frequently added to systems of a complex ionic nature. Reduction in the solubility of

10.5 Chelation and other forms of complexation

The term *chelation* (derived from the Greek *chele* meaning lobster's claw) relates to the interaction between a metal atom or ion and another species, known as the *ligand*, by which a heteroatomic ring is formed. Chelation changes the physical and chemical characteristics of the metal ion and of the ligand. It is simplest to consider the ligand as the electron-pair donor and the metal the electron-pair acceptor, the donation establishing a coordinate bond. Many chelating agents act in the form of anions which coordinate to a metal ion. For chelation to occur there must be at least two donor atoms capable of binding to the same metal ion, and ring formation must be sterically possible. For example ethylenediamine (1,2-diaminoethane, $NH_2CH_2CH_2NH_2$) has two donor nitrogens and acts as a bidentate (two-toothed) ligand.[13, 14] When a drug forms a metal chelate, the solubility and absorption of both drug and metal ion may be affected, and drug chelation can lead to either increased or decreased absorption. While the phenomenon can be useful in analytical procedures, in medicine it can lead to problems such as the binding of tetracyclines (which are chelators) to teeth. Deferiprone (**I**) chelates iron.

Tetracyclines have similar chelating groups in their structure.[15] Therapeutic chelators are used in syndromes where there is metal ion overload. EDTA (ethylenediaminetetraacetic acid) (**II**) as the monocalcium disodium salt is used in the treatment of lead poisoning, the calcium avoiding problems of calcium depletion.

Tetracyclines

Probably the most widely quoted example of complex formation leading to decreased drug absorption is that of tetracycline chelation with metal ions. Polyvalent cations such as Fe^{2+} and Mg^{2+}, and anions such as the trichloracetate or phosphate interfere with absorption in both model and real systems.[14] Fig. 10.9 shows the effect of a dose of 40 mg ferrous ion on the serum levels following 300 mg of tetracycline. As can be seen from this figure, the nature of the iron salt ingested is important. Ferrous sulfate has the greatest inhibitory effect on tetracycline absorption, perhaps because it dissolves in water more quickly than organic iron compounds. The ability of the various iron compounds to liberate ferrous or ferric ions in the upper part of the gastrointestinal tract before tetracycline is absorbed would therefore seem to be an essential step in the interaction. The order of activity of the different iron salts in the chelation process *in vivo* turns out to be the same as the order of the intestinal absorption of these iron compounds. All the active tetracyclines form stable chelates with Ca^{2+}, Mg^{2+} and Al^{3+}. The antibacterial action of the tetracyclines depends on their metal-binding activity, as their main site of action is on the ribosomes, which are rich in magnesium.

The tetracyclines have an avidity for divalent metals similar to that of glycine (**III**) but they have a greater affinity for the trivalent metals with which they form 3 : 1 drug–metal chelates. Therapeutically active tetracyclines form 2 : 1 complexes with cupric, nickel and zinc ions while inactive analogues form only 1 : 1 complexes.

Structure I Deferiprone

Structure II EDTA

Structure III The 1 : 1 copper–glycine chelate

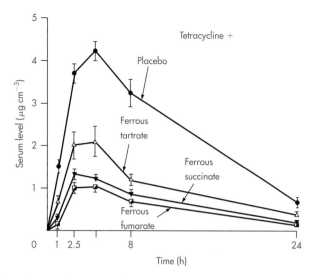

Figure 10.9 The effect of simultaneous ingestion of various iron salts (dose equivalent to 40 mg elemental iron) and tetracycline hydrochloride (500 mg) on serum levels of tetracycline (mean levels in 6 patients).
Reproduced from P. J. Neuvonen and H. Turakka, *Eur. J. Clin. Pharmacol.*, 7, 357 (1974).

The complexing of tetracyclines with calcium poses a problem in paediatric medicine. Discoloration of teeth results from the formation of a coloured complex with the calcium in the teeth; the deposition of drug in the bones of growing babies can lead to problems in bone formation. Table 10.4 reveals that there is no correlation between the binding capacity of a tetracycline with iron and that with calcium, suggesting different modes of complexation. The *in vitro* data are simpler to interpret: the serum levels are the result of two processes, the chelation of the tetracycline and the partitioning of the chelate. Table 10.4 demonstrates the affinities of different tetracyclines for metallic ions. Clinical studies have shown that the absorption of doxycycline is not significantly affected by milk in conditions where the absorption of tetracycline is reduced.

The structures of some tetracyclines are reproduced in Table 10.5, together with their pK_a values; from these data it should be possible to determine something of the relative

Table 10.4 Relative calcium-binding capacities of tetracycline derivatives and decreases in serum levels after 200 mg ferrous sulfate

Tetracycline	Calcium binding[a] (%)	Decrease in serum concentration (%) after 200 mg ferrous sulfate
Demecloclycline	74.5	n.s.[b]
Chlortetracycline	52.7	n.s.[b]
Tetracycline	39.5	40–50
Methacycline	39.5	80–85
Oxytetracycline	36.0	50–60
Doxycycline	19–22	80–90

[a] Percentage of dissolved antibiotic (5 mg/50 cm^3 H$_2$O) bound to calcium phosphate after overnight shaking. From the *US Dispensatory*, 27th edn, p. 1155ff.

[b] ns. = not studied.

Table 10.5 Structures and pK_a values for some tetracyclines

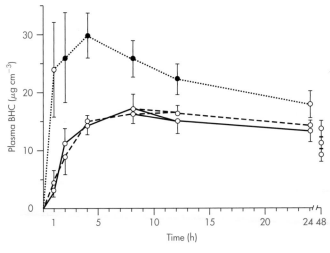

	R¹	R²	R³	R⁴	pK_{a1}	pK_{a2}	pK_{a3}
Chlortetracycline	Cl	Me	OH	H	3.27	7.43	9.33
Oxytetracycline	H	Me	OH	OH	3.5	7.6	9.2
Tetracycline	H	Me	OH	H	3.33	7.7	9.5
Demeclocycline	Cl	H	OH	H	3.3	7.16	9.25
Doxycycline	H	Me	H	OH	3.4	7.7	9.7

affinities of the tetracyclines for metal ions. One piece of evidence relating to the site of chelation is that isochlortetracycline, which lacks the C-11,C-12 enolic system, does not chelate with Ca²⁺ ions.

The highly coloured nature of the tetracycline complexes such as the uranyl ion–tetracycline complex may be utilised in analytical procedures.

Four criteria have been put forward for determining whether chelate formation has occurred:[16] coloured product, decreased aqueous solubility, a drop in pH during chelate formation, and the absence of metal ions in solution after chelate formation. The decreased aqueous solubility of chelates suggests increased lipophilicity but, in the case of the tetracycline chelates, precipitation would decrease the biological activity of the drug as it would be less available for transport across membranes; the larger volume of the chelate would also prevent easy absorption in the intact form.

There is evidence for complex formation of a coumarin derivative with magnesium ions

Figure 10.10 Plasma levels of bishydroxycoumarin (BHC), also known as dicoumarol, in 6 subjects after a 300 mg oral dose with water (solid line), magnesium hydroxide (dotted line) or aluminium hydroxide (dashed line). Closed data points represent a significant difference from control.
Reproduced from reference 17.

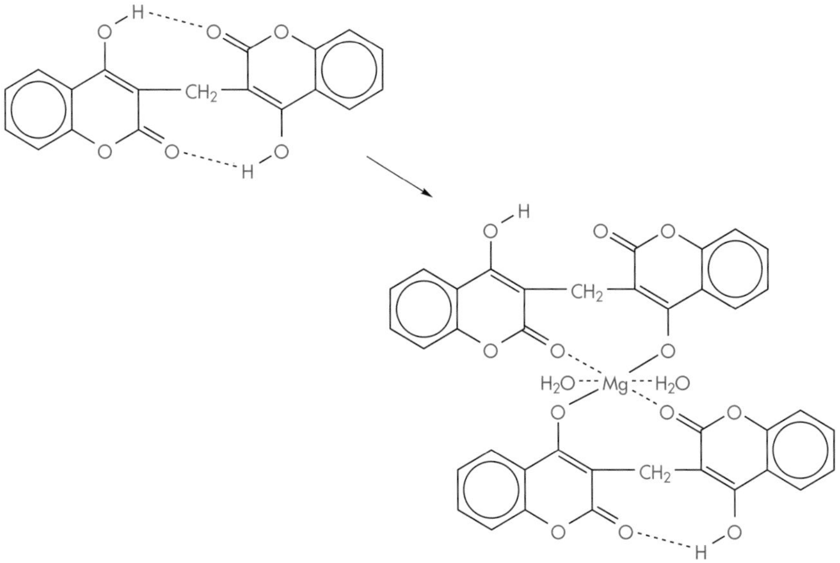

Structure IV Suggested form of the bishydroxycoumarin–Mg chelate. From L. D. Bighley and R. J. Spirey, *J. Pharm. Sci.,* 66, 124 (1977)

present in antacid formulations. In this case the formation of a more absorbable species is indicated since plasma levels of bishydroxycoumarin are elevated in the presence of magnesium hydroxide but are unaffected by aluminium hydroxide; neither antacid influenced warfarin absorption.[17] A magnesium–bishydroxycoumarin chelate having the structure (**IV**) has been isolated. Adsorption may counteract a chelate-mediated increase in absorption, so the adsorptive properties of aluminium hydroxide may be responsible for the lack of effect of this antacid on the absorption of the drug. Results are shown in Fig. 10.10. It has been suggested that the more rapid and complete absorption of warfarin makes it less susceptible to interactions of this type.[17]

Chelation of ciprofloxacin (**V**) by aluminium hydroxide and calcium carbonate reduces bioavailability, as seen in Fig. 10.11. Other quinolones (**VI–IX**), undoubtedly suffer the same fate.

Following treatment of acrodermatitis enteropathica with diiodohydroxyquinolone (**X**) the absorption and retention of dietary zinc and other trace metals has been found to be greater than in subjects not receiving the

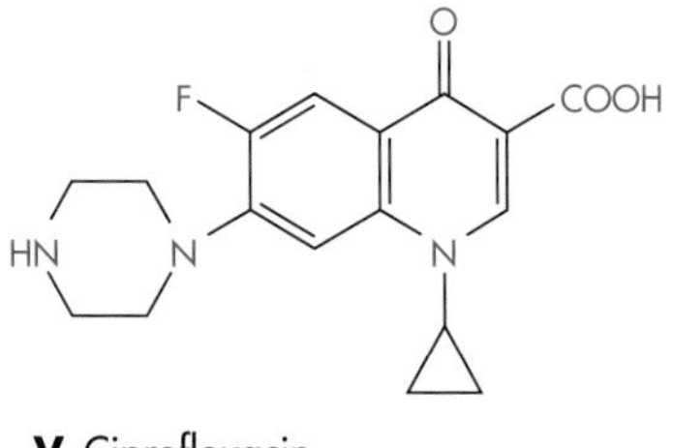

Structure V Ciprofloxacin

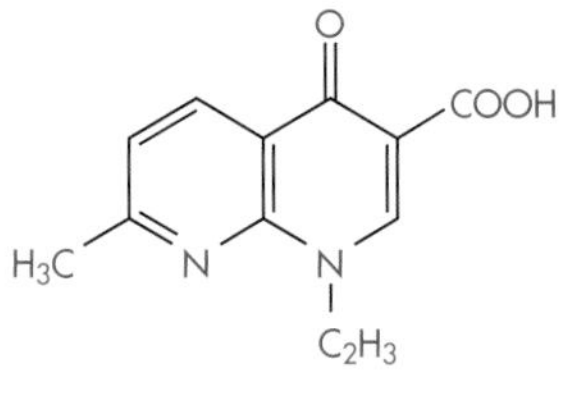

Structure VI Nalidixic acid

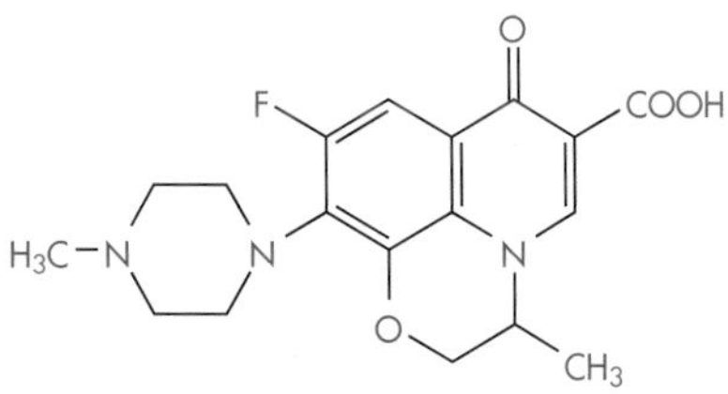

Structure VII Ofloxacin

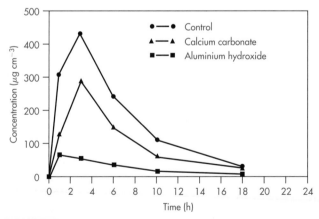

Structure VIII Enoxacin

Structure IX Norfloxacin

5, 7 - diiodo-8-hydroxyquinoline

Structure X Suggested form of chelate of zinc–diiodo-hydroxyquinolone

drug. Chelation of zinc and other trace metals by the drug could have resulted in the increased absorption from the intestinal lumen.

Desferrioxamine (as the mesylate) is used as a drug to sequester iron in iron poisoning or chronic iron overload; penicillamine is similarly used to aid the elimination of copper in Wilson disease. Chelation is also used for the safe delivery of toxic ions such as gadolinium (Gd^{3+}), which is used as a magnetic resonance imaging enhancing agent. One such preparation is gadobenic acid (**XI**) which is a gadolinium-BOPTA (**XIa**) octodentate chelate.

10.6 Other complexes

Molecular complexes of many types may be observed in systems containing two or more drug molecules. Generally, association follows from attractive interactions (hydrophobic, electrostatic or charge-transfer interactions) between two molecules. In the charge transfer system one component is usually an aromatic compound; the second may be a saturated moiety containing a long electron pair (donor atom) or a weakly acidic hydrogen (acceptor

Figure 10.11 Concentrations of ciprofloxacin in the urine following administration of 50 mg to 12 healthy volunteers in a three-way randomised crossover design by R. W. Frost *et al.* (*Antimicrob. Agents Chemother.*, 36, 830 (1992)), who write: 'The precise conditions required for ciprofloxacin to form chelate complexes with other cations have not been fully elucidated, but the carboxyl group seems to be the most likely site for chelation. Thus, the gastric pH would need to be elevated sufficiently to ionise the carboxyl group. Therefore, the lack of interaction with dairy products might be attributable to a gastric pH that was not elevated sufficiently to ionise the carboxyl group. Alternatively, it could be due to a decrease in the availability of calcium to chelate ciprofloxacin because of a lipid barrier.'

Gadobenic acid   (Meglumine)

Structure XI Gadobenic acid

Structure X1a BOPTA (benzyloxypropionic tetraacetate)

atom). The interaction therefore takes place between electron-rich donors and electron-poor acceptors. Interactions between aromatic rings in which there is a parallel overlap of π-systems fall into this category, as in the following example involving nicotinamide (acceptor) and the indole moiety of tryptophan (donor) (**XII**).

The imidazole moiety (**XIII**) is involved in many interactions; it is regarded as aromatic and the molecule is planar. Not surprisingly, caffeine (**XIV**) and theophylline (**XV**) are frequently implicated in interactions with aromatic species. Caffeine not only increases the solubility of ergotamine but also that of benzoic acid. The marked difference in the solubilising properties of caffeine and dimethyluracil (**XVI**) towards substances such as benzoic acid suggests that the imidazole ring of the xanthine nucleus is the portion involved in the interaction. In the main, 1 : 1 complexes are formed but 2 : 1 drug–caffeine complexes may also be found. Hydrophobic interactions are also implicated in the interaction since caffeine has a greater solubilising capacity than theophylline, which, as can be seen, lacks the N–CH$_3$ group in the imidazole nucleus.

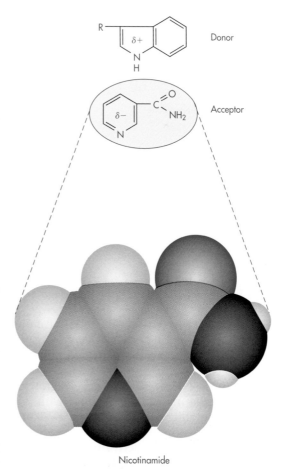

Nicotinamide

Structure XII Example of donor–acceptor interaction between tryptophan (donor) and nicotinamide

can accept protons
(moderately
strong base)

can lose proton
(weakly acidic)

Structure XIII Imidazole

Structure XIV Caffeine

Structure XV Theophylline

Structure XVI Dimethyluracil

10.6.1   Interaction of drugs with cyclodextrins

Compounds which have interior cavities which are large enough to incarcerate organic 'guest' molecules have been named *molecular container compounds*.

Over the last decade there has been growing interest in the interaction of drugs with one group of container compounds, the α-, β- and γ-cyclodextrins (cyclic D-glucose oligomers) and their now myriad derivatives. The cyclodextrin molecules have cyclic structures with internal diameters of 0.6–1 nm (see section 5.6). The interior cavity of the cyclodextrin ring is hydrophobic in nature and binds a hydrophobic portion of the 'guest' molecule, usually forming a 1 : 1 complex. The possible structure of β-cyclodextrin complexes of aspirin shown in Fig. 10.12.

Inclusion of some drugs (including peptides) into cyclodextrins increases their solubility, chemical stability and absorption. The solubilising effect of β-cyclodextrin on flufenamic acid suggests that a 1 : 1 complex is formed in aqueous solution. A relationship between the oil/water partition coefficient of a drug and its tendency to form inclusion complexes has generally been found.[18] This indicates that the hydrophobic cavity of the cyclodextrin 'eye' is more attractive to lipophilic guest molecules. The formation constants for mefenamic acid and meclofenamic acid were, however, lower than expected from the Me or Cl *ortho* substituent. α-Cyclodextrin showed no appreciable interaction with these anti-inflammatory acids, suggesting that its cavity is not large enough to contain the drug molecules.[19]

The altered environment of the drug molecules leads to changes in stability. The cyclodextrins catalyse a number of chemical reactions such as hydrolysis, oxidation and decarboxylation.[20] Although interactions between drugs and cyclodextrins have been mostly the result of deliberate attempts to modify the behaviour or properties of the drug, they are included here to illustrate an additional mode of interaction with other

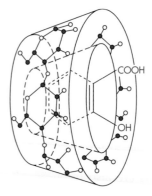

Figure 10.12 Schematic drawing of an aspirin-β-CD complex.
Reproduced from T. Loftsson and M. Masson, *Int. J. Pharm.*, 225, 15–30 (2001).

components which may well occur inside the body as well as in the laboratory.

The use of cyclodextrins as formulation aids is discussed in Chapter 5.

10.6.2   Ion-exchange interactions

Ion-exchange resins are now being used medicinally and as systems for modified release of drugs (see Fig. 10.13). Colestyramine and colestipol are insoluble quaternary ammonium anion-exchange resins which, when administered orally, bind bile acids and increase their elimination because the high molecular weight complex is not absorbed. As bile acids are converted *in vivo* into cholesterol, colestyramine is used as a hypocholesteraemic

agent. When given to patients receiving other drugs as well, the resin would conceivably bind anionic compounds and reduce their absorption. Phenylbutazone (**XVII**), warfarin (**XVIII**), chlorothiazide (**XIX**) and hydrochlorothiazide are bound strongly to the resin *in vitro*.

Structure XVII   Phenylbutazone

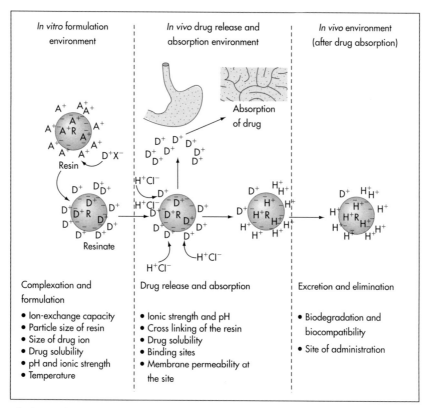

Figure 10.13   The basis of the ion-exchange process in drug delivery with factors affecting the therapeutic efficacy of the system at each stage. R and a blue circle represents resin; a minus sign depicts the integral ion of the resin, and A^+ is the counterion. D is the drug ion, X^- is the ion associated with drug cation and H^+Cl^- is hydrochloric acid. Ions inside and outside the resin indicate ions adsorbed at the surface, as well as in the interior, of the resin structure.
Reproduced from V. Anand, R. Kandarapu and S. Garg, *Drug Discovery Today*, 6, 905–915 (2001).

Structure **XVIII** Warfarin

Structure **XIX** Chlorothiazide

Colestyramine had no effect in animal experiments on the blood levels of these drugs. However, 95% of both warfarin and phenylbutazone were bound and peak blood levels of the latter were halved, although the same total amount was eventually absorbed. A single dose of resin did not significantly reduce the pharmacological effect of warfarin. Nevertheless, it is prudent to administer drugs orally a short time before colestyramine to preclude delay in the action of the drug through adsorption and slow leaching. Table 10.6 shows the effect of very high resin levels on the serum concentration of sodium fusidate. Since the binding is pH-dependent (Table 10.7) an ion-exchange resin can bind any drug with an appropriate charge under pH conditions in which both species are ionised. Decreased drug absorption caused by colestyramine or colestipol in the main has been

Table 10.6 The effect of colestyramine administration on sodium fusidate levels[a]

Resin dose (mg kg^{-1})	Mean serum conc. (μg cm^{-3})
0	3.7
72	2.5
215	1.9
356	0.8

[a] Reproduced from W. H. Johns and T. R. Bates, *J. Pharm. Sci.*, 61, 735 (1972).

Table 10.7 Binding of acetylsalicylic acid (aspirin) *in vitro* to colestyramine[a]

	Percentage binding			
	pH 2	pH 3	pH 5	pH 7.5
Buffer	5	–	6	6
Water	51	95	98	97

[a] Reproduced from K.-J. Halin *et al.*, *Eur. J. Clin. Pharmacol.*, 4, 142 (1972).

reported with thyroxine, aspirin, phenprocoumon, warfarin, chlorothiazide, cardiac glycosides, and ferrous sulfate as a consequence of binding. Absorption of vitamin K and vitamin B$_{12}$ is decreased indirectly by competition of the resin for binding sites on intrinsic factor molecules.[21, 22]

The influence of buffer ions on the binding of the drug in Table 10.7 indicates one of the problems of making *in vitro* measurements and attempting to assess the biological significance of the results. Binding of cefalexin, clindamycin (**XX**) and the components of cotrimoxazole to colestyramine has been measured; *in vivo* absorption of these substances in the presence of the resin is delayed and somewhat reduced, but the changed pattern of absorption is unlikely to affect therapeutic efficacy, except perhaps with cefalexin where it is more pronounced.

10.7 Adsorption of drugs

The process of adsorption and its medical and pharmaceutical applications have been dealt with in some detail in Chapter 6. The use of adsorbents to remove noxious substances from the lumen of the gut is considered there. Adsorbents generally are nonspecific so will adsorb nutrients, drugs and enzymes when given orally. It is not uncommon for adsorbents to be administered in combination with various drugs and it becomes a matter of practical importance to determine the extent to which adsorbents will interfere with the absorption of the drug substance from the gastrointestinal tract.

Several consequences of adsorption are possible. If the drug remains adsorbed until the preparation reaches the general area of the absorption site, the concentration of the drug presented to the absorbing surfaces will be much reduced. The driving force for absorption would then be reduced, resulting in a slower rate of absorption. During the course of absorption of the drug, it is probable that the adsorbate will dissociate in an attempt to re-establish equilibrium with drug in its immediate environment, particularly if there is competition for absorption sites from other substances in the gastrointestinal tract. As a consequence, the concentration of free drug in solution would be maintained at a low level and the absorption rate would be reduced. Alternatively, the release of drug from the adsorbent might be complete before reaching the absorption site, possibly hastened by the presence of electrolytes in the gastrointestinal tract, in which case absorption rates would be virtually identical to those in the absence of adsorbent. Figure 10.14 shows the reduced amounts of promazine excreted in the urine when the promazine was administered with activated charcoal – evidence of a reduced absorption rate of this drug in this situation.

A further example is the delayed absorption of lincomycin (**XX**) when administered with

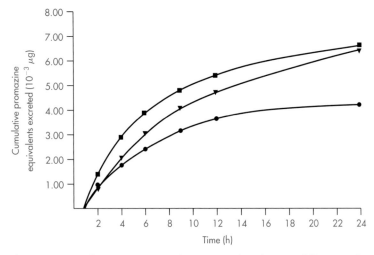

Figure 10.14 Cumulative amounts of promazine equivalents excreted in the urine following administration of various dosage forms to humans: (■), promazine in simple aqueous solution; (▼), promazine plus activated attapulgite; (●), promazine plus activated charcoal.
Reproduced from D. L. Sorby, *J. Pharm. Sci.*, 54, 677 (1965).

Structure XX Lincomycin (R = OH) and clindamycin (R = Cl)

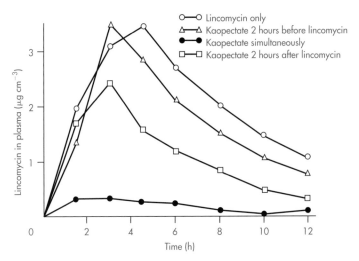

Figure 10.15 The influence of Kaopectate (kaolin and pectinic acid) on the absorption of lincomycin in humans after oral application; note the decrease in plasma levels caused by the simultaneous administration of the absorbent.
Reproduced from J. G. Wagner, *Can. J. Pharm. Sci.*, 1, 55 (1966).

kaolin and pectinic acid (Kaopectate) (Fig. 10.15). The dramatic effect of several antacids on the adsorption of digoxin from elixirs is shown in Fig. 10.16. In view of the relatively low doses of these glycosides, these adsorption effects are likely to have a significant impairing effect on digoxin bioavailability.

If the possibility of adsorption onto formulation ingredients is not kept in mind, erroneous conclusions may be drawn from bioavailability studies, as was the case in the suspected *in vivo* interaction between *p*-aminosalicylic acid (PAS) and rifampicin. It was thought that PAS impaired the intestinal absorption of rifampicin, reducing its serum levels to about half those occurring when it was administered by itself (Fig. 10.17). It was later found that bentonite, a naturally occurring mineral (montmorillonite), consisting chiefly of hydrated aluminium silicate present in the PAS granules was adsorbing the antibiotic and delaying its absorption[23] (Fig. 10.17). It can readily be seen how the initial erroneous conclusion was drawn.

Loss of activity of preservatives can arise from adsorption onto solids commonly used as medicaments. Benzoic acid, for example, can be adsorbed to the extent of 94% by sulfadimidine. Adsorption can be suppressed, however, with hydrophilic polymers. In solid

dosage forms, talc, a commonly used tablet lubricant, has been reported to adsorb cyanocobalamin and consequently to interfere with intestinal absorption of this vitamin.

10.7.1 Protein and peptide adsorption

Some properties of peptides and proteins are discussed in Chapter 11. We have previously

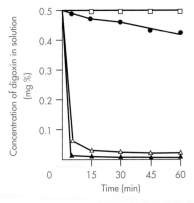

Figure 10.16 Adsorption of digoxin from Lanoxin paediatric elixir at 37 ± 0.1°C by: ●, Aluminium Hydroxide Gel BP (10% v/v); △, Magnesium Trisilicate Mixture BPC (10% v/v); ▲, Gelusil suspension (10% v/v); □, Lanoxin elixir diluted 1 : 10 with water.
Reproduced from S. A. H. Khalil, *J. Pharm. Pharmacol.*, 26, 961 (1974).

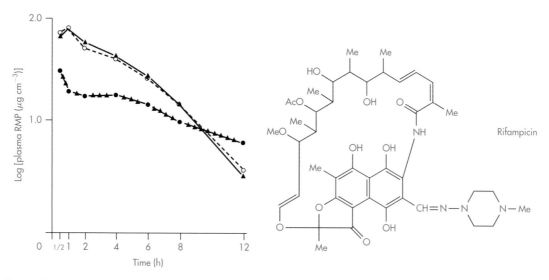

Figure 10.17 Plasma concentrations of rifampicin (RMP) after oral administration in solution (10 mg kg^{-1}) given alone (▲), with *p*-aminosalicyclic acid (PAS) granules (●), or with Na-PAS tablets (○); mean values (*n* = 6 patients) are indicated. Reproduced from reference 23.

(section 8.3.7) discussed the adsorptive loss of insulin from solution; adsorption can be a problem because of the amphipathic nature of many peptides, and becomes pharmaceutically important when they are present in low concentrations in solution. The adsorption of peptides onto glass has been ascribed to bonding between their amino groups and the silanol groups of the glass. A decapeptide derivative of LHRH, the natural luteinising hormone releasing hormone, has two basic amino groups positively charged at low pH, providing an opportunity for binding to silanol groups.[24] Siliconisation of the glass did not inhibit adsorption completely, suggesting that ionic binding was not the only mechanism of interaction. Phosphate buffer at 0.1 mol dm^{-3} concentration and acetate ions at 0.16 mol dm^{-3} concentration (both at pH 5) were most effective in preventing adsorption.

10.8 Drug interactions with plastics

In section 8.3.7 we discussed the adsorption of insulin on to glass and plastic materials used in syringes and giving sets. The plastic tubes

and connections used in intravenous containers and giving sets can adsorb or absorb a number of drugs (Fig. 10.18), leading to significant losses in some cases. Those drugs which show a significant loss when exposed to plastic, in particular poly(vinyl chloride) (PVC), include insulin, glyceryl trinitrate, diazepam, chlormethiazole, vitamin A acetate, isosorbide dinitrate and a miscellaneous group of drugs such as phenothiazines, hydralazine hydrochloride and thiopental sodium.

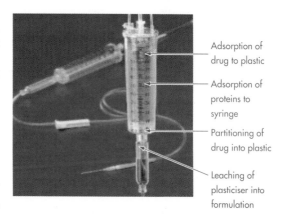

Adsorption of drug to plastic

Adsorption of proteins to syringe

Partitioning of drug into plastic

Leaching of plasticiser into formulation

Figure 10.18 The possible modes of interaction between a drug and the plastic of a giving set.

A theoretical treatment to account for the loss of glyceryl trinitrate from solution to plastic containers has been developed,[25] see Box 10.1.

Some idea of the rate and extent of disappearance of warfarin sodium from PVC infusion bags can be gained from Fig. 10.19. The marked effect of pH is seen. Losses can

---

Box 10.1   Adsorption of glyceryl trinitrate onto plastic containers

Considering a two-stage loss of drug:

$$A \underset{k_2}{\overset{k_1}{\rightleftharpoons}} B \overset{k_3}{\rightarrow} C$$

Where A = Glyceryl trinitrate in aqueous solution

Where B = Adsorbed glyceryl trinitrate

Where C = Glyceryl trinitrate dissolved in the matrix

Therefore,

$$\frac{dA}{dt} = -k_1 A + k_2 B \qquad (10.3)$$

$$\frac{dB}{dt} = -k_1 A - k_2 B - k_3 B \qquad (10.4)$$

and

$$\frac{dC}{dt} = k_3 B \qquad (10.5)$$

It is found that $dB/dt \gg dC/dt$. At steady state,

$dB/dt = 0$, and at $t = 0$, $A = A_0$, $B = 0$ and $C = 0$. Rate constant k_1 is a function of the amount of drug in solution, the surface area available for adsorption and the nature of the plastic, and k_3 is a function of the volume of the plastic matrix and the solubility of the glyceryl trinitrate in the plastic matrix. The ratio k_3/k_2 describes the partitioning of the drug between the plastic and the aqueous phase. So, if P is the partition coefficient,

$$\frac{k_3}{k_2} = aP \qquad (10.6)$$

a being a proportionality constant related to the mass of the plastic, the volume of the solution and other parameters. The ratio k_1/k_2 can be related to a Langmuir type of adsorption constant.

The final form of the equation accurately predicts the glyceryl trinitrate remaining in solution (A):

$$A = 8.957e^{-0.028t} + 14.943e^{-0.235t} \qquad (10.7)$$

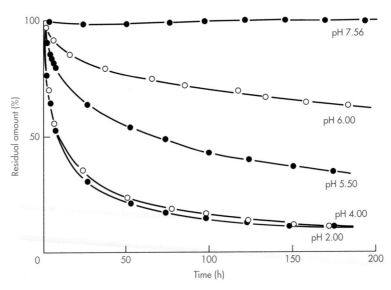

Figure 10.19   Disappearance of warfarin sodium from aqueous buffered solutions stored in 100 cm^3 PVC infusion bags at room temperature.
Reproduced from reference 26 with permission.

Table 10.8   Loss of drugs from normal saline solutions in poly(vinyl chloride)(PVC) bags stored at 22°C for 8 h[a]

Drug	Initial solute conc. (μg cm^{-3})	% loss	
		PVC (100 cm^3)	PVC (500 cm^3)
Diazepam	40	60	31
	120	58	31
Medazepam	40	76	–
Oxazepam	40	22	12
Nitrazepam	40	15	10
Warfarin sodium[b]	20	49	–
Warfarin sodium	20	29	–
Glyceryl trinitrate	200	54	–
Thiopental sodium[c]	30	25	–
Pentobarbital sodium	30	0	0
Hydrocortisone acetate	20	0	0

[a] Reproduced from E. J. Lien, J. Kuwahara and R. T. Koda, *Drug Intell. Clin. Pharm.*, 8, 470 (1974).
[b] At pH 2 and pH 4.
[c] At pH 4.0 and pH 7.2.

obviously be significant. When medazepam is present at an initial concentration of 40 μg cm^{-3} in 100 cm^3 normal saline stored in similar bags, a 76% loss of the drug occurs in 8 h at 22°C (Table 10.8).[26]

Preservatives such as the methyl and propyl parabens present in formulations can be sorbed into rubber and plastic membranes and closures, thus leading to decreased levels of preservative and, in the extreme, loss of preservative activity.

10.9   Protein binding

This is a topic which requires a chapter to itself for full coverage. Here we have space only for a treatment of mechanisms of protein binding which might enable readers to recognise molecules likely to be protein-bound.

High levels of protein binding alter the biological properties of the drug as free drug concentrations are reduced. The bound drug assumes the diffusional and other transport characteristics of the protein molecule. In cases where drug is highly protein-bound (around 90%), small changes in binding lead to drastic changes in the levels of free drug in the body. If a drug is 95% bound, 5% is free. Reduction of binding to 90% by, for example, displacement by a second drug, doubles the level of free drug. Such changes are not evident when binding is of a low order.

Most drugs bind to a limited number of sites on the albumin molecule. Binding to plasma albumin is generally easily reversible, so that drug molecules bound to albumin will be released as the level of free drug in the blood declines. Drugs bound to albumin (or other proteins) are attached to a unit too large to be transported across membranes. They are thus prevented from reacting with receptors or from entering the sites of drug metabolism or drug elimination, until they dissociate from the protein.

Plasma albumin consists of a single polypeptide chain of molecular weight of 67 000 ± 2000. Human albumin contains between 569 and 613 amino acid residues. It is a globular molecule with a diameter of 5.6 nm (calculated assuming the molecule to be an anhydrous sphere). With an isoelectric point of 4.9, albumin has a net negative charge at pH 7.4, but it is amphoteric and capable of binding acidic and basic drugs. Subtle structural changes can occur on binding small molecules. Fatty acid binding produces a volume increase and a decrease in the axial ratio. This is due primarily to nonpolar interaction between the hydrocarbon tail of the fatty acid molecule and the binding site, and reflects the adaptability of the albumin molecule. When a hydrophobic chain penetrates into the interior of the globular albumin molecule, the helices of the protein separate, producing a small change in the tertiary structure of the protein.

What are the binding sites? Organic anions are thought to bind to a site containing the amino acid sequence Lys-Ala-Try-Ala-Val-Ala-Arg (see Chapter 11). The five nonpolar side-chains of these residues form a hydrophobic 'pool'. A cationic group is present at each end. It has been proposed that the ε-amino group of lysine is the point of attachment for anionic drugs. Albumin is, however, capable of binding molecules that are not ionised at all, such as cortisone or chloramphenicol. Acidic drugs such as phenylbutazone, indometacin and the salicylates may establish primary contact with the albumin by electrostatic interactions, but the bond can be strengthened by hydrophobic interactions. The dual interaction would therefore limit the number of possible binding sites for anionic organic drugs. In spite of electrostatic interactions a number of drugs bind to albumin according to their degree of lipophilicity. Evidence for the importance of the hydrophobic interaction has been obtained from studies of the binding of phenol derivatives, which depend mainly on the hydrophobic character of the substituent, the phenolic hydroxyl group playing no significant role in the binding process. Similarly, penicillin derivatives and phenothiazines bind in a manner that depends on the hydrophobic characteristics of side-chains. It has been concluded that binding to albumin is a process comparable to partitioning of drug molecules from a water phase to a nonpolar phase. The hydrophobic sites are not

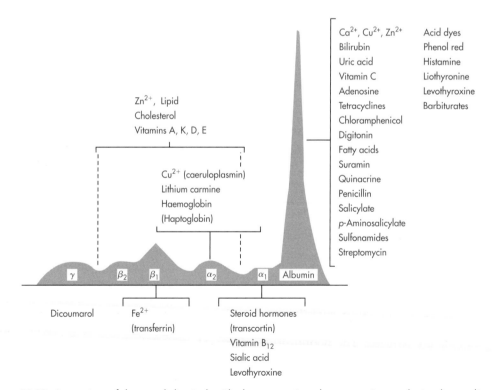

Figure 10.20 Interactions of drugs and chemicals with plasma proteins; plasma proteins are depicted according to their relative amounts.
Modified from F. W. Putnam, *The Proteins*, 2nd edn, vol. 3 (ed. H. Neurath), Academic Press, New York, 1965.

necessarily 'preformed'. Fatty acids and warfarin are both capable of inducing conformational changes which result in the formation of hydrophobic 'pools' in the protein.

Plasma proteins other than albumin may also be involved in binding; examples of such interactions are shown in Fig. 10.20. Blood plasma normally contains on average about 6.72 g of protein per 100 cm³, the protein comprising 4.0 g of albumin, 2.3 g of globulins and 0.24 g of fibrinogen. Although albumin is the main binding protein, dicoumarol is also bound to β- and γ-globulins, and certain steroid hormones are specifically and preferentially bound to particular globulin fractions.

An expression allowing the determination of the fraction of drug bound to a protein can be derived as shown in Box 10.2.

10.9.1 Thermodynamics of protein binding

Estimation of the thermodynamic parameters of binding allows interpretation of the mechanisms of interaction. Table 10.9 gives the thermodynamic parameters of binding of a number of agents to bovine serum albumin. The negative value of ΔG implies that binding is spontaneous. ΔH is negative, signifying an exothermic process and a reduction in the strength of the association as temperature increases. ΔS is positive, most likely signifying loss of structured water on binding. A diagrammatic representation of this last process is shown in Fig. 10.21. This diagram shows the change in the ordered water in the hydrophobic cavity of the albumin and around the nonpolar portion of the drug. The loss of the

---

Box 10.2   Estimation of the degree of protein binding

Protein binding can be considered to be an adsorption process obeying the law of mass action. If D represents drug and P the protein we can write

$D + P \rightleftharpoons (DP)$ (protein–drug complex)

At equilibrium,

$$D_f + (P_t - D_b) = D_b \qquad (10.8)$$

where D_f is the molar concentration of unbound drug, P_t is the total molar concentration of protein, and D_b is the molar concentration of bound drug (= molar concentration of complex). If one assumes one binding site per molecule, the equilibrium constant, K, is given by

$$K = \frac{k_1}{k_{-1}} = \frac{\text{rate constant for association}}{\text{rate constant for dissociation}} \qquad (10.9)$$

From equation (10.8),

$$K = \frac{D_b}{D_f(P_t - D_b)} \qquad (10.10)$$

It is obvious that $k_1 > k_{-1}$. The rate constant for dissociation, k_{-1}, is the rate-limiting step in the exchange of drug between free and bound forms. From equation (10.10) we obtain

$$KD_f P_t - KD_f D_b = D_b \qquad (10.11)$$

That is,

$$KD_f P_t = D_b + KD_f D_b = D_b(1 + KD_f) \qquad (10.12)$$

Therefore,

$$\frac{KD_f P_t}{1 + KD_f} = D_b \qquad (10.13)$$

or

$$\frac{D_b}{P_t} = r = \frac{KD_f}{1 + KD_f} \qquad (10.14)$$

where r is the number of moles of drug bound to total protein in the system. If there are not one, but n, binding sites per protein molecule, then

$$r = \frac{nKD_f}{1 + KD_f} \qquad (10.15)$$

or

$$\frac{1}{r} = \frac{1}{n} + \frac{1}{nKD_f} \qquad (10.16)$$

Protein binding results are often quoted as the fraction of drug bound, β. This fraction varies generally with the concentration of both drug and protein, as shown in equation (10.17), which relates β with n, K and concentration:

$$\beta = \frac{1}{1 + D_f/(nP_t) + 1/(nKP_t)} \qquad (10.17)$$

Table 10.10 Protein binding and other characteristics of some penicillins and cephalosporins[a]

Antibiotic	Log P[b]	Serum protein binding (%)	Serum concentration ($\mu g\ cm^{-3}$) during continuous infusion (500 mg h^{-1})		Peak serum levels after 500 mg kg^{-1}	
			Total	Free	Total	Free
Dicloxacillin	3.24	96–98	25	1	15	0.3
Cloxacillin	2.49	94–96	15	0.9	–	–
Oxacillin	2.38	92–94	10	0.8	15	0.8
Nafcillin	–	89–90	9	0.9	6	0.6
Benxylpenicillin	1.72	59–65	16	5.6	4.5	1.6
Methicillin	1.06	37–60			16	10
Ampicillin	–	20–29	29	23.2	12	9
Carbenicillin	–	50	73	36.5	–	–
Ceftriaxone	–	95	–	–	–	–
Cefazolin[c]	–	89	–	–	–	–
Cefditoren	–	88	–	–	–	–
Cefalotin	0.5	65	18	6.3	7.6	2.6
Cefaloridine	–	20	24.7	19.7	18.5	14.8
Cefalexin	0.7	15	27	23	–	–
Cefradine[c]	–1.2	14	–	–	–	–

[a] Reproduced from E. J. Lien, J. Kuwahara and R. T. Koda, *Drug Intell. Clin. Pharm.*, 8, 470 (1974).
[b] log P values from A. Ryrfeldt, *J. Pharm. Pharmacol.*, 23, 463 (1971) and D. B. Jack, *Handbook of Chemical Pharmacokinetic Data*, Macmillan, London, 1992.
[c] Additional values from S. M. Singhri et al., *Chemotherapy*, 24, 121 (1978).

little bound drug in extravascular regions. There is, however, no correlation between the degree of protein binding and peak serum levels of the penicillins and cephalosporins of Table 10.10; other factors such as rates of elimination also determine the peak levels. Protein binding will affect transport into other tissues, however, as the gradient that determines movement is the gradient caused by free drug. Both ampicillin (50 mg kg^{-1} every 2 h) and oxacillin (50 mg kg^{-1} h^{-1}) produced similar peak levels in the serum given as repeated intravenous boluses. Levels of free drug are markedly different, however, as oxacillin is 75% bound and ampicillin is 17.5% bound in rabbit serum.

10.9.3 Penetration of specialised sites

Muscle, bone, and synovial and interstitial fluid are readily accessible to intravascular antibiotics by way of aqueous pores in the capillary supply. The CSF, brain, eye, intestines and prostate gland lack such pores, and entry into these areas is by way of a lipoidal barrier. There is evidence that extensive protein binding may prevent the access of antibiotics into the eye and the inflamed meninges.

The level of free drug in serum is important in determining the amount of drug which reaches tissue spaces.[27] The total concentration of a drug in tissue fluid can be predicted from the serum concentration, the extent of serum protein binding, and the protein binding in the tissue fluid. Equation (10.18) has been shown to be highly predictive under equilibrium conditions:[27]

$$C_t + \frac{C_s f_s}{f_t} \tag{10.18}$$

where C_t is the tissue fluid drug concentration, C_s is the serum drug concentration, and f_s and f_t are the free fractions of drug in serum and tissue fluid, respectively. If protein binding in the serum and tissue fluid is identical then, provided the same proteins are present in both 'phases', the tissue fluid drug concentration will equal the serum concentration; this is true for both high and low protein-containing extravascular fluid.

When attempting to medicate a specialised compartment in the body separated from plasma by a lipoprotein membrane, it is vital to achieve therapeutic concentrations of drug, without achieving toxic levels. An example is in the treatment of bacterial prostatitis; most currently available antibiotics do not readily pass across the prostatic epithelium. The pH of the prostatic fluid is lower than that of plasma, being around 6.6; milk has a pH of 6.8. In passage of drugs both into prostatic fluid and into milk, the degree of dissociation of the drug appears to be the most important factor determining the degree of penetration. The partition coefficient plays a secondary role. When the prostatic fluid/plasma ratios of sulfonamides were studied it was found that the results could be predicted more closely from the ratio of undissociated/dissociated drug rather than from $\log P$ values. It is probable that this is because lipophilic drugs will be highly protein-bound and thus unable to penetrate the boundary membranes.

Summary

This chapter has dealt with the wide range of physicochemical factors that might cause changes in formulations or drug absorption processes. These have included effects of pH and solvent, interactions between cations and anions, salting-in and salting-out, ion-exchange reactions, adsorption and interactions with plastics, as well as protein binding often mediated by hydrophobic interactions. It is, as always, difficult to anticipate the exact quantitative nature of the events that follow from these effects, especially in the body, where there are many compensating and contradictory influences. However, a knowledge of the theoretical possibilities allows us to rationalise what has been observed. By analogy we should therefore be able to predict likely effects in new drugs. One has to be cautious, aware that what we anticipate theoretically may not take place *in vivo*, where a dynamic situation exists. But the physicochemical basis of interactions and incompatibilities must be appreciated if we are to rationalise interactions.

Appendix: Drug interactions based on physical mechanisms

The following information was taken originally from a comprehensive listing of drug interactions published in New Zealand (R. Ferguson. *Drug Interactions of Clinical Significance*, I.M.S., New Zealand, 1977). **This selection is intended for illustrative purposes only and must *not* be used as a definitive source**.

A: Interactions affecting absorption of drugs

Drugs	Effect	Mechanism/Note	Recommendation
Calcium therapy + aluminium hydroxide	Chronic aluminium hydroxide antacid intake (600 cm³ weekly) can cause osteomalacia	Calcium absorption is prevented	Use alternative antacid. Especial care should be taken with people with calcium deficiency
Chlorpromazine + aluminium hydroxide, magnesium oxide, magnesium trisilicate	Reduced blood levels of chlorpromazine, with possible inhibition of therapeutic effect	Possibly due to alteration of GI pH by the antacid	Doses should be spaced by 2–3 h

continued

B: Interactions involving protein binding (*continued*)

Drugs	Effect	Mechanism/Note	Recommendation
Dicoumarol, warfarin + p-aminosalicyclic acid	Increased anticoagulant serum levels with risk of haemorrhage	Displacement from protein	Monitor anticoagulant effect, especially with initiation or cessation of therapy
Dicoumarol, warfarin + paracetamol	With especially large doses, increase in anticoagulant effect	Possibly displacement from protein. Depression of clotting factor synthesis	Use low doses of paracetamol. Probably the safest mild analgesic to use with oral anticoagulants
Dicoumarol, warfarin + sulfadimethoxine, sulfamethoxypyridazine, sulfaphenazole	Increased anticoagulant blood levels with risk of haemorrhage	Displacement from protein by strongly bound sulfonamide	Use alternative chemotherapy. Monitor patient with initiation of cessation of therapy
Methotrexate + salicylates	Potentiation of methotrexate toxicity	Displacement of methotrexate from protein binding sites	Owing to severity of methotrexate toxicity, salicylates should not be given to patients receiving methotrexate
Methotrexate + sulfonamides	Potentiation of methotrexate with high risk of toxicity	Displacement from protein binding (sulfafurazole reduces methotrexate binding from 70% to 28%)	Owing to severity of methotrexate toxicity, sulfonamides that are protein-bound should never be administered
Penicillin + probenecid	Threefold increase in serum penicillin level with increase also in spinal fluid levels but decreased brain level	Displacement from protein binding, decreased renal tubule secretion and decrease biliary excretion	Combination can be used when high serum and spinal fluid levels are required
Thyroid hormones, levothyroxine + phenytoin	Rise in thyroxine blood levels with reported tachycardia	Displacement of thyroxine by phenytoin from protein binding	Great care should be taken in administering parenteral phenytoin to people on thyroid therapy
Warfarin + aspirin	Significant increase in anticoagulant effect with possible severe GI blood loss	Displacement from protein	Combination should be avoided if possible. Use alternative analgesic such as paracetamol or pentazocine
Warfarin + clofibrate	Higher blood levels of warfarin with risk of haemorrhage	Displacement from protein	Warfarin dose may require a reduction of one-third to one-half according to coagulation test
Warfarin + etacrynic acid	Increased blood level of warfarin with haemorrhage risk	Displacement from protein	Monitor patient with initiation and cessation of therapy
Warfarin + mefenamic acid	Enhanced anticoagulant blood levels with risk of haemorrhage and enhanced risk of GI bleeding	Displacement from protein	Concurrent administration is best avoided. If necessary, coagulation times should be monitored

continued

provided the same proteins are present in both 'phases', the tissue fluid drug concentration will equal the serum concentration; this is true for both high and low protein-containing extravascular fluid.

When attempting to medicate a specialised compartment in the body separated from plasma by a lipoprotein membrane, it is vital to achieve therapeutic concentrations of drug, without achieving toxic levels. An example is in the treatment of bacterial prostatitis; most currently available antibiotics do not readily pass across the prostatic epithelium. The pH of the prostatic fluid is lower than that of plasma, being around 6.6; milk has a pH of 6.8. In passage of drugs both into prostatic fluid and into milk, the degree of dissociation of the drug appears to be the most important factor determining the degree of penetration. The partition coefficient plays a secondary role. When the prostatic fluid/plasma ratios of sulfonamides were studied it was found that the results could be predicted more closely from the ratio of undissociated/dissociated drug rather than from $\log P$ values. It is probable that this is because lipophilic drugs will be highly protein-bound and thus unable to penetrate the boundary membranes.

Summary

This chapter has dealt with the wide range of physicochemical factors that might cause changes in formulations or drug absorption processes. These have included effects of pH and solvent, interactions between cations and anions, salting-in and salting-out, ion-exchange reactions, adsorption and interactions with plastics, as well as protein binding often mediated by hydrophobic interactions. It is, as always, difficult to anticipate the exact quantitative nature of the events that follow from these effects, especially in the body, where there are many compensating and contradictory influences. However, a knowledge of the theoretical possibilities allows us to rationalise what has been observed. By analogy we should therefore be able to predict likely effects in new drugs. One has to be cautious, aware that what we anticipate theoretically may not take place *in vivo*, where a dynamic situation exists. But the physicochemical basis of interactions and incompatibilities must be appreciated if we are to rationalise interactions.

Appendix: Drug interactions based on physical mechanisms

The following information was taken originally from a comprehensive listing of drug interactions published in New Zealand (R. Ferguson. *Drug Interactions of Clinical Significance*, I.M.S., New Zealand, 1977). **This selection is intended for illustrative purposes only and must *not* be used as a definitive source**.

A: Interactions affecting absorption of drugs

Drugs	Effect	Mechanism/Note	Recommendation
Calcium therapy + aluminium hydroxide	Chronic aluminium hydroxide antacid intake (600 cm^3 weekly) can cause osteomalacia	Calcium absorption is prevented	Use alternative antacid. Especial care should be taken with people with calcium deficiency
Chlorpromazine + aluminium hydroxide, magnesium oxide, magnesium trisilicate	Reduced blood levels of chlorpromazine, with possible inhibition of therapeutic effect	Possibly due to alteration of GI pH by the antacid	Doses should be spaced by 2–3 h

continued

A: Interactions affecting absorption of drugs (*continued*)

Drugs	Effect	Mechanism/Note	Recommendation
Dicoumarol, warfarin + colestyramine	Anticoagulant absorption is reduced and slowed (25% lower blood levels)	Binding to colestyramine	Space doses by 2–3 h
Dicoumarol, warfarin + laxatives	Chronic laxative administration may cause loss of anticoagulant control	Two possible effects: lubricant oil action may cause decreased absorption of anticoagulant; decreased absorption of vitamin K, particularly with oils and emulsions	Periodic long-term monitoring of prothrombin times in all suspect patients
Dicoumarol + magnesium hydroxide, magnesium oxide	Opposite effects have been reported: (i) Decreased absorption and lower blood levels (up to 75%) of dicoumarol (ii) Increased absorption	Possibly adsorption on drug leading to decreased absorption. Chelation might lead to more lipophilic species and increased absorption	Space doses by 2–3 h
Digitalis glycosides + docusate sodium (DOSS)	Increased absorption of digitalis to a possibly toxic level	Surface-active properties of DOSS increases wetting and perhaps solubility and absorption of poorly absorbed digitalis	Space doses by 2–3 h
Digoxin, digitoxin + colestyramine	Greatly reduced absorption of digitalis alkaloids with concurrent administration	Binding effect (anionic resin)	Space doses by about 8 h
Digoxin + disodium edetate	Disodium edetate chelates calcium ions thus antagonising the action of digoxin	Chelation of digoxin in the plasma	May be necessary to monitor blood calcium levels
Digoxin + magnesium trisilicate	Absorption of digoxin reduced by up to 90%	Surface absorption effect	Space doses 2–3 h. Use alternative antacid
Lincomycin + kaolin	Reduced GI absorption of lincomycin by up to 90%	Absorption of drug to kaolin	Space doses by 2–3 h
Oxyphenonium bromide + magnesium trisilicate	Reduced blood levels of oxyphenonium with reduced effect	Oxyphenonium adsorbed on to the surface of magnesium trisilicate, reducing availability	Space doses by at least 2–3 h
p-Aminosalicyclic acid (granule formulation) + rifampicin	Reduced blood levels of rifampicin and hence impaired effect	Impaired GI absorption of rifampicin due to binding to bentonite	Space doses by 8–12 h (see text)
Propantheline bromide + magnesium trisilicate	Reduced blood levels (with reduced action) of propantheline	Adsorption of propantheline to magnesium trisilicate, reducing availability for absorption	Space doses by 2–3 h

continued

A: Interactions affecting absorption of drugs   (continued)

Drugs	Effect	Mechanism/Note	Recommendation
Salicylates + colestyramine	Greatly decreased absorption of salicylates	Adsorption to ion-exchange resin	Space doses by 4–5 h
Tetracycline + iron preparations	Lower blood levels of tetracycline, possibly below minimal active concentration	Chelation effect (see text)	Either space doses at least 2–3 h or alternative antibiotic therapy
Tetracycline + milk products, aluminium, bismuth, calcium and magnesium ions	GI absorption of tetracycline and blood levels of tetracycline greatly reduced	Chelation effect (see text)	Space doses by 2–3 h; possible exception minocycline
Tetracycline + sodium bicarbonate (NB: Sodium bicarbonate is present in many antacid and effervescent preparations)	Impaired absorption of tetracycline	pH increase in GI tract prevents dissolution of complete dose	Space doses by 2–3 h
Thiazide diuretics + colestyramine	Decreased absorption and effect of diuretic	Colestyramine can bind thiazide	Space doses by 2–3 h
Thyroid hormones + colestyramine	Absorption of thyroid hormone prevented	Thyroid hormones become bound to the anionic resin	Space doses by 2–3 h

B: Interactions involving protein binding

Drugs	Effect	Mechanism/Note	Recommendation
Chlorpropamide, tolbutamide + sulfonamides	Increased blood level of hypoglycaemic drug. Hypoglycaemic shock reported	Displacement from protein binding and possible metabolic inhibition, competition for excretion	Not reported with sulfadimethoxine, sulfafurazole, sulfamethoxazole. Monitor patient
Chlorpropamide, tolbutamide + salicylates	Introduction of oral salicylate therapy can result in a hypoglycaemic reaction	Displacement from protein binding, salicylates increase tissue glucose uptake	Warn patients against high dose or chronic salicylate therapy. With long-term salicylate therapy patients should be monitored and restabilised if necessary
Dicoumarol, warfarin + indometacin	Possible elevated blood levels of anticoagulant with risk of haemorrhage. Risk of GI bleeding	Displacement from protein	This combination best avoided
Dicoumarol, warfarin + methandienone, norethandrolone, oxymetholone	Increased hypoprothrombinaemia with several reported cases of - haemorrhage	Possibly due to displacement from protein	If combination is definitely indicated, patients should be carefully monitored

continued

B: Interactions involving protein binding (continued)

Drugs	Effect	Mechanism/Note	Recommendation
Dicoumarol, warfarin + p-aminosalicyclic acid	Increased anticoagulant serum levels with risk of haemorrhage	Displacement from protein	Monitor anticoagulant effect, especially with initiation or cessation of therapy
Dicoumarol, warfarin + paracetamol	With especially large doses, increase in anticoagulant effect	Possibly displacement from protein. Depression of clotting factor synthesis	Use low doses of paracetamol. Probably the safest mild analgesic to use with oral anticoagulants
Dicoumarol, warfarin + sulfadimethoxine, sulfamethoxypyridazine, sulfaphenazole	Increased anticoagulant blood levels with risk of haemorrhage	Displacement from protein by strongly bound sulfonamide	Use alternative chemotherapy. Monitor patient with initiation of cessation of therapy
Methotrexate + salicylates	Potentiation of methotrexate toxicity	Displacement of methotrexate from protein binding sites	Owing to severity of methotrexate toxicity, salicylates should not be given to patients receiving methotrexate
Methotrexate + sulfonamides	Potentiation of methotrexate with high risk of toxicity	Displacement from protein binding (sulfafurazole reduces methotrexate binding from 70% to 28%)	Owing to severity of methotrexate toxicity, sulfonamides that are protein-bound should never be administered
Penicillin + probenecid	Threefold increase in serum penicillin level with increase also in spinal fluid levels but decreased brain level	Displacement from protein binding, decreased renal tubule secretion and decrease biliary excretion	Combination can be used when high serum and spinal fluid levels are required
Thyroid hormones, levothyroxine + phenytoin	Rise in thyroxine blood levels with reported tachycardia	Displacement of thyroxine by phenytoin from protein binding	Great care should be taken in administering parenteral phenytoin to people on thyroid therapy
Warfarin + aspirin	Significant increase in anticoagulant effect with possible severe GI blood loss	Displacement from protein	Combination should be avoided if possible. Use alternative analgesic such as paracetamol or pentazocine
Warfarin + clofibrate	Higher blood levels of warfarin with risk of haemorrhage	Displacement from protein	Warfarin dose may require a reduction of one-third to one-half according to coagulation test
Warfarin + etacrynic acid	Increased blood level of warfarin with haemorrhage risk	Displacement from protein	Monitor patient with initiation and cessation of therapy
Warfarin + mefenamic acid	Enhanced anticoagulant blood levels with risk of haemorrhage and enhanced risk of GI bleeding	Displacement from protein	Concurrent administration is best avoided. If necessary, coagulation times should be monitored

continued

B: Interactions involving protein binding   (*continued*)

Drugs	Effect	Mechanism/Note	Recommendation
Warfarin + nalidixic acid	Possible hypothrombinaemia with associated haemorrhage risk	Displacement from protein (NB: *In vitro* evidence)	Combination administration should be used with care and patient coagulation monitored
Oral anticoagulants + naproxen	Increased anticoagulant effect and risk of GI bleeding	Naproxen has ulcerogenic potential. Displacement from protein	Best to avoid concurrent administration. Monitor patient

Reminder: Use this appendix only to illustrate the range of problems that may arise from physicochemical interactions *in vivo*. Ivan Stockley's book[28] is an authoritative source of information on interactions between drugs.

References

1. C. L. J. Coles and K. A. Lees. *Pharm. J.*, 206, 153 (1971)

2. B. Lynn. [Letter] *Pharm. J.*, 206, 154 (1971)

3. K. A. Fitzgerald and M. W. MacKay. Calcium and phosphate solubility in neonatal parenteral nutrient solutions containing TrophAmine. *Am. J. Hosp. Pharm.*, 43, 88–93 (1986)

4. G. Levy and B. A. Hayes. Physicochemical basis of the buffered acetylsalicylic acid controversy. *N. Engl. J. Med.*, 262, 1053–8 (1960)

5. J. H. Lipton. Incompatibility between sulfamethizole and methenamine mandelate. *N. Engl. J. Med.*, 268, 92–3 (1963)

6. W. J. Jusko, M. Gretch and R. Gassett. Precipitation of diazepam from intravenous preparations. *J. Am. Med. Assoc.*, 225, 176 (1973)

7. D. E. Langdon, J. R. Harlan and R. L. Bailey. Thrombophlebitis with diazepam used intravenously *J. Am. Med. Assoc.*, 223, 184–5 (1973)

8. E. Tomlinson. Rx: never mix a cation with an anion? *Pharm. Int.*, 1, 156–8 (1980)

9. T. R. Marshall, J. T. Ling, G. Follis and M. Russell. Pharmacological incompatibility of contrast media with various drugs and agents. *Radiology*, 84, 536–9 (1965)

10. M. A. El-Nakeeb and R. T. Yousef. Influence of various materials on antibiotics in liquid pharmaceutical preparations. *Acta Pharm. Suec.*, 5, 1–8 (1968)

11. G. M. Irwin, H. B. Kostenbauder, L. W. Dittert, *et al.* Enhancement of gastrointestinal absorption of a quaternary ammonium compound by trichloroacetate. *J. Pharm. Sci.*, 58, 313–15 (1969)

12. A. C. Barbara, C. Clemente and E. Wagman. Physical incompatibility of sulfonamide compounds and polyionic solutions. *N. Engl. J Med.*, 274, 1316–7 (1966)

13. C. F. Bell. *Metal Chelation*, Clarendon Press, Oxford, 1977

14. P. R. Klink and J. L. Colaizzi. Effect of trichloroacetate anion on partition behavior of tetracyclines. *J. Pharm. Sci.*, 62, 97–100 (1973)

15. A. R. Sanchez, R. S. Rogers and P. J. Sheridan. Tetracycline and other tetracycline-derivatives staining of the teeth and oral cavity. *Int. J. Dermatol.*, 43, 709–15 (2004)

16. A. E. Martell and M. Calvin. *Chemistry of the Metal Chelate Compound*, Prentice-Hall, New York, 1952, p. 54

17. J. J. Ambre and L. J. Fischer. Effect of coadministration of aluminum and magnesium hydroxides on absorption of anticoagulants in man. *Clin. Pharm. Ther.*, 14, 231–7 (1973)

18. K. Ikeda, K. Uekama and M. Otagiri. Inclusion complexes of β-cyclodextrin with antiinflammatory drugs fenamates in aqueous solution. *Chem. Pharm. Bull.*, 23, 201–8 (1975)

19. K. Ikeda, K. Uekama, M. Otagiri and M. Hatano. Circular dichroism study on inclusion complexes of β-cyclodextrin with antiinflammatory fanamates. *J. Pharm. Sci.*, 63, 1168–9 (1974)

20. D. E. Tutt and M. A. Schwartz. Model catalysts which simulate penicillinase. V. The cycloheptaamylose-catalyzed hydrolysis of penicillins. *J. Am. Chem. Soc.*, 93, 767–72 (1971)

21. L. Gross and M. Brotman. Hypoprothrombinemia and hemorrhage associated with colestyramine therapy. *Ann. Intern. Med.*, 72, 95–6 (1970)

22. A. Coronato and G. B. J. Glass. Depression of the intestinal uptake of radio-vitamin B_{12} by colestyramine. *Proc. Soc. Exp. Biol. Med.*, 142, 1341–4 (1973)

23. G. Boman, P. Lundgren and G. Stjernstrom. Mechanism of the inhibitory effect of PAS [*p*-aminosalicylic acid] granules on the absorption of rifampicin. Adsorption of rifampicin by an excipient, bentonite. *Eur. J. Clin. Pharm.*, 8, 293–9 (1975)

24. S. T. Anik and J.-Y. Hwang. Adsorption of D-Nal(2)⁶LHRH, a decapeptide, onto glass and other surfaces. *Int. J. Pharm.*, 16, 181–90 (1983)

25. A. W. Malick, A. H. Amann, D. M. Baask and R. G. Stoll. Loss of nitroglycerin from solutions to intravenous plastic containers: a theoretical treatment. *J. Pharm. Sci.*, 70, 798–801 (1981)

26. L. Illum and H. Bundgaard. Sorption of drugs by plastic infusion bags. *Int. J. Pharm.*, 10, 339–51 (1982)

27. L. R. Peterson and D. N. Gerding. Protein binding and antibiotic concentrations *Lancet*, 312, 376 (1978)

28. I. H. Stockley (ed.), *Stockley's Drug Interactions*, Pharmaceutical Press, London, 2002

Further reading

L. A. Trissel. *Handbook on Injectable Drugs*, 12th edn. American Society of Health-System Pharmacists, Bethesda, MD, 2003. [This book deals with virtually all examples of incompatibilities of drug combination used in injectables.]

11

Peptides, proteins and other biopharmaceuticals

An increasing proportion of the pharmaceutical armamentarium comprises peptides and proteins, whether natural or synthetic in origin or, more likely, produced by recombinant DNA technology or from transgenic animals. Most peptides and proteins are not absorbed to any significant extent by the oral route and the most available formulations of protein pharmaceuticals are therefore parenteral products for injection or inhalation (Table 11.1). DNA, RNA and various oligo-nucleotides are being used increasingly in gene therapy. These share some of the problems of proteins as therapeutic agents, principally owing to their high molecular weight, relative fragility and ionic nature.

The object of this chapter is to provide some background for the appreciation of the pharma-ceutics of proteins, peptides DNA, oligonucleotides and monoclonal antibodies as therapeutic entities. From an understanding of the nature of amino acids and their physical properties comes an appreciation of the physical nature and properties of peptides, polypeptides and proteins, defined below. The solution properties of proteins in simple and complex media should be under-stood, together with the factors affecting the stability of proteins in solution. Problems in the formulation of proteins to be overcome will then become clearer.

Some definitions for proteins or peptides:[1]

- *Peptide*: a short chain of residues with a defined sequence; there is no maximum number of residues in a peptide, but the term is appropriate to a chain if its physical properties are those expected from the sum of its amino acid residues and if there is no fixed three-dimensional conformation.
- *Polypeptide*: a longer chain, usually of defined sequence and length.

Table 11.1 Some therapeutic proteins and peptides, their molecular weights and actions[a]

Protein/peptide	Size (kDa)	Use/action
Oxytocin	1.0	Uterine contraction
Vasopressin	1.1	Diuresis
Leuprolide acetate	1.3	Prostatic carcinoma therapy
LHRH analogues	~1.5	Prostatic carcinoma therapy
Somatostatin	3.1	Growth inhibition
Calcitonin	3.4	Ca^{2+} regulation
Glucagon	3.5	Diabetes therapy
Parathyroid hormone (1–34)	4.3	Ca^{2+} regulation
Insulin	6	Diabetes therapy
Parathyroid hormone (1–84)	9.4	Ca^{2+} regulation
Interferon gamma	16 (dimer)	Antiviral agent
TNF-α	17.5 (trimer)	Antitumour agent
Interferon α-2	19	Leukaemia, hepatitis therapy
Interferon β-1	20	Lung cancer therapy
Growth hormone	22	Growth acceleration
DNase	~32	Cystic fibrosis therapy
α_1-Antitrypsin	45	Cystic fibrosis therapy
Albumin	68	Plasma volume expander
Bovine IgG	150	Immunisation
Catalase	230	Treatment of wounds and ulcers
Cationic ferritin	400+	Anaemias

[a] Reproduced from R. W. Niven, *Pharmaceutical Technology*, 72(July) (1993).

- *Polyamino acids*: random sequences of varying lengths generally resulting from nonspecific polymerisation of one or more amino acids. One such is available as a drug for the treatment of multiple sclerosis – glatiramer (Copaxone).
- *Protein*: a term usually reserved for those polypeptides that occur naturally and have a definite three-dimensional structure under physiological conditions.

and for nucleic acids:

- *Nucleotide* – the building block of a nucleic acid, consisting of a five-carbon sugar covalently bonded to a nitrogenous base (adenine, thymine, guanine, cytosine, or uracil) and a phosphate group.
- *Oligonucleotide* – a short (10–25) sequence of nucleotides.
- *Plasmid DNA* – a circular piece of DNA that exists apart from the chromosome and replicates independently of it. Plasmids are often used in genetic engineering.

Other oligomeric substances such as the antisense oligonucleotides and DNA fragments are being used therapeutically and, for these as with proteins, no systematic approaches to their pharmacy yet exist. New modes of delivery of many or all of these agents will need to be developed if they are to be used to their maximal advantage. It is certainly misleading to assume, because many are either natural substances or their close analogues, that they are safe. Injection of abnormal doses even of endogenous agents at sites where they do not naturally exist can often induce bizarre side-effects. Hence the need for optimised formulations, delivered in appropriate ways to the most appropriate sites.

Development of improved formulations and delivery systems requires a good understanding of the physical pharmacy of these molecules if we are to avoid typical problems of degradation, unwanted adsorption to glassware and plastics and aggregation in delivery devices such as reservoirs or pumps.

11.1 Structure and solution properties of peptides and proteins

11.1.1 Structure of peptides and proteins

The *primary* structure of a protein is the order in which the individual amino acids are sequenced. This tells us little about the shape that the protein will assume in solution, although the primary structure naturally determines the *secondary, tertiary* and even *quaternary* forms. These amino acid building blocks (Table 11.2) give the key to structure and behaviour. The standard three-letter (Glu, Arg, Trp, etc.) and one-letter (E, R, W, etc.) abbreviations for amino acids are also listed: their use makes structural descriptions more accessible.

Secondary structures include the coiled α-helix, and pleated sheets, discussed below and shown in Figs. 11.1 and 11.2. Chain folding, arising from crosslinking through hydrogen bonding or disulfide bridges, leads to a definition of tertiary structure, and aggregation of these structural units leads to quaternary forms of the protein.

Representations in a stylised diagrammatic form of three proteins (interleukin-1β, zinc insulin dimers, and the Fc fragment of immunoglobulin) are shown in Fig. 11.3. The nature of the three-dimensional structure shows how difficult it is to define proteins in conventional ways, and how they must be considered in a new light as pharmaceutical entities. Loss of the unique tertiary or quaternary structure, through *denaturation*, can occur from a variety of insults that would not affect smaller molecules.

Complex structures are formed in solution because of interactions between the structural amino acids. Unfortunately, knowing the amino acid sequence of a protein is not enough to enable us to predict its behaviour. Function is determined by the way the linear chains of amino acids fold in solution to give specific three-dimensional structures comprising the coils, sheets and folds (shown in Figs. 11.1 and 11.2). It is not yet possible for these to be predicted *a priori*, although strides are being made in understanding the 'grammar' of protein folding, through the synthesis of synthetic peptides and sequences and observation of their structures.

Some of the primary structures are so complex that it is not possible to predict their physicochemical properties, although modern molecular modelling techniques have made great inroads into understanding tertiary structure and behaviour.[2, 3]

11.1.2 Hydrophobicity of peptides and proteins

Amino acids have a range of physical properties, each having a greater or lesser degree of hydrophilic or hydrophobic nature. Naturally, if amino acids are spatially arranged in a molecule so that distinct hydrophobic and hydrophilic regions appear, then the polypeptide or

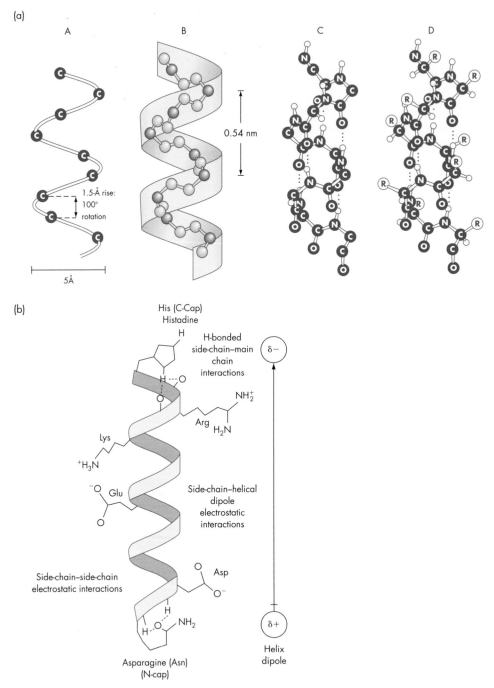

Figure 11.1 (a) The α-helix forms because —NH and —C=O groups interact through hydrogen bonding pulling the backbone into a spiral, as shown in this diagram in a 9-amino peptide: (A) here only the central carbon atoms are shown for clarity; in (B) the nitrogen and carbons of the backbone are shown and in (C) the oxygen and hydrogen atoms have been added. All the —NH groups point in the same direction 'up' and the —C=O groups point 'down' to allow the formation of —C=O⋯H—N— bonds. In (D) the side-chains are added and point outwards from the α-helix. Hydrophobic interactions between some helix-promoting side-chains (the more hydrophobic chains, see Table 11.3) help to stabilize the helix. (Modified from reference 3, with permission).

Table 11.2 Nomenclature and structure of the principal amino acids. The common name, the three-letter code and the single-letter code are given

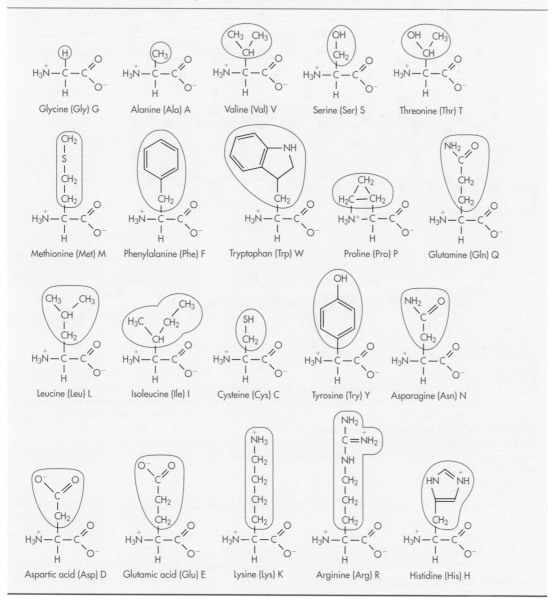

Figure 11.1 (*continued*) (b) An idealised α-helix, drawn as a ribbon showing typical stabilising intrahelical interactions. Specific hydrogen-bonded interactions are said to 'cap' the ends of the chain, known specifically as the N-terminal and C-terminal ends of the helix. Free energies (ΔG) of the interactions, compared to the free energy of hydrophobic bonding involving an isobutyl side-chain (-4.18 kJ mol^{-1}) are:

N-cap 4.2–8.4 kJ mol^{-1}
C-cap ~2 kJ mol^{-1}
Side-chain–side-chain electrostatic interactions ~2 kJ mol^{-1}

(Reproduced from J. W. Bryson, S. F. Betz and H. S. Lu *et al.*, *Science*, 270, 935 (1995).)

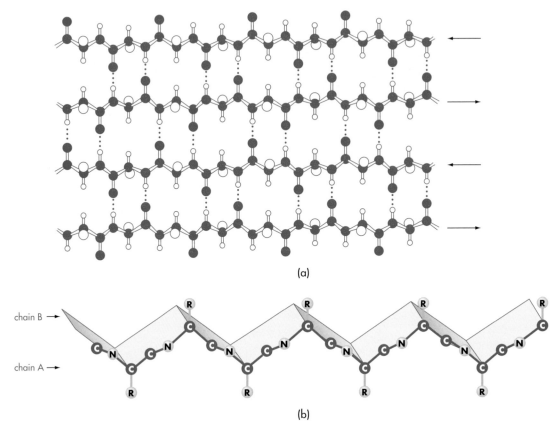

Figure 11.2 (a) A representation of β-sheet formation by four antiparallel polypeptide chains (to be visualised as being in and out of the plane on the paper). The interactions which determine β-sheet stability are more variable than those determining α-helix stability. Different amino acids have different propensities for forming β-sheets. (Reproduced from reference 3, with permission.) (b) A representation of the concertina shape of a β-sheet showing two antiparallel polypeptide chains, A and B, associated by hydrogen bonding as in (a). Exposed amides at the edge of a β-sheet can hydrogen-bond to other sheets, leading to the formation of insoluble aggregates. (Reproduced from J. W. Bryson, S. F. Betz, H. S. Lu, et al., *Science*, 270, 935 (1995).)

protein will have an amphiphilic nature. Table 11.3 lists the relative hydrophobic character of a range of amino acids, where Gly is considered to have a value of zero. The amino acids range from very hydrophobic to very hydrophilic. The side-chains of selected amino acids are shown in the table and demonstrate clearly their order in the table. Some values of log *P* (octanol/water) are given, demonstrating the trend in hydrophobic parameters.

An idea of the overall hydrophobicity of a peptide or protein may be gained from the use of indices of the hydrophobicity of the individual amino acids. Secondary and tertiary structures are important in determining the

actual hydrophobic nature of the polypeptide, however, and this complicates the prediction of their physicochemical properties such as solubility and adsorption.

If alternating hydrophilic and hydrophobic amino acid sequences in synthetic peptides are at the right distances in space, the molecule coils with the hydrophobic amino acids on the inside of each coil and the hydrophilic ones to the outside. There are still, however, many structural mysteries: the interior of many protein structures with myriads of side-chains, and the way in which metal ions can stabilize three-dimensional structures, have been likened to a *terra incognita*.

(a)   (b)

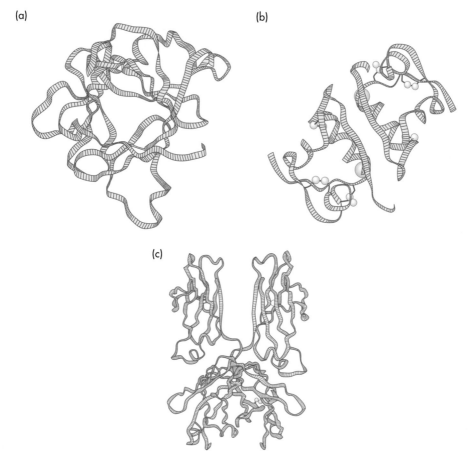

(c)

Figure 11.3 Ribbon diagrams of (a) interleukin 1-β, (b) zinc-insulin dimer and (c) the Fc fragment of immunoglobulin.
Reproduced from A. M. Lesk, *Protein Architecture*, IRL Press, Oxford, 1991.

11.1.3 Solubility of peptides and proteins

In physiological conditions the aqueous solubilities of proteins vary enormously from the very soluble to the virtually insoluble. In section 5.2.4 we discussed the solubility profiles of zwitterions, including tryptophan, which all have biphasic solubility–pH profiles. One would expect proteins with terminal —NH$_2$ and —COOH groups to behave similarly, although the effect will be complicated by the behaviour of the multitude of the intermediate amino acids, as can be seen from the pH–solubility profile of insulin in Fig. 9.20. Figure 11.4 shows the general solubility behaviour of a protein as a function of pH at two ionic strengths.

The solubility of globular proteins increases as the pH of the solution moves away from the *isoelectric point* (IP), which is the pH at which the molecule has a net zero charge and does not migrate in an electric field. Some examples of the IPs of amino acids are shown in Table 11.4. At its IP a protein has no net charge and, therefore, has a greater tendency to self-associate. As the net charge increases, the affinity of the protein for the aqueous environment increases and the protein molecules also exert a greater electrostatic repulsion. However, extremes of pH can cause protein unfolding which, not infrequently, exposes further nonpolar groups.

The relative hydrophilicities of the side-chains of the amino acids correlate well with

Table 11.3 Relative hydrophobic character of amino acid side-chains (Gly = 0)

Side-chain	Amino acid	Hydrophobic character[a]	Log P[b]
(Most hydrophobic)			
$CH_3CH_2CH(CH_3)-$	Isoleucine	1.83	−1.72
$CH_3CH(CH_3)CH_2-$	Leucine	1.80	−1.61
$C_6H_5CH_2-$	Phenylalanine	1.69	
(indole CH_2- structure)	Tryptophan	1.35	
$CH_3CH(CH_3)-$	Valine	1.32	
$CH_3-S-CH_2CH_2-$	Methionine	1.10	−2.08
(proline ring structure)	Proline	0.84	
$HSCH_2-$	Cysteine	0.76	
$HOC_6H_5CH_2-$	Tyrosine	0.39	
CH_3-	Alanine	0.35	−2.89
(Standard)	Glycine	0	
$CH_3CH(OH)-$	Threonine	−0.27	
$HOCH_2-$	Serine	−0.63	
(imidazole CH_2 structure)	Histidine	−0.65	
$H_2NCOCH_2CH_2-$	Glutamine	−0.93	
H_2NCOCH_2-	Asparagine	−0.99	
$H_2NCH_2CH_2CH_2-$	Ornithine	−1.50	
$H_3N^+-CH_2CH_2CH_2CH_2-$	Lysine	−1.54	−3.31
$HOOCCH_2-$	Aspartic acid	−2.15	−3.38
(Least hydrophobic)			

[a] High positive values indicate very hydrophobic amino acids, and negative values indicate amino acids with hydrophilic character. From reference 3.
[b] From V. Pliska et al., J. Chromatogr., 216, 79 (1981).

the hydration of the side-chain; proteins are surrounded by a hydration layer, equivalent to about 0.3 g H_2O per gram of protein, which represents about two water molecules per amino acid residue. Disturbing this layer has serious consequences.

The phase behaviour of protein solutions is affected by pH, ionic strength and temperature.

Protein–water solutions sometimes exhibit critical solution temperatures (see Chapter 5 for a discussion of phase separation). Phase transitions are important not only in manufacture and formulation, but also because they have some pathophysiological implications. Because of the involvement of phase separation in the opacification of the lens of the eye in certain cataracts, the phase separation of the γ-crystallins has been studied. Figure 11.5 shows the phase diagram obtained.

In section 5.2.3 we discussed the effect of salts on the solubility of organic electrolytes. The parabolic effects of salts on protein solubility (Fig. 11.6) might, at first sight, seem unexpected. Data, produced over 70 years ago, on haemoglobin solubility (Fig. 11.6b) shows a general increase in solubility with increasing ionic strength of salts such as NaCl, KCl and

Table 11.4   Values of pK and isoelectric point (IP) of common L-amino acids

Amino acid	pK_1 (COOH)	pK_2 (NH_3^+)	pK_3	IP
Alanine	2.34	9.69	–	6.00
Asparagine	2.02	8.80	–	5.41
Aspartic acid	1.88	3.65 (COOH)	9.60(NH_3^+)	2.77
Cysteine	1.96	8.18	10.28 (SH)	5.07
Glutamic acid	2.19	4.25 (COOH)	9.67 (NH_3^+)	3.22
Glutamine	2.17	9.13	–	5.65
Glycine	2.34	9.60	–	5.97
Histidine	1.82	6.00(imidazole)	9.17 (NH_3^+)	7.59
Isoleucine	2.36	9.68	–	6.02
Leucine	2.36	9.60	–	5.98
Lysine	2.18	8.95(a)	10.53(ε-NH_3^+)	9.74
Methionine	2.28	9.21	–	5.74
Phenylalanine	1.83	9.13	–	5.48
Proline	1.99	10.96	–	6.30
Serine	2.21	9.15	–	5.68
Threonine	2.71	9.62	–	6.16
Tryptophan	2.38	9.39	–	5.89
Tyrosine	2.20	9.11	10.07 (OH)	5.66
Valine	2.32	9.62	–	5.96

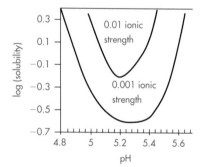

Figure 11.4   A plot of the logarithm of the aqueous stability of β lactoglobulin versus pH at two different ionic strengths, 0.001 and 0.01 mol kg^{-1}. When the protein is charged at pH values below and above pH 5.3, solubility increases from its lowest point at the isoelectric point. Increased ionic strength shifts the isoelectric point to lower pH values, around 5.2. See also Fig. 11.6.

$(NH_4)_2SO_4$, with a decrease in solubility occurring at higher ionic strengths – a salting-out effect. Several effects are responsible: (i) the preferential interaction of salts with bulk water, and (ii) the effect of the salts on the surface tension of water, which is related to the energy of cavity formation. The degree to

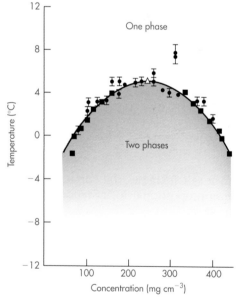

Figure 11.5   The temperature-concentration phase diagram for aqueous γ-crystallin (MW ~20 000) systems (pH = 7, I = 0.24 mol kg^{-1}) ●, cloud point measurements; ■, concentration measurements of separated phases; △ = critical point.

Reproduced from J. A. Thompson et al., Proc. Natl. Acad. Sci. USA, 84, 7079 (1987).

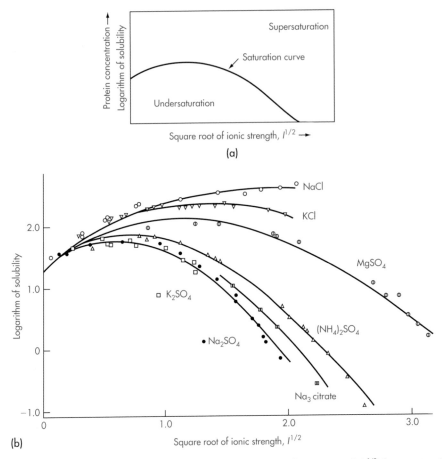

Figure 11.6 (a) A generic plot of log(solubility) as a function of square root of ionic strength ($I^{1/2}$) for proteins. (b) The plot for haemoglobin at 25°C, indicating the influence of the nature of the salt. Solubility is expressed as grams per 1000 grams H_2O.

Reproduced from A. A. Green, *J. Biol. Chem.*, 95, 47–66 (1932).

which a salt increases the surface tension of water is proportional to its tendency to salt-out proteins.

Organic solvents tend to decrease the solubility of proteins by lowering solvent dielectric constant, reducing the favourability of the protein–solvent interaction. The presence of other polymers in the solution will also tend to reduce protein solubility because of the volume exclusion effect: in extremes the addition of a water-soluble polymer (such as poly-oxyethylene glycol (PEG)) can lead to the formation of two distinct liquid phases, owing to changes in the energy required to accommodate the protein molecules and to the

unfavourable interaction of PEG with charges on the surface of the protein.

11.2 The stability of proteins and peptides

In Chapter 4 we examined how the stability of drug formulations may be improved from a knowledge of the principal routes of degradation and the kinetics of breakdown. It has been implicitly assumed that the drugs under discussion were typical low molecular weight compounds and it is clear that for this type of drug there is a large body of knowledge relating to all aspects of their stability. Far less is known of the way in which protein and peptide drugs degrade in solution and of the factors influencing their stability. Consequently, the formulation of this increasingly important class of compound presents more of a challenge.

Protein pharmaceuticals can suffer both physical and chemical instability: the major pathways are summarised in Fig. 11.7. Physical instability refers to changes in the higher-order structure (secondary and above), whereas chemical instability can be thought of as any kind of modification of the protein via bond formation or cleavage, yielding a new chemical entity. In this section we will examine aspects of both of these types of instability. For each degradation route we will look at the effect of formulation parameters such as pH and ionic strength on stability and also discuss the application of accelerated stability testing procedures.

11.2.1 Physical instability

Physical instability is a phenomenon which is rarely encountered with small organic molecules but arises in peptides and proteins because of the many conditions under which proteins can lose their native three-dimensional structure. Unfolding of stable forms can lead to adsorption, aggregation or further chemical reactivity. Aggregation can lead to precipitation. Loss of the unique biologically active three-dimensional structure (i.e. denaturation), can be caused by heating and, conversely, by cooling or freezing, extremes of pH, and contact with organic chemicals and denaturants. Most of these act through their influence on solubility or conformation, hence the importance of understanding protein–solvent interactions. It is generally thought that denaturation must first occur before the other processes such as aggregation, adsorption and precipitation can proceed.

Denaturation: reversible and irreversible

Denaturation refers to a disruption of the tertiary and secondary structure of the protein molecule. The denaturation can be *reversible* or *irreversible*. Denaturation caused by, for example, an increase of temperature is said to be reversible if the native structure is regained on decreasing the temperature. Irreversible denaturation implies that the unfolding process is such that the native structure cannot be regained simply by lowering the temperature (although it may sometimes be possible to return the protein to its native state

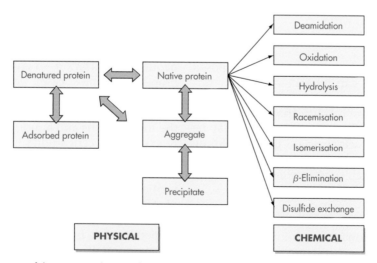

Figure 11.7 Schematic of the major pathways of protein degradation, which may be physical or chemical in origin.

by addition of a denaturant and subsequent dialysis). In many cases the protein may become more compact, exposing hydrophobic residues that are normally buried within its core. It is the interaction between these hydrophobic residues in the protein interior which determines the physical stability of the proteins. When they become exposed to the solvent these residues can interact with other hydrophobic surfaces such as the container walls or the exposed residues of other denatured proteins, leading to the localised accumulation of denatured protein molecules that results in the formation of aggregates. Increase of temperature results in greater flexibility of the proteins and an increased tendency for collision, leading to aggregate formation. An increase of the ionic strength may lead to neutralisation of the surface charge on the protein molecules which is responsible for their mutual repulsion, again resulting in aggregation. Charge neutralisation and subsequent aggregation can also occur when the pH of the solution approaches the isoelectric point of the protein. In both cases, molecules in the aggregated state can undergo denaturation with time as a result of subtle changes in their conformation and the aggregation process becomes irreversible.

Two basic pathways have been observed for proteins during denaturation and folding. The simplest is a two-state model. If we refer to the native state as N and the unfolded, denatured state as D, we can write

$$N \rightleftharpoons D$$

Once critical hydrophobic residues are exposed to solvents they can interact with other surfaces (containers or the air/water interface). The process may involve the formation of intermediate conformations (I) which may be stable and may self-associate during folding. The second general pathway for denaturation includes these stable intermediate species and may be written

$$N \rightleftharpoons I_n \rightleftharpoons \cdots \rightleftharpoons I_2 \rightleftharpoons I_1 \rightleftharpoons D$$

The equation shows the unfolding of a native protein to form an intermediate, I_n, which then unfolds to form other intermediates. If

the two-state model is assumed, the concentration of denaturant required to achieve equal concentrations of N and D will give some indication of the process. If the fraction of denatured protein, f_d, is calculated under given conditions (temperature, concentration of additive, etc.) we can write

$$f_d = \frac{[D]}{[N] + [D]} = \frac{K_{ND}}{1 + K_{ND}} \tag{11.1}$$

where K_{ND} is the equilibrium constant for denaturation $(K_{ND} = [D]/[N])$, related to the free energy of denaturation $\Delta G_{ND}^{\ominus}$ by

$$K_{ND} = \exp\left(\frac{-\Delta G_{ND}^{\ominus}}{RT}\right) \tag{11.2}$$

Hence,

$$\Delta G_{ND}^{\ominus} = -2.303 RT \log K_{ND} \tag{11.3}$$

When 50% of the molecules are unfolded [D] = [N] and $K_{ND} = 1$, therefore $\Delta G_{ND}^{\ominus} = 0$. The temperature at which this occurs is referred to as the melting temperature, T_m. An increase of T_m is indicative of an increase of stability; for example, T_4 lysozyme (lysozyme from bacteriophage T4) is more stable at pH 6.5 where T_m is 65°C than at pH 2 where T_m is 42°C.

Aggregation

Some proteins self-associate in aqueous solution to form oligomers. Insulin, for example, exists in several associated states; the zinc hexamer of insulin is a complex of insulin and zinc which dissolves slowly into dimers and eventually monomers following its subcutaneous administration, so giving it long-acting properties. In most cases, however, it is desirable to prevent association such that only monomeric or dimeric forms are present in the formulations and a more rapid absorption is achieved. Recent studies have been directed towards engineering insulin molecules which are not prone to association,[4-6] or the prevention of association through the addition of surfactants.[7] Protein self-association is a reversible process, i.e. alteration of the solvent properties can lead to the re-formation of the monomeric native protein. There is an important distinction between this *association* process and the *aggregation* of proteins, which relates to the usually nonreversible interaction of protein molecules in their denatured state. Aggregation therefore implies that the proteins have undergone some form of denaturation prior to their interaction.

If an intermediate forms that has a solubility less than that of N or D this can lead to aggregation and eventually to precipitation. For example, the addition of moderate amounts of denaturant to bovine growth hormone (bGH) can generate a partially unfolded intermediate of low solubility which aggregates. Similarly, γ-interferon (IFN-γ) is inactivated by acid treatment or by the addition of salt because the dimeric native state is converted into monomers, which are partially denatured. For both proteins the formation of intermediates leads to inactivation.

Surface adsorption and precipitation

The adsorption of proteins such as insulin on surfaces such as glass or plastic in giving sets is important as it can reduce the amount of agent reaching the patient. It can also lead to further denaturation, which can then cause precipitation and the physical blocking of delivery ports in insulin pumps, for example. Insulin adsorption on the surface of the containers and the subsequent 'frosting' effect, due to the presence of a finely divided precipitate on the walls, is accelerated by the presence of a large headspace allowing a greater interaction of the insulin with the air/water interface, which facilitates denaturation.

11.2.2 Formulation and protein stabilisation

There are several possible ways in which the physical stability of the protein can be improved through formulation. We will examine methods for minimising this and chemical degradation in the following sections.

Prevention of adsorption

Some measures can be taken to eliminate, or at least minimise, protein denaturation resulting from surface adsorption. The surface of glass is conducive to adsorption and it is preferable in principle to use more hydrophilic surfaces, although this may not be feasible in practice. Alternatively, when the use of glass cannot be avoided, components may be added to the protein solution to prevent adsorption to the glass surface. These additives can act by coating the surface of glass or by binding to the proteins. For example, serum albumin can be included in the formulation since this will compete with the therapeutic protein for the binding sites on the glass surface and so reduce its adsorption. A similar effect can be achieved by the addition of surfactants such as poloxamers and polysorbates to the protein solution. Consideration must, however, be given to the effects of the surfactants on the pharmacology of the protein and to the toxicological effects of the surfactant itself.

Minimisation of exposure to air

Significant denaturation of proteins can occur when the protein solutions are exposed at the air/solution interface. In this respect the air interface is behaving as a hydrophobic surface and the extent of denaturation is found to be dependent on the time of exposure of the protein at the interface. Agitation of protein solutions in the presence of air or application of other shear forces, such as those which occur when the solutions are filtered or pumped, may also cause denaturation. Again, the inclusion of surfactants can reduce denaturation arising from these processes. Stability testing of protein-containing formulations often involves subjecting the solutions to shaking for several hours and the subsequent assessment of the protein configuration. If the protein has retained its native state and has not aggregated, the formulation is considered to be stable against surface or shear-induced denaturation.

Addition of cosolvents

Some excipients and buffer components added to the protein solution are able to minimise denaturation through their effects on solvation. These compounds, including poly-ethylene glycols and glycerol, are referred to as *cosolvents*. They may act either by causing the preferential hydration of the protein or alternatively by binding to the protein surface. Preferential hydration results from an exclusion of the cosolvent from the protein surface due to steric effects (as in the case of poly-ethylene glycols); surface tension effects (as with sugars, salts and amino acids) or some form of chemical incompatibility such as charge effects. As a result more water molecules pack around the protein in order to exclude the additive and the protein becomes fully hydrated and stabilised in a compact form (Fig. 11.8). Alternatively, the cosolvent may stabilise the protein molecule either by binding to it nonspecifically or by binding to specific sites on its surface.

Cosolvent effects such as this can be analysed from a thermodynamic point of view. Addition of cosolvents which cause preferential hydration of the protein stabilises the compact conformations of the protein because the cosolvent results in an increase in the free energy of the system. To reduce the free energy, the surface area of the protein is minimised.

Optimisation of pH

In order to avoid stability problems arising from charge neutralisation and to ensure adequate solubility, a pH must be selected which is at least 0.5 pH units above or below the isoelectric point. This is often difficult to achieve, however, since a pH range of 5–7 is usually required to minimise chemical breakdown and this frequently coincides with the isoelectric point.

Characterisation of degradation

Finally, if the formulation does not prevent denaturation and aggregation of the protein, then the pharmacology, immunogenicity, and toxicology of the denatured or aggregated protein must be studied to determine its safety and efficacy. Several studies must be performed to determine the extent of degradation that is acceptable for administration. If the aggregates are soluble there may be a significant effect on the pharmacokinetics and immunogenicity of the protein. On the other hand, insoluble aggregates are generally unacceptable and instructions are usually given

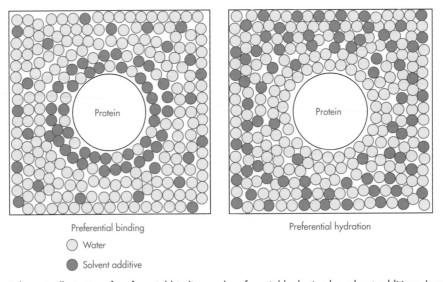

Preferential binding   Preferential hydration

○ Water

● Solvent additive

Figure 11.8 Schematic illustration of preferential binding and preferential hydration by solvent additives. In preferential binding the additive occurs in the solvation shell of the protein at a greater local concentration than in the bulk solvent, while preferential hydration results from the exclusion of the additive from the surface of the protein.
Reproduced from S. N. Timasheff and T. Arakawa, in *Protein Structure: A Practical Approach* (ed. T. E. Creighton), pp. 331–345, IRL Press, Oxford, 1989.

not to administer protein solutions containing precipitates.

11.2.3 Chemical instability

Chemical instability can involve one or more of a variety of chemical reactions including:

- *Deamidation*, in which the sole chain linkage in a glutamine (Gln) or asparagine (Asn) residue is hydrolysed to form a carboxylic acid.
- *Oxidation*: the side-chains of histidine (His), methionine (Met), cysteine (Cys), tryptophan (Trp) and tyrosine (Tyr) residues in proteins are potential oxidation sites.
- *Racemisation*: all amino acid residues except glycine (Gly) are chiral at the carbon atom bearing the side-chain and are subject to base-catalysed racemisation.
- *Proteolysis*, involving the cleavage of peptide (ZCO–NHY) bonds.
- *Beta elimination*: high-temperature treatment of proteins leads to destruction of disulfide bonds as a result of β-elimination from the cystine residue.
- *Disulfide formation*: the interchange of disulfide bonds can result in an altered three-dimensional structure.

Table 11.5 lists the amino acids or sequences which are subject to chemical degradation and lists the formulation approvals used to overcome the problems.

Protein deamidation[8]

In the deamidation reaction, the side-chain amide linkage in a glutamine (Gln) or asparagine (Asn) residue is hydrolysed to form a free carboxylic acid; the Asn peptides being more susceptible to deamidation than the Gln peptides.

The deamidation of Asn and Gln residues of proteins is an acid- and base-catalysed hydrolysis reaction which can occur rapidly under physiological conditions. As with all acid–base catalysed reactions, there will be an optimum pH for stability; for example, the deamidation of glutaminyl residues of pentapeptides occurs at a minimum rate at pH 6. The rate of deamidation is strongly influenced by the sequence of residues in the peptide molecule. Different mechanisms are responsible for deamidation in neutral/alkaline and in acidic aqueous solution. The acid-catalysed deamidation reaction involves protonation of the amide leaving-group to form aspartate directly as the major degradation product, as outlined in Scheme 11.1. At neutral to alkaline pH, deamidation is believed to proceed through a cyclic imide intermediate by attack of the peptide nitrogen on the C-terminal side of the asparagine on the side-chain carbonyl group, producing isoaspartate and aspartate as outlined in Scheme 11.2.

The hydrolysis reactions are completely reversible, i.e. the final products of deamidation can interconvert through the cyclic imide

---

Table 11.5 Amino acids or sequences susceptible to chemical degradation, together with formulation strategies to reduce degradation[a]

Amino acid or sequence	Mechanism of degradation	Formulation strategy
Cysteine–cysteine	Aggregation	Addition of surfactants, polyalcohols and other excipients
Glutamine, asparagine	Deamidation	pH 3–5
Tryptophan, methionine, cysteine, tyrosine, histidine	Oxidation	pH < 7
Methionine	Oxidation	Protect from oxygen
Tryptophan	Photodecomposition	Protect from light
Lysine-threonine	Copper induced cleavage	Chelating agents
Asparagine-proline, asparagine-tyrosine	Hydrolysis	pH > 7

[a] Reproduced from D. A. Parkins, U. T. Lashmar, *PSST*, 3, 129–137 (2000).

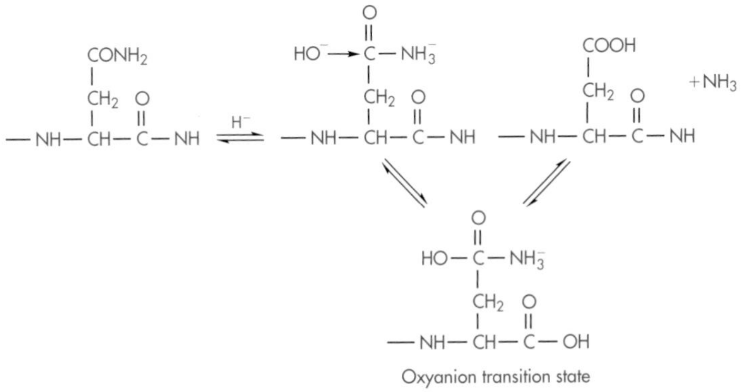

Scheme 11.1   General acid and base catalysis of deamidation. The tetrahedral oxyanion intermediate is inferred to be the transition state.

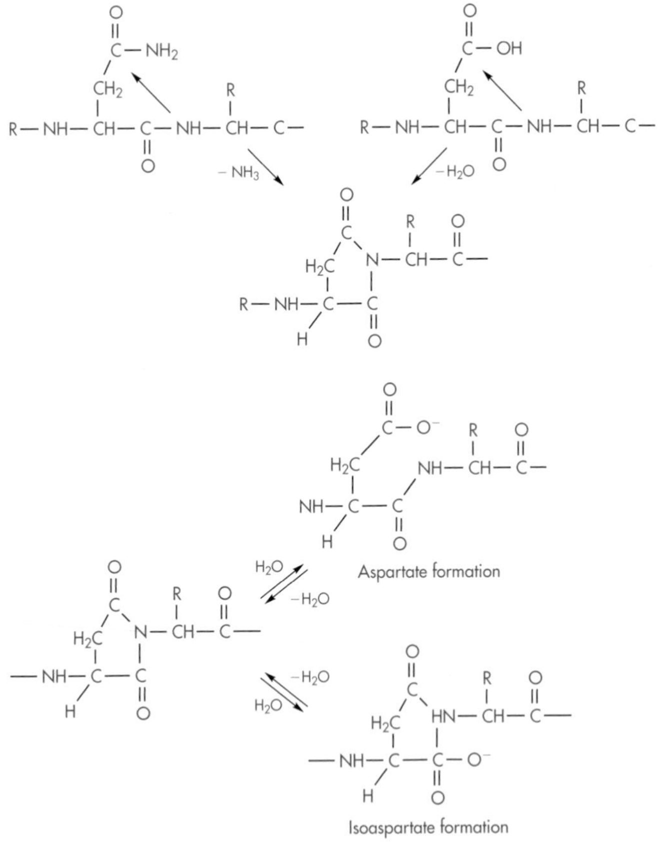

Scheme 11.2   Formation of a cyclic imide as a result of nucleophilic attack of asparagine by main-chain amide nitrogen on the carboxyl carbon of either the side chain amide or carboxylic acid groups and its subsequent hydrolysis to form either aspartate or isoaspartate.

intermediate. Since the succeeding amino acid is involved in the formation of the cyclic imide, the size and physicochemical properties of the neighbouring amino acid side-chain are expected to influence its rate of formation. Thus, the rate of cyclic imide formation of the Asn-Leu hexapeptide at pH 7 was approximately 50 times slower than for the Asn-Gly hexapeptide because of steric hindrance by the leucine (Leu) side-chain.[9]

The effect of deamidation on protein activity is generally unpredictable. For many proteins, including insulin and interleukin-1α, deamidation has no measurable effect. Other proteins such as cytochrome c, interleukin-1β, lysozyme and adrenocorticotropin exhibit a decrease of activity on deamidation. Consequently, for any particular protein it is necessary to determine experimentally the influence of deamidation on its therapeutic activity. Because of its effect on the surface charge of the protein at the site of modification, it is not surprising that deamidation can have pronounced effects on conformation. If deamidation results in irreversible unfolding of the protein molecule, there will be a greater susceptibility of that protein to irreversible aggregation. On the other hand, the modification of the charge following deamidation may result in greater repulsion of adjacent protein molecules and a reduced tendency for aggregation. As a general rule it is wise to consider means by which deamidation can be minimised in the protein formulation.

Prevention of deamidation

If the deamidation occurs by a general acid–base mechanism then the optimum pH for a peptide formulation will usually be about 6, where both rates are at their minimum. If the deamidation occurs through the cyclic imide intermediate it is, in principle, preferable to formulate at a low pH since this type of deamidation is base-catalysed. This may not be feasible in practice, however, since other routes of degradation tend to predominate at lower pH and a compromise must then be sought. It is well established that deamidation rate may be affected markedly by buffer components and hence care must be taken in the choice of buffer used in the control of pH. In general it is found that the phosphate anion is most problematic in its effect on the rates of deamidation.[10]

There have been relatively few reports of the influence of temperature on the rate of deamidation. Deamidation of peptides containing Gln and Asn[11] has been reported to proceed at a higher rate as the temperature was increased. From a study of the deamidation rates of an Asp residue in a model hexapeptide[12] it was concluded that the Arrhenius equation was obeyed over the temperature range 25–70°C at pH 5.0 and 7.5.

An increase of the ionic strength of aqueous solutions of glutaminyl and asparaginyl pentapeptides has been reported to result in an increased rate of deamidation.[11] Similar results have been noted in an earlier study on cytochrome c,[13] although a lack of effect of ionic strength on stability was observed[14] in a series of pentapeptides Val-Ser-Asn-X-Val and Val-X-Asn-Ser-Val, where X is an amino acid. The ionic strengths of most parenteral formulations of proteins in which sodium chloride is used to adjust the tonicity are sufficiently low that increased deamidation rates resulting from electrolyte addition will not be a major problem.

Studies of the rates of deamidation in a series of nonaqueous solvents have indicated a dependence of rate on the dielectric constant of the solvent. Although these experiments have generally involved solvents unsuitable for use in formulation, it is interesting to note a reported decrease of the rate of deamidation of N-terminal-blocked Boc-Asn-Gly-Gly in ethanol[11] (Boc = butoxycarbonyl). Similarly, the deamidation rate of the hexapeptide Val-Thr-Pro-Asn-Gly-Ala decreased with decrease in the dielectric constant of the solvent, an effect which was attributed to the destabilisation of the deprotonated peptide bond nitrogen anion which is involved in the formation of the cyclic imide intermediate.[15]

Protein oxidation

Oxidation is one of the major causes of protein degradation and has been widely studied. The side-chains of histidine (His), methionine (Met), cysteine (Cys), tryptophan (Trp) and tyrosine (Tyr) residues in proteins are potential oxidation sites. The reactive oxygen species include singlet oxygen $^1O_2$, superoxide radical O_2^-, alkyl peroxide ROOH, hydrogen peroxide H_2O_2, hydroxy radicals (HO$^\bullet$ or HOO$^\bullet$), and halide complexes (CLO$^-$).[16] The reactivity of these oxidants is:

$$\text{HO}^\bullet, \text{HOO}^\bullet > O_2^- > \text{ROOH}, H_2O_2 > \\ {}^1O_2, \text{CLO}^- > O_2$$

Although much is known about the reactive oxygen species, there are problems in predicting the probable extent of oxidation because it is often not known whether initiators are present.

Methionine is very susceptible to oxidation and reacts with a variety of oxidants to give methionine sulfoxide ($RS(OO)CH_3$) or, in highly oxidative conditions, methionine sulfone ($RS(O)CH_3$) (Scheme 11.3). Whether methionine residues are susceptible to oxidation depends to a large extent on their exposure to the solvent. In proteins such as myoglobin[17] and trypsin[18] these residues are buried within the hydrophobic regions of the protein and are relatively inert under conditions of mild oxidation. In contrast, in proteins such as ribonuclease A,[19] chymotrypsin,[20] pepsin[21] and lysosyme[22] the methionine residues are partially exposed to the solvent and the oxidation rate is very much faster.

The thiol group of cysteine readily reacts with oxygen to yield successively, sulfenic acid (RSOH), a disulfide (RSSH), a sulfinic acid (RSO_2H), and finally, a sulfonic (cystic) acid (RSO_3H) depending on reaction conditions. An important factor determining the extent of oxidation is the spatial positioning of the thiol groups in the proteins. Where contact between thiol groups within the protein molecule is hindered or when the protein contains only a single thiol group, intramolecular disulfide bonds are not formed. Factors that influence oxidation rate include the temperature, pH, the buffer medium, the type of catalyst and the oxygen tension.

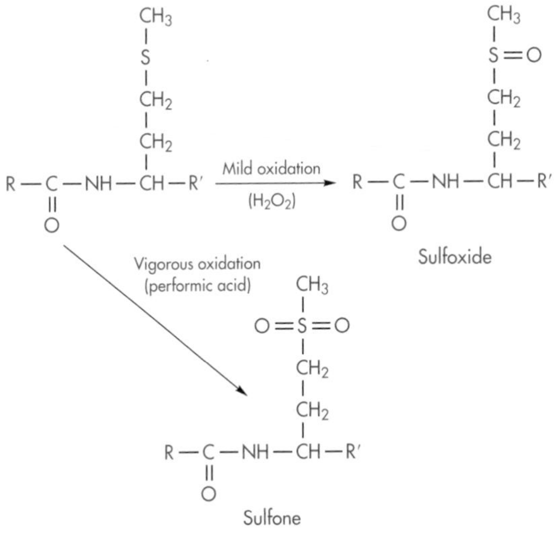

Histidine is susceptible to oxidation in the presence of metals, primarily by reaction with singlet oxygen, and this constitutes a major cause of enzyme degradation. Both histidine and tryptophan are highly susceptible to photooxidation.[23]

Prevention of oxidation

In most cases oxidation results in a complete or partial loss of activity, although antigenicity is not affected except in the relatively few instances in which the protein undergoes gross conformational changes. It is clear that minimising protein oxidation is essential for maintaining the biological activity of most proteins and avoiding the immunogenic response caused by degraded proteins.

A variety of measures may be employed to prevent protein oxidation in pharmaceutical formulations. Temperature reduction, either by refrigeration or by freezing, will generally minimise oxidation, although the effect may be small because of the low activation energies involved. There are exceptions to this; for example, the oxidation of proteins with cysteine residues may increase as a consequence of increased intra- or intermolecular disulfide exchange due to the increase in concentration of the protein by its exclusion from the ice matrix which forms during the freezing process. The rate of oxidation may be pH-dependent; for example, as the pH is decreased the rate of the hydrogen peroxide-catalysed oxidation of cysteine decreases whereas that of methionine oxidation increases.[24] The determination of the pH of maximum stability is of primary importance in the formulation of protein solutions, as is the obvious precaution of excluding oxygen from the headspace of the container. Antioxidants may be included in the formulation, where they may act by inhibition of oxidation, by removing trace metal ions or as scavengers of oxygen.

Scheme 11.3 Mechanism of oxidation of Met-containing peptide under mild and strong conditions to yield methionine sulfoxide or methionine sulfone respectively.

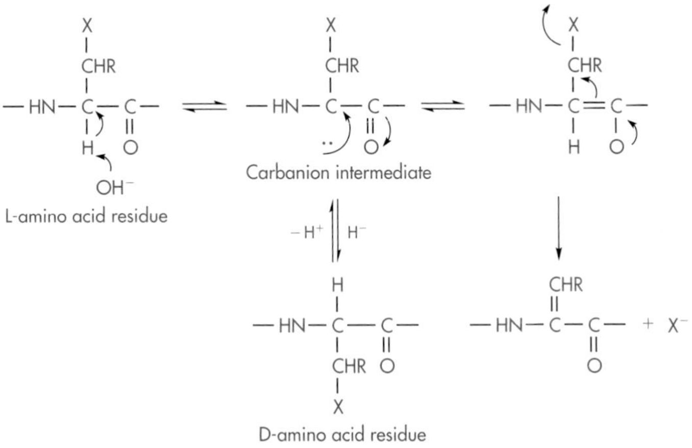

X = H, OH, O-glycosyl, O-phosphoryl, SH, SCH$_2$-R, aliphatic or aromatic residue. R = H or CH$_3$.

Scheme 11.4 Mechanism of beta-elimination and racemisation reactions in alkaline media.

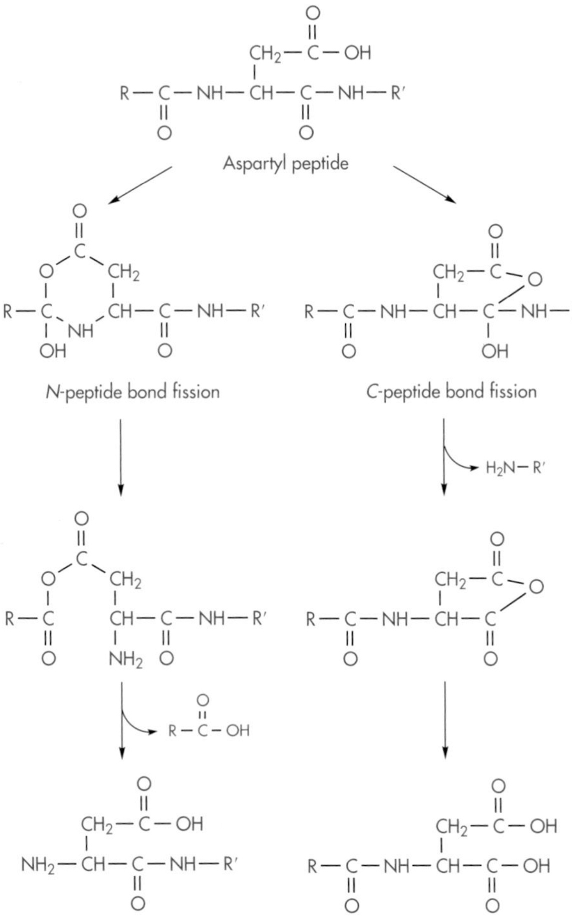

Scheme 11.5 Mechanism of degradation of aspartyl peptides in acidic media.

Racemisation

All amino acid residues except Gly are chiral at the carbon bearing the side-chain and are subject to base-catalysed racemisation. Scheme 11.4 shows the mechanism involved. In alkaline solution the hydrogen of the α-methine is removed by base to form a carbanion intermediate which can then generate D-enantiomers, which are nonmetabolisable, or create peptide bonds which are not broken down by proteolytic enzymes.

Proteolysis

The amino acid residue which is by far the most susceptible to proteolysis is Asp; the cleavage of the peptide bonds in dilute acid proceeds at a rate at least 100 times that for other peptide bonds. The hydrolysis can occur at the N-terminal and/or the C-terminal peptide bonds adjacent to the Asp residue (Scheme 11.5). Cleavage of the N-terminal peptide bond proceeds via an intermediate with a six-membered ring, while cleavage of the C-terminal peptide bond is thought to involve a five-membered ring. Such peptide bond cleavage can result in protein inactivation.

Beta-elimination

The inactivation of proteins at high temperatures is often due to β-elimination of disulfides from the cystine residue, although other amino acids including Cys, Ser, Thr, Phe, and Lys can be degraded via β-elimination, as seen from Scheme 11.4. The inactivation is particularly rapid under alkaline conditions and is also influenced by the presence of metal ions.

Disulfide formation

The interchange of disulfide bonds can result in incorrect pairings with consequent changes of three-dimensional structure and loss of catalytic activity. The mechanism is thought to be different in alkaline and acid conditions. In alkaline and neutral solutions the reaction involves the nucleophilic attack on a sulfur atom of the disulfide (Scheme 11.6a). This reaction is catalysed by thiols and can be prevented if thiol scavengers such as *p*-

(a) *Alkaline or neutral conditions:*

$$R'S^- + R''S{-}SR'' \rightleftharpoons R'S{-}SR'' + R''S^-$$
$$R''S^- + R'S{-}SR' \rightleftharpoons R''S{-}SR' + R'S^-$$

(b) *Acidic conditions:*

$$R'S{-}SR' + H^+ \rightleftharpoons \left[\begin{array}{c} R'S{-}SR' \\ | \\ H \end{array} \right]^+ \rightleftharpoons R'SH + R'S^+$$

$$R'S^+ + R''S{-}SR \rightleftharpoons R'S{-}SR + R''S^+$$
$$R''S^+ + R'S{-}SR' \rightleftharpoons R''S{-}SR' + R'S^+$$

Scheme 11.6 Mechanism of disulfide exchange in (a) alkaline or neutral media and (b) acidic media

mercuribenzoate, *N*-ethylmaleimide or copper ions are present. In acidic conditions the disulfide exchange takes place through a sulfenium cation, which is formed by attack of a proton on the disulfide bond (Scheme 11.6b). The sulfenium cation carries out an electrophilic displacement on a sulfur atom of the disulfide. Addition of thiols can inhibit this exchange by scavenging the sulfenium ions.

11.2.4   Accelerated stability testing of protein formulations

As we have seen from the above discussions, the processes involved in the degradation of proteins may be complex and highly dependent on the proximity of other functional groups in the molecule and also on the protein conformation. As a consequence, the mechanisms of degradation at higher temperatures may not be the same as at lower temperatures and the application of the Arrhenius equation in the prediction of protein stability will be more uncertain than with formulations of small-molecule drugs. Nevertheless, many workers have attempted to use the Arrhenius approach with some degree of success. In general, this approach appears to be applicable when only the activity is monitored. In most of these studies degradation was due to thermal denaturation, and loss of activity was a consequence of conformational changes rather than covalent chemical reaction. Although the product of this reaction may involve many different unfolded forms of the protein, these forms will be inactive and indistinguishable from each other by activity assay. Deviation from the Arrhenius equation occurs, however, if the protein exists in multiple conformational forms that retain activity during unfolding. Where degradation occurs by deamidation or oxidation, it may still be possible to apply the Arrhenius equation if protein activity only is monitored, since the final activity loss will be determined by the fastest reaction.

11.3   Protein formulation and delivery

It has been said[25] that 'drug delivery represents the potential Achilles' heel of biotechnology's peptide drug industry'. The reasons for this include the range of instabilities discussed above, the inherent low membrane transport by diffusion, because of molecular size and hydrophilicity, and often the need for temporal and site control of delivery.

11.3.1   Protein and peptide transport

For a series of 11 model peptides in an *in vitro* intestinal cell monolayer system, a good correlation was found between the permeability coefficient, P, and the log of the partition coefficient of the peptides between heptane and ethylene glycol (rather than octanol and water) (Fig. 11.9), results which also suggest that the principal deterrent to peptide transport is the breaking of hydrogen bonds.[26] Molecular volume (or size) will increasingly be a factor as the molecular weight of the peptide increases.

The diffusion of proteins and peptides in solution is dictated by the same considerations as those discussed in section 3.6. The rate of translational movement depends on the size of the molecule, its shape and interactions with solvent molecules. The rate of translational movement is often expressed by a frictional coefficient, f, defined in relation to the diffusion coefficient D, by equation (11.4):

$$f = \frac{k_B T}{D} \tag{11.4}$$

where k_B is the Boltzmann constant and T is the absolute temperature. Many proteins are nearly spherical in solution, but if their shape deviates from sphericity this is reflected in a frictional ratio, f/f_0, above unity, where f_0 is the rate of diffusion of a molecule of the same size but of spherical shape. The frictional ratio

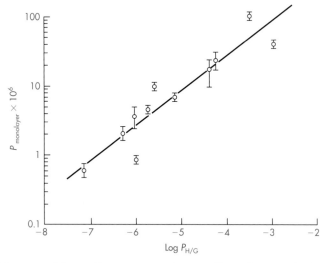

Figure 11.9 A plot of the permeability coefficient P across Caco-2 cell monolayers vs the log P (heptane/glycol) for a series of synthetic peptides to illustrate relationships between lipophilicity and transport.
Reproduced from reference 26.

of lysozyme is 1.24 and that of trypsin is 1.187. Globular proteins have values of f/f_0 in the range 1.05–1.38.

The diffusion coefficients and translational movements of proteins are important in considering the release of proteins from hydrogel matrix devices and other delivery vehicles, and in membrane transport, as far as this can be considered to be a passive diffusion process. Changes in shape during membrane transport in a lipid environment may also have to be considered. Table 11.6 gives some values of diffusion coefficient of a number of therapeutic peptides and proteins.

The key factors governing the design of formulations and delivery of drugs are summarised in the diagram in Fig. 11.10. Physicochemical factors are weighed along with biological data and the potential aggregation, deamidation, oxidation and other hazards are looked for, before deciding on strategies to overcome these problems. Freeze-drying (lyophilisation) is an obvious, but not straightforward, route, to provide a product with a long shelf-life.

11.3.2 Lyophilised proteins

Because of their potential instability in solution, therapeutic proteins are often formulated as lyophilised powders. Even in this state several suffer from moisture-induced aggregation. Proteins such as insulin, tetanus toxoid, somatotropin and human albumin aggregate in the presence of moisture, which can lead to reduced activity, stability and diffusion.

In the presence of water vapour at 37°C, lyophilised recombinant human albumin (rHA) experiences intermolecular thiol–disulfide interchange and forms high molecular weight, water-insoluble aggregates.[28] The use of excipients (low and high molecular weight sugars, organic acids, etc.) to prevent such effects leads to the conclusion that the stabilising effect is correlated with the ability of the additives to preferentially absorb water. Figure 11.11 illustrates the effects on rHA solubility and the influence of sorbitol on the changes in solubility.

11.3.3 Water adsorption isotherms

Because of the sensitivity of proteins to moisture, the ability to measure sorption of water is vital in preformulation. Water sorption isotherms from recombinant bovine somatotropin (rbST), a protein with 191 amino acids, molecular weight 22 000, show water content versus the relative vapour pressure (p/p_0) for the sodium salt and the 'internal' salt of rbST (Fig. 11.12). These were fitted to modified BET isotherms which have an additional state of interacting water intermediate to the free water and the strongly bound water states.[29, 30] Calculations reveal that a monolayer of water is formed from 88 moles of H_2O per mole of protein for the lyophilised Na^+ salt of rbST, which is equivalent to about 7.3 g per g of protein. The much higher apparent surface areas obtained using water, as opposed to nitrogen, adsorption isotherms (typically 264 m^2 g^{-1}, compared with 1.3 m^2 g^{-1} with nitrogen) suggest that water penetrates the powder and that the isotherm represents adsorption and absorption.

The practical implications of moisture load are seen in Fig. 11.13, which shows the rate of decomposition of rbST (albeit at 47°C) following incubation in sealed vials.

Table 11.6 Diffusion coefficients and molecular weights of peptides and proteins[a]

Compound	MW	$10^6 D$ (cm^2 s^{-1})
Oxytocin	1 007	4.30
Lys-vasopressin	1 056	4.18
Arg-vasopressin	1 084	4.27
Somatostatin	1 638	3.74
Calcitonin	3 418	2.76
Insulin	5 807	1.14
Calculated (insulin)		
Monomer	5 807	2.03
Hexamer	34 845	0.93

[a] Reproduced from O. Hosoya, et al., J. Pharm. Pharmacol., 56, 1501–150 (2004).

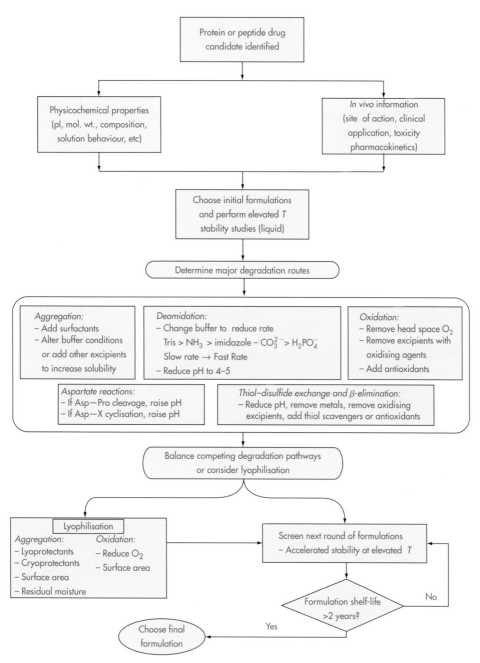

Figure 11.10 Process diagram for formulation development of proteins and peptides.
Reproduced from reference 27.

Considerations of solubility and stability have to be addressed, as well as the mode of delivery. The wide range of biodegradable polymers used for the controlled delivery of proteins and peptides include natural substances, starch, alginates, collagen and a variety of proteins such as crosslinked albumin, as well as a range of synthetic hydrogels, polyanhydrides, polyesters or orthoesters, poly(amino acids) and poly(caprolactones).   Poly(lactide-glycolide)

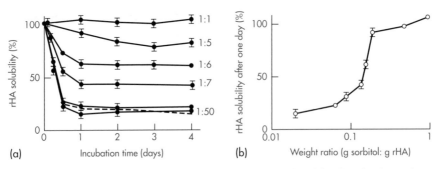

Figure 11.11 Stabilisation of rHA against aggregation afforded by co-lyophilised sorbitol. (a) The time-dependent change of solubility of rHA co-lyophilised with sorbitol at various sorbitol-to-rHA weight ratios, as indicated (the dashed line depicts the time course of rHA aggregation in the absence of sorbitol). (b) rHA solubility after a one-day incubation as a function of sorbitol-to-rHA weight ratio.
Reproduced from reference 28.

Table 11.7   Routes of delivery for proteins and peptides[a]

Delivery routes	Formulation and device requirements	Commercial products[b]
Invasive		
Direct injection: intravenous (i.v.), subcutaneous (s.c.), intramuscular (i.m.), intracerebral vein (i.c.v.)	Liquid or reconstituted solid, (syringe)	Activase (alteplase) Nutropin (somatrotropin) RecombiVax (hepatitis B vaccine)
Depot system (s.c. or i.m.)	Biodegradable polymers, liposomes, permeable polymers (not degradable) microspheres, implants	Lupron Depot (leuprolide) Zoladex (goserelin) Decapeptyl (triptorelin)
Noninvasive		
Pulmonary	Liquid or powder formulations, nebulisers, metered dose inhalers, dry powder inhalers	Pulmozyme (dornase alfa)
Oral	Solids, emulsions, microparticulates, with or without absorption enhancers	
Nasal	Liquid, usually requires permeation enhancers	Synarel (nafarelin)
Topical	Emulsions, creams or pastes (liposomes)	
Transdermal	Electrophoretic (iontophoresis), electroporation, chemical permeation enhancers, prodrugs, ultrasonics	
Buccal, rectal, vaginal	Gels, suppositories, bioadhesives, particles	

[a] Modified from reference 27.

[b] Activase (recombinant human tissue plasminogen activator), Nutropin (recombinant human growth hormone) and Pulmozyme (recombinant human deoxyribonuclease I) are all products of Genentech; RecombiVax (recombinant hepatitis B surface antigen) is produced by Merck; Lupron Depot (leuprolide acetate – PLGA) is a product of Takeda Pharmaceuticals; Zoladex (goserelin acetate – PLGA) is produced by AstraZeneca; Decapeptyl is produced by Debiopharm; Synarel (nafarelin acetate) is produced by Roche.

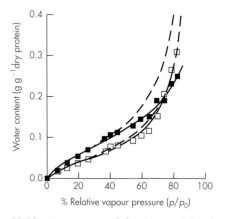

Figure 11.12 Comparison of fits obtained by the BET (dashed lines) and GAB (solid lines) models for the sorption isotherms of the sodium (■) and internal (□) salts of bovine somatropin.
Reproduced from reference 29.

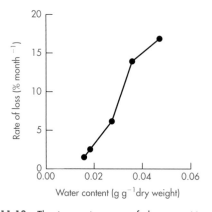

Figure 11.13 The increasing rate of decomposition of a lyophilised rbST formulation with increasing water content following incubation in sealed vials at 47°C.
Reproduced from reference 29.

(PLGA) is one of the commonest polymers used in microsphere form to deliver, *inter alia*, growth-hormone-releasing factor, a somatostatin analogue, ciclosporin, and LHRH antagonists.[27]

11.3.4   Routes of delivery

Table 11.7 summarises the invasive and non-invasive routes of delivery for peptides and proteins, involving direct injection of solutions, depot systems and a variety of oral, nasal, topical and other formulations.

11.4   A therapeutic protein and a peptide

11.4.1   Insulin

It is appropriate that the protein therapeutic substance with the longest pedigree is discussed here. There are three main types of insulin preparations:

- Those with a *short* duration of action which have a relatively rapid onset (soluble insulin, insulin lispro and insulin aspart)
- Those with an *intermediate* action (isophane insulin and insulin zinc suspension)
- Those with a slow action, slower in onset and lasting for *long* periods (crystalline insulin zinc suspension)

Some aspects of insulin were dealt with in section 9.4.4. Table 11.8 lists some of the insulin formulations designed to produce different durations of onset and action. Insulin is generally self-administered subcutaneously with injection pens, needle-free devices or pumps.

Precipitation of insulin and other proteins

Precipitation of insulin in pumps due to the formation of amorphous particles, crystals or fibrils of insulin can lead to changes in release pattern or to blockage which prevents insulin release. 'Amorphous' or 'crystalline' precipitates can be caused by the leaching of divalent metal contaminants or lowering of pH (due to CO_2 diffusion or leaching of acidic substances), but can be prevented. More difficult to solve is the tendency of insulin to form fibrils as illustrated in Fig. 11.14.

It appears that the interactions leading to fibril formation result from the monomeric form, and from change in monomer conformation and hydrophilic attraction of the parallel β-sheet forms. Fibril formation is also encouraged by contact of the insulin solution with hydrophobic surfaces. Contact with gamma-irradiated PVC leads to instability, apparently induced by chemical changes in the insulin.

Table 11.8 Effect of insulin formulation on its pharmacokinetics after subcutaneous injection

Product[a]	Formulation	Pharmacokinetics[b]
Humulin R Novolin R	Zinc-insulin crystalline suspension (acid regular)	Rapid onset, short duration Start, 0.5 h; peak, 2.5–5 h; end, 8 h
Humulin N Novolin N	Isophane suspension protamine, zinc crystalline insulin (buffer water for injection)	Intermediate-acting, slower onset, longer duration than regular insulin Start, 1.5 h; peak, 4–12 h; end, up to 24 h
Humulin 70/30[c] Novolin 70/30[c]	70% isophane suspension 30% zinc crystalline	Intermediate-acting, faster onset, longer duration Start, 0.5 h; peak, 2–12 h; end, up to 24 h
Humulin U	Extended zinc-insulin suspension – all crystalline	Slow-acting, slow onset, longer, less-intense duration than R or N forms
Humulin L Novolin L	70% zinc-insulin crystalline suspension 30% amorphous insulin (cloudy suspension)	Intermediate-acting, slower onset, longer duration Start, 2.5 h; peak, 7–15 h; end, 22 h
Humulin BR	Zinc crystalline insulin dissolved in sodium diphosphate buffer	Rapid onset, short duration; use in pumps only

[a] Humulin products (Eli Lilly & Company) contain recombinant human insulin derived from *Escherichia coli*; Novolin products (Novo Nordisk) are recombinant human insulin derived from *Saccharomyces cerevisiae*; both companies also sell other forms of recombinant human insulin and may have additional forms (formulations or new drugs) in clinical trials.

[b] The pharmacokinetics of each formulation may vary greatly among different individuals; the onset of therapeutic levels of insulin is referred to as the start of the effect, the maximum serum level of insulin is denoted the peak, and the time at which the insulin levels are below therapeutic levels is listed as the end of the therapeutic time course.

[c] Solution consists of 70% N form and 30% R form for both products.

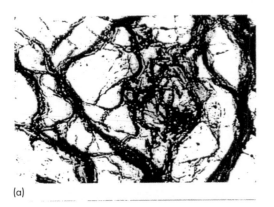
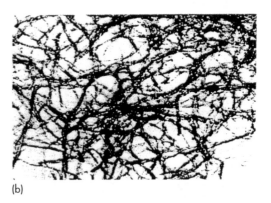

(a)   (b)

Figure 11.14 Transmission electron micrographs of insulin fibrils formed (a) at 37°C, (b) at 80°C (×100 000). Reproduced from J. Brange, *Galenics of Insulin*, Springer, Berlin, 1987.

Propylene glycol, glycerol, nonionic and ionic surfactants and calcium ions have been used in formulations to achieve greater stability, reducing fibril formation, but the most successful strategy is the addition of calcium ions or zinc, which appear to protect the hexameric form of the insulin (see section 9.4.4).

Recombinant human insulin: insulin lispro and insulin aspart

Chemical modifications to an endogenous protein, however minor, can lead to significant differences in properties and activity. Species differences can also be great. Salmon calcitonin is ten times more potent than human calcitonin, for example. Recombinant human protein analogues may be subtly different, as in the case of insulin lispro (Lilly) in which the sequence of proline and lysine at positions 28 and 29 in the B protein chain has been reversed (Fig. 11.15). This sole difference leads to hexamers which more rapidly dissociate to monomers on injection, giving a faster onset of action than human insulin in which the B28 is proline and B29 is lysine (such as the recombinant product Humulin S, which is injected up to an hour before meals).

As we have discussed, peptides become less soluble the closer they are to their isoelectric point. The first attempt to use this principle to prolong insulin action (*circa* 1988) was unsuccessful owing to injection site reactions and variable bioavailability.

Insulin glargine (Lantus, Aventis) has two arginines added to the B30 position (Fig. 11.15). Its isoelectric point changes from a pH of 5.4 to 6.7, making it a soluble (and thus clear) solution in the acid medium of pH 4 in which it is supplied. When it is injected subcutaneously, however, glargine precipitates at the physiological pH of 7.4, thereby delaying its absorption and prolonging its action. Substituting glycine for asparagine at the A21 position and adding zinc stabilises the hexamer and delays absorption further.

Glargine has a similar insulin receptor affinity as NPH (Neutral Protamine Hagedorn, an intermediate-acting insulin that initially achieves slower action through the addition of protamine to short-acting insulin) so that once absorbed in the circulation, glargine is

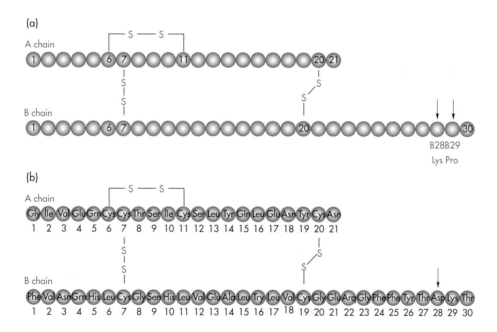

Figure 11.15 (a) Insulin lispro, a product of recombinant DNA technology, is an analogue of human insulin in which the natural sequence of proline and lysine at positions B28 and B29 (shown arrowed) of human insulin has been reversed. (b) Insulin aspart (Novo Nordisk) has an aspartame at B28 (see arrow) replacing the proline of the natural insulin. Insulin glargine has a glycine at position A21 and two arginines at B30.

NovoLog is a sterile, aqueous, clear, and colourless solution that contains insulin aspart 100 units cm^{-3}, glycerin 16 mg cm^{-3}, phenol 1.50 mg cm^{-3}, metacresol 1.72 mg cm^{-3}, zinc 19.6 μg cm^{-3}, disodium hydrogen phosphate dihydrate 1.25 mg cm^{-3}, and sodium chloride 0.58 mg cm^{-3}. NovoLog has a pH of 7.2–7.6. Hydrochloric acid 10% and/or sodium hydroxide 10% may be added to adjust the pH.

equipotent to NPH. The result is a relatively constant supply of insulin with an onset of approximately 2 h and a duration of action of approximately 24 h.

Small changes in the chemistry of large proteins such as insulin can lead to changes in stability, conformation and dissociation which might affect biological performance. There is as yet no simple way to predict the consequence of these subtle changes in structure.

11.4.2 Calcitonin

Calcitonin, a peptide hormone of 32 amino acids having a regulatory function in calcium and phosphorus metabolism, is used in various bone disorders such as osteoporosis. Salmon, human, pig and eel calcitonin are used therapeutically. Species differences may be significant – salmon calcitonin is ten times more potent than human calcitonin, for example. Human calcitonin (hCT) has a tendency to associate rapidly in solution and, like insulin, form fibrils, resulting in a viscous solution.[31] The fibrils are 8 nm in diameter and often associate with one another. Heating fibrillated hCT solutions in 50% acetic acid–water converts the system back to soluble monomers. hCT has a pK of 8.7, while salmon calcitonin (SCT) has a pK of 10.4. This accounts for the high stability of SCT at pH 7.4, as electrostatic interactions between calcitonin monomers play a role. At pH 7.4, SCT monomers will be charged and will repel each other. At 20 mg mol^{-1} in Tris buffer at 22°C and pH 7.4 the fibrillation time for hCT is 1 minute, whereas for SCT it is of the order of 21 days.

11.5 DNA and oligonucleotides

11.5.1 DNA

DNA of varying molecular weights is used in gene therapy. Figure 11.16 shows the well-known primary structure of DNA and the

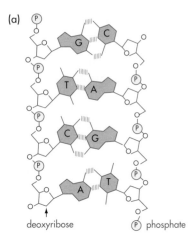

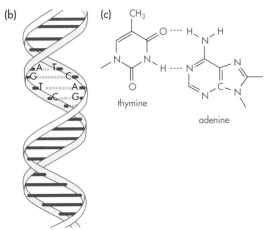

Figure 11.16 (a) Diagrammatic representation of the interactions between two oligonucleotide strands. ////// represents hydrogen-bonding interactions between the base pairs G–C, T–A, C–G, A–T. P represents the phosphate groups which confer the negative charge in the molecule. (b) Representation of the double helix again illustrating the hydrogen-bonding interaction that is key to the helical conformation. (c) The detailed primary structure showing the phosphate-deoxyribose base point sequence for T–A.

charge-determining phosphate groups connected to the deoxyribose rings. As DNA is a large hydrophilic, polyanionic and sensitive macromolecule, its successful delivery to target cells and the nucleus within these cells is an issue. Shearing of high molecular weight DNA while stirring in solution can lead to breakage of the molecule. One approach to delivery is to complex the DNA with polymers or particles of opposite charge to produce, by condensation, more compact species. Many studies have been conducted to condense the DNA with cationic polymers (e.g. polylysine and chitosan), cationic liposomes and dendrimers, to produce nano-sized complexes which retain an overall positive charge and which are able to transfect cells more readily than native or naked DNA. The interaction of DNA with polycationics like chitosan is akin to a coacervation process[32] (Fig. 11.17).

Through the formation of particulates (Fig. 11.18) cell-uptake characteristics and stability are improved, although transfection inside the cell depends ultimately on the successful release of DNA from the complex and its uptake into the nucleus.

11.5.2 Oligonucleotides

Antisense oligonucleotides (used for the sequence-specific inhibition of gene expression) are polyanionic single-strand molecules comprising between 10 and 25 nucleotides. They resemble single-stranded DNA or RNA. They have molecular weights ranging from 3000 to 8000 and are hydrophilic, having a

$\log P$ of approximately -3.5. Like DNA they clearly do not have the appropriate properties for transfer across biological membranes. They are also sensitive to nucleases and nonspecific adsorption to biological surfaces, and hence require to be formulated to achieve delivery and nuclear uptake. Chemical modification of oligonucleotides, which is outside of the scope of this book, increases the stability and activity of the molecules.

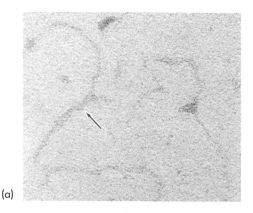

(a)

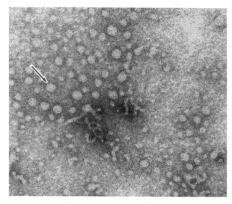

(b)

Figure 11.18 (a) Electron micrograph of naked plasmid DNA; (b) the same sample after condensation with a cationic partial dendrimer (Ramaswamy and Florence, *J. Drug Det. Sci. Technol.*, 15, 307–311 (2005)). The size, shape, charge and stability of such complexes depend on the ionic strength of the medium, lipid composition, lipid/DNA ratio and concentration, and even on mixing procedures. Manufacturing issues include those of reproducibility, avoiding aggregation of the resulting colloidal suspension and lyophilisation, as discussed in R. I. Mahato *et al.*, Cationic lipid-based gene delivery systems: pharmaceutical perspectives, *Pharm. Res.*, 14, 853–859 (1997).

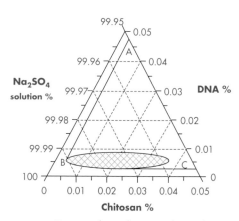

Figure 11.17 Ternary phase diagram of complex coacervation between pRE-luciferase plasmid and chitosan at 55°C in 50 mmol dm^{-3} Na$_2$SO$_4$. Sodium sulfate solution was regarded as one component, since the concentration change in the experiment range was minimal. The region to the right of line the ABC depicts the conditions under which phase separation occurs. The concentration ranges in the small grid area yield distinct particles.

Reproduced from H.-Q. Mao *et al.*, *J. Control. Release*, 70, 399–421 (2001).

11.6 Therapeutic monoclonal antibodies[33]

There are now a number of monoclonal antibodies (antibodies produced from a single clone of cells) available for use in the clinic. Although they have been available since the mid 1970s, there have been problems, not least with their poor distribution and tissue penetration. They are large molecules and diffuse slowly in tissues, especially tumours or inflamed sites. The intravenous route has been most commonly used, so formulations have so far been linked to the development of stable solutions. Physical chemistry can explain in part their mechanism of action, which includes[33] blocking or through steric hindrance the action of target antigens, binding to an antigen, diffusion and translocation in tissues. The literature seems sparse on these topics.

Summary

This chapter has not attempted to provide a complete overview of proteins and peptides and other complex therapeutics such as DNA, oligonucleotides and monoclonal antibodies. That would require a whole textbook in itself. It has tried to give some feeling for the properties of peptides and proteins and how their physical properties are dictated not only by the properties of their individual amino acids but also by the spatial arrangement of the amino acids in their polypeptide chains. Hydrophobic amino acids alternating with hydrophilic, or charged amino acids can produce tertiary and quaternary structures which are quite different from those induced by the spatial separation of hydrophobic and hydrophilic amino acids. The stability of proteins and peptides is of prime pharmaceutical significance. Maintenance of chemical and physical stability is a prerequisite for clinical use. The macromolecular and generally hydrophilic character of all but the smallest peptides makes this class of compound one which is challenging in terms of delivery for therapeutic ends. Some of the issues involved in the formulation of proteins are discussed in the chapter.

DNA and oligonucleotides provide similar challenges – large hydrophilic molecules with no propensity for movement across cell walls and prone to degradation physically and chemically.

Monoclonal oligonucleotides were deprived of their early promise by their size, adverse properties and poor diffusion characteristics, but if monoclonal antibodies are used by the intravenous route they can exert powerful effects *in vivo*.

References

1. T. E. Creighton. *Proteins*, 2nd edn, W. H. Freeman, New York, 1993

2. F. Flam. Molecule makers learn the rules of a crooked game. *Science*, 263, 1563–4 (1994)

3. D. Dressler and H. Potter. *Discovering enzymes*. Scientific American, New York, 1991

4. J. Brange, D. R. Owens, S. Kang and A. Volund. Monomeric insulins and their experimental and clinical implications. *Diabetes Care*, 13, 923–54 (1990)

5. J. Brange, K. Drejer, J. F. Hansen, *et al*. Design of novel insulins with changed self-association and ligand binding properties. In *Advances in Protein Design, International Workshop 1988* (ed. H. Blocker, J. Collins, R. D. Schmid and D. Schomburg), Chemie Weinheim, Basel, 1989, pp. 139–44

6. D. N. Brems, P. L. Brown, C. Bryant, *et al*. Altering the self-association and stability of insulin by amino acid replacement. In *Protein Folding: In Vivo and In Vitro* (ed. J. Cleland), ACS Symposium Series vol. 526, American Chemical Society, Washington, DC, 1993, pp. 254–69

7. Z. Shao, Y. Li, R. Krishnamoorthy, *et al*. Differential effects of anionic, cationic, nonionic, and physiologic surfactants on the dissociation, alpha-chymotryptic degradation, and enteral absorption of insulin hexamers. *Pharm. Res.*, 10, 243–51 (1993)

8. A. B. Robinson and C. J. Rudd. Deamidation of glutaminyl and asparaginyl residues in peptides and proteins. In *Current Topics in Cellular Regulation* (ed. B. L. Horecker and E. R. Stadtman), vol. 8, Academic Press, New York, 1974, pp. 247–95

9. T. Geiger and S. Clarke. Deamidation, isomerization, and racemization at asparaginyl and aspartyl residues in peptides. Succinimide-linked reactions that contribute to protein degradation. *J. Biol. Chem.*, 262, 785–94 (1987)

10. S. Capasso, L. Mazzarella and A. Zagari. Deamidation via cyclic imide of asparaginyl peptides: dependence on salts, buffers and organic solvents. *Peptide Res.*, 4, 234–8 (1991)

11. J. H. McKerrow and A. B. Robinson. Deamidation of asparaginyl residues as a hazard in experimental protein and peptide procedures. *Anal. Biochem.*, 42, 565–8 (1971)

12. K. Patel and R. T. Borchardt. Chemical pathways of peptide degradation. II. Kinetics of deamidation of an asparaginyl residue in a model hexapeptide. *Pharm. Res.*, 7, 703–11 (1990)

13. T. Flatmark. Heterogeneity of beef heart cytochrome *c*. III. Kinetic study of the nonenzymic deamidation of the main subfractions (cytochrome I–cytochrome III). *Acta Chem. Scand.*, 20, 1487–96 (1966)

14. R. Tyler-Cross and V. Schirch. Effects of amino acid sequence, buffers, and ionic strength on the rate and mechanism of deamidation of asparagine residues in small peptides. *J. Biol. Chem.*, 266, 22549–56 (1991)

15. T. V. Brennan and S. Clarke. Spontaneous degradation of polypeptides at aspartyl and asparaginyl residues: Effects of the solvent dielectric. *Protein Sci.*, 2, 331–8 (1993)

16. B. Halliwell and J. M. C. Gutteridge. Role of free radicals and catalytic metal ions in human disease: an overview. In *Free Radicals and Metal Ions in Human Disease*, Methods in Enzymology, vol. 186, Academic Press, New York, 1990, pp. 1–85

17. C. M. Harris and R. J. Hill. The carboxymethylation of human metmyoglobin. *J. Biol. Chem.*, 244, 2195–203 (1969)

18. V. Holeysovsky and M. Lazdunski. Structural properties of trypsinogen and trypsin. Alkylation and oxidation of methionines. *Biochim. Biophys. Acta*, 154, 457–67 (1968)

19. T. P. Link and G. R. Start. *S*-Methylmethionine-29 ribonuclease A. I. Preparation and proof of structure. *J. Biol. Chem.*, 243, 1082–8 (1968)

20. W. J. Ray Jr and D. E. Koshland Jr. Comparative structural studies of phosphoglucomutase and chymotrypsin. *Brookhaven Symp. Biol.*, 13, 135–50 (1960)

21. K. Kido and B. Kassel. Oxidation of methionine residues of porcine and bovine pepsins. *Biochemistry*, 14, 631–5 (1975)

22. J. Jauregui-Adell and P. Jolles. The active center of lysozyme of hen egg white. Action of iodoacetic acid at pH 5.5. *Bull. Soc. Chim. Biol.*, 46, 141–7 (1964)

23. J. D. Spikes and R. Straight. Sensitized photochemical processes in biological systems. *Annu. Rev. Phys. Chem.*, 18, 409–36 (1967)

24. G. E. Mears and R. E. Feeney. *Chemical Modification of Proteins*, Holden-Day, San Francisco, 1971, p. 35

25. B. M. Wallace and J. S. Lasker. Stand and deliver: getting peptide drugs into the body. *Science*, 260, 912–3 (1993)

26. D. A. Paterson, R. A. Conradi, A. R. Hilgers, *et al.* A nonaqueous partitioning system for predicting the oral absorption potential of peptides. *Quantitative Structure–Action Relationships*, 13, 4–10 (1994)

27. J. L. Cleland and R. Langer. Formulation and delivery of proteins and peptides: design and development strategies. In *Formulation and Delivery of Proteins and Peptides* (ed. J. L. Cleland and R. Langer), American Chemical Society, Washington DC, 1994, pp. 1–19

28. J. R. Costantino, R. Langer and A. M. Klibanov. Aggregation of a lyophilized pharmaceutical protein, recombinant human albumin: effect of moisture and stabilization by excipients. *Biotechnology*, 13, 493–6 (1995)

29. M. J. Hageman, P. L. Possert and J. M. Bauer. Prediction and characterization of the water sorption isotherm for bovine somatotropin. *J. Agric. Food Chem.*, 40, 342–7 (1992)

30. G. Zografi. States of water associated with solids. *Drug. Dev. Ind. Pharm.*, 14, 1905–26 (1988)

31. T. Arvinte, A. Cudd and A. F. Drake. The structure and mechanism of formation of human calcitonin fibrils. *J. Biol. Chem.*, 268, 6415–22 (1993)

32. H. Q. Mao, K. Roy, *et al.* Chitosan–DNA nanoparticles as gene carriers: synthesis, characterisation and transfection efficiency. *J. Control. Release*, 70, 399–421 (2001)

33. F. C. Breedveld. Therapeutic monoclonal antibodies. *Lancet*, 355, 735–40 (2000)

12

In vitro assessment of dosage forms

This chapter presents the basics of some *in vitro* tests which can be applied to pharmaceutical products, using the background physical chemistry discussed in earlier chapters. In particular, we will examine how we can measure the influence of some of the key parameters of pharmaceutical systems, such as particle size, viscosity, adhesion or formulation in general on drug release or performance. It is necessary to appreciate the importance of *in vitro* testing in formulation development and in batch-to-batch control but also in assessing defects in products. *In vitro* tests might be preferred to *in vivo* measures when there is a good correlation between *in vitro* and *in vivo* behaviour, but it should be appreciated that such correlations and physiological verisimilitude are not essential for validity in quality control, where reproducibility of a product is in itself a goal.

12.1 Dissolution testing of solid dosage forms

Equations cannot readily be applied to deal with the situation of tablet and capsule dissolution because of the constantly changing surface area of the disintegrated tablet components and because of the presence of additives which may alter solubility and wettability. However, the rate of solution of a solid drug substance from a granule or a tablet is dependent to a large extent on its solubility in the solvent phase and its concentration in that phase. The rationale of testing solid dosage forms *in vitro* will not be considered here. Suffice it to say that the test conditions should provide a reasonable challenge to the dosage form in terms of degree of agitation, temperature, volume and pH of the dissolution medium. *In vitro* tests provide the opportunity to make precise and reproducible release measurements to distinguish between different formulations of the same drug or the same formulation after ageing or processing changes or during production, i.e. batch-to-batch variation. They do not replace the need for clinical work, but an *in vitro* test can pinpoint formulation factors during development which are of importance in determining drug release.

The physicochemical factors which point to the need for dissolution testing include:

- *Low drug solubility* – evidence that the drug has a low aqueous solubility
- *Poor product dissolution* – evidence from the literature that the dissolution of one or more marketed products is poor when tested by an official compendial test procedure (BP or USP)
- *Drug particle size* – evidence that particle size may affect bioavailability
- *The physical form of drug* – evidence that certain polymorphs, solvates or complexes have poor dissolution characteristics and hence bioavailability may be affected

- *Presence of specific excipients* – evidence that specific excipients may alter dissolution or absorption.
- *The nature of tablet or capsule coating* – evidence that coating may interfere with the disintegration or dissolution of the formulation

In vitro methods may be divided into two types, involving either natural convection or forced convection. Most practical methods fall into the latter category, as there is a degree of

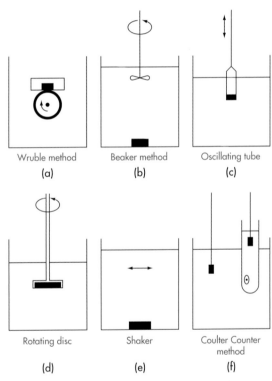

Figure 12.1 Six configurations of simple dissolution test apparatus: (a) the Wruble method in which the dose form is rotated in a container of solvent; (b) a simple beaker method; (c) an apparatus in which the dosage form is in a cradle which oscillates vertically; (d) the rotating disc method to determine the intrinsic dissolution characteristics of a compressed powder; (e) method in which the dosage form is placed in a medium which is shaken and (f) a method in which the decreasing size of suspensions is measured on dissolution.

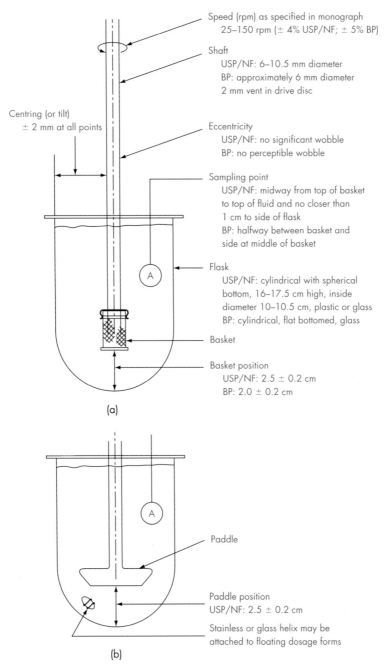

Figure 12.2 The rotating basket and rotating paddle versions of the official method for dissolution testing of solid oral dosage forms. (a) The rotating basket – method 1, USP/NF. This method is official for USP/NF and BP. Current specifications describing geometry and positions for each compendium are shown. (b) The rotating paddle – method 2, USP/NF.

agitation *in vivo*. In natural-convection methods in which, for example, a pellet of material is suspended from a balance arm in the dissolution medium, the conditions are unnatural. In forced-convection methods a degree of agitation is introduced. These can, in turn, be divided into those that employ nonsink conditions and those that achieve sink conditions in the dissolution medium. Figure 12.1 illustrates methods involving forced convection and nonsink conditions, that is where there is no mechanism for replenishing the solvent, so that for most drugs the concentration in solution will increase rapidly to approach C_∞. Most methods rely on the assay of the dissolution medium for drug content, although particle sizing techniques (such as the Coulter Counter method) can directly measure the change in particle size as dissolution (and disintegration of granules) occurs.

12.1.1 Pharmacopoeial and compendial dissolution tests

The dissolution method now widely used and adopted by the British Pharmacopoeia is a variant of the rotating basket method (Fig. 12.2a). Tablets or capsules are placed in a basket of wire mesh, the mesh being small enough to retain broken pieces of tablet but large enough to allow entry of solvent without wetting problems. The basket may be rotated at any suitable speed but most USP monographs specify 50, 100 or 1500 rpm. In all the methods the appropriate pH for the dissolution medium must be chosen, and a reasonable degree of agitation in those techniques which allow it. The considerable effect of rotation speed on the dissolution profile of a sulfamethizole formulation is shown in Fig. 12.3, an effect which would be predicted from our understanding of particle dissolution.[2]

With drugs of very low solubility it is sometimes necessary to consider the use of *in vitro* tests which allow sink conditions to be maintained. This generally involves the use of a lipid phase into which the drug can partition; alternatively, it may involve dialysis or physical replacement of the solvent phase. Mixed-solvent systems such as ethanol–water or surfactant systems may be used to enhance the solubility of sparingly soluble drugs, but some prefer the use of flow-through systems in these cases.

12.1.2 Flow-through systems

A variant on the dissolution methods discussed uses neither basket nor paddle. Convection is achieved by solvent flow through a chamber such as that drawn in Fig. 12.4. Dissolution data obtained from such a system where continuous monitoring of drug concentration is achieved must be interpreted with care as the concentration–time profile will be dependent on the volume of solvent, its flow rate and the distance of the detection device from the flow cell, or rather the void volume of solvent.

This emphasises that there is no absolute method of dissolution testing. With whatever form of test is adopted, results are really only useful on a comparative basis – batch vs batch, brand vs brand, or formulation vs formulation.

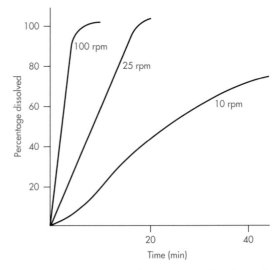

Figure 12.3 Single-tablet dissolution profiles for sulfamethizole formulation in dilute HCl with USP XVIII method at three stirring rates.
Reproduced from reference 2.

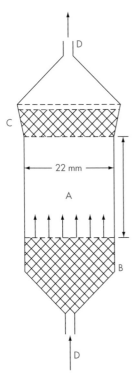

Figure 12.4 A recommended standard design for a flow-through cell: the cell is cylindrical in shape and constructed of glass or other suitable material. A, an internal volume not exceeding 20 cm³ between barrier and filter. B, a bottom barrier of either a porous glass plate or a bed of 1 mm diameter glass beads designed to disperse flow and provide uniform distribution over the dosage chamber A. C, a suitable filter of approximately 25 mm diameter. D, fluid flow from bottom to top.

Factors affecting the release of drugs from other dosage forms can usefully be examined. These include suppositories, topical ointment and cream preparations, and transdermal devices.

12.2 *In vitro–in vivo* correlations

Some factors that influence the sensitivity and degree of *in vitro–in vivo* correlations are shown in Scheme 12.1. Some relate to the dissolution method, some to the dosage form and some, of course, to *in vivo* behaviour.

12.3 *In vitro* evaluation of nonoral systems

12.3.1 Suppository formulations

Suppositories are probably more difficult to study *in vitro* than many other dosage forms because it is not easy to simulate the conditions in the rectum. In one system,[3] shown in Fig. 12.5, a suppository is placed in a pH 7.8 buffer in a dialysis bag. This bag is placed in a second dialysis bag filled with octanol, the whole is suspended in a flow system at 37°C, and the amount of drug released into the outer liquid is monitored. The results from this set-up must be interpreted with care as it is possible for substances that complex with the drug to reduce transport across the dialysis membrane – something which may or may not happen in the body.

A variant on this arrangement was used[4] to obtain the data shown in Fig. 12.6 illustrating the reduction in aminophylline release from Witepsol H15 bases on ageing of the product.

12.3.2 *In vitro* release from topical products and transdermal systems

In vitro testing of the lot-to-lot uniformity of semisolid dosage forms of creams, ointments and lotions is gaining in importance in quality control. Ointments and transdermal systems encounter little water in use but, in the spirit of using release tests to compare basically similar products, useful data can be obtained by measuring release into aqueous media, and sometimes this information can be predictive of *in vivo* performance. Sometimes an attempt can be made to simulate a lipid biophase. Steroid formulations can be tested clinically using the vasoconstrictor activity of the steroid to quantitate the results. In a few cases it is feasible to measure quantities of drug reaching the systemic circulation after topical application. An *in vitro* system[5] using isopropyl myristate as the 'solvent phase' or 'biophase' is shown in Fig. 12.7. The amount of drug released in 7 h in this

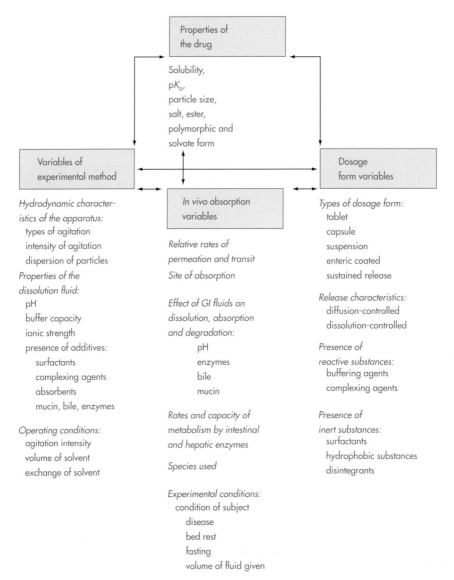

Properties of the drug

Solubility,
pK_a,
particle size,
salt, ester,
polymorphic and
solvate form

Variables of experimental method

Hydrodynamic character-istics of the apparatus:
  types of agitation
  intensity of agitation
  dispersion of particles
Properties of the dissolution fluid:
  pH
  buffer capacity
  ionic strength
  presence of additives:
    surfactants
    complexing agents
    absorbents
    mucin, bile, enzymes

Operating conditions:
  agitation intensity
  volume of solvent
  exchange of solvent

In vivo absorption variables

Relative rates of permeation and transit
Site of absorption

Effect of GI fluids on dissolution, absorption and degradation:
  pH
  enzymes
  bile
  mucin

Rates and capacity of metabolism by intestinal and hepatic enzymes

Species used

Experimental conditions:
  condition of subject
    disease
    bed rest
    fasting
    volume of fluid given

Dosage form variables

Types of dosage form:
  tablet
  capsule
  suspension
  enteric coated
  sustained release

Release characteristics:
  diffusion-controlled
  dissolution-controlled

Presence of reactive substances:
  buffering agents
  complexing agents

Presence of inert substances:
  surfactants
  hydrophobic substances
  disintegrants

Scheme 12.1 Some interacting variables which influence the sensitivity and degree of *in vivo* correlation of *in vitro* methods for measuring drug release and dissolution.
Modified from W. H. Barr, *Pharmacology*, 8, 55 (1972).

system correlates with the vasoconstriction index for four formulations of fluocinonide. Vasoconstriction evidenced by skin blanching correlates with steroid potency in topical preparations.

A variant of this simple apparatus is that shown in Fig. 12.8 based on the Franz diffusion cell, which has been used to measure the release rate of tacrolimus from an ointment.[6]

When a restraining membrane has to be employed, as with suppositories and most semisolids, the retarding properties of the membrane have to be considered and the amount of formulation applied in the test apparatus must be considered before the key parameters, such as particle size of the drug, are determined. Examples in Fig. 12.9 demonstrate in one test system how the influence of

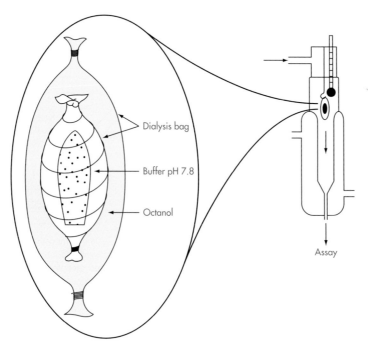

Figure 12.5 An *in vitro* system for studying drug release from suppositories. The suppository is placed in a buffer with a dialysis bag which itself resides in a dialysis bag containing octanol to simulate partitioning into tissue. The amount of drug which is eluted into a flowing aqueous phase is then measured.
Modified from reference 3.

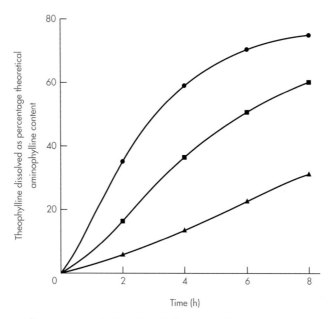

Figure 12.6 Dissolution profiles for aminophylline (theophylline and ethylenediamine mixture) suppositories stored at 35°C: ● 2 months old; ■ 8 months old; ▲ 12 months old.
Reproduced from reference 4 with permission.

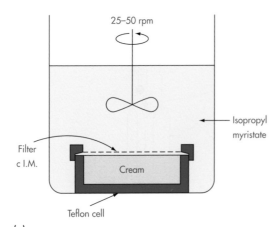

(a)

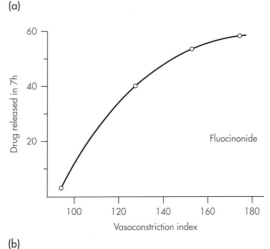

(b)

Figure 12.7 (a) An apparatus for the examination of the release of a steroid from a cream formulation: the cream is placed in a Teflon receptacle and covered with a membrane impregnated with isopropyl myristate, and the concentration of fluocinonide is monitored in the bulk isopropyl myristate layer. (b) Release *in vitro* compared with results of vasoconstrictor tests on four formulations.
Modified from reference 5.

total drug loading and mean particle size can be illustrated, in this case with terconazole.[7]

Using a rotating bottle apparatus, release of glyceryl trinitrate from Deponit transdermal patches gives the results shown in Fig. 12.10.[8] The influence of temperature and pH on release was examined using the same technique, the results confirming that release is essentially determined by the diffusion of drug in the adhesive layer of the product (see section 9.5) but is clearly proportional to surface area, as

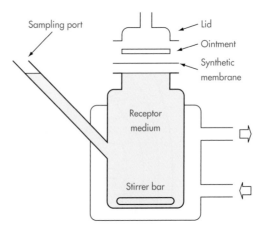

Figure 12.8 A system to measure the release of drug from an ointment via a synthetic membrane into a temperature-controlled and stirred receptor medium.
Reproduced from reference 6.

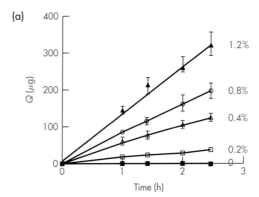

(a)

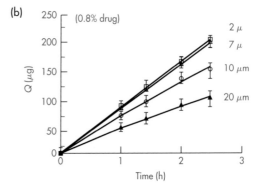

(b)

Figure 12.9 An illustration of the usefulness of *in vitro* tests in drug formulation development: the effect on terconazole release rate *in vitro* of (a) drug loading and (b) particle size.
Reproduced from reference 7.

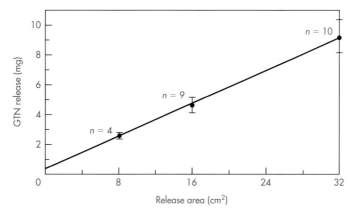

Figure 12.10 In vitro glyceryl trinitrate (GTN) release (24 h) into 80 cm^3 isotonic NaCl versus release area of Deponit TTS.
Reproduced from reference 8 with permission.

expected. Release increases as temperature increases; between 32 and 37°C an increase in release rate of between 1 and 2 μg cm^{-2} h^{-1} is detected. The BP specifies a distribution (release) test for transdermal patches based on the paddle apparatus for tablet and capsules.

12.4 Rheological characteristics of products

The rheological behaviour of liquids and semi-solids can be described as discussed in sections 7.3.10 and 7.4.4 of Chapter 7. Viscosity monitoring can be used as a quality control procedure, but some very practical rheological tests may be carried out. Some are discussed here.

The injectability of nonaqueous injections, which are often viscous and thus difficult to inject, can be assessed by a test for syringeability. Sesame oil has a viscosity of 56 cP, but added drugs and adjuvants can increase the viscosity of such vehicles.

The desired physical properties of various topical preparations are listed in Table 12.1. The terms 'soft and unctuous' and 'hard and stiff' are difficult to quantify, but it is useful at least to consider the variety of descriptions that may be applied in a consistency profile of an external pharmaceutical product. Scheme 12.2 lists these comprehensively, dividing them into primary, secondary and tertiary characteristics. The tertiary properties are probably the most elusive.

Table 12.1 Properties of some topical preparations[a]

Class	Nature	Required physical properties
1	Ophthalmic ointments	Softest type of ointment
2	Other commonly used ointments	Soft and unctuous, but stiff enough to remain in place when applied
3	Protective ointments, e.g. zinc oxide paste	Hard and stiff; remain in place when applied to moist ulcerated areas

[a] Reproduced from P. Sherman, *Rheol. Acta*, 10, 121 (1971).

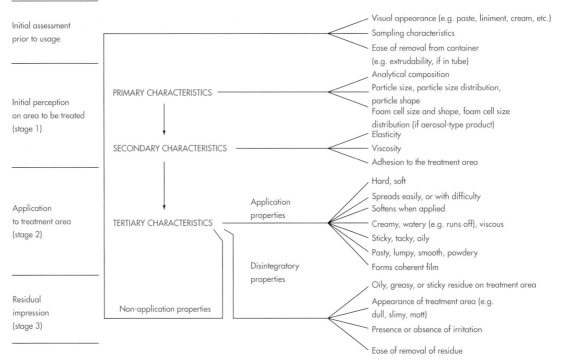

Scheme 12.2   Consistency profile for pharmaceuticals employed externally.
Reproduced from P. Sherman, *Rheol. Acta*, 10, 21 (1971).

12.5   Adhesivity of dosage forms

Interest in the adhesion of dosage forms to epithelial surfaces has been aroused by the possibility of deliberate contact between oral dosage forms and the gut wall to retard the rate of transit down the gastrointestinal tract, but also by the possibility of dosage forms accidentally adhering to the oesophagus or other epithelial surfaces. Adhesive preparations have been formulated for diverse tasks such as the topical treatment of stomatitis and the administration of insulin. The adhesive nature of transdermal patches is important, as is the adhesion of film coats to tablet surfaces. Adhesion of erythrocytes and bacterial cells to polymer surfaces is also of importance in the understanding, respectively, of blood compatibility of polymers and bacterial infection mediated by catheters.

Some examples of solid–solid adhesion processes are shown diagrammatically in Fig.

12.11. Peeling tests for film coats are a part of pharmaceutical development and similar tests for the adhesion of transdermal particles to skin have been used.

Several methods of testing oral dosage forms for adhesivity are in use. One[9] involves the raising of the dosage form through an *ex vivo* porcine oesophagus (Fig. 12.12). Another method assesses the adhesion of a moistened capsule or tablet to a surface using a strain gauge[10] (Fig. 12.13). The effects of polymer concentration and composition and of additives on the adhesivity of film coating materials can be studied using this apparatus, and the force, *f*, required to separate tablet from substrate can be measured. In this apparatus, the force per unit area required to separate two circular plates of radius *r* initially in contact through a liquid layer of thickness *h* and viscosity η over time *t* is

$$f = \frac{3k'}{4t}\left[\frac{r^2\eta}{h^2}\right] \tag{12.1}$$

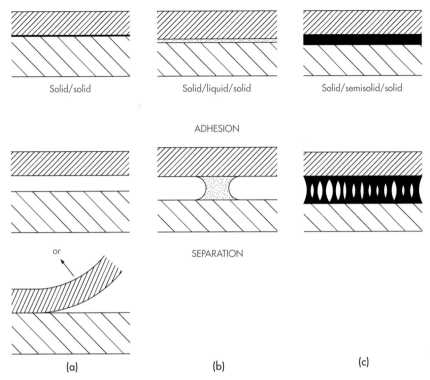

Figure 12.11   Diagrammatic representation of adhesion between solid surfaces at rest: (a) no adhesive layer; (b) a viscous liquid at the interface; and (c) a semisolid adhesive layer. On separation, the nature of the intervening film is shown: (a) no film, (b) a necking filament of liquid, (c) multiple filaments of the semisolid layer

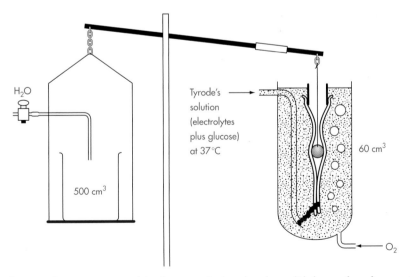

Figure 12.12   A system for measurement of the force required to detach a solid dosage form from an isolated porcine oesophagus.
Reproduced from reference 9.

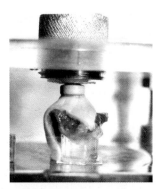

Figure 12.13 A device to measure the force of detachment of tablets or capsules from porcine oesophageal tissue, used to determine the values given in Fig. 12.14.

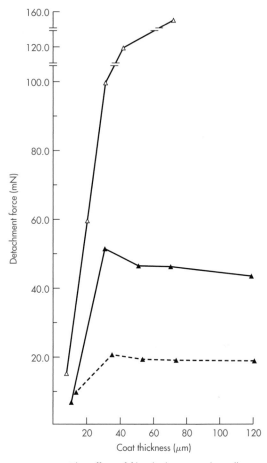

Figure 12.14 The effect of film thickness on the adhesiveness of tablets coated with HPMC-606 from a 4% solution (△) and in the presence of 4% PEG 6000 (– ▲ –) and 6% PEG 6000 (··· ▲ ···), i.e. 1 : 1 and 1 : 1.5 ratios of HPMC to PEG respectively.
Reproduced from reference 12 with permission.

where k' is a constant. This equation applies only when the surfaces are pulled apart slowly.

Clearly the viscosity of the liquid is a determinant of the force of separation; it is less obvious why the thickness of the layer has the effect shown by the equation. The 'tackiness' of a system is not, however, simply related to viscosity.[11] High molecular weight materials must be present in aqueous solutions at least to provide an elastic element to the viscous flow. Rubbery polymers which have partly liquid and partly elastic characteristics are employed as adhesives in surgical dressings and adhesive tapes. What factors influence the adhesivity of high molecular weight soluble polymers such as hydroxypropylmethylcellulose (HPMC) is still unclear. HPMC is a component of film coating materials. Figure 12.14 shows the detachment force required to separate tablets from a glass surface when coated with HPMC-606 from a 4% solution, shown here as a function of the thickness of the film coat.[12] The effect of the presence of high concentrations of polyoxyethylene glycol 6000 is to reduce adhesivity, presumably because the glycol solution is less tacky.

The variables likely to affect the process of adhesion of coated tablets to mucosal surfaces are shown in diagrammatic form in Fig. 12.15: film coat thickness, the nature of the film coat, its rate of solution or hydration, the rheology of the solution formed, its surface tension and its elongational characteristics. Eight stages have been identified. Stage I

(before contact occurs) defines the system and the variables of film coating thickness, the nature of the coating and the nature of the tissue surface. In stage II the presence of moisture or water is postulated, and here the wetting characteristics of the film will be important. In stage III the film coat begins to dissolve and we assume that contact is made, or is about to be made with the tissue; the forces bringing the tablet and the tissue together are not controllable because contact is made by collision and is dependent to some extent on the ratio of tablet size to oesophageal diameter. Stage IV represents

VARIABLES

Thickness of film coat
Nature of coating material

Hydrophobicity of film coat
(i.e. is the coat wetted?)

Rate of coat hydration or
dissolution
Nature of contacting surface

Geometry of contact with tissue;
tablet size and shape

Rheology of solution of film coating
material

Surface tension of film coating
material in solution

Elongational characteristics and
critical rupture thickness of filament

Forces leading to separation

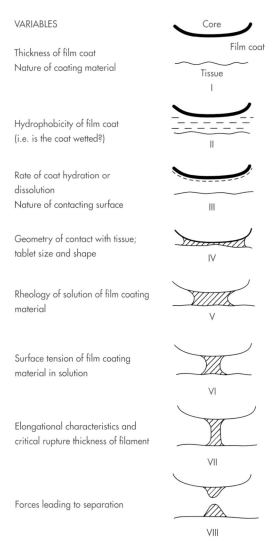

Figure 12.15 Diagrammatic representation of the possible sequence of events in the adhesion of a tablet to the mucosal surface and its subsequent separation, with a partial listing of the many variables in the process.
Reproduced from A. T. Florence and E. G. Salole, *Formulation Factors in Adverse Reactions*, Wright, London, 1990.

contact, when the angle of approach, together with the tablet size and shape, will determine the opportunity for adhesion. Stages V to VIII represent the detachment process initiated, for example, by swallowing food or water or dry swallowing; here the rheological and elongational characteristics of the adhesive material are important. The process is complex and is the subject of much research.

12.6 Analysis of particle size distribution in aerosols

Analysis of particle size distribution of aerosol formulations during formulation, development and clinical trial or after storage is of obvious clinical relevance (see section 9.9). Aerosols are not easy to size, primarily because they are dynamic and inherently unstable systems. Methods of sampling may be divided into techniques which utilise a cloud, and dynamic methods in which particles are carried in a stream of gas. In cloud methods, sedimentation techniques based on Stokes' law are applied and the usual detection system is photometric. The Royco sizer is a commercially available instrument which measures individual particles in a cloud (it is used to monitor the air of 'clean rooms'). This instrument can be used to size particles in aerosol clouds provided that the particle size distribution does not change during the time of the analysis either by preferential settling of larger particles or by coagulation. Dynamic methods depend on the properties of particles related to their mass. Instruments utilise both sedimentation and inertial forces.

Probably the most widely used instrument in categorising airborne particles is the cascade impactor, in which large particles leave the airstream and impinge on baffles or on glass microscope slides. The airstream is then accelerated at a nozzle, providing a second range of smaller sized particles on the next baffle and so on (Fig. 12.16). Progressively finer particles are collected at the successive stages of impingement owing to jet velocity and decreasing jet dimension. Shearing action of the jets may lead to the break-up of aggregates.

For more routine examination of medicinal aerosols, 'artificial throat' devices are useful. With these, comparative studies of the behaviour of aerosols can be carried out. In these devices the particles are segregated according to size. Analysis of the collecting layers at the several levels of the device allows the monitoring of changes in released particle size. In devices with an artificial mouth, this

(a)

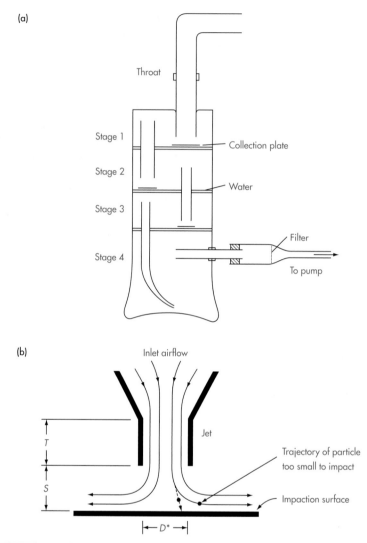

(b)

Figure 12.16 (a) The multistage liquid impinger. (Reproduced from G. W. Hallworth. *Br. J. Clin. Pharm.*, 4, 689 (1977).) (b) The principal features affecting the performance of inertial impactors: air flow, the dimensions S and T, the diameter of the jet, D^*, the density, ρ, and the diameter of the particles, d. The trajectory of particles which are too small to deposit is shown.

Reproduced from G. W. Hallworth, in *Drug Delivery to the Respiratory Tract* (ed. D. Ganderton and T. Jones), Ellis Horwood, Chichester, 1987.

can be washed to reveal the extent of fall-out of large particles. The smallest particles of all reach the collecting solvent.

Because of the need for standardisation of test equipment, the British Pharmacopoeia and other compendia have adopted detailed specifications for impinger devices. Two impinger devices have been adopted by the British Pharmacopoeia. Apparatus 'A' is shown in Fig. 12.17. All these operate by

dividing the dose emitted from an inhaler into the respirable and nonrespirable fractions. The device in Fig. 12.17 employs the principle of liquid impingement and has a solvent in both chambers to collect the aerosol. Air is drawn through the system at $60 \ dm^3 \ min^{-1}$ and the inhaler is fired several times into the device. There are several impaction surfaces at the back of the glass throat about 10 cm away from the activator

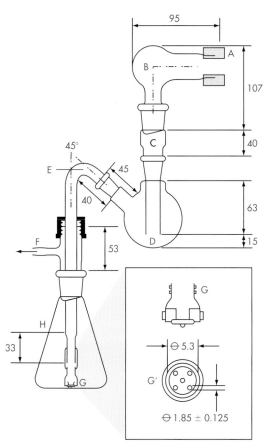

Figure 12.17 Impinger apparatus A, showing dimensions (mm) in order to ensure indenticality between equipment used in quality control.
Source: British Pharmacopoeia.

25% and 20% respectively, while estimates of the percentage of the dose reaching the lung were 12.0% and 8.8% respectively.

Many other tests could have been included to demonstrate the value of *in vitro* tests in quality control. Some, such as multistage impingers for aerosols, can be predictive of *in vivo* behaviour, or at least give an assurance of consistency of effect. An interesting test system for evaluating inhaled nasal delivery systems (Fig. 12.18) combines a physical device with cultured cells so that the interaction of microparticles with living cells can be studied directly. As new delivery systems appear, new tests will be required – as will ingenuity.

(a)

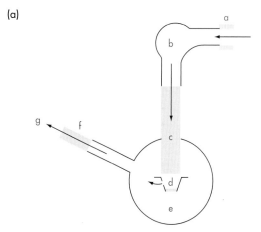

(b)

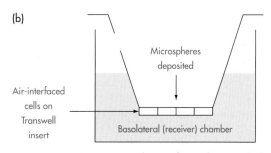

Figure 12.18 An *in vitro* technique for evaluating inhaled nasal delivery systems in which particles/microspheres are deposited on a cell monolayer. Drug that is absorbed through the monolayer can be arranged in the basolateral chamber.
Reproduced from B. Forbes, S. Lim, G. P. Martin and M. B. Brown, *STP Pharma Sci.*, 12, 75–79 (2002).

(similar to human dimensions). The upper impinger has a cut off at a particle size of ~6.4 μm, with the first impact surface known as stage 1 and the last impact surface being in the lower impinger (stage 2), which is considered to be the respirable fraction.

Apparatus B (not illustrated) is made of metal and can be engineered to finer tolerances than the glass apparatus A; it is considered to be a superior apparatus for quality control testing and product release.

Typical of the result achieved with Apparatus B are those for two Intal formulations, Intal 1 and Intal 5. Intal 1 delivers 1 mg per shot and Intal 5 delivers 5 mg per shot. *In vitro* the respirable fraction was found to be

Summary

In this chapter:

- We have seen a selection of tests which can be conducted to measure the key parameters of a variety of formulations.
- These tests are not necessarily predictive of performance *in vivo*, but can be used to ensure batch-to-batch consistency.
- When good *in vitro–in vivo* correlations have been established, laboratory based tests can be predictive of performance.
- Release tests can be applied to rectal and transdermal products by adapting methods used for oral products, altering the receptor phase to mimic the medium in which the formulation resides *in vivo*.
- Key parameters are different for different routes of delivery and different formulations: particle size is a key factor in inhalation products and in topical preparations where the drug is dispersed rather than dissolved in the vehicle.
- Adhesivity of oral dosage forms may be a factor in determining their efficacy (buccal delivery) or in causing adverse events (as in oesophageal injury); adhesion of transdermal patches to the skin is clearly important.
- The rheological properties of topical preparations and formulations for nasal delivery are important, and a key factor is the syringeability of injectables.

Finally, no laboratory test can mimic the complexity of the biological environment and the dynamic factors involved in drug absorption in patients, but well-designed *in vitro* experiments can elucidate whether different formulations are comparable in terms of their key features. At best, *in vitro* tests are predictors of quality of performance in the patient; at the least they can ensure consistency of response; where, for example, chemical assays of drug content in generic products may give identical results, release studies may show differences due to drug–excipient interactions which may be of significance.

References

1. W. A. Hanson. *Handbook of Dissolution Testing*, 2nd edn, Aster Publishing Group, Eugene, OR, 1991

2. G. L. Mattock and I. J. McGilveray. Comparison of bioavailabilities and dissolution characteristics of commercial tablet formulations of sulfamethizole. *J. Pharm. Sci.*, 61, 746–9 (1972)

3. W. A. Ritschel and M. Banarer. Correlation between *in vitro* release of proxyphylline from suppositories and in vivo data obtained from cumulative urinary excretion studies. *Arzneim Forsch.*, 23, 1031–5 (1973)

4. J. B. Taylor and D. E. Simpkins. Aminophylline suppositories: *in vitro* dissolution and bioavailability in man. *Pharm. J.*, 227, 601–3 (1981)

5. J. A. Ostrenga, J. Haleblian, B. Poulsen, *et al.* Vehicle design for a topical steroid, fluocinolide. *J. Invest. Dermatol.*, 56, 392–9 (1971)

6. H. Yoshida, S. Tamura, T. Toyoda, *et al. In vitro* release of Tacrolimus from Tacrolimus ointment and its speculated mechanism. *Int. J. Pharm.*, 270, 55–64 (2004).

7. M. Corbo, T. W. Schultz, *et al. Pharm Tech. Int.*, 17(9), 112 (1993)

8. M. Wolff, G. Cordes and V. Luckow. *In vitro* and *in vivo*-release of nitroglycerin from a new transdermal therapeutic system. *Pharm.Res.*, 1, 23–9 (1985)

9. M. Marvola, K. Vahervuo, A. Sothmann, *et al.* Development of a method for study of the tendency of drug products to adhere to the esophagus. *J. Pharm. Sci.*, 71, 975–7 (1982)

10. H. Al-Dujaili, A. T. Florence and E. G. Salole. *In vitro* assessment of the adhesiveness of film-coated tablets. *Int. J. Pharm.*, 34, 67–74 (1986)

11. M. Marvola, M. Rajaniemi, E. Marttila, *et al.* Effect of dosage form and formulation factors on the adherence of drugs to the esophagus. *J. Pharm. Sci.*, 72, 1034–6 (1983)

12. H. Al-Dujaili, A. T. Florence and E. G. Salole. The adhesiveness of proprietary tablets and capsules to porcine esophageal tissue. *Int. J. Pharm.*, 34, 75–9 (1986)

Index